Clinical Biomechanics
of the Spine

Clinical Biomechanics
of the Spine

AUGUSTUS A. WHITE III, M.D., D.Med.Sci.
Professor of Orthopaedic Surgery
Harvard Medical School;
Orthopaedic Surgeon-in-Chief
Beth Israel Hospital
Boston, Massachusetts

MANOHAR M. PANJABI, Ph.D., D.Tech.
Associate Professor of Biomechanics in Surgery
Director of Bioengineering Research
Yale University School of Medicine
New Haven, Connecticut

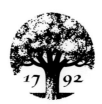

J. B. Lippincott Company
PHILADELPHIA · TORONTO

ISBN 0 397 50388 1

Library of Congress Catalog Card Number 78-15708

Printed in the United States of America

5 6 4

Library of Congress Cataloging in Publication Data

White, Augustus A
  Clinical biomechanics of the spine.

  Includes bibliographical references and indexes.
  1. Spine—Abnormalities. 2. Spine—Wounds and injuries. 3. Spine—Surgery. I. Panjabi, Manohar M., joint
author. II. Title. [DNLM: 1. Spine. 2. Biomechanics.
WE725 W582c]
RD768.W43   617'.375   78-15708
ISBN 397-50388-1

To

Alissa	*Arvind*
Anita	*Gita*
Atina	*Elisabeth*
Augustus Jr.	*Dadanbai*
Vivian	*Murlidhar*

Martin Luther King, Jr., and Mohandas Karamchand Gandhi

Foreword

The human spine, an ingenious mechanical structure, serves many purposes: It combines weight bearing with physiologic motion and, at the same time, offers protection to the spinal cord and nerves. It is therefore natural that through the ages this structure has received much attention from physicians, as well as technicians. Unfortunately, however, much anecdotal observation was presented, with little scientific data to support various points of proposed importance for health and disease.

Only during the last century (and mainly during the last two decades) have scientists from various fields begun to gather enough data on the mechanical behavior of the spine; mostly, these relate to properties of its different parts.

The obvious reason for this interest in the fundamental mechanical behavior, the biomechanics of the spine, is, of course, the increasing number of injuries and diseases afflicting the structure. To understand and treat spinal disorders, a thorough knowledge of spine biomechanics is necessary.

Hitherto, this field has been poorly covered in text books on the spine. Most review articles discuss only the biomechanics of selected parts of the spine in relation to certain aspects of spine pathology. In the past, interested readers have had to consult articles often published in obscure and highly specialized scientific journals. Augustus A. White III, the orthopaedic surgeon, and Manohar M. Panjabi, the mechanics engineer, have now presented the first comprehensive text on what is really known about measured behavior of the spine as a whole and in its various parts.

They have succeeded in presenting all important information with extensive references in a book that is written in a language readily understandable to every practicing physician. In essence then, they have succeeded in presenting *clinical* biomechanics of the spine.

Their own long-standing cooperative scientific efforts in the field have made them internationally well known and respected in orthopaedic and bioengineering circles; also, they are aware of the importance of simple and intelligible language, especially in this interdisciplinary field.

The authors have created a text of fundamental importance for everyone concerned with disorders of the back, from a clinical or engineering point of view.

In my eyes, this book is the most important contribution to the literature on spinal diseases since Schmorl and Junghanns' book, *Die Gesunde und die Kranke Wirbelsäule in Röntgenbild und Klinik*, which appeared in 1932.

At long last, we have a scientific back book.

ALF NACHEMSON
Professor and Chairman
Department of Orthopaedic Surgery
University of Göteborg
Göteborg, Sweden

Foreword

CLINICAL BIOMECHANICS OF THE SPINE is a comprehensive study of biomechanics of the spine in health, trauma, and disease.

The unique approach, made possible by the combined talents of a practicing orthopaedic surgeon and a biomechanical engineer, adds a new dimension to the understanding of spinal physiology and pathology. The practical application of the many principles described in this book will greatly assist in the management of patients with problems related to the axial skeleton and its supporting and controlling mechanisms.

Chapters 1 and 2 deal with the normal spine and prepare the reader for Chapters 3 and 4, concerning spinal injuries, and Chapters 5 through 8, concerning treatment.

The book contains a wealth of information gleaned from the literature and the authors' extensive personal, clinical, and research experience. The clear, concise text is further clarified by well constructed and easily understood drawings and augmented by clinical examples.

Ruptures of the transverse ligament of the atlas, "hangman's fracture," vertebral body compression, the behavior of the intervertebral disc in health and disease, and the pathophysiology of mechanical stress on the spinal cord are explained biomechanically. Various surgical fusions are described in relation to their ability to support the injured spine.

An extensive glossary of biomechanical terms is available at the end of the book for ready reference.

The authors' great theoretical and practical knowledge, their dedication to spinal biomechanics, and their ability for understandable expression is clearly evident. This book, the first of its type devoted entirely to the spine, adds greatly to our knowledge and will serve as a model for similar future publications.

BILL FIELDING

Foreword

Although backache is second only to upper respiratory infection as a cause of time lost from work, surprisingly, little fundamental research has been carried out on the etiology of this irksome burden of modern-day society. Most of our knowledge has been gleaned solely from clinical impressions.

It has been recognized that backache is a symptom, not a disease, and that the cause of the pain may lie outside the spine. It is accepted that spondylogenic backache may be due to bony lesions or to malfunction of the supporting soft tissues. The bony lesions are easily recognizable upon radiographic examination, and methods of treatment are well established. However, because the pathogenesis of the symptoms resulting from soft-tissue lesions is still largely a matter of conjecture, clinical examination and treatment must, perforce, be empirical.

If the clinician questions himself honestly, he cannot help but be astonished at our remarkable and disturbing ignorance.

In 1934 Mixter and Barr stated that a ruptured intervertebral disc was one of the causes of sciatic pain. Although their observation has been amply confirmed through the years by clinical experience, we still do not know why pressure on a nerve root by a ruptured disc gives rise to pain. Pressure on peripheral nerves gives rise to paresthesia. It has been shown experimentally that applying pressure to a normal lumbar nerve root by inflation of a Fogarty catheter gives rise to paresthesia and not to pain. However, if this experiment is repeated with the catheter placed under an "inflamed" nerve root previously compressed by a ruptured disc, upon distention of the catheter, pain is produced. Why?

Upon clinical examination, patients suffering from an acute rupture of a lumbar intervertebral disc demonstrate "marked spasm" of the sacrospinalis muscles, associated with *an obliteration of the normal lumbar lordosis*. The sacrospinalis muscles are extensors of the spine. Why is the lumbar lordosis obliterated when they are in spasm?

In a patient suffering from lumbar nerve root compression, why is the sciatic pain reproduced by straight leg raising, aggravated by forced dorsiflexion of the ankle? Surely, this is not due to stretching of the posterior tibial nerve as it courses around the medial malleolus. One must remember that the anterior tibial nerve would be stretched by forced plantar flexion of the ankle!

Clinicians throughout the world have learned that with the onset of disc degeneration, the involved segment may become unstable or may "sag into" hyperextension. These mechanical changes have been cited as a cause of mechanical low back pain resulting from damage to the related zygoapophyseal joints.

Specific radiological changes demonstrating segmental instability have been described: disc narrowing, rocking on flexion-extension films; the traction spur; gas in the disc; and posterior joint subluxation. When a patient crippled by low back pain demonstrates these radiological changes, it is generally acknowledged that the cause of the pain has been clearly demonstrated. However, a year later, after the patient has been able to engage in unrestricted activities over the last 9 months without any discomfort at all, additional radiographs demonstrate the same phenomena: disc narrowing and abnormal mobility; traction spurs; the Knuttson phenomenon; and persisting posterior joint subluxation. What, then, is the significance of these radiographic findings?

With advancing age, the incidence of radiological changes indicative of disc degeneration increases exponentially, whereas the incidence of discogenic back pain reaches a maximum at the age of 45 and declines thereafter. Here again, the following question is raised: What is the significance of the radiological changes? Or, perhaps, what is the significance of disc degeneration?

When considering surgical procedures, one must remember that in some health centers, cervical disc degeneration is treated by anterior discectomy without fusion, with results that are equivalent to those produced by the more commonly practiced technique of anterior cervical discectomy and fusion. Other health centers have reported spontaneous fusion after anterior cervical discectomy alone. What evidence have we that a bone graft following anterior cervical discectomy has any function at all?

Though we have stumbled from hunch to hunch, we have made gratifying progress in our philosophy of the management of low back pain, if not in our scientific understanding of the underlying problems. We must acknowledge the fact that it would be very easy to ask a different question every day for 3 years about the pathogenesis of symptoms, the significance of findings on examination, and the rationale of the chosen method of treatment, whether operative or nonoperative. We have reached a stage at which it is of vital importance to stop, to think, and to ask.

This is exactly what Drs. White and Panjabi have done in their book. This is why their analysis of clinical biomechanics of the spine constitutes such an important step in our continuing search for knowledge.

IAN MACNAB, F.R.C.S.

Preface

We define *clinical biomechanics of the spine* as that body of knowledge that employs mechanical facts, concepts, principles, terms, and mathematics to interpret and analyze normal and abnormal human anatomy and physiology so as to better understand and treat the problems that patients have with their spines. Our purpose in writing this book is to advance that body of knowledge by presenting a comprehensive review and analysis of the clinical and clinically relevant scientific data on the mechanics of the human spine. Emphasis has been placed on making an accessible and useful presentation for those who work with the spine but do not have a broad background in the engineering sciences.

During the course of our experience with the biomechanics of the spine, we became aware of the value of the team approach, that of an orthopaedic surgeon working closely with a mechanical engineer. This approach was beneficial in the improvement of research techniques and the application of engineering theory for a better understanding of clinical problems in the human spine. We also recognized that a considerable amount of biomechanical information concerning the mechanical behavior of the spine and its components is based on reliable research that may be applied to the patient by the clinician. There are many general engineering theories and principles that are crucial to the basic understanding of the normal and abnormal functioning of the spine. This information is useful in the understanding and treatment of patients with diseases of the spine, and it can aid the surgeon in his evaluation and management of certain clinical problems. A good deal of this information is directly applicable to patient care, provided that it is presented in a clinical context, and not purely in advanced engineering and mathematical language. Our goal is to present this information in a manner that is understandable and useful to the clinician who may not be a student of biomechanics. In doing so, we hope to make some small contribution to the progression toward a stronger scientific basis for the practice of this particular aspect of clinical medicine.

Since the clinician increasingly employs biomechanical terms and interprets his problems with the assistance of the engineer, and since biomechanical engineers are showing more interest in the field of spine orthopaedics, it is important to bridge the communication gap between the two groups. This book is particularly designed to improve the accuracy and effectiveness of communications between the clinician and the engineer.

The text is written so that it can be read at two levels without loss of continuity. It is designed for the clinician who is not interested in complex principles of engineering, but it also contains ample quantitative data, explanatory notes, and advanced references for more thorough study.

Chapters 1 and 2 deal with physical properties and kinematics of the spine; together they may be regarded to constitute the basic science of spine biomechanics. These chapters constitute a review of the literature and the authors' selective interpretation and analysis of the most reliable information that is important clinically, now or in the foreseeable future. Chapter 1 describes physical properties of structures that are responsible for the behavior of the spine; it relates to the patient in terms of practical application or fundamental understanding of clinical phenomena. Care has been taken not to oversimplify these data and material. However, we have avoided discussing facts that have no obvious clinical application. An attempt has been made to combine these data and to provide a biomechanical analysis for a better understanding of the basic functional mechanics of the human spine.

Chapter 2 is a comprehensive presentation of what is known about the kinematics of the spine. Here we have sought to weigh the data according to our best interpretation of their validity and reliability and to offer an overview of the kinematic function of the entire spine.

Much of clinical spine work is based on engineering principles, stated or unstated. We have endeavored to explain and clarify some of these principles. Chapters 3 through 8 are devoted to specific clinical problems, the understanding and treatment of which are largely based on the clinical biomechanics of the spine.

Chapter 3 is unique in that it attempts to collect all of the scientific, mechanical, and clinical studies on scoliosis and to offer an overview of the problem.

In Chapter 4, we evaluate a number of well recognized fracture patterns, from occiput to sacrum, and offer a practical theoretical analysis and interpretation of the mechanisms of these fractures. In addition to this, the clinical literature is reviewed, and we recommend methods of management for these fractures.

Chapter 5 combines anatomic biomechanical data with clinical data in a comprehensive method that will facilitate clinical management and decision making. In addition, checklists for evaluation and diagnosis of clinical stability are provided, and a flow diagram that may be helpful in subsequent management determination is constructed.

Chapter 6 reviews the literature on spine pain. This chapter attempts to collect and integrate the various facets of this problem and discuss them from a biomechanical perspective. Biomechanics is involved in the epidemiology, diagnosis, and treatment of spine pain. This has been presented and analyzed in considerable detail: The question of spinal manipulation, spinal traction, and

physical therapy; the biomechanics that may be involved in diagnostic procedures; and the biomechanical effects of surgical procedures are evaluated scientifically.

In Chapter 7, the basic principles and mechanics of orthotic devices are discussed. This is followed by a clinical review of virtually all spinal braces.

In Chapter 8, all surgical spinal procedures are studied in a special manner. Traditionally, surgical procedures have been described in terms of the anatomic approach, the surgical technique, and the clinical results. In this chapter we include some of the preceding information, but, in addition, there are *mechanical analyses* of the *surgical contructs* that are employed in spine surgery. This chapter also analyzes the mechanical advantages of polymethylmethacrylate in spine surgery.

Although the Appendix, a glossary of over 100 terms, cites many examples that relate to the spine, the terms have been selected to cover any type of orthopaedic biomechanics. Most of the important biomechanical concepts and terminology are included. Each entry is first defined in scientific terms and is followed by at least one lay- or clinical example. Most are accompanied by an illustration. When relevant, the term is further discussed and mathematical formulas are given in the form of explanatory notes. We hope that this format allows easy and rapid assimilation of each definition and enriches the reader with general orthopaedic biomechanical knowledge.

The Appendix:Glossary is also designed for two levels of interest and reading. It has been written for the reader who is primarily interested in a fundamental understanding of biomechanical terms and for individuals who seek a more detailed and mathematical grasp of the terms. The Appendix:Glossary is designed to be helpful in the understanding of this book, as well as any works referred to therein.

Each chapter has a section called Clinical Biomechanics that summarizes the salient practical clinical features. Explanatory notes also appear at the end of each chapter; they clarify biomechanical concepts by application of mathematical formulas and, in some instances, by citing clinical examples. They are indicated by superscripted letters in the text. A partially annotated bibliography and a topically organized reference section are also included.

The general approach to both the scientific and the clinical aspects of the book is to review the literature, to bring forth the valid trends, and to provide some clinical examples and practical applications. We have endeavored to point out salient unanswered questions or unresolved conflicts and to separate fact, reasoned hypothesis, theory, and speculation.

Although we have tried to be as precise and scientific as possible, for pedagogic reasons we have taken the liberty to interpret and present the information in a teleological context. We trust that this will not offend the pure scientist or distract from our attempts at objectivity.

The authors trust that this integration of theory, fact, and practice involving the biomechanics of the spine will aid both the clinician and the basic scientist in treating and studying the problems of the human spine.

AUGUSTUS A. WHITE III
MANOHAR M. PANJABI

Acknowledgments

To the late Professor Carl Hirsch and his many colleagues, we offer our gratitude and respect. Their inspired investigations have provided a nucleus of information on the biomechanics of the spine. We also wish to express our appreciation to Professor Wayne Southwick, who encouraged us and allowed us to spend the necessary time during the 6 years of preparation that were required to complete this work.

In addition, our thanks are extended to the Medical Illustration Unit at Yale Medical School. A large majority of the illustrations were produced by Mr. Pat Lynch. They reflect his intelligent understanding of the subject matter and his superb perceptual abilities. Mrs. Virginia Simon, the head of the Unit, was most supportive and extremely helpful. Mrs. Gertrude Chaplin, Mr. Tom McCarthy, Dr. Claudia Thomas, Dr. Leon Kier, Mrs. Viola Jacobs, Mrs. Anita White, and Miss Roseann Perito were all most helpful in a variety of ways with the production of illustrations. The Yale Medical Library and its staff lent great assistance. This work has been supported in part by USPHS Grant NS10174.

A number of friends sacrificed their time to read ponderous interim drafts and to offer valuable suggestions; our thanks to Drs. Ben Bradburn, Robert Bucholtz, Donald Chrisman, Edmund Crelin, George Dohrmann, Alan Goodman, Willard Greenwald, Tom Johnson, Peter Jokl, Martin Krag, Robert Margolis, Henry Moss, Lutz Schlicke, John Wolf, and John Fulkerson.

We are ever grateful to Miss Mary Carroll, Mrs. Audrey Mendel, and Miss Joan Mihalakos, who so carefully and laboriously typed several drafts of the manuscript.

Gratitude is also extended to Mr. Lewis Reines for his cooperation, encouragement, and understanding and to Mr. Kenneth Cotton for his precise and conscientious editing skills.

Others who have also been most helpful in a variety of endeavors include Drs. William Fielding, Alf Nachemson, William Collins, Richard Brand, David Keller, Carlton West, and Jeffrey Hausfeld and Mrs. Jacqueline Koral, Mr. Bennie Mayes, and Mr. Donald Summers.

Thank you all.

AUGUSTUS A. WHITE III
MANOHAR M. PANJABI

Contents

8. Biomechanical Considerations in the Surgical Management of the Spine (*Continued*)

1 Physical Properties and Functional Biomechanics of the Spine

It is a capital mistake to theorize before one has data.
Sir Arthur Conan Doyle

This chapter is a review of the literature of what may be thought of as the *basic science* of spine mechanics. It is scientifically rather than clinically oriented and offers thorough knowledge and understanding of the biomechanics of the spine. As such, we believe that it will be helpful to the reader in the evaluation and assimilation of subsequent chapters which are more clinically oriented. We have attempted to present the material so that it is palatable and understandable to those who do not have a special interest in the mechanics of the spine. The in-depth reader is encouraged to refer frequently to the Appendix: Glossary, where all of the biomechanical terms used are defined. Although reading this chapter is not required for comprehension of succeeding chapters, we suggest that it be read and/or referred to as background material for the rest of the book.

The spine is a mechanical structure. The vertebrae articulate with each other in a controlled manner through a complex system of joints, ligaments, and levers. The long, slender, ligamentous, bony structure is markedly stiffened by the rib cage. Although the spine has some inherent ligamentous stability, the major portion of the mechanical stability exhibited is due to highly developed, dynamic neuromuscular structures and a control system. The spine structure is designed to protect the spinal cord, which lies at its center.

The spine has at least three fundamental biomechanical functions. First, it transfers the weights and the bending moments of the head and trunk to the pelvis. Second, it allows sufficient physiologic motion between these three body parts. Finally and most importantly, it protects the delicate spinal cord from potentially damaging forces or motions produced by trauma. These functions are accomplished through the highly specialized mechanical properties of the normal spine anatomy.

We have treated the components of the spine with degrees of detail depending upon the clinical importance and the availability of data. While presenting the experimental data, emphasis has been placed on what was found in a given experiment and how it relates to the biomechanical functions of the spine. Although the experimental techniques are discussed, the details are not given. References are provided for those with a more specific interest.

How should the experimental results be presented? Mere description is not enough.

I often say that when you can measure what you are speaking about and express it in numbers you know something about it: but when you cannot measure it, when you cannot express it in numbers, your knowledge is of a meagre and unsatisfactory kind. (Kelvin, 1891)

However, to keep a logical flow of ideas, an attempt has been made to present as few numbers as possible within the text. The remainder have been collected together and are presented in tabular format throughout the chapter.

BIOMECHANICALLY RELEVANT ANATOMY

The spine consists of seven cervical vertebrae, twelve thoracic vertebrae, five lumbar vertebrae, five fused sacral vertebrae, and three to four fused coccygeal segments. As the spine is viewed in the frontal plane, it generally appears straight and symmetrical. In some individuals there may be a slight right thoracic curve, which may be due either to the position of the aorta or to the increased use of the right hand. In the lateral or sagittal plane there are four normal curves. These curves are convex anteriorly in the cervical and lumbar regions and convex posteriorly in the thoracic and sacral regions. There is a mechanical basis for these normal anatomic curves; they give the spinal column increased flexibility and augmented, shock-absorbing capacity, while at the same time maintaining adequate stiffness and stability at the intervertebral joint level.

The thoracic curve is structural and is due to the lesser vertical height of the anterior thoracic vertebral borders, as opposed to the posterior borders. This is also true of the sacral curve. Curvature of the cervical and lumbar regions is largely due to the wedge-shaped intervertebral discs. Consequently, when distracting forces are applied to the entire spine, there is a greater flattening of the cervical and lumbar lordosis as compared to the thoracic kyphosis.

INTERVERTEBRAL DISC

The intervertebral disc, which has many functions, is subjected to a considerable variety of forces and moments. Along with the facet joints it is responsible for carrying all the compressive loading to which the trunk is subjected.[43,85] When a person is standing in anatomic position, the forces to which a disc is subjected are much greater than the weight of the portion of the body above it. In fact, Nachemson and his associates have determined that the force on a lumbar disc in a sitting position is more than three times the weight of the trunk.[A,65,69] In addition, with any activity where dynamic loads are involved (e.g., jumping and trauma) the actual loads on the intervertebral disc are much higher, perhaps up

to twice as high as those in the static positions. These are mainly compressive loads, producing compressive stresses in the disc. The disc is also subjected to other types of loads and stresses. Tensile stresses are produced in certain portions of the disc during physiologic motions of flexion, extension, and lateral bending. Axial rotation of the torso with respect to the pelvis causes torsional loads which result in shear stresses in the disc. Because rotation and bending are known to be coupled, the stresses in the disc are a combination of tensile, compressive, and shear stresses.

The loads to which the disc is subjected may be divided into two main categories according to the time duration of application: short duration—high amplitude loads (e.g., jerk lifting) and long duration—low magnitude loads due to more normal physical activity. This division is important, since the disc has certain time-dependent properties, such as fatigue and viscoelasticity characterized by hysteresis, creep, and relaxation.

Short duration loading causes irreparable structural damage of the intervertebral disc when a stress of higher value than the ultimate failure stress is generated at a given point. The mechanism of failure during long duration loading of relatively low magnitude is entirely different and is due to fatigue failure. A tear develops at a point where the nominal stress is relatively high (but much less than the ultimate or even yield stress), and it eventually enlarges and results in complete disc failure.

Biomechanically Relevant Anatomy

The intervertebral disc has probably received as much attention as any anatomic structure in the entire spine complex, with the exception of the spinal cord. It constitutes 20 to 33 per cent of the entire height of the vertebral column. The intervertebral disc is comprised of three distinct parts: the nucleus pulposus, the annulus fibrosus, and the cartilaginous end-plates.

The nucleus pulposus is a centrally located area composed of a very loose and translucent network of fine fibrous strands that lie in a mucoprotein gell containing various mucopolysaccharides. The water content ranges from 70 to 90 per cent. It is highest at birth and tends to decrease with age. The lumbar nucleus fills 30 to 50 per

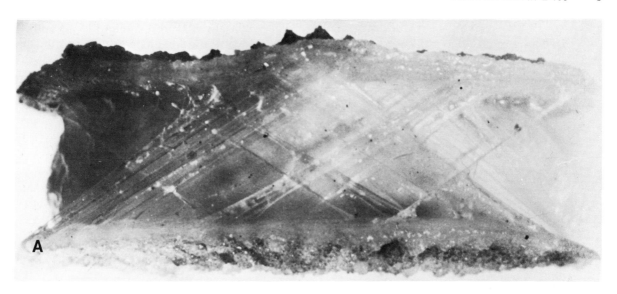

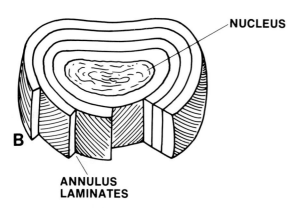

NUCLEUS

ANNULUS
LAMINATES

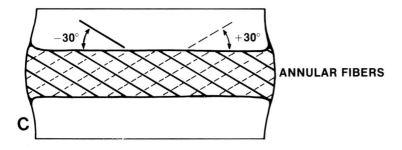

−30° +30°

ANNULAR FIBERS

Fig. 1-1. Intervertebral disc. (*A*) A photograph of a disc clearly shows the annular fibers and their orientation. (*B*) The disc consists of a nucleus pulposus surrounded by the annulus, made of concentric laminated bands of annular fibers. In any two adjacent bands the fibers are oriented in opposite directions. (*C*) The fibers are oriented at about ±30 degrees with respect to the placement of the disc. (Photograph courtesy of Dr. Leon Kazarian.)

cent of the total disc area in cross-section. In the low back, the nucleus is usually more posterior than central and lies at about the juncture of the middle and posterior thirds of the sagittal diameter. The size of the nucleus as well as its capacity to swell is greater in the cervical and lumbar regions.

The annulus fibrosus is a portion of the intervertebral disc which gradually becomes differentiated from the periphery of the nucleus and forms the outer boundary of the disc. This structure is composed of fibrous tissue in concentric laminated bands (Fig. 1-1A, B). The fibers are arranged in a helicoid manner. They run in about the same direction in a given band but in opposite directions in any two adjacent bands. They are oriented at 30 degrees to the disc plane and therefore at 120 degrees to each other in the adjacent bands (Fig. 1-1B, C). The annulus fibers are attached to the cartilaginous end-plates in the inner zone, while in the more peripheral zone they attach directly into the osseous tissue of the vertebral body and are called Sharpey's fibers. This attachment to the vertebra is a good deal stronger than the other more central attachments, which is a useful characteristic in the clinical evaluation of spine trauma, clinical stability, and surgical constructs.

The cartilaginous end-plate is composed of hyaline cartilage that separates the other two components of the disc from the vertebral body. Comparatively little is known about this structure.

BIOMECHANICS OF THE INTERVERTEBRAL DISC

Compression Characteristics

The compression test has been the most popular mechanical test for study of the disc, probably because the disc is the major compression-carrying component of the spine. Many experiments have been done to determine the compressive properties of the disc.[18,27,43,45,87,100]

It may be helpful to know how such a test is actually performed. Typically, a test specimen or a construct consists of a lumbar disc with anterior and posterior longitudinal ligaments, intact, and a thin slice of bone on either side. The specimen is placed in a compression testing machine (Instron type) that is capable of applying large, controlled compressive loads. The load applied to the test specimen and the deformation produced are recorded continuously. The load (y-axis) and deformation (x-axis) curve has been found to be very useful in documenting the physical behavior of test specimens. The specimens for the compression tests of the disc have greatly varied in different experiments, from a disc with thin slices of vertebrae on each side, to a disc with two whole vertebral bodies. Typically, the load displacement curve is of a sigmoid type, with concavity toward the load axis initially, followed by a straight line, and convexity toward the load axis in the final phase, just prior to failure. Such a curve implies that the disc provides very little resistance at low loads. But as the load is increased, the disc becomes stiffer. Thus, it provides flexibility at low loads and stability at high loads.

Virgin observed that although discs were subjected to very high loads and showed permanent deformation on removal of the load, there was no herniation of the nucleus pulposus due to compressive load.[100] Even when a longitudinal incision was made in the posterolateral part of the annulus fibrosus all the way to the center and the specimen was loaded in compression, there was very little change in the elastic properties and definitely no disc herniation. This has been substantiated by further experiments by Hirsch[43] and Markolf and Morris.[62]

To compare the relative strength of the disc to that of the vertebral body in supporting compressive loads, static tests were conducted by Brown and colleagues on motion segments (without posterior elements) of the lumbar region.[18] They found that the first component to fail in such a construct was the vertebra, due to fracture of the end-plates. No failure of the disc ever took place. The mode of failure was solely dependent on the condition of the vertebral body. Osteoporotic vertebrae showed extensive collapse of the end-plate and the underlying bone at relatively low loads. Brown and colleagues observed that there were no differences between the vertebrae with "normal" and degenerated discs. Farfan, to the contrary, proved by his large number of tests that the degenerated disc was actually stronger than the normal disc when subjected to compression,[27] a factor that may be related to the clinical observation of frequent disc rupture and herniation in older age-groups (i.e., 50 and above). Experiments were conducted on lumbar spine specimens utilizing discography to demonstrate the movements of the nucleus pulposus under compressive loading. After the first cracks were heard indicating fracture of the vertebral end-plates, the nucleus was found to migrate into the bodies,

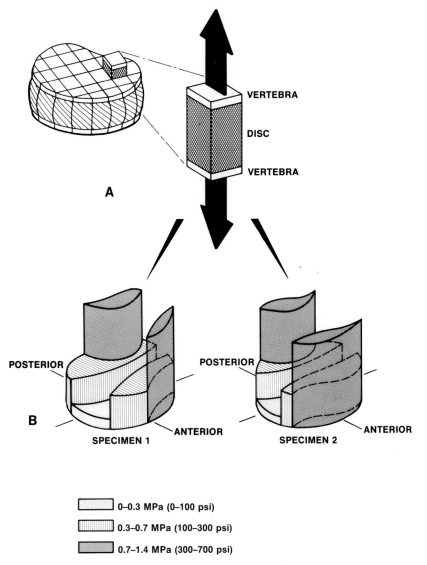

Fig. 1-2. Tensile strength of disc material. (*A*) For the tensile test, the disc specimens were obtained by dividing the vertebra-disc-vertebra construct into longitudinal sections. (*B*) The results of the tensile tests performed on two specimens are depicted in the form of contour maps, where the height represents the strength in tension at that point. The disc is strongest in the anterior and posterior regions, the center being the weakest. (Based upon the findings of Brown, T., Hanson, R., and Yorra, A.: Some mechanical tests on the lumbosacral spine with particular reference to the intervertebral discs. J. Bone Joint Surg., 39A: 1135, 1957.)

resembling Schmorl's nodes. These observations suggest that disc herniation is not caused by excessive compressive loading, although Schmorl's nodes may be the result of such a loading.

With central compressive loading, the disc was observed to bulge in the horizontal plane, but not in any particular direction.[18] This implies that the tendency for the disc to herniate posterolaterally, as seen in the clinical situation, is *not* inherent to the structure of the disc, but must depend upon

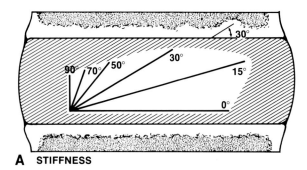

A STIFFNESS

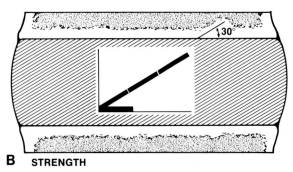

B STRENGTH

Fig. 1-3. Disc anisotropy. (A) Stiffness of the disc annulus in different directions is shown. The stiffness is highest along a direction 15 degrees to the disc plane and lowest along the disc axis. (B) The strength of the annulus along two directions is compared. Samples taken along the direction of the annulus fiber were found to be about three times as strong as those taken along the horizontal direction. (Results based upon data from Galante, J. O.: Tensile properties of the human lumbar annulus fibrosis. Acta Orthop. Scand., *100* [Suppl.], 1967.)

certain loading situations other than compression (assuming that uniform stress prevails in the disc under compressive loading).

Tensile Properties

Axial tensile stresses are produced in the annulus fibrosus of the disc during physiologic flexion, extension, and lateral bending. The instantaneous axes of rotation (IAR) for these motions lie in a frontal plane that divides the disc into two equal halves. Their exact position, which has not been precisely determined, depends upon the type and amount of motion and, probably, upon the region of the spine. Due to rotation about the instantaneous axes, some part of the disc is always subjected to axial tensile stresses during these

activities. Axial rotation of the spine also produces tensile stress, but at 45 degrees to the spine axis. Finally, compressive loading also produces tensile stresses (Figs. 1-8, 1-9). Thus, it may be concluded that the disc is subjected to tensile stresses in all different directions under various loading situations.

Two types of studies have been conducted on the tensile properties of the disc: mapping out the strength of disc material at different locations and orientations; and determining the mechanical properties of the intact disc. Strength of disc material was studied by cutting the disc-vertebrae construct into multiple, axially oriented, rectangular sections (Fig. 1-2A). The specimens were stretched to failure in a testing machine, and the load-displacement diagrams were recorded. Failure load values were collected from various samples and were put together as axial tensile strength maps of the disc. Results for the two discs tested by Brown and colleagues are shown in Figure 1-2B. We note that although there is some variation between the strength maps of the two discs, in general, the anterior and posterior regions are stronger than the lateral region, and the central region, consisting of the nucleus pulposus, is the weakest. This distribution may be "nature's attempt" to provide strength where most of the failures and herniations tend to occur.

What is the strength along directions other than axial? With this question in mind, Galante performed extensive biomechanical tests of the disc material.[35] He cut the disc annulus into thin samples (1 × 2 mm) along different orientations and subjected these samples to tensile loads. His results for stiffness[B] of the disc are summarized in Figure 1-3A. The stiffness was found to vary to a great extent with the orientation of the samples; the axial samples were the most flexible, while the samples taken at 15 degrees to the horizontal plane were the stiffest.

Since the loads applied in these experiments were rather low, separate experiments were performed to determine the strength. Samples were taken from only two directions. The samples were loaded until failure occurred. The results are presented in Figure 1-3B. Comparing the results of the samples taken along the horizontal direction with those taken along the fiber direc-

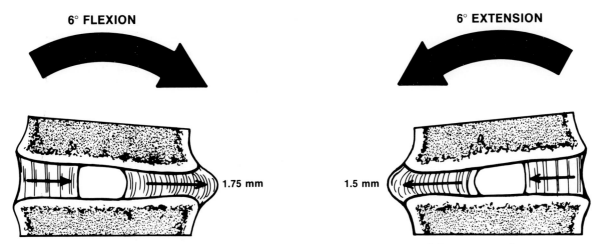

6° FLEXION

6° EXTENSION

1.75 mm

1.5 mm

Fig. 1-4. Disc protrusion with bending. Flexion as well as extension of the spine produces motion of the disc in the horizontal plane. In both cases of bending there is bulging of the disc on the concave side and contraction on the convex side. In a pathologic case the expansion of the disc during physiologic bending may stretch or impinge the nerve root. (Based upon the data of Brown, T., Hanson, R., and Yorra, A.: Some mechanical tests on the lumbosacral spine with particular reference to the intervertebral discs. J. Bone Joint Surg., 39A:1135, 1957.)

tion, the latter were found to be about three times as strong as the former.

The results of tests of stiffness as well as strength clearly show that the disc is a highly anisotropic structure. This specialized structure has been optimized to resist certain kinds of loads in the most efficient manner. However, such specialization of the mechanical properties of the disc has a negative consequence; the disc is not able to resist other kinds of loads in an equally optimal manner.

The second type of study on the tensile properties of the disc as a structure was conducted by Markolf.[60] He loaded the vertebra-disc-vertebra specimens from the thoracic and lumbar regions in tension using an Instron testing machine. The disc was found to be less stiff in tension than under compression. This was attributed to the buildup of fluid pressure within the nucleus under compression loading.

Bending Characteristics

Bending and torsional loads are of particular interest, since experimental findings suggest that these and not the compression loads are the most damaging to the disc.[27]

Bending of 6 to 8 degrees in the sagittal, fron-

tal, and other vertical planes did not result in failure of the lumbar disc. However, after removal of the posterior elements and with 15 degrees of bending (anterior flexion), failure did occur.[18] A triangular piece of bone was avulsed from the posteroinferior aspect of the superior vertebra in this experiment. Other interesting findings concerned the bulging of the disc during normal physiologic motions. The disc bulged anteriorly during flexion, posteriorly during extension, and toward the concavity of the spinal curve during lateral bending. The disc contracted on the opposite sides (on the convexity of the curve). Very little motion took place in a direction perpendicular to the plane of motion. The results of flexion and extension showing sagittal plane expansion and contraction of the disc are depicted in Figure 1-4. These findings were confirmed by Roaf,[87] who noticed that the bulging of the annulus is always on the concave side of the curve, and that denucleation seemed to *increase* bulging. However, no exact measurements were given. With the help of nucleographs of the disc, Roaf found that during flexion/extension the nucleus pulposus does not change in shape or position. This information is useful and offers support to those who emphasize the importance

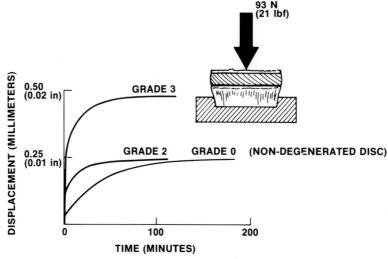

Fig. 1-5. Creep behavior of the disc. The creep behavior of a structure is documented by applying a sudden load and maintaining it. The deformation of the structure as a function of time is recorded. This behavior seems to correlate with the degree of degeneration of the intervertebral disc. A sample of creep curves for discs with different grades of degeneration are shown. The non-degenerated disc (Grade 0) has smaller overall deformation, and this deformation is reached over a relatively longer period as compared to the degenerated disc (Grade 3). (Based upon data of Kazarian, L. E.: Creep characteristics of the human spinal column. Orthop. Clin. North Am., 6:3, 1975.)

of a "flat back" or the maintenance of a slightly flexed lumbar spine as treatment and prophylaxis for patients with low back pain or sciatica.

Torsional Behavior

The hypothesis that torsion may be the major injury-causing load was put forward by Farfan in 1973.[27] It is based upon the earlier work by his group.[29] In the particular experiment, vertebra-disc-vertebra construct (including the posterior elements) was subjected to torsional loading around a fixed axis passing through the posterior aspect of the disc. Torque was applied, and continuous record was made of the applied torque and the angle of deformation until the failure occurred. The torque angle curves were found to be of sigmoid shape, with three distinct phases. In the initial phase, 0 to 3 degrees of deformation could be produced by very little torque. In the intermediate phase, consisting of 3 to 12 degrees of rotation, there was a linear relationship be-

tween the torque and the angular deformation. In the final phase, about 20 degrees of rotation was generally required to produce the failure. The angle of failure was somewhat less for degenerated discs. Sharp, cracking sounds emanating from the specimen were always noted before failure occurred. On close examination, no failure of the end-plates was found. It is believed that the cracking sounds came from the injuries to the annulus. This is reminiscent of the crack or snap that is sometimes felt or heard when patients report acute low back injuries.

Farfan and colleagues[29] tested a total of 21 normal and 14 abnormal discs from the lumbar region, according to the technique described above. They found that the average failure torque for the normal discs was 25 per cent higher than that for the abnormal discs. The average angle at failure for the normal discs was 16 degrees, and that for the abnormal discs was 14.5 degrees. Generally, a large disc exhibited large torsional

Table 1-1. Stiffness Coefficients of the Intervertebral Disc (Average Values)

AUTHORS	STIFFNESS COEFFICIENT*	MAXIMUM LOAD*	SPINE REGION
Compression (−Fy†)			
Virgin, 1951	2.5 MN/m	4500 N	Lumbar
Hirsch & Nachemson, 1954	0.7 MN/m	1000 N	Lumbar
Brown, et al., 1957	2.3 MN/m	5300 N	Lumbar
Markolf, 1970	1.8 MN/m	1800 N	Thoracic & lumbar
Tension (+Fy†)			
Markolf, 1970	1.0 MN/m	1800 N	Thoracic & lumbar
Shear (Fx, Fz†)			
Markolf, 1970	0.26 MN/m	150 N	Thoracic & lumbar
Axial Rotation (My†)			
Farfan, 1970	2.0 N m/deg	31 N m	Lumbar

* N = newton, kN = 1000 newton, MN = 1,000,000 newton
To convert to the inch-pound system, multiply by the following numbers:

(MN/m) × 5600 = lbf/in   (N m/deg) × 0.738 = in lbf/deg
(N) × 0.225 = lbf   (N m) × 0.738 = in lbf

† See Figure 1-23.

strength. A round disc was found to be stronger than an oval disc.

Shear Characteristics

Experiments on torsion of the disc provide important information regarding the torsional strength of the disc *as an intact structure.* Although the disc is subjected to shear stresses during torsional loading, the stresses are not uniformly distributed. They are high along the periphery and low in the center. Therefore, the torsional experiments do not provide precise information about the horizontal shear charcteristics of the disc. Experiments were performed to study the lumbar disc in direct shear. The shear stiffness in the horizontal plane (anteroposterior and lateral directions) was found to be about 260 N/mm.[60] This is a high value and is clinically significant, showing that a large force is required to cause an abnormal horizontal displacement of a normal vertebral disc unit. This means that it is relatively rare for the annulus to fail clinically due to pure shear loading. Most likely, clinical evidence of annular disruption implies that the disc has failed due to some combination of bending, torsion, and tension. Numerical values for stiffness properties of the disc for various physiologic motions have been collectively provided in Table 1-1.

Creep and Relaxation

The intervertebral disc exhibits creep and relaxation.[45] Markolf and Morris studied creep under the application of three different loads and made observations up to 70 minutes.[62] The higher loads produced greater deformation and faster rates of creep. Kazarian performed creep tests on spine motion segments and classified the discs of the specimens into four grades, from 0 to 3 according to their degree of degeneration.[46] (This classification is similar to the one used by Rolander.[89]) He observed that the creep characteristics and the disc grades are related, as shown in Figure 1-5. Note that the shapes of the curves are different. The non-degenerated discs (Grade 0) creep slowly and reach their final deformation value after considerable time, as compared to the degenerated discs (Grades 2 and 3). The Grade 0 curve is characteristic of a more viscoelastic structure as compared to the curves of Grades 2 and 3. Thus, the process of degeneration makes the discs less viscoelastic. This implies that as the disc degenerates, it loses the capability to attenuate shocks and to distribute the load uniformly over the entire end-plate.

Hysteresis

All viscoelastic structures, including the disc and motion segment, exhibit hysteresis. It is a phenomenon in which there is loss of energy when a structure is subjected to repetitive load and unload cycles. When a person jumps up or down, the shock energy is absorbed on the way from the feet to the brain by the discs and vertebrae due to hysteresis. It may be thought of as a protective mechanism. This phenomenon was first observed in the discs by Virgin.[100] Hysteresis seems to vary with the load applied and the age of the disc, as well as its level. The larger the load, the greater the hysteresis. It is largest in very young people and least in the middle-aged. Virgin observed that the lower thoracic and upper lumbar discs showed less hysteresis than the lower lumbar discs. He also observed that hysterresis decreased when the same disc was loaded a second time. This may imply that we are less protected against repetitive loads. Epidemiologic studies show people who drive motor vehicles have a higher incidence of herniated discs.[48] The repetitive axial vibrations may be a factor.

Fatigue Tolerance

Fatigue tests of the disc are important for establishing the number of load cycles which can be tolerated before radial and circumferential tears develop. As the biologic capacity for repair and regeneration of the disc is thought to be low, its fatigue properties are rather important. Unfortunately, very little is known about this subject. Brown and colleagues performed a single fatigue test on the disc by applying a small constant axial load and a repetitive forward bending motion of 5 degrees.[18] The disc showed signs of failure after only 200 cycles of bending, and it completely failed after 1000 cycles. This indicates that the fatigue life is low under such experimental conditions in vitro. The fatigue tolerance of the disc in vivo is not known.

Intradiscal Pressure

There are very few precise studies on the behavior of the spine components in vivo. Most of the work is done on cadaver materials. Although these studies have provided large amounts of valuable information, the magnitude of the loads applied to the disc cannot be determined in vitro. Nachemson and his associates determined for the first time the actual loads to which a disc is sub-

jected in vivo.[69] They utilized the concept of nucleus pulposus as a load transducer. By means of in vitro experiments on vertebra-disc-vertebra preparations, they found that the fluid pressure within the nucleus is directly related to the axial compression applied to the disc (Fig. 1-6A). The pressure was measured by a transducer in the form of a special needle, carrying a miniature electronic pressure gauge at its tip. Thus, by measuring the pressure within the nucleus, they could compute the load on the disc.

This technique was utilized by Nachemson[65] and Rolander[89] to measure the prestress present in the discs. They measured the nucleus before and after cutting the posterior elements. A pressure of 0.07 MPa (10 psi) was found in the intact motion segment, while there was none when the arch was removed. This corresponds to a compressive prestress of about 120 N (26 lbf).

Having developed the technique, Nachemson and his group have measured the in vivo loads to which the lumbar discs are subjected when a person is resting in different body postures or performing a certain task.[66,67,69] A sample of the results of their work is shown in Figure 1-6B. Observe that the load carried by the discs is rather large. Although the portion of the body about the L3 disc constitutes 60 per cent of the total body weight, the load on the L3 disc, in sitting and standing positions with 20 degrees of flexion, is 200 per cent. It becomes 300 per cent with the addition of 20 kg (44 lb) of weight in the hands. A biomechanical analysis of the high load to which the disc is subjected is depicted in Figure 1-24 and is discussed in the Notes.[1]

"Self Sealing" Phenomenon

Since the intervertebral disc lacks a direct blood supply, which is essential for any normal reparative process in the body to take place, another kind of repair mechanism is most likely.[44] There is some experimental evidence which suggests that the construction of the disc is such that when an intact disc is injured, some type of immediate "self sealing" mechanism takes place.

Markolf and Morris reported the results of an experiment with compression loading of injured discs.[62] Their basic specimen consisted of a motion segment which had been modified by saw-

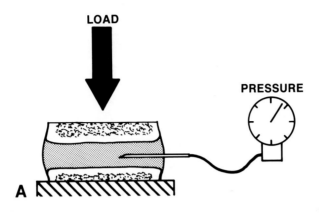

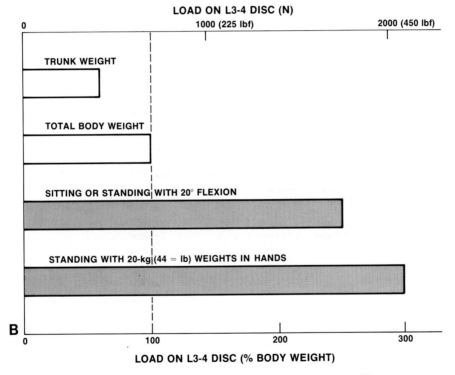

Fig. 1-6. Interdiscal pressure and loads on the disc. (A) The needle pressure transducer is calibrated by introducing it into the nucleus pulposus of a cadaveric motion segments. A correlation is obtained between the compressive load applied and the pressure within the nucleus. (B) Using the same needle transducers, in vivo measurements were made at the L3-4 disc in volunteers performing physiologic tasks. The bar graphs record the compressive load on the disc. Note that the disc load while standing with a 20-kg weight in the hands is about three times the weight of the whole body. (Results based upon those of Nachemson, A.: Electromyographic studies on the vertebral portion of the psoas muscle. Acta Orthop. Scand., 37:177, 1966.)

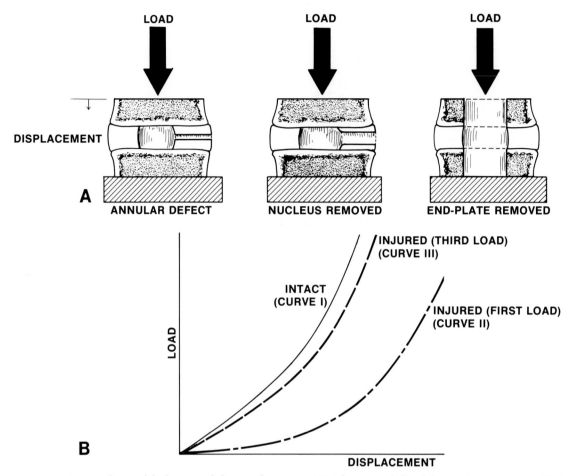

Fig. 1-7. Biomechanical behavior of disc with injury. (*A*) Three models of disc injury were studied. An annular defect involved puncturing the posterolateral wall of the annulus, producing a vent 3 to 4 mm in diameter. A nucleus defect was created by entirely removing the nucleus by way of a tunnel through the annulus. End-plate removal was accomplished by removing the nucleus, and the end-plates and the supporting bone directly above and below it. (*B*) The behavior of three disc injury models under the application of compressive load was similar. A typical set of load-deflection curves is shown. Curve I is for an intact disc specimen, and Curve II is for the same specimen after injury. Note the decrease in stiffness as shown by the lower slope of this curve as compared to that of Curve I. The same injured specimen when loaded a third time (after two load/unload cycles) exhibited Curve III. Note how similar Curves I and III are. (Results from Markolf, K. L., and Morris, J. M.: The structural components of the intervertebral disc. J. Bone Joint Surg., 56A:675, 1974.)

ing off the posterior elements at the pedicles. Three models of injury were studied: a radial hole (3–4 mm in diameter through the annulus), discectomy, and an axial hole through the entire construct, removing the central portion of the end-plates and the nucleus pulposus. These are graphically depicted in Figure 1-7A. Each specimen was tested twice, once before and once after the experimental injury. The test after injury involved three load/unload cycles. The mechanical characteristics recorded were the load-deflection curve, the creep behavior, and the relaxation test, all under compressive loading.

With the first loading cycle and with subsequent injury results showed that there were definite changes in the mechanical characteristics of an intact specimen. But a remarkable "self sealing" process came into play when the specimen was loaded for a second and third time. During the third loading cycle, the motion segment showed near "intact" behavior again. This was found to be independent of the type of injury. A total of 18 specimens were tested, consisting of normal as well as degenerated discs. Figure 1-7B shows three typical load-deformation curves of a specimen that was injured and subsequently loaded three times. Curve I was obtained when the specimen was intact. Curve II shows the load-deflection relationship of the specimen, with injury during the first loading cycle. Note the definite shift of the curve. Finally, Curve III shows the same relationship but under the third loading cycle. Note the similarity between Curves I and III.

This experiment suggests that there is a repair or an adjustment mechanism in the disc which is mechanical in nature. It has been shown that a defect in the annular ring alters the mechanical characteristics of the disc and the adjustment is such as to restore near pre-injury disc function. Since the specimens were taken from younger and older people, with normal as well as degenerative discs, these results are not dependent on the viscosity or softness of the nucleus. However, there are at least two unmentioned qualifying issues. First, these tests were done with only one kind of loading, compression. How does the sealing mechanism work with other physiologic loads, such as bending and torsion? Secondly, how is the *immediate* repair mechanism maintained or modified by time and in vivo? The answers to these questions await further experimental studies.

Functional Biomechanics of Disc

Conclusions drawn from the analyses in this section are based upon experimental observations,[18,43,87,89,97] as well as on sophisticated computer simulations.[52,53,96] Although in vivo the loads applied to the disc are certainly very complex, for the sake of understanding each is discussed separately.

Compression. The compressive load is transferred from one vertebral end-plate to the other by way of the nucleus pulposus and the annulus

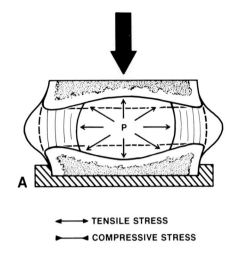

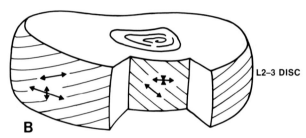

Fig. 1-8. Non-degenerated disc under compression. (A) Pressure within the nucleus is produced due to compression. This pressure pushes the disc annulus and the two end-plates outward. The disc bulges out in the horizontal plane, and the end-plates deflect in the axial direction. (B) The annulus is subjected to varying amounts of stresses in different directions and at different depths. On the outer layers there is a large tensile stress in the tangential peripheril direction, a large tensile stress along the annulus fibers, and a relatively small tensile stress in the axial direction. In the inner layers of the annulus the stresses are generally smaller in magnitude but of the same type, except for the axial stress, which is now compressive. (Based upon mathematical simulations by Kulak, R. F., Belytschko, T. B., Schultz, A. B., and Galante, G. O.: Non-linear behavior of the human intervertebral disc under axial load. J. Biomech., 9:377, 1976.)

fibrosus. In early years of life (up to age 25 to 30), the nucleus has sufficient moisture to act like a gelatinous mass.[13,71,86] As the load is applied, a certain pressure is developed within the nucleus. This fluid pressure pushes the surrounding structures in all directions away from the nucleus center (Figure 1-8A). In other words, the central

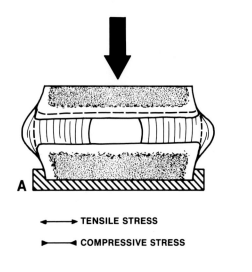

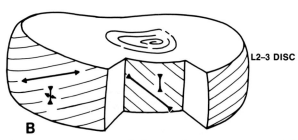

Fig. 1-9. Degenerated disc under compression. (*A*) The compressive load is carried through a different mechanism. The load is transferred from one end-plate to the other by way of the annulus only, thus loading the end-plates at the periphery. (*B*) The stresses in the degenerated disc annulus are significantly different as compared to those in the non-degenerated disc (Fig. 1-8B). In the outer layers of the disc the tangential (peripheral) stress is much smaller while the annulus fibers are subjected to nearly twice as much stress. Further, the axial stress is smaller but compressive. In the inner layers the fiber stress remains very high but now it is compressive. (Based upon mathematical simulations by Kulak, R. F., Belytschko, T. B., Schultz, A. B., and Galante, G. O.: Non-linear behavior of the human intervertebral disc under axial load. J. Biomech., 9:377, 1976.)

portions of the two vertebral end-plates are pushed away from each other, and the annular ring is pushed radially outward. The compression produces complex stresses within the annular ring. Stresses along various directions in the outer and inner laminae of the annulus are shown in Figure 1-8B. The length of an arrow approxi-

mately corresponds to the relative magnitude of the stress. In the outer layer there is tension in all directions, but it is significantly greater in the circumferential than in the axial direction. Also depicted is the stress along the direction of the annular fibers. Arrangement of the fibers at ±30 degrees accommodates absorption of tensile stresses, as shown by the high value of stress along these directions. The innermost lamina of the annulus is subjected to somewhat different stresses. The circumferential stress is lower as is the fiber stress, and the axial stress is now compressive. In addition, there is fluid pressure of the nucleus that supports the inner laminae. The orientation of annular fibers and the nucleus play important roles in transferring the compressive loads from one vertebra to another.

The situation is quite different when the nucleus is dry (Fig. 1-9A). The load-transferring mechanism is significantly altered because the nucleus is not capable of building sufficient fluid pressure. As a result, the end-plates are subjected to less pressure at the center, and the loads are distributed more around the periphery. The stresses in the annular ring are also changed. Compare Figure 1-9B and 1-8B. In the outer layers of the annulus of a degenerated disc there is less peripherial tension, more axial stress and much larger fiber stress. Note that the axial stress is now compressive. In the inner layers of the annulus the fiber stress is still large but changes direction and becomes compressive, while the axial compressive stress remains constant throughout the annulus, and the peripheral stress nearly vanishes. These findings are based upon computer simulations of an L2–L3 intervertebral disc, subjected to compression by Kulak and colleagues.[53]

Tension. A detailed computer simulation of the disc under tensile loading has not been carried out. We present a highly simplified analysis. To find out the mechanism by which the disc is able to carry tensile loads, imagine the disc being cut by a plane that is perpendicular to the fiber directions of an annular lamina. (This is the technique of free body analysis.) To support the tensile loads, there are two types of stresses that are produced within the annulus, normal and shear, respectively perpendicular and parallel to the cut surface. The shear stresses are relatively larger in magnitude. Although the normal stresses are nicely absorbed by the alternating layers of annular fibers, there is no provision for resisting the shear stresses. Thus the risk of disc failure is greater with tensile loading as compared to compressive loading. Another difference between the two types of loading is the change in the horizontal dimensions of the disc. Due to Poisson's effect, the disc bulges during compression and contracts in tension.

Bending. The spine is subjected to tension on its convex side and compression on its concave side when bending loads are applied during flexion, extension, and lateral bending. One part of the disc is subjected to compression, while the other part is loaded in tension, as depicted in Figure 1-10A. Thus, bending loads can be thought of as somewhat of a combination of tensile and compressive loads, each applied to about one-half of the disc.[c] The effect on the disc is, then, a combination of the effects due to the two types of load. The side of the annulus subjected to tension contracts in the horizontal plane, while the side under compression bulges out. The annular fibers resist the compressive and tensile loads by the mechanisms already described. The complete mathematical stress analysis of the intervertebral disc subjected to bending has not been performed. However, a simplified version is presented in Figure 1-10B. The instantaneous axis of rotation separates the compressive and the tensile stress zones. Note the increase in stress from the inner towards the outer layers.

Torsion. When the disc is subjected to torsion, there are shear stresses in the horizontal as well as the axial plane. The magnitude of these stresses varies in direct proportion to the distance from the axis of rotation (Figure 1-11A). In planes between the horizontal and the axial, there are other combinations of stresses present. The stresses at 45 and 60 degrees to the horizontal plane are shown in Figure 1-11B. If the direction of the torque is reversed, the directions of all the stresses also reverse. As the orientation of the annular fibers is about ±30 degrees to the horizontal plane, these fibers, although not ideally suited, are capable of resisting the tensile stresses due to torsional loads. However, shear stresses

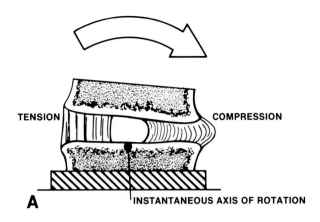

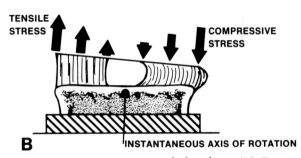

Fig. 1-10. Disc stresses with bending. (A) During bending (flexion, extension, and lateral bending) one side of the annulus is subjected to compression while the other side is put under tensile load. The instantaneous axis of rotation separates the two zones. On the compression side the disc bulges, while it contracts on the tension side. (B) The stresses vary in magnitude from maximum in the outer laminae of the annulus to zero at the instantaneous axis of rotation.

that are perpendicular to the fiber direction may produce disc failure.

Shear. This is the type of force that acts in the horizontal plane, perpendicular to the long axis of the spine. It produces shear stresses that are about equal in magnitude over the entire annulus and are parallel to the applied shear force. There are also tensile and compressive stresses at ±45 degrees to the horizontal plane. These are similar to those for the torsional load shown in Figure 1-11B.

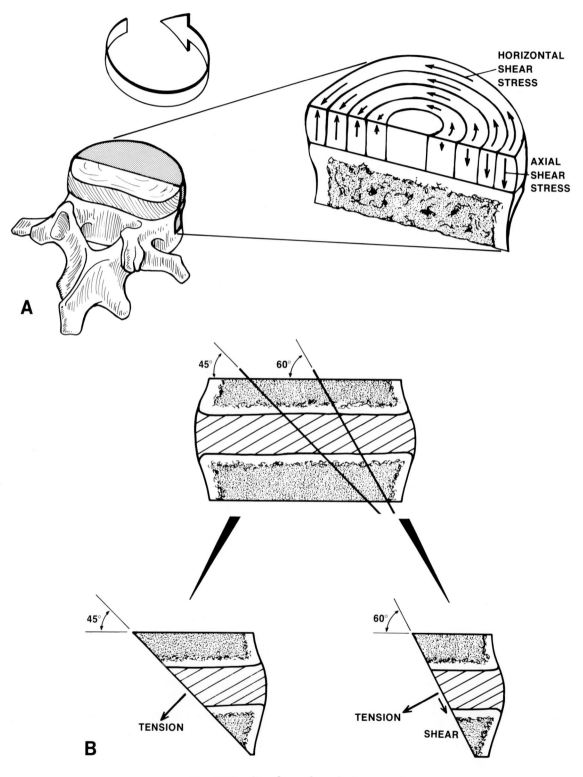

Fig. 1-11. (See legend on facing page.)

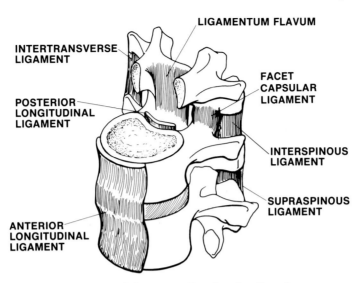

LIGAMENTUM FLAVUM

INTERTRANSVERSE
LIGAMENT

POSTERIOR
LONGITUDINAL
LIGAMENT

FACET
CAPSULAR
LIGAMENT

INTERSPINOUS
LIGAMENT

SUPRASPINOUS
LIGAMENT

ANTERIOR
LONGITUDINAL
LIGAMENT

Fig. 1-12. Ligaments of the spine. Besides the disc, there are seven ligaments that connect one vertebra to the next. Contribution to the spine stability by an individual ligament is dependent upon its cross-section, its distance from the instantaneous axis of rotation, and its orientation in space. The anatomy of the ligaments is such as to collectively provide stability to the spine in its various physiologic motions.

These free body analyses show how various combinations of functional loading patterns and torsion and bending modalities have the potential to exert the greatest tensile stresses in the annular fibers. This mechanism of mechanical failure of annular fibers fits best with what is known about the biomechanical, structural, and anatomic characteristics of the intervertebral disc.

SPINE LIGAMENTS

Ligaments are uniaxial structures; they are most effective in carrying loads along the direction in which the fibers run. In this respect, they are much like rubber bands. They readily resist tensile forces but buckle when subjected to compression. Nature has designed the spine motion segments in such a way that when the motion segment is subjected to different complex force and torque vectors, the individual ligaments, providing resistance to the loads, experience only the tensile forces.

The ligaments have many different functions, some of which may seem to be in opposition to others. First, the ligaments must allow adequate physiologic motion and fixed postural attitudes between vertebrae, with a minimum expenditure of muscle energy. Secondly, they must protect the spinal cord by restricting the motions within well-defined limits. Finally, they must protect the spinal cord in traumatic situations where high loads are applied at fast speeds. In these highly dynamic situations, not only is the displacement to be restricted within safe limits, but large amounts of energy that are suddenly applied to the spine must also be absorbed.

Fig. 1-11. Disc stresses with torsion. (*A*) Application of a torsional load to the disc produces shear stresses in the disc. These are in the horizontal plane as well as in the axial direction and both are always of equal magnitude. However, they vary at different points in the disc in proportion to the distance from the instantaneous axis of rotation. (*B*) At 45 degrees to the disc plane, the stresses are normal (i.e., there are no shear stresses). However, at 60 degrees to the disc plane, perpendicular to the annular fibers, both types of stresses are present, normal as well as shear. The normal stresses are efficiently taken up by the annular fibers.

Biomechanically Relevant Anatomy

There are seven ligaments of the spine (Fig. 1-12). A short description of each of the ligaments arranged from anterior to posterior follows:

The anterior longitudinal ligament is a fibrous tissue structure which arises from the anterior aspect of the basioccipital and is attached to the atlas and the anterior surfaces of all vertebrae, down to and including a part of the sacrum. It attaches firmly to the edges of the vertebral bodies but is not so firmly affixed to the annular fibers of the intervertebral disc. The width of the anterior longitudinal ligament is diminished at the level of the disc. It is narrower and thicker in the thoracic region.

The posterior longitudinal ligament arises from the posterior aspect of the basioccipital, covers the dens and the transverse ligament (where it is called the membrana tectoria), and runs over the posterior surfaces of all the vertebral bodies down to the coccyx. It too is thicker in the thoracic region. It has an interwoven connection with the intervertebral disc. In contradistinction to the anterior longitudinal ligament, it is wider at the disc level and narrower at the vertebral body level.

The intertransverse ligaments pass between the transverse processes in the thoracic region and are characterized as rounded cords, intimately connected with the deep muscles of the back.

The capsular ligaments are attached just beyond the margins of the adjacent articular processes. The fibers are generally oriented in a direction perpendicular to the plane of the facet joints. They are shorter and more taut in the thoracic and lumbar regions than in the cervical region.

The ligamenta flava extend from the anterior inferior border of the laminae above to the posterior superior border of the laminae below. They connect the borders of adjacent laminae from the second cervical vertebra to the first sacral vertebra. The yellow ligaments are thicker in the thoracic region. Although they seem to be paired due to a midline cleavage, each is rather like a single structure that extends from the roots of the articular process on one side to the corresponding process on the other. The ligament is composed of a large amount of elastic fibers and represents the most pure elastic tissue in the human body. It has been noted, however, that with aging there is an increase in the relative amount of fibrous tissue.

The interspinous ligaments connect adjacent spines, and their attachments extend from the root to the apex of each process. They are narrow and elongated in the thoracic region, broader and thicker in the lumbar region, and only slightly developed in the neck.

The supraspinous ligament originates in the ligamentum nuchae and continues along the tips of the spinous processes as a round, slender strand down to the sacrum. It is thicker and broader in the lumbar region than in the thoracic region.

BIOMECHANICS OF SPINE LIGAMENTS

Anterior and Posterior Longitudinal Ligaments

The anterior and posterior ligaments lie on the anterior and posterior surfaces of the disc and are attached to both the disc and the vertebral bodies. Therefore, these ligaments deform not only due to the relative separation between the two adjacent vertebrae but also due to bulging of the disc.

Several functions and characteristics have been attributed to the longitudinal ligament. Traction at the attachment points may produce "anterior lipping" of the vertebrae, as seen clinically.[3] Longitudinal ligaments degenerate with age, as does the disc.[8,39] Roaf claimed that it is not possible to disrupt the anterior longitudinal ligament by flexion or extension of the spine, although it could be accomplished by rotation.[87]

Tkaczuk did an extensive study (484 samples) of the tensile characteristics of both the anterior and posterior longitudinal ligaments of the lumbar spine with the purpose of examining the influence on the biomechanical properties due to degeneration and age.[99]

In one set of experiments, specimens of a standard size were used.[D] These samples were loaded up to one-third of the failure load, and the load-deformation curves were plotted. Three parameters were measured: the maximum deformation, the residual or permanent deformation, and the energy loss of hysteresis. All the biomechanical parameters were found to decrease with age. The greatest decrease was found in the energy absorption values. This documents the decrease in the shock-absorbing characteristics of the ligaments with age. Regarding the degenerative changes, Tkaczuk found that the maximum, as well as the residual, deformations were lower for the degenerated discs.

In another set of experiments, intact ligament samples were tested to failure.[D] The load-deformation curves were found to be similar in shape to the stress-strain curves of the ligamentum flavum.[68] This implies that the functional design of the spinal ligaments are similar. The anterior longitudinal ligament was found to be twice as strong as the posterior ligament. But, the *material* properties of the two ligaments were nearly the same, as shown by the strength values of the samples of *equal* cross-section (failure stress) taken from the two ligaments. Just as in the ligamentum flavum, there was some pre-tension present in these ligaments. It was estimated to be about one-tenth of that of the ligamentum flavum. Measurements of the physical properties of anterior and posterior longitudinal ligaments are given in Table 1-2.

Intertransverse and Capsular Ligaments

The physical properties of the intertransverse and capsular ligaments have yet to be determined. The intertransverse ligaments may have some significant effect on the mechanics of the spine because of the large lever arms of these ligaments with respect to the instant centers of motion in lateral bending and axial rotation. The contribution of the capsular ligaments has been proven in the cervical spine.[78,105] It has also been shown that under certain conditions of axial loading, such as in pilot ejections from aircrafts, the capsular ligaments are stretched.[85]

Ligamentum Flavum

The function and importance of the ligamentum flavum in humans has been a matter of discussion from the beginning of this century.[31,98] Although there have been some studies where the biomechanical aspects have been explored,[2,74]

Table 1-2. Physical Properties of Spine Ligaments

Ligamentum Flavum*		
	YOUNG† (< 20 years)	OLD† (> 70 years)
Resting force	18 N	5 N
Failure stress	10 MPa	2 MPa
Extension at failure	70%	30%

Anterior and Posterior Longitudinal Ligaments‡		
	ANTERIOR†	POSTERIOR†
Pretension (non-degenerated)	1.8 N	3.0 N
Pretension (degenerated)	1.2 N	1.8 N
Failure load	340 N	180 N
Failure stress	21 MPa	20 MPa

* Adapted from Nachemson, A., and Evans, J.: Some mechanical properties of the third lumbar inter-laminar ligament (ligamentum flavum). J. Biomech., *1*:211, 1968.
† 1 MPa = 1,000,000 N/m² = 145 lbf/in²
  1 N = 0.225 lbf
‡ Adapted from Tkaczuk, H.: Tensile properties of human lumbar longitudinal ligaments. Acta Orthop. Scand., *115* [Suppl.], 1968.

there has been only one study where modern tissue handling techniques and mechanical testing machines have been utilized.[68] In that study, ten specimens of ligamentum flavum and attached laminae, from the L3–4 motion segments, were tested. The specimens were loaded in tension along the spine axis, and the tests were performed at slow speed in an Instron testing machine.

While separating the vertebral laminae from the bodies, Nachemson and Evans found the ligamentum flavum to have pre-tension (the tension present in situ when the spine is in neutral position). This "resting" tension in the ligament produces "resting" compression of the disc. The value of these resting forces was found to decrease with age from about 18 N (4.5 lbf) in the young (< 20 years) to about 5 N (1.1 lbf) in the older (> 70 years) subjects. These "resting" forces most probably have some function. Perhaps they prevent protrusion of the ligament into the spinal canal during full extension of the spine when the ligamentum flavum is slack. Also, the resting compression in the disc may add some stability to the spine. Detailed physical properties of this ligament are given in Table 1-2.

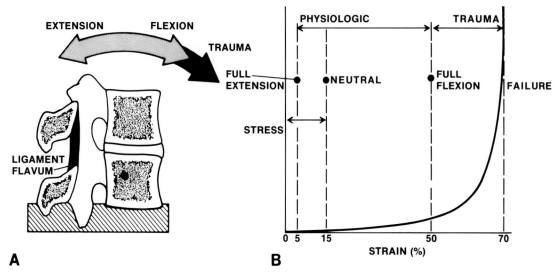

Fig. 1-13. Ligamentum flavum in flexion/extension. (*A*) The functional biomechanics of a ligament are exemplified by the ligamentum flavum undergoing spine motion. In flexion of the spine, the ligamentum flavum is stretched, and in extension it contracts. This is due to its location with respect to the instantaneous axes of rotation during these motions. In hyperflexion such as trauma this ligament may be stretched beyond its elastic limit to failure. (*B*) A stress-strain curve of deformation of the ligamentum flavum. In the neutral position of the spine, the ligamentum flavum has 15 per cent of pre-tension or pre-strain (i.e., if the ligamentum flavum is transected in situ it will contract by about 15 per cent of its length). During full extension, the ligamentum flavum contracts about 10 per cent, resulting in decrease of the pre-tension to 5 per cent. During full flexion of the spine from the neutral position, the ligamentum flavum is additionally stretched by 35 per cent of its length. Thus, within the physiologic range, the strain in the ligamentum flavum varies from 5 per cent to 50 per cent. Loaded beyond its physiologic range due to trauma, the ligamentum flavum fails at about 70 per cent of stretch. The values of elongation were calculated based upon the experimental findings of Nachemson, A., and Evans, J.: Some mechanical properties of the third lumbar inter-laminar ligament (ligamentum flavum). J. Biomech., *1:*211, 1968.)

Histologically, the ligamentum flavum has the highest percentage of elastic fibers of any tissue in the body.[19,68] This allows a large amount of extension of the ligament without permanent (residual) deformation. Clinically, this is an important characteristic. In a situation when the spine suddenly goes from full flexion (ligament stretched) to full extension (ligament relaxed), the high elasticity of the yellow ligament, together with its pre-tension, minimizes the chances of any impingement of the spinal cord.

Interspinous and Supraspinous Ligaments

There are no experimental studies dealing with the physical properties of these ligaments, and there is only one in vivo study in humans that attempted to measure the tension in these liga-

ments resulting from flexion of the spine.[95] The tension was measured by inserting pins under local anesthesia into the supraspinous and interspinous ligaments between L3 and L4, from the posterior direction, in the sagittal plane. The amount of sideways motion of the pin under the application of a given force was taken as a measure of the tension in the ligaments. It was found that the tension gradually increased as the spine was flexed, reaching its maximum at full flexion. The physical properties of other ligaments have not been reported in the literature.

Ligament vs. Bone Failure

The ligaments transfer tensile loads from one bone to another. When they are subjected to large loads in situ, the failure may occur either within the ligaments or in the bone at the point of attachment. On what factors does this pattern of failure depend? To our knowledge there are no studies specifically conducted in the spine that have addressed this question. Noyes and colleagues have reported, utilizing cruciate ligaments of the Rhesus monkey, that the failure pattern (ligament vs. bone) depends upon the rate of application of the loads and the status of the bone.[72,73]

They conducted tensile tests to failure on bone-cruciate ligament-bone preparations. The tests compared slow to fast rates of loading, and specimens from normal animals to those immobilized for 6 months. In specimens from normal animals, more often bone failed at slow rates of loading, and ligament failed at high rates of loading. The preparations taken from immobilized animals, tested only at the fast loading rate, always failed by bone avulsion. The general concept here is that in any series structure like the bone-ligament-bone preparation, failure occurs at the single weakest point. It has been well documented that the bone and ligament strengths increase with the rate of loading.[59,72,79] We may conclude that there is a relatively greater increase in strength for the bone than for the ligament with an increase of the rate of loading, accounting for the ligament failure at higher rates of loading. Further, immobilization decreases the strength of the bone to a greater degree than that of the ligament, leading to bone failure in the experiments.

Functional Biomechanics of the Ligaments

The anterior and posterior ligaments, as well as the ligamentum flavum, have similar biomechanical characteristics, as shown by their load-deformation curves. The curve is nonlinear and the slope increases with load. A theoretical analysis, based upon the special shape of this curve, is presented here with the purpose of explaining the three biomechanical functions of a ligament. The analysis is limited to sagittal plane motion and uses the ligamentum flavum as an example. The conclusions of the analysis, with some modifications, can be applied to other ligaments.

A typical stress-strain curve for the ligamentum flavum, reported by Nachemson and Evans,[68]

Table 1-3. Mechanical Parameters of the Ligamentum Flavum in the Various Ranges of Motion *

	PHYSIOLOGIC RANGE		TRAUMA RANGE
	EXTENSION	FLEXION	
Average Force	25	100	1750
Energy Absorbed	23	100	680
Average Stiffness	30	100	7500

* Data based upon the results of Nachemson, A., and Evans, J.: Some mechanical properties of the third lumbar inter-laminar ligament (ligamentum flavum). J. Biomech., *1*:211, 1968.

is shown in Figure 1-13. The stress is the load applied per unit area. The strain is the percentage of elongation of the ligament from its unstretched length. Motions of the spine and corresponding deformations of the ligamentum flavum are depicted in Figure 1-13A and B, respectively.

Because the ligamentum flavum is located posterior to the axes of rotation of flexion/extension, it contracts with extension of the spine and elongates with flexion of the spine. Calculations show that with full extension of the spine from the neutral position, there is decrease in the length of ligamentum flavum by 10 per cent. Because the ligamentum flavum has 15 per cent of pre-tension, it does not buckle into the spinal canal with extension. Full flexion of the spine from the neutral position results in a 35 per cent increase in its length. This is the total physiologic range. An additional 20-per cent lengthening of the ligament, due to further flexion of the spine during trauma, results in failure.

From the curve, the average values of three parameters have been calculated: the force required, the energy absorbed, and the stiffness of the ligament during the various ranges of motion. Assigning a value of 100 to the average magnitudes of these quantities during flexion, the relative values for extension and trauma ranges are given in Table 1-3.

The numbers in the table clearly show that during physiologic ranges of motion, very small force (25–100) is required to move the spine. There is not much resistance (stiffness 30–100) and not much energy (23–100) is expanded to produce this useful motion. However, this smooth and efficient motion is effectively limited

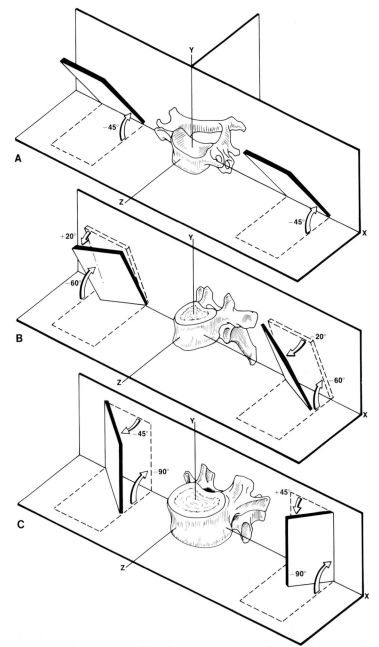

Fig. 1-14. Orientation of the facet joints. A graphical representation of the facet joint inclinations in various regions of the spine is obtained by rotating two cards lying in the horizontal plane through two consecutive angles, x-axis rotation followed by y-axis rotation. Typical values for the two angles for the three regions of the spine are as follows—(*A*) Cervical spine: −45 degrees followed by 0 degrees. (*B*) Thoracic spine: −60 degrees followed by +20 degrees for right facet, or −20 degrees for left facet. (*C*) Lumbar spine: −90 degrees and −45 degrees for right facet, or +45 degrees for left facet. These are only rough estimates. There are variations within the regions of the spine and between different individuals.

by the sharp increase in stiffness as the curve leaves the physiologic range. This is shown by the average stiffness in the trauma range, which is 75 times that in the flexion range. Thus, the two functions required of ligaments in the physiologic range are accomplished by the design of the load-deformation curve. When large flexion loads are applied to the spine so that a traumatic situation exists, the design of the curve is such that large amounts of energy are absorbed before failure. Nearly seven times more energy is absorbed in the trauma range as compared to the flexion range.

This analysis clearly shows the means by which the ligamentous mechanism enables the spine to perform two quite different roles: allowing smooth motion within the physiologic range, with a minimum of resistance and expenditure of energy; and at the same time providing a maximum of protection to the spinal cord in traumatic situations.

THE VERTEBRA

Probably the earliest biomechanical study concerning the human spine is that of the strength measurements of the vertebrae, conducted by Messerer nearly 100 years ago.[63] Since that time a good deal more has been learned about the mechanical properties of the human vertebrae.

Biomechanically Relevant Anatomy

A vertebra consists of an anterior block of bone, the body, and a posterior bony ring, known as the neural arch, containing articular, transverse, and spinous processes. The vertebral body is a roughly cylindrical mass of cancellous bone contained in a thin shell of cortical bone. Its superior and inferior surfaces, slightly concave, are the vertebral end-plates. The neural arch consists of two pedicles and two laminae, from which arise seven processes.

Although the basic design of the vertebrae in the various regions of the spine is the same, the size and mass of the vertebrae increases all the way from the first cervical to the last lumbar vertebra. This is a mechanical adaptation to the progressively increasing loads to which vertebrae

are subjected. There are also other differences. In the cervical region of the spine, there are foramina for the vertebral arteries; the thoracic vertebrae have articular facets for the ribs, and the lumbar spine has mammary processes. Of course, the sacral spine, being fused, is unique.

The pattern of movements of the spine are dependent upon the shape and position of the articulating processes of the diarthrodial joints. It is the orientation of these joints in space that determines their mechanical importance. Figure 1-14 helps to visualize the changing pattern of these orientations. Two cards are initially placed in the horizontal plane. A sequence of rotations of the cards about the various axes of the coordinate system show the orientation of the facet joints they represent.

In the cervical spine the inclination of the facet joint plane is simulated by first placing the two cards in the horizontal plane and subsequently rotating them through an angle of −45 degrees around the x-axis (Fig. 1-14A). In this position they represent the inclination of the right as well as the left facet joints, C2–3 to C7–T1.

Orientation of the thoracic facet joints, T1–T2 to T11–T12, is depicted in Figure 1-14B. Again starting with the horizontal plane, a rotation of −60 degrees about the x-axis is followed by a 20-degree rotation about the y-axis. The latter rotation is positive for the right facet joint and negative for the left facet joint.

The facets of the lumbar region are not plane, but have curved mating surfaces; the inferior facets are convex, while the superior facets are concave. Average planes of inclination of the facet joints, T12–L1 to L5–S1, are depicted in Figure 1-14C. The horizontal cards are first given a negative rotation of about 90 degrees around the x-axis. This is followed by a 45-degree rotation about the y-axis. This last rotation is positive for the left and negative for the right facet joint.

It should be emphasized that these orientations are only approximate. We do not know of any studies where precise measurements have been made. There is a considerable variation within specific regions of the spine, and transition from one inclination to another does not always coincide with transition from one region of the spine to another. For example, the transition vertebra

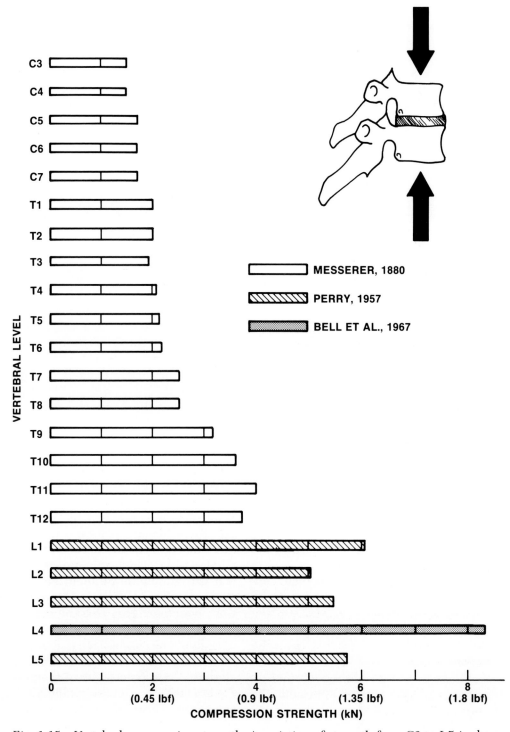

Fig. 1-15. Vertebral compression strength. A variation of strength from C3 to L5 is shown.

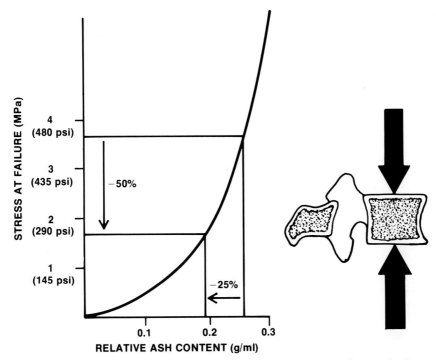

Fig. 1-16. Relationship between osseous tissue and vertebral strength. A 25 per cent decrease in the osseus tissue of the vertebra causes a much larger (50%) decrease in the vertebral strength. This has to do with the load-carrying capacity of vertical and horizontal trabeculae. (See Fig. 1-21; data by Bell, G. H., Dunbar, O., Beck, J. S., and Gibb, A.: Variation in strength of vertebrae with age and their relation to osteoporosis. Clacif. Tissue Res., *1:*75, 1976.)

between the thoracic and lumbar regions could be any vertebra from T9 through L1.

BIOMECHANICS OF THE VERTEBRA

Vertebral Body

Determination of compression strength of the human vertebrae has been the subject of research from the early days of biomechanics. One of the driving forces behind the research has been the problem of pilot ejection. Basically, it involves ejecting the pilot from the high speed aircraft with the help of a rocket attached to the seat. To minimize the injury to the spine at the time of ejection, it is necessary to use a safe ejection acceleration. This requires a knowledge of the strength thresholds of the vertebrae.

We do not know the design of the experimental set-up or the conditions of the cadaver material used by Messerer in 1880,[63] but his is the only data available, even to this day, which gives strength values of the *cervical* vertebrae. Ruff, in his classical paper on the experiments in connection with the pilot ejection problem, reports the results obtained by Geartz.[91] More recently, Perry performed static compression tests on 40 lumbar spine motion segments in order to study the endplate fractures.[83] Bell and colleagues also performed similar tests on 32 L4–5 motion segments.[15] The results of some of these studies, in the form of strength vs. vertebral level, are summarized in Figure 1-15. The trend seems to be clear, although there is some variation between the results of different authors, probably due to differences in the experimental design, testing

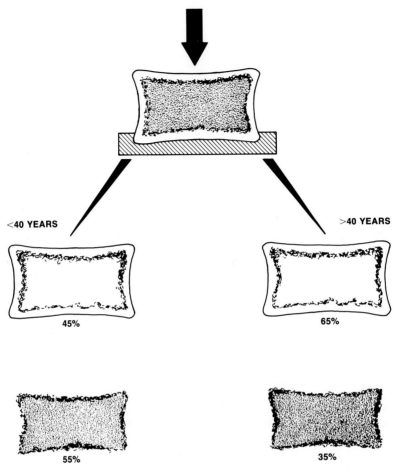

Fig. 1-17.   Relative compressive load-carrying capacity of two components of the vertebral body: cortical shell and cancellous core. Below 40 years of age, the former carries 45 per cent and the latter 55 per cent of the share. Above 40 years, the corresponding numbers are 65 per cent and 35 per cent. (Based upon data by Rockoff, S. D., Sweet, E., and Bleustein, J.: The relative contribution of trabecular and cortical bone to the strength of human lumbar vertebrae. Calcif. Tissue Res., 3:163, 1969.)

conditions, and age of the cadaver specimens. Weaver has shown by the strength measurements of vertebral cancellous bone cubes that the material properties of L3, L4, and L5, at least of the cancellous portion, are about the same.[102] Therefore, the variation in the vertebral strength with the spine level is most probably due to the size of the vertebrae only.

In general, the vertebrae decrease in strength with age, especially beyond 40 years. Bell and colleagues have shown that there is a definite relationship between the strength (stress of fail-

ure) and relative ash content or osseous tissue of the vertebrae (Fig. 1-16).[15] The graph indicates that vertebral strength is lost with age, and this loss is due to the decrease in the amount of osseous tissue. Another important point reported by Bell and colleagues is that a small loss of osseous tissue produces considerable loss in the vertebral bone strength. From the graph in Figure 1-16, we see that a 25 per cent decrease in the osseous tissue results in a larger than 50 per cent decrease in the strength of a vertebra. This has to do with the column-like design of the trabecular

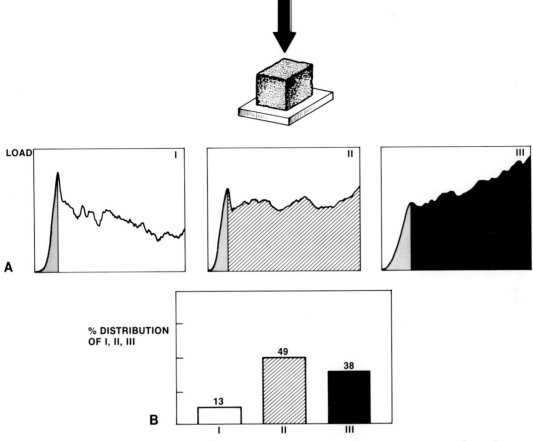

Fig. 1-18. Cancellous bone failure patterns. (A) Cancellous bone samples of vertebrae when subjected to compression fail in three different ways, as shown by the load-deformation curves, Types I, II, and III. It is the latter part of the curve, after the first peak is reached, which differentiates the three types. (B) The majority of the curves were found to be of Type II, followed by Types III and I. (Based upon data by Lindahl, O.: Mechanical properties of dried defatted spongy bone. Acta Orthop. Scand., 47:11, 1976.)

mesh that forms the central part of the vertebra. An analysis of this phenomenon is depicted in Figure 1-21 and given in the Notes.[H] In a recent study of the lumbar vertebrae, Hanson and co-workers have shown that there is a high correlation between the bone-mineral content, as measured by photon absorptiometry, and mechanical strength.[38a] It is hoped that such a method may be utilized clinically to assess the vertebral strength in vivo.

Cortical Shell vs. Cancellous Core

Although the facets carry some compressive loads, it is the vertebral body that carries the ma-

jor share in most physiologic situations. This load is transmitted from the superior end-plate of a vertebra to the inferior end-plate by way of two paths, the cortical shell and the cancellous core.

What is the relative share of the load carried by the two paths? The literature concerning this is conflicting. One study concluded that the load-supporting part of a vertebral body is the compact rather than the spongy bone.[25] According to others, the outer wall of a vertebra, unlike that of a long bone, is very thin and can make only a small contribution to its strength.[12,15] To resolve this conflict, a study was conducted by Rockoff and colleagues.[88] To appreciate their findings, a

Table 1-4. Compressive Strength Properties of Cancellous Bone of Vertebrae[*]

PHYSICAL PROPERTY	MAGNITUDE
Proportional-limit stress[†]	4.0 MPa
Compression at proportional limit	6.7%
Modulus of elasticity	55.6 MPa
Failure stress	4.6 MPa
Compression at failure	9.5%

[*] Based on data from Lindahl, O: Mechanical properties of dried defatted spongy bone. Acta Orthop. Scand., 47:11, 1976.

[†] A point on the load-deformation curve beyond which the elastic portion of the curve is no longer linear.

short description of the experimental procedure is in order.

Vertebrae without posterior elements were taken from the lumbar spine of cadavers. Nondestructive tests for compression strength were carefully performed on each vertebra, and the specimens were then divided into two groups. In one group, the vertebral bodies were hollowed out with the help of a rotating burr, introduced into the bodies by way of the basivertebral vien canal. This produced a vertebra with only the cortical shell left intact. In the second group, the outer shell was carefully ground away, leaving only the cancellous core. The vertebrae of the two groups were again subjected to the same nondestructive test. The resulting loss in strength of a specimen, as compared to its intact strength, represented the contribution of the trabecular bone in the first group and the cortical bone in the second group. Other complimentary tests, such as bone density, bone volume, and ash content, were also performed. The effects of age were included.

In general, there was a decrease in strength of the intact vertebrae with age.[E] A rapid rate of decrease was observed from 20 to 40 years, while the strength remained more or less constant after 40. This finding is supported by bone strength measurements of Bartley and colleagues,[12] and Weaver,[102] histologic findings of bone quantity by Bromley and colleagues,[17] and bone surface area measurements by Dunnhill and colleagues.[24]

In addition, Rockoff and colleagues found that under compressive load, the trabecular bone contributes 25 to 55 per cent of the strength of a lumbar vertebral body, depending upon the ash content of the bone.[88] Regarding variation with age, they found that under 40 years of age 55 per cent of load is carried by the trabecular core, while after 40 years, this share decreases to about 35 per cent. This is depicted in Figure 1-17.

Cancellous Core

Spongy bone of vertebrae has other interesting aspects. In a recent paper by Lindahl, the mechanical properties of this part of the vertebra were studied in detail.[55] He subjected small cubic blocks of the trabecular bone from L2 to L4 to compressive loads until failure occurred, while recording the load-deformation curves. The shape of these curves indicated some remarkable characteristics of the spongy bone. Three types of curves, distinguished by the latter portions, were identified (Figure 1-18A). Type I shows *decreasing* strength after the maximum load is reached. Type II *maintains* its strength, and Type III shows *increasing* strength after the failure point. Decreasing strength (Type I) was exhibited by only 13 per cent of the specimens tested. About half of the specimens showed constant strength after failure (Type II), and in 38 per cent of the cases, the strength kept increasing after the "failure" (Type III). These results are depicted graphically in Figure 1-18B. Lindahl further reported that vertebrae with a Type III curve, which are biomechanically the superior of the three,[F] were found most frequently in males under 40 years of age and least frequently in women over 40. These findings may have some relation to the probability of progressive collapse following vertebral compression injuries.

Although there was much variation in the latter part of the curves of different specimens, the mechanical properties represented by the early part of the load-deformation curve were quite consistent. These properties have been quantified and are presented in Table 1-4. Note that the cancellous bone of a vertebra undergoes large compressive deformation, up to 9.5 per cent, before it fails. The corresponding deformation for the cortical bone is less than 2 per cent. Therefore, in vertical compressive loading, injury pain is more likely to be the result of cortical plate

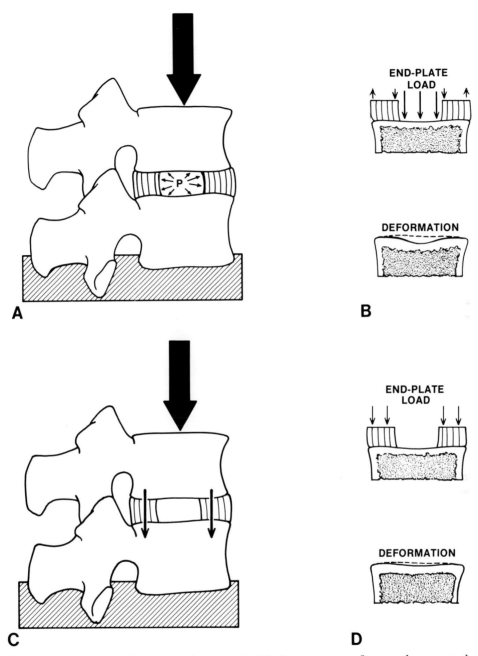

Fig. 1-19. End-plate failure mechanism. *(A, B)* Compression of a non-degenerated disc produces pressure within the nucleus, which results in compression at the middle of the end-plate and some tension on its periphery. Loading of the end-plate in this manner produces deflection of the end-plate, so that high bending stresses occur in the center. The latter may cause central fractures of the end-plate and Schmorl's nodes. *(C, D)* In a degenerated disc the compressive load is mostly transferred from one end-plate to the other by way of the annulus. The nucleus does not carry any significant loads. The end-plate is loaded more at its periphery. The stresses are more evenly distributed within the entire end-plate. The failure is by fracture of the vertebral body.

fractures than of microfractures in cancellous bone. Obviously, if the magnitude of the force is large enough, then both types of fractures are likely to occur.

The study by Lindahl was done on trabecular samples from which the bone marrow had been removed. In a recent study by Hayes and Carter, they have proven that the shock-absorbing mechanism of trabecular bone is enhanced by the presence of bone marrow, especially in highly dynamic situations, such as traumatic injury.[41] Cylindrical specimens of subchondral trabecular bone of bovine femurs were loaded in a specially designed test fixture, with the specimen so confined that the fluid within the specimen could not leak out during the compression loading. They recorded the load-deformation curves at slow as well as very fast rates of loading. The curves were found to be mostly of Types II and III, as reported by Lindahl.[55] Type III curves were more often associated with the samples that had high apparent density. Hayes and Carter further reported that the presence of bone marrow significantly increased the compressive strength as well as the energy absorption capacity of the trabecular bone samples. This effect was more significant at higher rates of loading. The suggested mechanism of energy absorption by the cancellous bone was the collapse of an increasing number of intertrabecular spaces as the load was increased. This further constrained the movement of the bone marrow, providing a hydraulic cushion. Therefore, the function of the cancellous core seems to be not only to share the load with the cortical shell, but, at least at high rates of loading, to act as the main resistor of the dynamic peak loads. This is important to keep in mind in the analysis and understanding of vertebral trauma.

End-Plate

Let us take an empty tin can of relatively large diameter and small height, fill it with some water, and seal off its opening. When this can is heated, water is converted to steam, which applies pressure equally to the cylindrical walls as well as the lids. Engineering analysis shows that the stresses generated in the walls are much lower than those in the lids. The result is outward bulging of the lids, while the walls remain intact. The annulus and the end-plates may be visualized as the walls and the lids of a tin can, respectively. As the fluid pressure within the nucleus increases due to external load, the end-plates are subjected to large pressures.

Although failure of the end-plates under compressive loading has been observed by many research workers, it was Perry in 1957 who conducted exhaustive experiments to obtain the basic understanding of the end-plate failure mechanism.[83] His spine specimens were mostly from the lumbar region, with a few lower thoracic specimens also included. The age of the subjects varies from under 40 to over 60 years, covering a wide range of disc degeneration.

The experimental procedure involved an application of increasing compressive force to the intact motion segment specimens. The deformation produced and the force applied were continuously recorded. The end point was reached when the load suddenly decreased, indicating failure of the specimen. In these static tests, one-third of the specimens had end-plate fractures with herniation of the nucleus pulposus into the vertebral spongiosa. This fracture pattern was present more often in the younger age-group and in the upper lumbar vertebrae. There were no disc herniations. Generally, the strength of the motion segment was greater in the lower region than in the upper region of the lumbar spine. However, there was much greater variation due to age. Below 40 years, the motion segment could bear about 8000 N (1800 lbf) of compressive load. Between 40 and 60 years the strength decreased to about 55 per cent of this value and above 60 years, to 45 per cent.

Perry also performed high speed dynamic tests on 76 specimens. Again, there were no disc herniations. The failures of the specimens were either due to failure of the end-plate or the compression of the vertebra, depending upon the intensity of the load. In these dynamic tests lasting 0.006 seconds the loads applied were much higher, up to 13500 N (3030 lbf).

Basically, there were three failure patterns of the end-plate observed by Perry: central, periph-

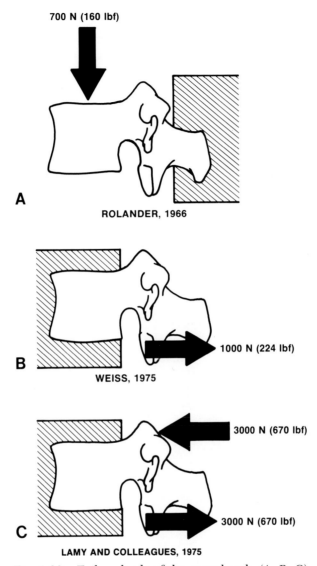

700 N (160 lbf)

A

ROLANDER, 1966

B

1000 N (224 lbf)

WEISS, 1975

3000 N (670 lbf)

3000 N (670 lbf)

C

LAMY AND COLLEAGUES, 1975

Fig. 1-20. Failure loads of the neural arch. (*A*, *B*, *C*) The variation in the failure loads is representative of the differing methods of load application in the three experiments.

eral, and one involving the entire end-plate. The central fractures were more often present in the specimens with non-degenerated discs. The opposite was true for the peripheral fractures. The fractures encompassing the whole of the end-plate were the result of higher loads. We can look at these failure mechanisms in some detail.

Figure 1-19A shows a motion segment with a non-degenerated jelly-like nucleus. When the compression load is applied, there is a buildup of pressure within the nucleus. This produces tension in the outer fibers of the annulus and a central compressive loading on the end-plate (Fig. 1-19B). Also shown is the deflection curve of the end-plate. As the stresses are in direct proportion to the bending moment, the fracture will

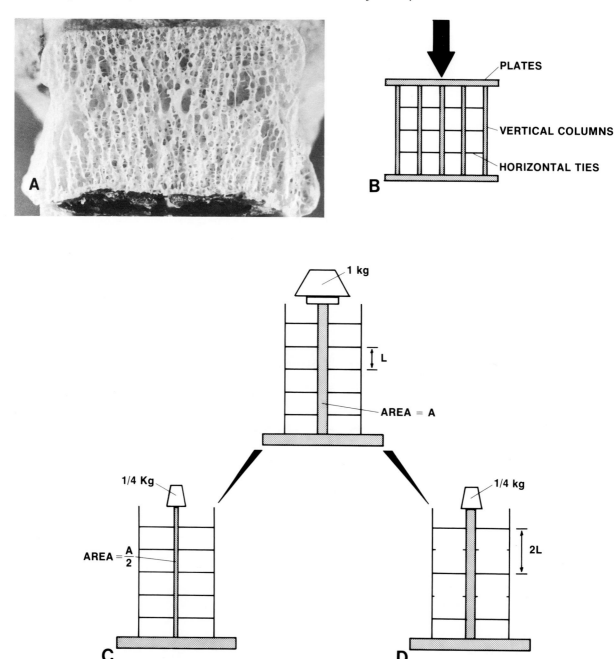

Fig. 1-21. Biomechanical analysis of vertebral failure in osteoporosis. (*A*) A photograph of a longitudinal section through a vertebral body shows the dominant vertical and horizontal arrangement of the trabeculae of the cancellous bone. (*B*) A model representing the trabecular pattern of the vertebra. Horizontal ties effectively reduce the free length of the vertical columns, thus providing support. (*C, D*) Based on Euler's formula the model predicts that the compression strength of the cancellous part of the vertebra will decrease to 25 per cent of its original value when either there is a 50 per cent decrease in the cross-sectional area of the vertical trabeculae or there is loss of horizontal trabeculae, so that the free length of the vertical trabeculae is effectively increased by 100 per cent.

most probably start in the center of the end-plate, where the bending moment is maximum under these circumstances.

A completely different situation arises when the nucleus is not jelly-like, and it is not able to build up any significant fluid pressure. This is depicted in Figure 1-19C. The compressive load is mostly transferred directly from one vertebra to the other by way of the annulus. The annulus is mostly under compression and so is the periphery of the end-plate, with much less deflection at its center (Fig. 1-19D). The failure of the vertebra is due to the fracture of the periphery of the end-plate.

Rolander and Blair[90] did experiments similar to those done by Perry, but in addition they measured the deflection of the center of the end-plate.[G] Results showed that the end-plates did indeed buckle away from the disc, increasing the disc height at the center by about 0.6 mm (0.024 in) just prior to the failure. In all the specimens tested, there were fractures of one or both end-plates. None of the failures were due to compression of the vertebral body.

Neural Arch

There are no biomechanical studies that have treated the components of the neural arch separately, although there is a definite need for better understanding of this aspect of spine function. The studies discussed here have all considered the neural arch as a single unit. A total of three biomechanical studies have been reported.[54,89,103] The methods of loading have varied greatly among the authors, which is a reflection of our very imprecise knowledge at the present time concerning the loads applied to the neural arch in vivo. The methods of loading and the average failure loads are depicted in Figure 1-20.

Most failures occurred through the pedicles. In the experiments by Lamy and colleagues about one-third of the failures were through the pars interarticularis.[54] This number increased when the tests were conducted at higher rates of loading. The strength was found to be the same for male as well as female subjects and for those with normal and degenerated discs. However, it decreased with age.

Facets

Nachemson, utilizing his needle pressure transducer, measured the nucleus pressures (and therefore, the disc loads) of an intact motion segment and of a motion segment in which the posterior elements had been removed. He concluded that the facets carry about 18 per cent of the total compressive load borne by a motion segment.[65]

Recent dynamic studies of whole cadavers by King and colleagues have shown that the mechanism of load sharing between the facets and the disc is rather complex. Using cadavers fitted with a special load-measuring device in place of a disc, the facet and disc loads could be separated. The cadavers were subjected to caudocephalad accelerations of varying degrees. After extensive measurements, they concluded that, depending upon the spine posture, the share of the load carried by the facets could be anywhere from 33 per cent to zero. In certain spinal postures, the facets were unloaded and the capsular ligaments were put under tension.[50]

In a comparative study of the various components of a motion segment with respect to their contribution towards the torsional strength, Farfan found that the disc and the longitudinal ligaments shared equally with the two facets including the capsular ligaments, about 45 per cent each. The remaining 10 per cent of the torsional strength was contributed by the interspinous ligaments.[27]

White and Hirsch studied the role played by the facets and the posterior ligamentous complex in restricting the physiologic motions of the spine.[104a] Using thoracic motion segments, they measured the various ranges of motion of intact motion segments and of segments with posterior elements removed. In the upper thoracic region there was a 50- to 80-per cent increase (greatest during flexion/extension and least during lateral bending). In the lower thoracic motion segments, the increase was only 15 per cent during flexion/extension and lateral bending, and 40 per cent in axial rotation.

In a study of the flexion/extension stability of the cervical spine in vitro, the various components of the motion segment were transected in two different sequences under simulated flexion and extension.[78,105] The transaction sequences were either anterior to posterior or posterior to anterior. Under the application of a flexion producing a load equivalent of up to one-third body weight, the transection of the disc and the longitudinal ligaments produced a 33-per cent increase in the horizontal translation as compared to the intact motion segment. When the facets were transected next, the corresponding increase was 140 per cent. Thus, the facets provide significant stability to the spine in flexion, especially when the disc is already ruptured.

The importance of facet orientation for the pathology of the intervertebral disc has been well documented by Farfan and Sullivan.[30] Using radiographic measurements, they studied 45 patients admitted for low back pain with sciatica and who were treated conservatively. In addition, there were 52 patients who were ultimately treated surgically. From radiographic measurements and operating room findings of these patients, they established a highly significant correlation between the asymmetry of the facet joints and the level of disc pathology, and between the side of the more oblique facet orientation and the side of sciatica.

Functional Biomechanics of the Cancellous Bone

In osteoporosis there is reduction in osseous tissue (ash content).[11,14] There is also a decrease in vertebral strength with age as observed by Perry[83] and Bell and colleagues.[15] Proportionally, there is much greater decrease in strength as compared to the loss in the osseous tissue (Fig. 1-16).[15] Utilizing a model described subsequently, one may explain these changes in the mechanical strength on the basis of engineering principles.

The cancellous part of the vertebral body (Fig. 1-21A) may be thought of as an engineering structure composed of vertical trabeculae (vertical columns) joining the two end-plates and horizontal trabeculae (horizontal ties) supporting the columns from the sides (Fig. 1-21B).[37] This pattern has been observed by Casuccio,[21] Atkinson,[10] and Amstutz and Sissons.[4]

According to a well established engineering principle, Euler's formula, the compressive strength of a column is in direct proportion to the square of the area of its cross section and in inverse proportion to the square of its unsupported length.[H] In other words, reduction of the area by 50 per cent while keeping the length constant decreases the strength to one-quarter of its original value (Fig. 1-21C). Alternatively, the same weakening could also be obtained by doubling the length of the column by removing some horizontal ties and keeping the original area unchanged (Fig. 1-21D).

In osteoporosis, the decrease in the amount of osseous tissue of a vertebra may result in a decrease in sectional area of the vertical trabeculae (columns) and/or a breakdown of horizontal trabeculae (ties). A decrease in mass for a column of a given length may result in an equal decrease in area. Thus, a 50 per cent decrease in the mass results in one-quarter of the original strength (Fig. 1-21C). On the other hand, breakdown of horizontal ties effectively increases the unsupported length. If 50 per cent of the horizontal ties (i.e., every alternate tie) were removed, the strength of the structure would be reduced to one-quarter of its original value (Fig. 1-21D). This reduction in strength would be even greater if adjacent ties instead of the alternate ties were removed.

Atkinson did a histologic study of the vertebral trabeculae and its changing patterns with age. The earliest change seen was the loss of the horizontal trabeculae. However, this was accompanied by simultaneous thickening of some of the vertical trabeculae; although there was no appreciable loss of osseous tissue on the whole until the age of 50, there was nonetheless a substantial decrease in the mechanical strength. The biomechanical analysis nicely shows the high sensitivity of the strength to the loss of the horizontal trabeculae.[10]

Another observation by Atkinson was that with age there was a loss of horizontal trabeculae in the central region of the vertebral body, while those in the peripheral regions remained unaltered. This implies that the loss of strength with age occurs preferentially in the middle of the vertebrae. This seems to fit nicely with the clinical observations of central collapse of the vertebral body in patients with osteoporosis.

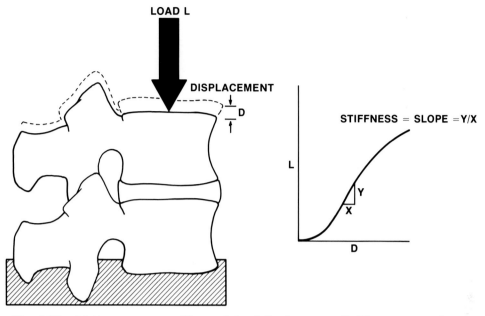

Fig. 1-22. Motion segment stiffness. A load-displacement (L-D) curve provides information about the stiffness of a structure. The stiffness is defined as the ratio of the load applied to the displacement produced. The slope of the L-D curve is a measure of the stiffness. Generally, the L-D curve for a motion segment is nonlinear, and therefore its slope and stiffness of the motion segment are different for different values of the load.

FUNCTIONAL SPINAL UNIT AND MATHEMATICAL MODELS

The functional spinal unit, or the motion segment as it is popularly called, is the smallest segment of the spine that exhibits biomechanical characteristics similar to those of the entire spine. It consists of two adjacent vertebrae and the connecting ligamentous tissues. In the thoracic region, costovertebral articulations are also included. For its biomechanical characterization, the lower vertebra is fixed while the loads are applied to the upper vertebra, and its displacements are measured. The behavior of a motion segment is dependent upon, among other things, the physical properties of its components, such as the intervertebral disc, ligaments, and articulating surfaces. Because the spine may be considered as a structure composed of multiple motion segments connected in series, its total behavior is a composite of the individual motion segments.

Mathematical Models

One of the goals of a mathematical model is to link the basic physical properties of individual components of a structure to the total behavior of the structure itself. By utilizing the physical properties, data of the motion segments, and the mathematical modeling techniques, it is then possible to recreate the behavior of the entire spine. Even the effects of the rib cage and spine musculature may be incorporated by using the mathematical modeling process.

The mathematical model can simulate behavior of the spine in situations where other means of investigation are not feasible. Clinical investigations are restricted to studies where the subjects are not put in danger. Animal models are limited by the anatomic differences between the animal and the human spines. In vitro experiments using human cadavers are free from the restrictions of the clinical and animal studies, but they are expensive to conduct, provide limited

Table 1-5. Stiffness Coefficients of the Motion Segment (Average Values)

AUTHORS	STIFFNESS COEFFICIENT*		MAXIMUM LOAD*†		SPINE REGION
Compression (−Fy‡)					
Hirsch & Nachemson, 1954	3.0	MN/m	4.5	kN	Lumbar
Rollander, 1966	2.0	MN/m	1.0	kN	Lumbar
Panjabi, et al., 1976	1.3	MN/m	160	N	Thoracic
Tension (+Fy‡)					
Panjabi, et al., 1976	0.80	MN/m	160	N	Thoracic
Shear (Fx, Fz‡)					
Liu, et al., 1976	0.55	MN/m	450	N	Lumbar
Panjabi, et al., 1976	0.10	MN/m	160	N	Thoracic
Flexion (+Mx‡)					
Markolf, 1972	2.0	N m/deg	7	N m	T7–8/L3–4
Panjabi, et al., 1976	2.6	N m/deg	8	N m	Thoracic
Extension (−Mx‡)					
Markolf, 1972	2.6	N m/deg	7	N m	T7–8/L3–4
Panjabi, et al., 1976	3.2	N m/deg	8	N m	Thoracic
Lateral Bending (Mz‡)					
Markolf, 1970	1.8	N m/deg	7	N m	Thoracic
Panjabi, et al., 1976	2.9	N m /deg	8	N m	Thoracic
Axial Rotation (My‡)					
Markolf, 1970	6.0	N m/deg	7	N m	Thoracic
Farfan, 1970	4.0	N m/deg	8	N m	Lumbar
Panjabi, et al., 1976	2.5	N m/deg	8	N m	Thoracic

* For units and conversion to inch-pound system, see footnote to Table 1-1.
† Failure load.
‡ See Figure 1-23.

information, and cannot simulate the muscle structures and the neuromusculature controls present in vivo. The mathematical models, which have been thoroughly validated for their accuracy, need not have any of these restrictions. In theory at least, they have the potential for truly simulating the biomechanical behavior of the human spine in vivo. However, one must be careful to interpret the results of mathematical models in an appropriate biological and clinical perspective before the results are applied to patients.

Utilizing high speed modern computers, such models, once validated by experiments and clinical applications, can become powerful tools in the understanding, prevention, and treatment of disorders of the spine. Scoliosis serves as an important example. A suitable mathematical model may provide insight into the probable etiology by showing which mechanical anomalies (e.g., disc wedging, rib resection, and asymmetrical bone or muscle development) must be present to produce scoliosis. The methods of present treatment,

such as the Milwaukee brace, Harrington rods, and the Dwyer procedure, can be evaluated and optimized. New treatment methods (e.g., correction of scoliotic deformity by stimulation of selective back muscles) can be analyzed.[92] In general, computer simulations are more economical, safer, and should precede the clinical trials.

Some of the recent mathematical models that have the capability to simulate the three-dimensional behavior of the spine are by Belytschko and coworkers,[15a] and by Panjabi.[75a] The former model has been successfully tested in the simulation of scoliosis as seen clinically. The latter model, although it has potential for greater validity, has not yet been tested. It can incorporate more complex and realistic sets of spine data, but unfortunately such data is not readily available at this time.

Stiffness Measurements

Stiffness is that property of a structure by which resistance is offered to an imposed load. *Flexibility* is the ability of the structure to deform

Table 1-6. Coupled Motions*

APPLIED LOAD†	MAIN MOTION†	COUPLED MOTIONS†	
A. Thoracic Motion Segments			
Comp./ten.	Axl. trn. (Ty)‡	A-P trn.§ & sag. rot.	(Tz & Rx)‡
A-P shear	A-P trn. (Tz)	Sag. rot.	(Rx)
Lat. shear	Lat. trn. (T.x)	Frn. rot.	(Rz)
Axl. torsion	Axl. rot. (Ry)	Frn. rot.	(Rx)
Flx./ext.	Sag. rot. (Rx)	A-P trn.	(Tz)
Lat. bending	Frn. rot. (Rz)	Lat. trn.	(Tx)
B. Lumbar Motion Segments			
Comp./ten.	Axl. trn. (Ty)	Sag. rot.	(Rx)
A-P shear	A-P trn. (Tz)	Sag. rot.	(Rx)
Lat. shear	Lat. trn. (Tx)	Frn. rot., sag. rot.	(Rz & Rx)
Axl. torsion	Axl. rot. (Ry)	Frn. rot.§, sag. rot.	(Rz & Rx)
Flx./ext.	Sag. rot. (Rx)	A-P trn.§	(Tz)
Lat. bending	Frn. rot. (Rz)	Lat. trn., axl. rot. & sag. rot.	(Tx, Ry, Rx)

* Adapted from Krag, M. H.: Three dimensional flexibility measurements of preloaded human vertebral motion segments [thesis]. Yale University School of Medicine, New Haven, 1975; Panjabi, M. M., Brand, R. A., and White, A. A.: Mechanical properties of the human thoracic spine: as shown by three-dimensional load-displacement curves. J. Bone Joint Surg., 58A: 642, 1976.

† Comp. = compression   Ten. = tension
   Axl. = axial   Lat. = lateral
   A-P = anterior-posterior   Ext. = extension
   Flx. = flexion   Rot. = rotation = R
   Trn. = translation = T   Frn. = frontal
   Sag. = sagittal

‡ These symbols refer to Figure 1-23.
§ Highly coupled motion.

under the application of a load. To quantitate these structural qualities, the concepts of coefficients of stiffness and flexibility have been evolved. The *coefficient of stiffness* is defined as the ratio of the amount of load applied to the displacement produced. The *coefficient of flexibility* is defined as the ratio of the displacement produced to the load applied. The first is the inverse of the second. This is illustrated by an example of a typical load-displacement curve of a motion segment in Figure 1-22. The slope of the curve at any point is y/x and this is the measure of the coefficient of stiffness. The reciprocal of the slope is x/y, which is the coefficient of flexibility. Generally, the load displacement curve is nonlinear, which means that the slope varies with the amount of the load applied. Therefore, it is necessary to specify not only the stiffness and flexibility coefficients, but also the load at which these were obtained.

To determine stiffness and flexibility coefficients requires the simultaneous measurement of the load as well as the displacement. Only a few studies have met this requirement. The results reported here relate to the thoracic and lumbar regions. The cervical spine has not yet been studied. The results are described in the following text, while the specific values for the stiffness coefficients have been collected in Table 1-5.

Compression, Tension, and Shear

Compression loading, again because of its assumed clinical importance and simplicity of testing, has dominated the studies of stiffness of the spine.[26,45,63,76,83,89] Tension and shear, on the other hand, are probably the least studied.[56]

Experiments have shown that the spine motion segments are stiffer under compression than in tension in both the thoracic and lumbar regions. We found that, in the thoracic region, the com-

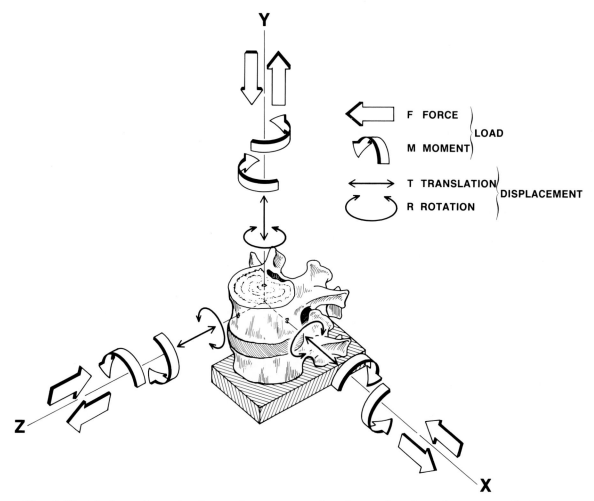

Fig. 1-23. A three-dimensional coordinate system has been placed at the center of the upper vertebral body of a motion segment. The coordinate system is fixed in space. To document the complete mechanical behavior of the spine motion segment, six forces along and six moments or torques about the three axes of the coordinate system are applied. These twelve load components are depicted. The application of any one of the load components produces displacement of the upper vertebra with respect to the lower vertebra. The displacement consists of translation and rotation. These two motions can be further divided with respect to the coordinate axes. Thus, the three-dimensional displacement has six components, three translations along and three rotations about the three axes of the coordinate system. These are also shown.

pressive stiffness was about 60 per cent higher than the tensile stiffness.[76] The higher value for compression is probably due to the hydrostatic pressure within the disc and the loading of the facets. The spine becomes stiffer at higher loads, shown by studies of Hirsch and Nachemson and Rolander.[45,89]

The shear stiffness, at least in the thoracic region, seems to be about equal in the horizontal plane in all directions (e.g., anterior, posterior, or lateral).[76] However, in the lumbar region the shear stiffness is about twice as high in the lateral direction as compared to the anteroposterior direction.[56] However, in two newly released studies by Lin and coworkers,[55a] and Berkson and colleagues,[15b] it was found that even in the lumbar spine the differences in the shear stiffness between the lateral and the anteroposterior directions are not large. The latter study found the lumbar motion segments to be stiffest during posterior shear. Again, there is no consistent pattern of change with the levels of the spine. In general, the spine was found to be much more flexible during shear. As compared to the axial compression stiffness, the shear stiffness was only 8 per cent in the thoracic region[76] and 15 per cent in the lumbar region.[15a]

Flexion, Extension, and Lateral Bending

Although the compression behavior of the motion segments has been more thoroughly studied, it has yet to be related to the clinically observed failures of disc herniation.[18,83,100] Bending and other rotatory loads, on the other hand, may easily produce disc failures.[18,27] Only two studies have reported the spine stiffness behavior in bending.[61,76]

The spine seems to be more flexible (or less stiff) in flexion than in extension. The increased flexibility is about 25 to 30 per cent. On removal of the posterior elements, the extension flexibility increased so that there was no more difference between the flexion and extension flexibility and stiffness values. No such difference was found for flexion when the posterior elements were removed.[61] This implies that the posterior elements play a part in resisting extension but not flexion. There was no consistent variation of these properties within the thoracic region with the level of the motion segments. This is confirmed by Schultz and coworkers.[94a]

Stiffness in lateral bending was about the same as that for flexion. Similarly, removing the posterior elements had no effect, and the stiffness T1 and L4.[61] Again, similar findings were observed by Schultz and coworkers while studying the lumbar motion segments.[94a]

Axial Rotation

This motion is probably more dangerous to the disc than any other, except for a combination of axial rotation and lateral bending.[27] The characteristics of the stiffness properties of axial rotation are markedly different from those of the other rotatory motions. The torsional stiffness within the upper thoracic region is more or less constant, its value being about the same as that

for flexion and lateral bending. But, from T7–8 to L3–4, there is a continuous increase in the torsional stiffness.[61] The value at L3–4, for example, is about nine times as large as that at T7–8. Special mention must be made of the stiffness at the thoracolumbar junction. This level was found to have the highest torsional stiffness, about eleven times that of T7–8. The effect of removal of the posterior elements on the torsional stiffness properties has also been studied. Although only small change occurred in the upper thoracic region, the effect was marked from T7–8 to L3–4. For example, the stiffness of L3–4 motion segment was reduced to almost one-fourth of its intact value. In a study of a large number of motion segments from the L1 to L4 region, removal of the posterior elements increased the rotation by 150 per cent for the same torque.[94a]

Combined Loads

In a recent study Lin and coworkers have performed mechanical tests on the lumbar motion segments to which combined loads were applied.[55a] For example, in one test compression, shear and bending were simultaneously applied. Such tests, in general, are better representatives of the situations in vivo. The difficulty in such tests lies in choosing a certain combination of the loads that is representative of reality, because the loads in vivo are not known. One of the interesting findings of Lin and coworkers was that the motion segment provides greater resistance to failure when the loads are applied centrally rather than eccentrically or at some inclination. Further, they found the lamina to be highly strained when the spine was inclined anteriorly and less so when inclined posteriorly. These finds would suggest that in lifting a weight the spine should be kept, as much as possible, in the vertical position.

Combined Physiologic Motions

Each of the physiologic motions of the spine, such as bending and rotation, has been described separately for the sake of simplicity. However, they are inherently connected. This phenomenon, which is called *coupling,* is due to the geometry of the individual vertebrae and the connecting ligaments, as well as the curvature of the spine. Mathematical models may be used to account for the curvature of the spine, but the coupled behavior must be studied while determining the physical properties of the motion segments.

Coupling Effects. The phenomenon of coupling has been well documented experimentally. It occurs in the thoracic spine,[76,104] but it is more common in the cervical spine[58] and the lumbar segments.[51,77] It has also been observed clinically. Two or more individual motions are said to be coupled (e.g., lateral bending and rotation) when it is not possible to produce one without producing the other at the same time. Therefore, the physical properties of the coupled motions must be measured simultaneously to provide valid representation of the actual behavior of the spine.

Some recent studies have taken into account the coupling phenomenon while measuring the stiffness properties of the thoracic and lumbar motion segments.[51,76] In the first study, thoracic motion segments were tested. Twelve forces and moments were applied, and six translations and rotations of the upper vertebra in three-dimensional space were measured (Fig. 1-23). Without going into the details of the complicated techniques of load application, motion measurement, and data analysis, some conclusions regarding the coupling phenomenon are presented in Table 1-6A, B. The applied loads are the physiologic forces and moments. The main motion is in the same direction as the applied load. The coupled motions are all other motions that take place beside the main motion.

In the thoracic region there is strong coupling between all motions in the sagittal plane (e.g., translation and rotation). The coupling of axial rotation to lateral bending is much stronger in the lumbar region than in the thoracic region. In addition, the lumbar region shows certain cross coupling of all three rotations. In other words, when the lumbar motion segment is axially rotated, it bends in the frontal and sagittal planes. Also, when bent laterally, it simultaneously bends in the sagittal plane and rotates axially. However, bending in the sagittal plane does not produce two other rotations. This phenomenon of coupling can be visualized with the help of a curved bar. Application of either an axial torque or a lateral bending moment produces twisting and bending in a three-dimensional space. However, bending in the plane of curvature produces motion only in that plane and, therefore, no lateral bending or axial rotation.

Preload Effects. In situ the motion segment is subjected to the physiologic loads of motion during normal activities. In addition, there are much larger loads present due to body posture. Nachemson and Morris found these so-called compressive preloads at the L3–4 motion segment to be very high, about twice the body weight when standing in the normal anatomic posture.[69] In our experimental study of the lumbar spine, we found unexpectedly that the addition of preload greatly affected certain stiffness values, while hardly changing others. Furthermore, of those values affected, some were increased while others were decreased with the preload.[77] For example, the spine became less stiff in flexion and more stiff in axial rotation due to the addition of the preload. We may conclude by saying that the true stiffness and flexibility properties of the spine should be measured in the presence of suitable preload, so as to simulate, as closely as possible, the conditions in vivo.

The Analysis of Preload. The preload in situ, such as the axial load on the disc or the motion segment due to body posture, has two origins. First, there is the direct compressive load due to the weight of the body part above the motion segment (Fig. 1-24A); for example, the lumbar motion segments are subject to the weight of the entire torso. Secondly, because the position of the center of gravity of the supported weight is anterior to the spine, the motion segment is also subjected to large flexion bending moments which are counterbalanced by the ligament and back muscle forces. These ligament and muscle forces, in turn, apply compression to the motion segment. All of these forces and moments which act on the disc-vertebra are shown on the free-body diagram in Figure 1-24B and are analysed.[1]

Facets and Motion Segment Behavior

The torsional stiffness of the spine is largely determined by the design of the facet joints. The observations by Markolf of increasing torsional

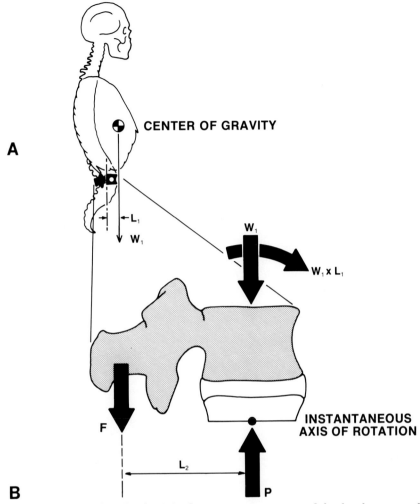

CENTER OF GRAVITY

A

L_1

W_1

W_1

$W_1 \times L_1$

F

**INSTANTANEOUS
AXIS OF ROTATION**

L_2

B

P

Fig. 1-24. Analysis of preloads. (A) The motion segments of the lumbar spine have been observed to bear very large compressive loads (preloads). A simple mechanism of this phenomenon is depicted here. The center of gravity of the weight of the body parts above the motion segment is anterior to the instantaneous axis of rotation of the motion segment. (B) A free-body diagram of the motion segment is shown. The external loads are the weight of the body parts W_1 and the flexion bending moment $W_1 \times L_1$. The internal loads are the ligamentous and muscle forces F and the compressive reaction force acting at the instantaneous axis of rotation in the vertebra (i.e., the preload P). Length L_2 is the lever arm for the force F to the instantaneous axis of rotation.

stiffness from T7–T8 to L3–L4, with the peak at T12–L1, and subsequent decrease in these values with the removal of the facet joints,[61] can be explained on the basis of the changing patterns of the facet joints.

Two examples of facet joints are shown in Figure 1-25. When the plane of the facet joint is such as to allow nearly unhindered rotation of one vertebra with respect to the other, the motion segment has low rotatory stiffness, which is dependent on the contributions of the ligamentous structures only. The facets do not play any significant role. Such a case is that of the T5–T6 motion segment (Fig. 1-25A). On removal of the facet joints, there is minimal change in the motion segment mechanics (Fig. 1-25B). On the other hand, the T12–L1 motion segment has facet joints that effectively hinder the relative axial rotation (Fig. 1-25C). Here the facet joints play an important role. When they are intact they provide high resistance to axial torsion, and their removal significantly decreases the stiffness (Fig. 1-25D). The same mechanism is present to varying degrees in the other motion segments of the spine.

A sudden change in the stiffness properties of a structure at a given point implies a stress concentration at that point, which will eventually lead to mechanical failure. Such a point in the spine is represented by the T12–L1 motion segment. This hypothesis is well supported by experimental studies[47] as well as clinical observation.[38] The highest frequency of spine injury is in the region of the thoracolumbar junction. As the above analysis showed, the abnormally high stiffness is the result of special orientation of the articulating facets. Anatomically, this articulation (of highest stiffness) may vary among individuals from T9 to L1.

Age, Sex, Degeneration, and Motion Segment Behavior

It is sometimes assumed that with age the disc space narrows and the discs become stiffer; it is also assumed that a herniated disc is biomechanically unsound.[39] In a carefully conducted study of lumbar cadaveric motion segments, Nachemson and colleagues made the following observations.[69a] The disc height, even in a group of grossly degenerated specimens, was found to be average. In general, age was not related to the mechanical behavior of the motion segment in any pronounced manner. The same was true for the disc level within the lumbar region. However, females were found to have more flexible spines as compared to males. The most interesting finding, however, concerned the disc degeneration: No consistent correlation was observed between disc degeneration and the mechanical behavior. In a specimen with a grossly herniated disc, the mechanical tests showed it to have near normal behavior. We would like to make one comment about these quite interesting findings. This study measured only the elastic behavior. The viscoelastic behavior may turn out to be a more significant factor. As reported elsewhere,

Kazarian found a relationship between disc degeneration grade and the viscoelastic creep behavior obtained under compression loading.[46]

THE RIB CAGE

The rib cage has several important biomechanical functions related to the spine. It is a protective barrier for any traumatic impact directed from the anterior or the sides. It stiffens and strengthens the spine, thus providing greater resistance to displacement, which is advantageous when the spine is injured or has been disrupted by a disease. The stiffening effect of the rib cage is two-fold. The costovertebral joint provides additional ligamentous structures that contribute to spinal stiffness. But the more important biomechanical aspect of the rib cage is its moment of inertia. The transverse dimensions of the thoracic spine are increased manifold by the inclusion of the ribs and the sternum. The increased moment of inertia stiffens the spine when it is subjected to any kind of rotatory forces such as bending moments and torques. Because the rib cage is part of the spine structure, it provides additional strength and energy absorbing capacity during trauma.

Biomechanically Relevant Anatomy

The ribs are curved bones of elliptical cross section joining the vertebral column to the sternum and, thus, forming a closed cylindrical cavity, the thorax. The first seven ribs join the sternum by means of individual costal cartilages, the next three by means of a fused costal cartilage, and the last two are free floating, ending in the muscles of the abdominal wall.

The ribs articulate with the vertebrae at both the heads and tubercles. The head of the rib articulates with the sides of the corresponding vertebra and the one above, forming the costovertebral joint. This synovial joint has an articular capsule that is strengthened by the radiate ligament, which spreads from the head to the vertebrae and corresponding disc. The tubercle of the rib articulates with transverse processes of the corresponding vertebra, forming the costotransverse joint. Although the articular capsule of the

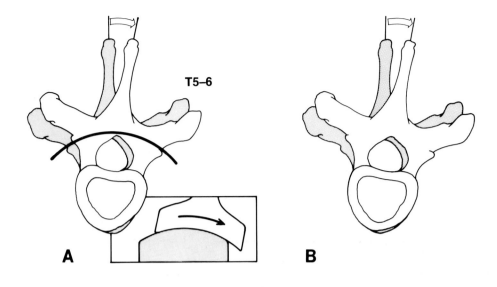

T5–6

A   **B**

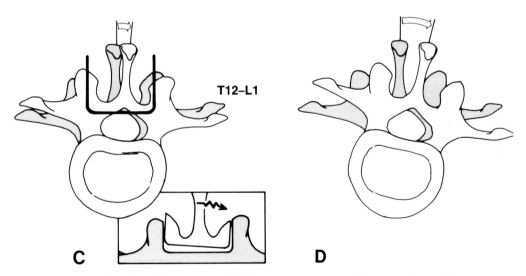

T12–L1

C   **D**

Fig. 1-25. The role of facet joints. (A) The axial rotation of the vertebra with respect to the other of a T5–T6 motion segment is unhindered by the facet articulation. This is due to the orientation of the plane of the facet joints with respect to the instantaneous axis of rotation. For a given torque, a certain axial rotation is produced. (B) On removal of the facet joints there is no significant change in the axial rotational stiffness of a T5–T6 motion segment. For the same torque as in A, about the same rotation is produced. (C) It is quite different for a motion segment in which the facet joint articulation is oriented so that the two facets impinge on each other when the segment is subject to axial torsion. An example of this type of motion segment is that of T12–L1, which has been found to have the highest rotatory stiffness of any motion segment. Thus, for the same torque as in A, a smaller rotation is produced. (D) On removal of the facets of the T12–L1 motion segment, the motion is unhindered and there is a significant change in the axial rotational stiffness. For the same torque as in A, much greater rotation is produced.

Table 1-7. Stiffness Properties of the Human Ribs*

Load Directions[†]	R-2[‡]	R-4 to R-8[‡]	R-10[‡]
	(N/mm)§	(N/mm)§	(N/mm)§
Anterior/Posterior, ±z	1.50	0.75	0.30
Lateral/Medial, ±x	0.75	0.40	0.25
Superior/Inferior, ±y	0.40	0.25	0.20

* Data adapted from Schultz, A. B., Benson, D., and Hirsch, C.: Force deformation properties of human ribs. J. Biomech., 7:303, 1974.
† These directions refer to Figure 1-23.
‡ These are average stiffness values measured with a load of 7.5 N (1.7 lbf). The load and deformation point was at the head of the rib, while the other end of the rib was fixed. The ribs were much stiffer when the load direction was anterior compared to posterior.
§ 1 N/mm = 5.6 lbf/in

joint is weak, it is greatly strengthened by three costotransverse ligaments. The medial and lateral costotransverse ligaments extend from the tip of the transverse process to the neck and lateral aspect of the rib, respectively. The superior costotransverse ligament extends from the neck to the transverse process of the vertebra above.

The end of the rib joins its costal cartilage by means of the costochondral joint. The costal cartilage articulates with the sternum in several ways. The first rib is joined firmly to the manubrium by a cartilaginous joint. The cartilage of the second rib articulates with demifacets on both the manubrium and the body of the sternum by way of the synovial joints. The cartilages of the third to seventh ribs have small synovial joints with the body of the sternum.

BIOMECHANICS OF THE RIB CAGE

The Ribs

The only physical property of the ribs that has been studied is stiffness, by Schultz and colleagues.[93] In this study the ribs were fixed at the heads, and loads were applied to the free ends of the costal cartilage in six different directions: anterior, posterior, lateral, medial, superior, and inferior. The deformations of the loading point were measured and are summarized in Table 1-7. The highest stiffness was exhibited by the shortest rib (R-2) when pulled in the anterior direction, while the lowest stiffness (the highest flexibility) was shown by the longest rib (R-10) when loaded in the superior and inferior directions.

All ribs exhibited higher stiffness in the anterior direction as compared to the posterior direction. Generally, the ribs were highly flexible: a 10 N-load (2.2 lbf) produced a deformation of 25 mm (1 in). The ribs also exhibited coupling effects, as are seen in motion segments. For example, superior loading not only produced superior displacement but also posterior and medial displacements. This was probably due to the curved geometry of the ribs. Although other coupled motions such as rotation were probably present, they were not measured.

Costovertebral and Sternocostal Joints

There is only one study that has measured the physical properties of the costovertebral and sternocostal articulations.[94] The results of stiffness of the two joints measured in various directions are shown in Table 1-8. The costovertebral joint, especially for the middle ribs, exhibited the highest stiffness in the lateral direction, while the lowest stiffness resulted from loads applied in the superior and inferior directions. Highly nonlinear behavior was observed. Initial motions about the neutral position could be accomplished by very small forces, while beyond this range there was a sudden increase in stiffness. The sternocostal joints, on the other hand, provided maximum resistance when loaded in the superior and inferior directions, especially for the joint of the second rib. The least resistance was offered by the inferior joints in the anterior and posterior directions.

In a recent study Panjabi and coworkers found the costovertebral joint to play a pivotal role in providing stability to the motion segment of the thoracic spine.[76a] When flexion was simulated and all posterior elements, the posterior longitudinal ligament, and the posterior half of the disc were cut, the spine was on the verge of instability. Subsequent transection of the costovertebral joint consistently produced failure. When extension was simulated, the spine was found to be on the border of instability when the anterior longitudinal ligament, the disc, and the costovertebral joint were transected. Therefore, in the clinical situation if there is evidence of the destruction of the costovertebral joint, one should sus-

*Table 1-8. Stiffness Properties of Costovertebral and Sternocostal Joints**

LOAD DIRECTION†	COSTOVERTEBRAL JOINTS‡			STERNOCOSTAL JOINTS§		
	R-2	R-4 TO R-8	R-10 TO R-12	R-2	R-4	R-6 TO R-10
	(N/mm)	(N/mm)	(N/mm)	(N/mm)	(N/mm)	(N/mm)
Lateral, ±x	2.50	5.00	2.50	—	—	—
Anterior/Posterior, ±z	1.50	1.75	1.50	2.50	2.5	0.50
Superior/Inferior, ±y	0.75	1.50	1.00	3.0	1.50	0.75

* Data adapted from Schultz, A. B., Benson, D., and Hirsch, C.: Force deformation properties of human ribs. J. Biomech., 7:303, 1974. The values are average stiffness, measured with a load of 7.5 N (1.7 lbf).
† These directions refer to Figure 1-23.
‡ The load and deformation point was on the rib just beyond the costovertebral joint. The vertebra was fixed.
§ The load and deformation point was on the rib just medial to the sternocostal joint. The sternum was fixed.

pect the ability of the spine to carry normal physiologic loads.

Functional Biomechanics of the Rib Cage

Agostoni and colleagues[1] subjected the relaxed rib cage of live subjects to a lateral squeezing force and measured the resulting changes in the lateral and frontal diameters. Patrick and colleagues[81] and Nahum and colleagues[70] studied the load-displacement behavior of the thorax for an anterior to posterior load applied at the sternum. On the average, the stiffness was found to be 10 to 20 times that of a single rib. From these studies, however, it is not possible to determine the contribution of the rib cage or its components to the stiffness and stability of the spine.

Although the individual components of the rib cage (ribs and their joints) are quite flexible, the rib cage as a whole greatly enhances the stiffness of the spine. Utilizing a mathematical model of the thoracic and lumbar spine and the rib cage, Andriacchi and colleagues[7] performed computer simulations to determine the effect of the rib cage on: (A) the stiffness properties of the normal spine during flexion, extension, lateral bending, and axial rotation; (B) the stability of the normal spine under axial compression; and (C) the scoliotic spine subjected to traction. Also studied were the effects of removing one or two ribs or the entire sternum from an intact thorax. The mathematical model was validated by its ability to simulate reasonably well the experimental results of Agostoni, Patrick, and Nahum.[1,70,81] The findings of the model regarding stiffness, stability, and scoliosis were as follows:

(A) The stiffness properties of the spine were found to be greatly enhanced by the presence of the rib cage for all the four physiologic motions, especially for extension (Fig. 1-26). Here, the stiffness with the thorax was nearly 2.5 times that of the ligamentous spine alone during extension.

Removal of the sternum from the rib cage, on the other hand, had a profound effect, almost completely destroying the stiffening effect of the thorax (Fig. 1-26A). The stiffness in all four types of physiologic motion decreased to values that were representative of the ligamentous spine without the thorax. This effect can be illustrated by the behavior of a thin-walled cylinder, subjected to bending and torsion loads, before and after a narrow longitudinal strip is removed.[J] Removal of one or two ribs, as is sometimes carried out in a scoliosis operation to obtain optimum correction, did not affect the stiffness properties significantly.

(B) The rib cage was found to increase the axial mechanical stability of the spinal column in compression by four times. This relative increase can be put into perspective by the fact that without the muscles and the rib cage, a ligamentous spine in upright position could support an axial compressive load of only 20 N (4 lbf).[57]

(C) Finally, the application of traction to the spine was simulated by the computer model for both the normal and scoliotic spines. Although the axial stiffness of the normal spine increased by 40 per cent due to the presence of a rib cage, there was no corresponding increase for the scoliotic spine. In addition, the scoliotic spine was found to be about 2.5 times as flexible as the

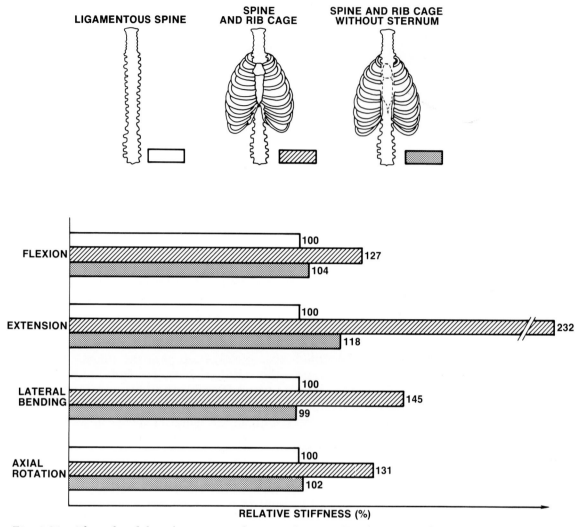

Fig. 1-26. The role of the rib cage in enhancing the overall stability of the spine is depicted. The stiffness values were computed for each of the three structures during four different physiologic motions: flexion, extension, lateral bending, and axial rotation. The results of the relative stiffness values for the three structures are presented here in the form of horizontal bar graphs. For each motion the "ligamentous spine" has been assigned a value of 100 per cent. Note that the significant increase in stiffness achieved during all four physiologic motions due to the addition of the rib cage is entirely lost when the sternum is removed. (Results based upon mathematical model by Andriacchi, T. P., Schultz, A. B., Belytscko, T. B., and Galante, J. O.: A model for studies of mechanical interactions between the human spine and rib cage. J. Biomech., 7:487, 1974.)

normal spine when both were subjected to traction (Fig. 1-27). Although the authors of the paper do not comment upon this finding, we believe it has the following biomechanical explanation. The extra mobility of the scoliotic spine in the axial direction was probably due to the additional curvature in the frontal plane that is present in a scoliotic spine. These curves straighten when the axial load is applied, giving the impression of a more flexible spine. (This is similar to the axial stiffness of a straight steel wire as compared to that of a spiral spring made of the same wire.) In the computer simulation of scoliosis, the physical properties of the ligaments were not

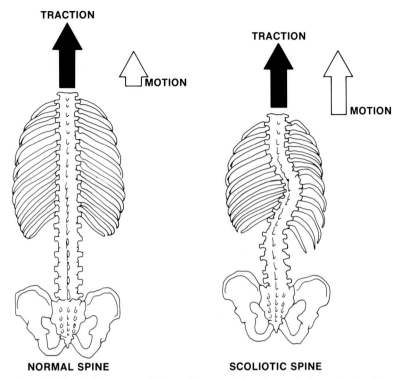

Fig. 1-27. Relative flexibility of a normal and scoliotic spine in the axial direction is depicted in this diagram. Under the application of the same amount of traction force to the two spines, the motion produced at T1 with respect to the pelvis was found to be about 2.5 times for the scoliotic spine as compared to that for the normal spine. (Results based upon computer simulation by Andriacchi, T. P., Schultz, A. B., Belytscko, T. B., and Galante, J. O.: A model for studies of mechanical interactions between the human spine and rib cage. J. Biomech., 7:487, 1974.)

altered.[K] Therefore, the observed flexibility was due to the abnormal geometric curvature of the spine only.

THE MUSCLES

The spine, with its ligaments intact but devoid of muscles, is an extremely unstable structure. We have stated previously that a fresh cadaveric spine (without the rib cage), oriented vertically and fixed at the sacrum, could carry a maximum load of 20 N (4 lbf) placed centrally at T1.[57] Any additional load would permanently displace the spine from its central position. The muscles and complex neuromusculature controls are required to provide stability of the trunk in a given posture and to produce movements during physiologic activity. The muscles may also play a role in protecting the spine during trauma in which there is time for voluntary control and possibly in the post-injury phase.

Biomechanically Relevant Anatomy

The muscles that directly control the movements of the vertebral column may be divided into categories according to their position, postvertebral and prevertebral.[36]

The postvertebral muscles may be further divided into three groups, deep, intermediate,

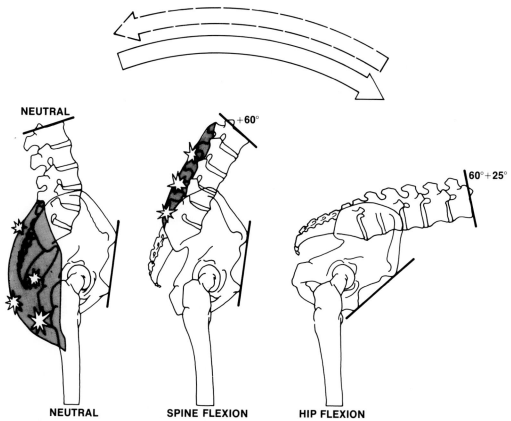

Fig. 1-28.   Muscle activity in forward bending. Bending forward is a two part movement involving both the spine and the pelvis. In the first 60 degrees of movement the pelvis is locked by the gluteal muscles, while the lumbar spine is gradually flexed, with the accompanying increasing activity of the erector spinae and superficial muscles of the back. In the second phase there is additional motion of about 25 degrees which is obtained by relaxation of the pelvis with respect to the femurs. In the fully flexed position all the muscles are relaxed, and the weight of the trunk is borne by the ligaments and passive extension of the muscles. Extension from the fully flexed position to the neutral position is achieved in the reverse order; the pelvis extension is followed by extension of the lumbar spine.

and superficial. The deep muscles consist of short muscles that connect adjacent spinous processes, *musculi interspinales;* adjacent transverse processes, *musculi intertranversarii;* transverse processes below to laminae above, *musculi rotatores;* and in the thoracic region, transverse processes to the ribs, *musculi levatores costarum.* The intermediate muscles are more diffused but certain components can be identified. These muscles arise from the transverse processes of each vertebra and attach to the spinous process of the vertebra above. According to the regions, they are the *multifidus* (lumbosacral),

semispinalis thoracis, semispinalis cervicis, and *semispinalis capitis.* Finally, the superficial postvertebral muscles, collectively called the *erector spinae,* are the *iliocostalis* (most laterally placed), the *longissimus,* and the *spinalis* (most medially placed).

The prevertebral muscles are the four abdominal muscles. Three of the muscles encircle the abdominal region. They are the *external oblique, internal oblique,* and *transversus abdominis.* The fourth muscle is the *rectus abdominis,* located anteriorly at the midline. The four muscles are arranged in distinctly different directions.

The results of various experiments, conducted to determine the electrical activities of the muscles while the subject is performing a given task, follow. Standard techniques of electromyography using the surface and/or needle electrodes have been utilized. It should be emphasized that the results presented are only for those muscles which were studied in a given experiment.

BIOMECHANICS OF THE MUSCLES

Posture

In the relaxed standing posture, the activity of the back muscles is generally low, especially in the cervical and lumbar regions. Slight activity of the abdominal muscles has been reported, but not simultaneously with activity of the back muscles.[9] Some activity in the vertebral portion of the psoas major muscle has also been measured.[66] These findings can be explained biomechanically. The ligamentous spine supporting the weight of the trunk is inherently unstable in its central position. A shift of the center of gravity of the trunk in the horizontal plane requires an active, counterbalancing muscle force on the opposite side. Therefore, an anterior, posterior, and lateral shift of the center of gravity activates the back, abdominal, and psoas major muscles, respectively. Morris and colleagues found the longissimus dorsi and rotatores spinae to be continuously active during standing.[64]

In the unsupported sitting posture, the muscle activity in the lumbar region was found to be about the same as that in the standing posture. In the thoracic region, Andersson and Örtengren observed that there was somewhat higher activity of the back muscles compared to activity found in the standing posture.[5]

Flexion

Bending forward is a two-part movement involving both the spine and the pelvis. The first 60 degrees of movement, on the average, are due to flexion of the lumbar motion segments. This is followed by an additional movement at the hip joints of about 25 degrees (Fig. 1-28). In extension from the fully flexed position, the movement is reversed, so that at first the pelvis rotates back-

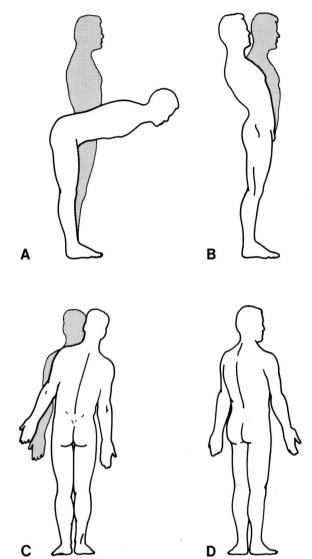

Fig. 1-29. Muscle activity during the four physiologic motions is presented in this composite diagram. (*A, B*) In flexion and extension, gluteus and erector spinae muscles are active. (*C*) Lateral bending is achieved by an imbalance of muscle forces on both sides of the back. There is greater muscle activity on the ipsilateral side. (*D*) During axial rotation erector spinae muscles on the ipsilateral side, the rotators and multifidi on the contralateral side, and the glueteals on both the sides were found to be active.

ward, followed by extension of the lumbar motion segments to the neutral position.[22,28]

The muscle activity closely follows the pattern of motion. Initially the pelvis is locked, as dem-

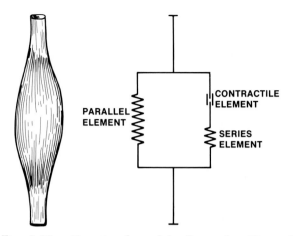

Fig. 1-30. Functional model of muscle. Physical properties of a muscle are quite different when it is in passive or in active state. Both these aspects of muscle behavior may be represented in a quantifiable manner by the three-element mathematical model shown on the right. The model consists of a parallel element, representing the passive elastic behavior of the muscle, and a series element which, together with a contractile element, represents the active elastic behavior of the muscle. The parallel and the series elements have constant stiffness values for a given muscle, while the contractile element is variable depending upon the activity of the muscle. Such models for individual muscles may be incorporated into the mathematical models of the spine to represent the total active behavior of the entire spine.

onstrated by strong myoelectric activity of the gluteus maximus and medius, and the hamstring muscles.[20] As flexion progresses, the increasing bending moment due to the weight of the trunk is balanced by the corresponding increase in the activity of the erector spinae muscles and the superficial muscles of the back.[6] However, on reaching full flexion, there is complete relaxation of these muscles (Fig. 1-28).[33] At this point the ligaments provide the major share of the required bending moment, while the passive extension of the muscles supplies the remainder. Morris and colleagues found most of the back muscles to be active during flexion. At full flexion, however, all muscles became inactive except the illiocostalis dorsi.

Extension

Myoelectric activity in the back muscles has been shown to occur at the beginning and at the completion of full extension from the neutral position, with only slight activity between these two extremes.[64] The abdominal muscles, on the other hand, show increasing activity while bending.[32] Extension of the trunk against load increased the activity of the back muscles of the lumbar region.[82]

Lateral Bending

With lateral bending, the activity of the back muscles increased on both sides of the spine, but mostly on the ipsilateral side.[64] Thus, the trunk is bent over to one side by the imbalance of forces. However, if the spine carrying a load is bent laterally, there is relatively higher activity registered in both the contralateral side of the lumbar region and ipsilateral side of the thoracic region.[6]

Axial Rotation

During axial rotation of the spine, erector spinae muscles on the ipsilateral side and musculi rotatores and multifidi on the contralateral side were found to be active.[64] However, Donish and Basmajian found the activity in the thoracic muscles of the back to be symmetrical, while that in the lumbar muscles was present only on the contralateral side.[23]

The abdominal muscles showed only a slight activity. But, strong activity was noticed in the gluteus medius and the tensor faciae latae muscles.[20] These findings are depicted graphically in Figure 1-29.

Biomechanical Function of a Muscle

The inactivated muscle has physical properties that are similar to those of other noncontractile soft tissues. The mechanical output of an active muscle is dependent upon the external load and the muscle length. The passive muscle resists, and the active muscle produces force that seems to be related to the cross-sectional area of the muscle.[40] A representation of the active muscle function by a mathematical model was proposed in 1939 by Hill.[42] A modified Hill's model that also includes the passive behavior of the muscle, according to Fung,[34] is diagrammed in Figure 1-30.

The model consists of three elements, two spring-like elastic elements (parallel and series), and one contractile element under the control of a neuromuscular signal. The passive behavior of the muscle is completely represented by the parallel element, since the contractile element is inactive, and therefore no force is transmitted by way of the series element. When a muscle is voluntarily contracted, it may either remain in a fixed position with no change of muscle length (isometric contraction), or it may contract and shorten (isotonic contraction) to provide work against an external load. In both situations, the series element shares the load together with the parallel element. This effectively increases the muscle stiffness. It should be emphasized that the mathematical model presented in Figure 1-30 is not a physical representation of a muscle, but it is a simple and precise way to describe the actual mechanical behavior of the muscle. Such models have recently been used to study the protective role of the back muscles of the spine in front-end auto collisions.[96]

In general, the purpose of a muscle force is to produce torque or moment across one or more joints. This force results in a torque that resists or does work against an external load. In addition, there are large compressive forces created at the joint between the two bones. This compressive, joint-reaction force is equal in magnitude to the vectorial sum of all the tensile muscle forces across the joint. An example of this is the large preload to which the spine motion segments are subjected in normal erect posture (Fig. 1-24).

Measurement of muscle action and forces may be documented by electromyographic studies. Although no definite relationship has been established between the electromyographic signal and the muscle tensile force, it is a monotonic relationship, implying an increasing signal with increasing muscle force.[75] Thus, with the present knowledge it is difficult to quantify the precise force a given muscle exerts. However, its electrical activity can be documented, and this signal gives some indication of the muscle forces.

THE SPINAL CORD

Although protection of the spinal cord is crucial to survival, little is known about the physical properties and the functional biomechanics of this vital structure. The delicate spinal cord is enclosed within the relatively hard spinal canal, made of rigid vertebrae connected end to end in space. The spinal canal changes in length due to physiologic flexion, extension, and lateral bending. Its effective cross-sectional area also undergoes changes with physiologic axial rotation and horizontal displacement. The spinal cord itself is supported and protected by surrounding soft-tissue structures: pia matter, dentate ligaments, the subarachnoid and subdural space filled with spinal fluid, and dura matter.

Biomechanically Relevant Anatomy

Three membranes cover the spinal cord. They are the dura mater, the pia mater, and the arachnoid (Fig. 1-31).

The dura mater is a long, cylindrically shaped sac of dense connective tissue that encloses the cord. It is separated from the periosteum lining the vertebral canal by epidural space containing fat and venous network. The dura also envelops the spinal roots, ganglia, and nerve as they pass through the intervertebral foramina.

The arachnoid is a very delicate cobweb-like membrane, consisting of fine, elastic, fibrous tissue. It follows the contours of the dura mater. It is separated from the dura by subdural space (moistened by fluid) and from the pia mater by subarachnoid space (filled with cerebrospinal fluid). The arachnoid is attached to the dura by thread-like subdural trabeculae. Strands of arachnoid traverse the subarachnoid space to become attached to the pia mater.[21a]

The pia mater is a vascular membrane covering the cord. Its inner layer is composed of a closely fitted network of five elastic fibers. Its outer layer is formed by a loose meshwork of collagenous fiber bundles, continuous with the arachnoid trabeculae.

In the cervical and thoracic region, the pia mater thickens between the anterior and posterior roots and on each side, forming the dentate ligaments. These tooth-like processes traverse the subarachnoid and dura spaces to become fixed to the inner side of the dura. There are 20 dentate ligaments, the last being at the level of the T12–L1.

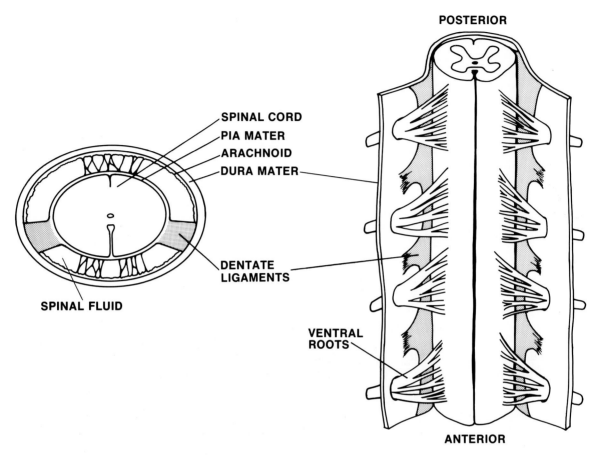

Fig. 1-31. Anatomy of the spinal cord and the surrounding structures.

BIOMECHANICS OF THE SPINAL CORD

There has been a single biomechanical study of the physical properties of the spinal cord, conducted by Brieg in 1960.[16] Most of the experimental findings presented here are taken from this investigation.

The spinal cord (cord and pia mater) is a structure with special biomechanical characteristics. When removed of circumferential attachments, nerves and dentate ligaments, and suspended from its upper end in vertical position, it lengthens due to its own weight by more than 10 per cent. This very flexible behavior changes suddenly into stiff resistance when attempt is made to produce any further deformation. In other words, the load-displacement curve of the spinal cord has two distinct phases: an initial phase where large displacement is obtained with very small forces, and a second phase where relatively large forces are required to produce relatively small deformations. There is an abrupt change from one phase to the other. The forces in the initial phase measured less than 0.01 N (0.04 oz), while in the second phase the spinal cord supported 20 to 30 N (4.5 to 6.7 lbf) before rupture. This behavior is qualitatively analogous to the behavior of the ligaments (Fig. 1-13).

Axial compression of the cord, however, did not show such abrupt change. When compression was applied to a spinal cord specimen, there was large initial deformation (with very small forces), followed by increasing elastic resistance until the specimen buckled. The spinal cord without the

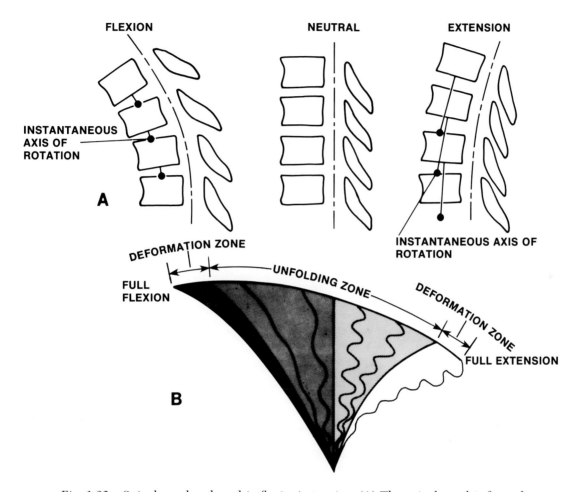

FLEXION　　　　**NEUTRAL**　　　　**EXTENSION**

INSTANTANEOUS
AXIS OF
ROTATION

INSTANTANEOUS AXIS OF
ROTATION

A

DEFORMATION ZONE

UNFOLDING ZONE

DEFORMATION ZONE

FULL
FLEXION

FULL EXTENSION

B

Fig. 1-32. Spinal canal and cord in flexion/extension. (A) The spinal canal is formed by a series of spaces of the neural arch. In flexion, from the neutral position, the length of the spinal canal increases. This is due to the location of the instantaneous axis of rotation, which is anterior to the canal. The greatest increase is at the posterior border of the canal. In extension the canal length decreases, again for the same reason. The greatest decrease is at the posterior border of the canal. (B) The spinal cord is required to follow the changes in length of the spinal canal during physiologic motions. This it does through two mechanisms, unfolding/folding and elastic deformation. In the neutral postion the cord is folded like an accordian and has slight tension. During flexion the spinal cord first unfolds, with a minimum of increase in its tension, followed by some elastic deformation near full flexion of the spine. During extension, the spinal cord first folds, with a minimum of decrease in the tension, followed by some elastic compression. (B is based upon expermental findings of Brieg, A.: Biomechanics of the Central Nervous System: Some Basic Normal and Pathological Phenomena. Stockholm, Almquist and Wiskell, 1960.)

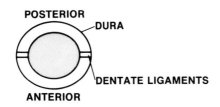

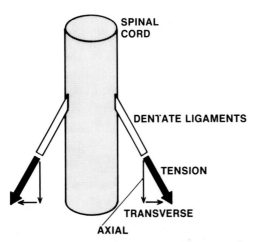

Fig. 1-33. Role of the dentate ligaments. Besides the support provided by the three meninges (pia mater, arachnoid, and dura mater) and the two fluid-filled spaces (subarachnoid and subdural), the spinal cord is stabilized in its central position within the dura by several pairs of dentate ligaments under tension. Due to inclination, the tension in these ligaments may be divided into axial and transverse components. Because the dentate ligaments come in pairs, the axial components are added, and together they balance the axial tension of the cord. The transverse forces of the two dentate ligaments balance each other and provide stability and protection.

pia mater was found to behave like a semifluid cohesive mass.

The large deformations with very small forces are probably due to the design of the spinal cord structure. The extreme mobility of the cord in the initial phase is achieved by folding and unfolding of the cord, much like an accordian. Beyond these limits of unfolding, the tissue is subjected to direct tensile forces. Thus, the second phase of the load-displacement curve truly represents the tissue properties of the spinal cord *material,* while the initial phase of extreme flexibility represents its accordian-like *structural design.*

The variation in length of the cord was accompanied by a change in its cross-sectional area, which increased under compression and decreased on extension. This is due to the incompressibility of the cord tissue. The cross-sectional area in situ was observed to change from a rounder to a more oval shape when the spine was bent from full flexion to full extension.

Functional Biomechanics of the Spinal Cord

The cervical, thoracic, and lumbar spinal canals are lengthened during flexion and shortened during extension.[16] The mechanism for these observations is shown in Figure 1-32A, in which the instantaneous axes of rotation (IAR) refer to the thoracic spine motion segments.[L,80] In flexion, the length of the canal as measured by its center line is increased in comparison to that of the neutral position. The anterior border of the canal also increases, but to a lesser extent. The maximum increase, however, is that for the posterior border of the canal. In extension, the canal is shortened as measured by the decrease in its anterior border, center line, and posterior border lengths. The maximum decrease is on the concave side of the curve, on the posterior border.

The changes in length of the bony canal are always followed by similar changes in the spinal cord. The mechanism of folding and unfolding is responsible for an estimated 70 to 75 per cent of the entire length change from full extension to full flexion (Fig. 1-32B). The rest of the change at the extremes of physiologic motions are due to the elastic deformation of the spinal cord tissue.[16]

The spinal cord folds like an accordian during extension. The folds are more distinct on its posterior surface, the place of maximum decrease in length, than on the anterior surface. Clinically, these folds are visualized on contrast radiographs as a series of protruberances. Yellow ligament encroachment may also contribute to these folds in older people, since this ligament becomes less elastic with age.

The spinal cord is suspended within the dura by the dentate ligaments, and the nerve roots may also provide some support. During full flexion the spinal cord, its nerve roots, and the dentate ligaments are under physiologic tension. Because the dentate ligaments are inclined inferiorly, the tensile force in the ligaments has two components with respect to the axis of the spinal cord (Fig. 1-33). The axial component balances the tension in the cord, probably reducing its magnitude. On the other hand, the transverse components balance each other in pairs to position the cord near the center of the canal and anchor it there. The central position of the spinal cord is advantageous because it provides maximum protection from bony impingement or shock during·trauma. (In the design of football and military helmets, a similar principle is utilized. The head is protected against trauma by suspending the helmet from the headband by several radially directed straps.)

There are two other substances that may offer mechanical protection to the spinal cord, namely the epidural fat and the spinal fluid. Very likely, these aid in reducing friction and in absorbing the energy from physiologic and other forces. The biomechanical and pathophysiological factors related to spinal cord trauma are reviewed in Chapter 4.

CLINICAL BIOMECHANICS

The Intervertebral Disc

When a vertebra-disc-vertebra unit is subjected to a compressive load, it fails by fracture of the end-plate or of the vertebral body, with no apparent damage to the disc.

Compression loading of the disc can not produce disc herniation. However, the disc bulges in the horizontal plane under such loading, with no propensity for posterolateral bulging.

During bending, the disc bulges on the concave side of the curve and collapses on the convex side. Thus, in flexion, the disc protrudes anteriorily and is depressed posteriorily.

The bending and torsional loads are probably more dangerous to the disc than is axial compression.

The intervertebral disc is viscoelastic and exhibits its creep and relaxation behavior. These phenomena may be advantageously utilized in traction and with the Harrington rod procedure.

There seems to be a correlation between the degree of disc degeneration and its creep characteristic. A degenerated disc exhibits less creep and thus has less capability to attenuate shocks and vibrations from the ground.

In vivo the loads on the disc are relatively very high. In a standing posture the compressive load is about two times the whole body weight.

An injury to the disc annulus or removal of the nucleus does not substantially alter the biomechanical behavior of the disc in vitro.

Under compression loading the disc is subjected to relatively much higher stresses when it is degenerated.

Spine Ligaments

In a physiologic range of motion of the spine, the vertebrae easily move with respect to each other (the spine is relatively flexible), and there is the least amount of energy expenditure. Further, beyond the physiologic range the ligaments provide substantial protection by resisting forces and absorbing large amounts of energy before failure.

A bone-ligament-bone system subjected to tensile loads fails either through the bone or through the ligament. At slow rates of loading, the failure is more often through the bone, and at high rates of loading, it is the ligament that fails.

The Vertebra

The compression strength of vertebrae increases from C1 to L5.

There is a sharp decrease in the vertebral strength with age beyond 40 years. However, the decrease is more gradual after 60 years.

In osteoporosis there is greater loss of horizontal trabeculae in comparison to the vertical trabeculae of cancellous bone of the vertebrae. This loss may not be easily visualized on the radiograph, however its effect on the strength of the vertebrae is considerable.

Under 40 years of age, the cancellous core of a vertebra provides 55 per cent of the vertebral strength. Over 40 years this contribution decreases to 35 per cent.

Half of the cancellous bone samples tested in an experiment were found to be *stronger* after the first fracture. Thus, a vertebra with the compression fracture may actually be able to carry equal or higher loads after a fracture.

Central fractures of the end-plates are more often associated with the nondegenerated discs. The opposite is true for peripheral fractures which were found to be related to degenerated discs.

The facet joints may carry large compressive loads (up to 33%) depending upon the body posture. They also provide, in equal proportion to the disc, 45 per cent of the torsional strength of a motion segment.

The Motion Segment

The highest torsional stiffness is typically exhibited at the thoracolumbar junction. This makes the T12–L1 motion segment the site of high stress concentration. The clinical observation of a higher incidence of spine fractures at this level may be related to this factor.

There is no consistent correlation between the elastic properties of a motion segment and its disc level, disc grade, or disc height, or the sex or age of the patient.

The Rib Cage

The rib cage substantially increases the stiffness of the spine in all physiologic motions. The removal of the sternum completely negates the stiffening effect of the rib cage.

A scoliotic spine is much more flexible in axial traction than is a normal spine. The additional flexibility is due to the more curved shape of the scoliotic spine.

The Muscles

Muscles are extremely important in maintaining the erect spine.

The first 60 degrees of flexion are achieved by locking the pelvis and flexing the lumbar spine. Release of the hip joint provides an additional 25 degrees of flexion.

Lateral bending of the spine is achieved by the imbalance of the forces exerted by the muscles on both the sides of the spine.

During axial rotation, the erector spinae on the ipsilateral side and musculi rotatores and multifidus on the contralateral side were found to be the most active.

The Spinal Cord

The spinal cord is very flexible when subjected to small loads. However, it provides considerable resistance before failure. In its unstretched position it is folded like an accordian, thus providing additional flexibility.

The spinal canal decreases in length when the spine is extended and increases in length when the spine is flexed.

The spinal cord follows this pattern easily because of its high flexibility. In flexion, the accordian-like spinal cord unfolds, and in extension, it folds.

The spinal cord is protected from traumatic forces due to its three membranes and two fluid-filled spaces. Dentate ligaments provide additional protection and stability to the spinal cord.

NOTES

[A] The main reason for the large magnitude of forces on a lumbar disc is that the center of gravity of the trunk is in front of the disc, causing a bending moment in the sagittal plane. To balance this, large muscular forces are required on the posterior elements. The reaction to these forces, in turn, is an equally large compressive disc load.

[B] Stiffness as used by Galante is the maximum load applied (0.5 N or 0.1 lbf) divided by the displacement produced in millimeters or inches. The load-displacement curve was found to be highly nonlinear; therefore, this stiffness represents an average value.

[C] The precise line of demarcation between the compressive and tensile zones will depend upon the location of the instantaneous axis of rotation. Shown in Figure 1-10B are an instantaneous axis of rotation and the corresponding distribution of the tensile and compressive stresses in a disc. The length of the vertical lines in the stress diagram represents the magnitude of the stress at a given location. As can be seen, the stresses are maximum at the periphery and decrease toward the line passing through the instantaneous axis of rotation.

[D] So that the important differences between the experiments on the longitudinal ligaments are appreciated, a short discussion of the concepts of material and structural properties is necessary. An intact ligament is a structure. It has shape, size, and a certain distribution of material. Because of these fundamental properties it performs its structural function of providing mechanical stability to the spine. When tests are performed on *intact* ligaments, the failure load in newtons (poundforce) and the load deformation curves represent the physical properties of the ligament as a *structure*. On the other hand, when samples of *standardized size*, obtained from a ligament, are tested, the failure load is presented as the breaking *stress* in newtons per square meter (poundforce) per square inch) and the load-deformation curves are shown as the *stress-strain* curves. These parameters represent the physical properties of the *material* of the ligament. For more information, see the italicized terms in the Appendix: Glossary.

[E] In the study by Rockoff and colleagues, *strength* was defined as a point on the load deformation curve where the curve departed from the linear behavior. This is not the true, ultimate strength. But it may be expected to correlate reasonably with it.

[F] For a given deformation, the area under the load-deformation curve represents the energy that has been absorbed to produce the deformation. Comparing the Type I curve with the Type III curve for a given deformation beyond the failure load (see Figure 1-18), it is seen that the Type III curve has the greatest reserve of energy. This energy may be advantageously utilized either during trauma, where the damage to the adjoining soft tissue is diminished, or during the recovery period, where it may serve as a safeguard against further increase in the deformity.

[G] Rolander and Blair took a motion segment and drilled an axial hole from the top in the center of the upper vertebral body and used a displacement gauge to measure the vertical motion of the lower end-plate of the upper vertebra. Another set of guages was arranged to measure the motion of the periphery of the same end-plate. The difference between the readings of the two sets of gauges represented the true deflection of the center of the end-plate.

[H] Euler's formula. The strength of a slender column of circular cross section under compressive load F is given by

$$F = \frac{\pi^2 \, E D^2}{16 \, L^2} \times A$$

where $\pi = 3.14$
    E = modulus of elasticity of the column material,
    D = diameter of the column,
    A = cross-sectional area of the column, and
    L = free length of the column.

This reduces to

$$F = \frac{\pi \, E}{4} \times \frac{A^2}{L^2}$$
$$= C \times \frac{A^2}{L^2}$$

where C is a constant for a column of a given material. Thus the strength of a column is directly proportional to the square of its cross-sectional area and inversely proportional to the square of its length.

[I] With reference to Figure 1-24, the computations of preload with the body in anatomic posture are as follows:

Sum of forces = $P - F - W_1 = 0$
Sum of moments = $W_1 \times L_1 - F \times L_2 = 0$

Solving for P, we get

$$P = (L_1 + L_2)W_1/L_2$$

Assuming that $L_1 = 80$ mm, $L_2 = 40$ mm and $W_1 = 0.6$ times body weight, we get

$$P = 1.8 \times \text{body weight}$$

(W_1 is the weight of the body portion above the motion segment; L_1 is the lever arm of this weight with respect to the instantaneous axis of rotation; F is the representative ligament and back muscle tension; L_2 is the lever arm of F; and P is the compressive load on the disc.)

[J] As a simple experiment, take the cylindrical core of a roll of paper towels. Subject it to bending and torsion with your hands and feel the resistance. Remove a longitundinal strip. Repeat the bending and torsion tests, and feel the enormous decrease in the resistance.

[K] Waters and Morris showed from their experiments that the tensile properties of the interspinous ligaments of idiopathic and other scoliotic spines are about the same.[101] Although they did not directly compare these results with those of the ligaments from normal spines, it was implied that the mechanical properties of the ligaments are not affected by the various diseases of scoliosis.

[L] The mechanism of lengthening of the spinal cord for the thoracic region is probably similar to that for other regions of the spine; although no precise information regarding the IAR in flexion/extension for other regions has been published, they are most likely anterior to the spinal cord.

CLASSIFICATION OF REFERENCES

Intervertebral disc 8, 18, 27, 29, 35, 39, 43, 44, 45, 46, 48, 52, 53, 60, 62, 63, 65, 67, 69, 71, 85, 86, 87, 89, 96, 97, 100
Spine ligaments 2, 3, 19, 31, 59, 68, 72, 73, 74, 78, 79, 85, 87, 95, 98, 99, 101, 105
Vertebra 4, 10, 11, 12, 14, 15, 17, 21, 24, 25, 27, 30, 37, 38a, 41, 50, 54, 55, 63, 65, 78, 83, 84, 88, 89, 90, 91, 102, 103, 104a, 105
Functional spinal unit (motion segment) 15b, 18, 26, 27, 38, 45, 47, 51, 55a, 56, 58, 61, 63, 69, 69a, 76, 77, 83, 89, 94a, 100, 104, 104a
Mathematical model of the spine 45a, 75a, 92
The rib cage 1, 7, 70, 76a, 81, 93, 94
The muscles 5, 6, 9, 20, 22, 23, 28, 32, 33, 34, 36, 40, 42, 57, 64, 66, 75, 82, 96
Spinal cord 16, 21a, 80

REFERENCES

1. Agostoni, E., Mognoni, G., Torri, G., and Miserocki, G.: Forces deforming the rib cage. Respir. Physiol., 2:105, 1966.
2. Akerblom, B.: Standing and sitting posture [thesis]. Stockholm, A/B Nordiska Bokhandelns Förlag, 1948.
3. Allbrook, D.: Movements of the lumbar spinal column. J. Bone Joint Surg., 39B:339, 1957.
4. Amstutz, H. C., and Sissons, H. A.: The structure of the vertebral spongiosa. J. Bone Joint Surg., 51B:540, 1969.
5. Andersson, G. B. J., and Örtengren, R.: Myoelectric back muscle activity during sitting. Scand. J. Rehab. Med., Suppl. 3:73, 1974.
6. Andersson, G. B. J., Örtengren, R., and Herberts P.: Quantitative electromyographic studies of back muscle activity related to posture and loading. Orthop. Clin. North Am., 8:85, 1977.
7. Andriacchi, T. P., Schultz, A. B., Belytscko, T. B., and Galante, J. O.: A model for studies of mechanical interactions between the human spine and rib cage. J. Bio-

mech., 7:497, 1974. (*Relevance of the rib cage to the entire spine is presented well through simulations of many clinically relevant situations.*)

8. Arutynow, A. J.: Basic problems of the pathology and surgical treatment of proplapsed intravertebral discs. Vopr. Neirokhir., 4:21, 1962.

9. Asmussen, E., and Klausen, K.: Form and function of the erect human spine. Clin. Orthop., 25:55, 1962.

10. Atkinson, P. J.: Variation in trabecular structure of vertebrae with age. Calcif. Tissue Res., 1:24, 1967. (*An interesting article describing the changes in the vertebral cancellous bone as a function of age.*)

11. Barnett, E., and Nordin, B. E. C.: The radiological diagnosis of osteoporosis. Clin. Radiol., 11:166, 1960.

12. Bartley, M. H., Arnold, J. S., Haslam, R. K., and Jee, W. S. S.: The relationship of bone strength and bone quantity in health, disease and aging. J. Gerontol., 21:517, 1966.

13. Beadle, O. A.: The intervertebral disc. Observations on their normal and morbid anatomy in relation to certain spinal deformities. Med. Res. Counc. Spec. Rep. Ser. (Lond.), No. 161, 1931.

14. Beck, J. S., and Nordin, B. E. C.: Histological assessment of osteoporosis by iliac crest biopsy. J. Pathol. Bacteriol., 80:391, 1960.

15. Bell, G. H., Dunbar, O., Beck, J. S., and Gibb, A.: Variation in strength of vertebrae with age and their relation to osteoporosis. Calcif. Tissue Res., 1:75, 1967.

15a. Belytschko, T., Andriacchi, T., Schultz, A., and Galante, J.: Analog studies of forces in human spine: computational techniques. J. Biomech., 6:361, 1973.

15b. Berkson, M. H., Nachemson, A. and Schultz, A. B.: Mechanical properties of human lumbar spine motion segments. Part II: Responses in compression and shear; influence of gross morphology. Journal of Biomechanical Engineering. [In Press].

16. Breig, A.: Biomechanics of the Central Nervous System: Some Basic Normal and Pathological Phenomena. Stockholm, Almquist & Wiksell, 1960. (*An important, thorough, and very well illustrated presentation of the biomechanical anatomy of the spinal cord.*)

17. Bromley, R. G., Dockum, N. L., Arnold, J. S., and Jee, W. S. S.: Quantitative histological study of human lumbar vertebrae. J. Gerontol., 21:537, 1966.

18. Brown, T., Hanson, R., and Yorra, A.: Some mechanical tests on the lumbo-sacral spine with particular reference to the intervertebral discs. J. Bone Joint Surg., 39A:1135, 1957. (*An important study of the physical behavior of the intervertebral disc under many different conditions of loading.*)

19. Buckwalter, J. A., Cooper, R. R., and Maynard, J. A.: Elastic fibers in human intervertebral discs. J. Bone Joint Surg., 58A:73, 1976.

20. Carlsöö, S.: The static muscle load in different work positions: an electromyographic study. Ergonomics, 4:193, 1961.

21. Casuccio, C.: An introduction to the study of osteoporosis. Proc. R. Soc. Med., 55:663, 1962.

21a. Crafts, R. C.: A Textbook of Human Anatomy. New York, Ronald Press, 1966.

22. Davis, P. R., Troup, J. D. G., and Burnard, J. H.: Movements of the thorax and lumbar spine when lifting: a chronocyclophotographic study. J. Anat., 99:13, 1965.

23. Donish, E. W., and Basmajian, J. V.: Electromyography of deep back muscles in man. Am. J. Anat., 133:25, 1972.

24. Dunnhill, M. S., Anderson, J. A., and Whitehead, R.: Quantitative histological studies on age changes in bone. J. Pathol. Bacteriol., 94:275, 1967.

25. Evans, F. G.: Stress and Strain in Bones. Charles C. Thomas, Springfield, Ill., 1957. (*A good reference book for the mechanical properties of bone tissue.*)

26. Evans, F. G., and Lissner, H. R.: Biomechanical studies on the lumbar spine and pelvis. J. Bone Joint Surg., 41A:273, 1959.

27. Farfan, H. F.: Mechanical Disorders of the Low Back. Philadelphia, Lea & Febiger, 1973. (*Biomechanical studies conducted by the author and his associates are presented well together with his hypothesis of disc degeneration due to mechanical factors.*)

28. ———: Muscular mechanism of the lumbar spine and the position of power and efficiency. Orthop. Clin. North Am., 61:135, 1975.

29. Farfan, H. F., Cossette, J. W., Robertson, G. H., Wells, R. V., and Kraus, H.: The effects of torsion on the lumbar intervertebral joints: the role of torsion in the production of disc degeneration. J. Bone Joint Surg., 52A:468, 1970.

30. Farfan, H. F., and Sullivan, J. D.: The relation of facet orientation to intervertebral disc failure. Can. J. Surgery, 10:179, 1967.

31. Fick, R.: Handbook der Anatomie und Mechanik der Gelenke. Jena, Verlag G. Fischer, 1904.

32. Floyd, W. F., and Silver, P. H. S.: Electromyographic study of patterns of activity of the anterior abdominal wall muscles in man. J. Anat., 84:132, 1950.

33. ———: Function of erectores spinae in flexion of the trunk. Lancet, 260:133, 1951.

34. Fung, Y. -C.: Mathematical representation of the mechanical properties of the heart muscle. J. Biomech., 3:381, 1970. (*An authoritative article on the mathematical modeling of muscle biomechanics.*)

35. Galante, J. O.: Tensile properties of the human lumbar annulus fibrosis. Acta Orthop. Scand., Suppl. 100:1, 1967.

36. Gardner, W. D., and Osburn, W. A.: Structure of the human body. Philadelphia, Saunders, 1973.

37. Gibb, A.: Appendix. *In* Bell, G. H., Dunbar, O., Beck, J. S., and Gibb, A.: Variation in strength of vertebrae with age and their relationship to osteoporosis. Calcif. Tissue Res., 1:75, 1967. (*The author presents a biomechanical hypothesis for osteoporosis in simple mathematics.*)

38. Griffith, H. B., Cleane, J. R. W., and Taylor, R. G.: Changing patterns of fracture in the dorsal and lumbar spine. Br. Med. J., 1:891, 1966.

38a. Hansson, T. H., Ross, B. O., and Nachemson, A. L.: The bone mineral content and biomechanical properties of lumbar vertebrae. Presented at the 24th annual meeting of Orthopaedic Research Society, Dallas, 1978.

39. Harris, R. I., and MacNab, I.: Structural changes in the lumbar intervertebral discs. Their relationship to low back pain and sciatica. J. Bone Joint Surg., 36B:304, 1954.

40. Haxtion, H. A.: Absolute muscle force in the ankle flexons in man. J. Physiol., 103:267, 1944.

41. Hayes, W. C., and Carter, D. R.: The effect of marrow on energy absorption of trabecular bone. Presented at the

22nd Annual Meeting of Orthopedic Research Society, New Orleans, 1976.

42. Hill, A. V.: Heat of shortening and dynamic constants of muscle. Proc. R. Soc. Lond., *B126:*136, 1939.

43. Hirsch, C.: The reaction of intervertebral discs to compression forces. J. Bone Joint Surg., 37A:1188, 1955.

44. Hirsch, C.: The mechanical response in normal and degenerated lumbar discs. J. Bone Joint Surg., 38A: 242, 1956.

45. Hirsch, C., and Nachemson, A.: A new observation on the mechanical behavior of lumbar discs. Acta Orthop. Scand., 23:254, 1954.

46. Kazarian, L. E.: Creep characteristics of the human spinal column. Orthop. Clin. North Am., 6:3, 1975.

47. Kazarian, L. E., Boyd, D. D., and Von Gierke, H. E.: The dynamic biomechanical nature of spinal fractures and articular facet derangement. Report Number AMRL-TR-71-7, Aerospace Medical Research Laboratory, Wright-Patterson Airforce Base, Ohio, 1971.

48. Kelsey, J. L., and Hardy, R. J.: Driving of motor vehicles as a risk factor for acute herniated intervertebral disc. Am. J. Epidemiol., 102:63, 1975.

49. Kelvin, W.: Popular Lectures and Addresses. *Vol. 1.* London, Macmillan, 1891.

50. King, A. I., Prasad, P., and Ewing, C. L.: Mechanism of spinal injury due to candocephalad acceleration. Orthop. Clin. North Am., 6:19, 1975.

51. Krag, M. H.: Three dimensional flexibility measurements of preloaded human vertebral motion segments [thesis]. Yale University School of Medicine, New Haven, 1975.

52. Kraus, H.: Stress analysis. *In* Farfan, H. E.: Mechanical Disorders of the Low Back. Philadelphia, Lea & Febiger, 1973.

53. Kulak, R. F., Belytschko, T. B., Schultz, A. B., and Galante, J. O.: Non-linear behavior of the human intervertebral disc under axial load. J. Biomech., 9:377, 1976. (*An advance mathematical model of the intervertebral disc.*)

54. Lamy, C., Bazergui, A., Kraus, H., and Farfan, H. F.: The strength of the neural arch and the etiology of spondylolysis. Orthop. Clin. North Am., 6:215, 1975.

55. Lindahl, O.: Mechanical properties of dried defatted spongy bone. Acta Orthop. Scand., 47:11, 1976. (*An important article describing experimental findings of increase in compressive strength after the initial failure.*)

55a. Lin H. S., Liu, Y. K., and Adams, K. H.: Mechanical response of the lumbar intervertebral joint under physiological (complex) loading. J. Bone Joint Surg., 60A:41, 1978.

56. Liu, K. Y., Ray, G., and Hirsch, C.: The resistance of the lumbar spine to direct shear. Orthop. Clin. North Am., 6:33, 1975.

57. Lucas, D., and Bresler, B.: Stability of ligamentous spine. Biomechanics Lab. Report 40, University of California, San Francisco, 1961.

58. Lysell, E.: Motion in the cervical spine. Acta Orthop. Scand., Suppl. *123,* 1969.

59. McHelhaney, J. H., and Edward, B. F.: Dynamic response of biological materials. Am. Soc. Mech. Engin. 65-WA/HUF-9, 1965. (*One of the first papers describing the increase in strength of bone when tested at higher rates of loading.*)

60. Markolf, K. L.: Stiffness and damping characteristics of the thoracic-lumbar spine. Proceedings of Workshop on Bioengineering Approaches to the Problems of the Spine, NIH, September, 1970.

61. ———: Deformation of the thoracolumbar intervertebral joint in response to external loads: a biomechanical study using autopsy material. J. Bone Joint Surg., 54A:511, 1972. (*A thorough examination of the stiffness properties of the thoracic and lumbar motion segments of the spine.*)

62. Markolf, K. L., and Morris, J. M.: The structural components of the intervertebral disc. J. Bone Joint Surg., 56A: 675, 1974.

63. Messerer, O.: Uber Elasticitat and Festigkeit der Meuschlichen Knochen. Stutgart, J. G. Cottaschen Buchhandling, 1880.

64. Morris, J. M., Benner, G., and Lucas, D. B.: An electromyographic study of intrisic muscles of the back in man. J. Anat., 96:509, 1962.

65. Nachemson, A.: Lumbar Interdiscal Pressure. Acta Otrhop. Scand., Suppl. *43,* 1960.

66. ———: Electromyographic studies on the vertebral portion of the psoas muscle. Acta Orthop. Scand., 37:177, 1966.

67. ———: The load on lumbar discs in different positions of the body. Clin. Orthop., 45:107, 1966.

68. Nachemson, A., and Evans, J.: Some mechanical properties of the third lumbar inter-laminar ligament (ligamentum flavum). J. Biomech., 1:211, 1968.

69. Nachemson, A., and Morris, J. M.: In vivo measurements of intradiscal pressure. J. Bone Joint Surg., 46:1077, 1964. (*An important paper describing the in vivo loads on the lumbar discs in different physiological postures and activities.*)

69a. Nachemson, A. L., Schultz, A. B., and Berkson, M. H.: Mechanical properties of human lumbar spine motion segments. Part III: Influences of age, sex, disc level and degeneration. [In Press].

70. Nahum, A. M., Gadd, C. W., Schneider, D. C., and Kroell, C. R.: Delfections of human thorax under sternal impact. International Automobile Safety Conference, Detroit and Brussels, 1970.

71. Naylor, A., Happey, F., and MacRae, T.: Changes in the human intervertebral disc with age: a biophysical study. J. Am. Geriatr. Soc., 3:964, 1955.

72. Noyes, F. R., DeLucas, J. L., and Torvik, P. J.: Biomechanics of anterior cruciate ligament failure: an analysis of strain-rate sensitivity and mechanisms of failure in primates. J. Bone Joint Surg., 56A:236, March 1974. (*Description of experimental finding that the ligaments have higher strength when tested at higher speeds.*)

73. Noyes, F. R., Torvik, P. J., Hyde, W. B., and DeLucas, J. L.: Biomechanics of ligament failure: an analysis of immobilization, exercise, and reconditioning effects in primates. J. Bone Joint Surg., 56A:1406, 1974.

74. Nunley, R. L.: The ligamenta flava of the dog: a study of tensile and physical properties. Am. J. Phys. Med., 37:256, 1958.

75. Örtengren, R., and Andersson, G. B. J.: Electomyographic studies of trunk muscles, with special reference to the functional anatomy of the lumbar spine. Spine, 2:44, 1977. (*A review article describing the presently available methodology of electromyography and some*

results concerning the muscles of the back. An excellent article for a researcher.)

75a. Panjabi, M. M.: Three-dimensional mathematical model of the human spine structure. J. Biomech., 6:761, 1973.

76. Panjabi, M. M., Brand, R. A., and White, A. A.: Mechanical properties of the human thoracic spine: as shown by three-dimensional load-displacement curves. J. Bone Joint Surg., 58A:642, 1976. (*A systematic determination of 36 load-displacement curves of each of the thoracic motion segments.*)

76a. Panjabi, M. M., Hausfeld, J., and White, A. A.: Experimental determination of thoracic spine stability. Presented at the 24th annual meeting of Orthopaedic Research Society, Dallas, 1978.

77. Panjabi, M. M., Krag, M. H., White, A. A., and Southwick, W. O.: Effects of preload on load displacement curves of the lumbar spine. Orthop. Clin. North Am., 88:181, 1977.

78. Panjabi, M. M., White, A. A., and Johnson, R. M.: Cervical spine mechanics as a function of transection of components. J. Biomech., 8:327, 1975.

79. Panjabi, M. M., White, A. A., and Southwick, W. O.: Mechanical properties of bone as a function of rate of deformation. J. Bone Joint Surg., 55A:322, 1973.

80. Panjabi, M. M., Wolf, J., Brand, R. A., and White, A. A.: Instant centers of the human thoracic spine. [In Press].

81. Patrick, L., Kroell, C., and Mertz, H.: Forces on the human body in simulated crashes. Proceedings 9th Stapp Car Crash and Field Demonstration Conference, p. 237, 1965.

82. Pauley, J. E.: An electromyographic analysis of certain movements and exercises. I. Some deep muscles of the back. Anat. Rec., 155:223, 1966.

83. Perry, O.: Fracture of the vertebral end-plate in the lumbar spine. Acta Orthop. Scand., 25 [Suppl.], 1957.

84. Perry, O.: Resistance and compression of the lumbar vertebrae. *In* Encyclopedia of Medical Radiology. New York, Springer-Verlag, 1974. (*A detailed and important study of the end-plate fractures of vertebrae.*)

85. Prasad, P., King, A. I., and Ewing, C. L.: The role of articular facets during +Gz acceleration. J. Appl. Mech. 41:321, 1974.

86. Puschel, J.: Der wassergehalt normaler und degenerierter zwischenwirbelscheiben. Bietr. Path. Anat., 84:123, 1930.

87. Roaf, R.: A Study of the Mechanics of Spinal Injuries. J. Bone Joint Surg., 42B:810, 1960.

88. Rockoff, S. D., Sweet, E., and Bleustein, J.: The relative contribution of trabecular and cortical bone to the strength of human lumbar vertebrae. Calcif. Tissue Res., 3:163, 1969. (*An interesting study of the relative role played by the cancellous core and cortical shell of a vertebra in bearing weight.*)

89. Rolander, S. D.: Motion of the lumbar spine with special reference to the stabilizing effect of posterior fusion [thesis]. Department of Orthopaedic Surgery, University of Gothenburg, Sweden, 1966.

90. Rolander, S. D., and Blair, W. E.: Deformation and fracture of the lumbar vertebral end-plate. Orthop. Clin. North Am., 6:75, 1975.

91. Ruff, S.: Brief acceleration: less than one second. *In* German Aviation Medicine in World War II. *Vol. 1.* Washington, D.C., U.S. Government Printing Office, 1950.

92. Schultz, A. B.: A biomechanical view of scoliosis. Spine, 1:162, 1976.

93. Schultz, A. B., Benson, D., and Hirsch, C.: Force deformation properties of human ribs. J. Biomech., 7:303, 1974.

94. Schultz, A., Benson, D., and Hirsch, C.: Force deformation properties of human costosternal and costovertebral articulations. J. Biomech., 7:311, 1974.

94a. Schultz, A. B., Warwick, D. N., Berkson, M. H., and Nachemson, A. L.: Mechanical properties of human lumbar spine motion segments. Part I: Responses in flexion, extension, lateral bending and torsion. J. Biomech. Engineering [In Press].

95. Silver, P. H. S.: Direct observations of changes in tension in the supraspinous and interspinous ligaments during flexion and extension of the vertebral column in man. J. Anat., 88:550, 1954.

96. Soechting, J. F., and Paslay, P. R.: A model for the human spine during impact including musculature influence. J. Biomech., 6:195, 1973.

97. Sonnerup, L.: A semi-experimental stress analysis of the human intervertebral disc in compression. Expl. Mech., 12:142, 1972.

98. Strasser, H.: Lehrbuch der Musker, und Gelenkmechanik. Berlin, Springer-Verlag, 1908.

99. Tkaczuk, H.: Tensile properties of human lumbar longitudinal ligaments. Acta Orthop. Scand., 115 [Suppl.], 1968.

100. Virgin, W.: Experimental investigations into physical properties of intervertebral disc. J. Bone Joint Surg., 33B:607, 1951.

101. Waters, R. L., and Morris, J. M.: An in vitro study of normal and scoliotic interspinous ligaments. J. Biomech., 6:343, 1973.

102. Weaver, J. K.: Bone: its strength and changes with aging and an evaluation of some methods for measuring its mineral content. J. Bone Joint Surg., 41A:935, 1966.

103. Weiss, E. B.: Stress at the lumbosacral junction. Orthop. Clin. North Am., 66:83, 1975.

104. White, A. A.: Analysis of the mechanics of the thoracic spine in man. Acta Orthop. Scand., 127 [Suppl.], 1969.

104a. White, A. A., and Hirsch, C.: The significance of the vertebral posterior elements in the mechanics of the thoracic spine. Clin. Orthop., 81:2, 1971.

105. White, A. A., Johnson, R. M., Panjabi, M. M., and Southwick, W. O.: Biomechanical analysis of clinical stability in the cervical spine. Clin. Orthop., 109:85, 1975.

2 Kinematics of the Spine

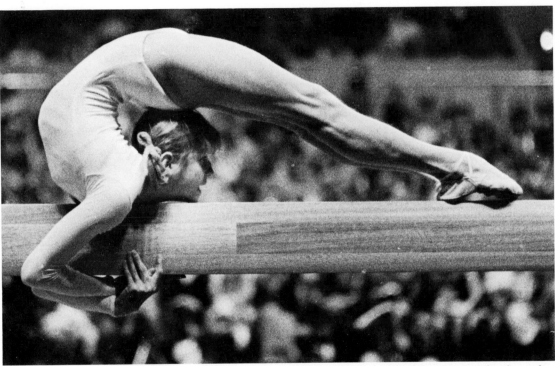

Fig. 2-1. This Olympic Gold Medal Winner represents the epitome of health. Her spinal column has no pathologic subluxations but represents the maximal range of motion as it is involved in this artistic and athletic form of normal kinematics. A keen appreciation of normal kinematics is basic to all aspects of the clinical care of the spine. (Courtesy of *San Francisco Examiner.*)

A comprehensive knowledge of spinal kinematics is of paramount importance for the understanding of all aspects of the clinical analysis and management of spine problems. This is true in the evaluation of radiographs, the understanding of clinical stability, spine trauma, scoliosis, the clinical effects of fusions, orthotic prescriptions, and the evaluation of surgical constructs. Much information is available on this complex topic.

TERMS AND DEFINITIONS

All terms and definitions in this section may also be found in the Appendix:Glossary.

Kinematics

Kinematics is that phase of mechanics concerned with the study of motion of rigid bodies, with no consideration of the forces involved.

Fig. 2-2. The suggested central coordinate system with its origin between the cornua of the sacrum is shown. Its orientation is as follows. The −y-axis is described by the plumb line dropped from the origin, and the +x-axis points to the left at a 90-degree angle to the y-axis. The +z-axis points forward at a 90-degree angle to both the y-axis and x-axis. The human body is shown in the anatomic position. There are some basic conventions that are observed which make this a useful system. *The planes* are as shown: The sagittal plane is the y, z plane; the frontal plane is the y, x plane; the horizontal plane is the x, z plane. *Movements* are described in relation to the origin of the coordinate system. The arrows indicate the positive direction of each axis. The origin is the zero point, and the direction opposite to the arrows is negative. Thus, direct forward translation is +z; up is +y; to the left is +x, and to the right is −x; down is −y; and backwards is −z. The convention for rotations is determined by imagining oneself at the origin of the coordinate system looking in the positive direction of the axis. Clockwise rotations are $+\theta$ and counterclockwise rotations are $-\theta$. Thus, $+\theta x$ is roughly analogous to flexion; $+\theta z$ is analogous to right lateral bending; $+\theta y$ is axial rotation towards the left. A coordinate system may be set up at any defined point parallel to the master system described above. The location of the coordinate system should be clearly indicated for precise, accurate communications. In spinal kinematics, the motion is usually described in relation to the subjacent vertebra. The secondary coordinate system may be established in the body of the subjacent vertebra. For in vivo measurements, the tip of its spinous process may be used. (Panjabi, M. M., White, A. A., and Brand, R. A.: A note on defining body parts configurations. J. Biomech., 7:385, 1974.)

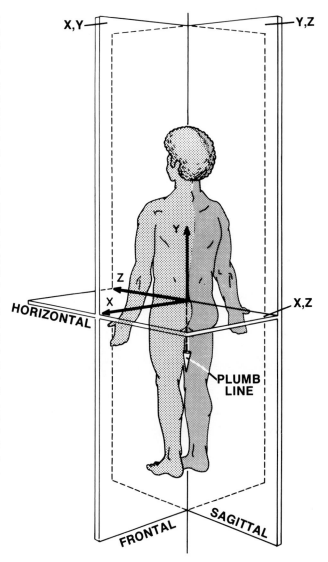

A Comprehensive Description of Kinematics of the Spine*

The important basic and clinical aspects of kinematics of the spine are as follows:

Range of motion for all six degrees of freedom
  Rotations
  Translations
Traditional physiologic patterns of motion
  Flexion/extension
  Lateral bending
  Axial rotation
Coupling characteristics and ratios
Instantaneous axes of rotation of motion segments in each of the traditional planes[B]
  Sagittal plane (y,z)
  Frontal plane (y,x)
  Horizontal plane (x,z)
Helical axes of motion located throughout the range of motion[B]
Functions of anatomic elements. A description of the roles played by the various anatomic elements in determining kinematic characteristics
Analysis of cephalocaudal variations within the regions
Analysis and comparison of the regional variations
  Occipital-atlanto-axial
  Lower cervical
  Thoracic
  Lumbar

* For a comprehensive review of the subject, the reader is referred to the works of Lysell,[51] Rolander,[70] Werne,[81] and White.[82]

Coordinate System

The coordinate system employed here is easy and efficient for accurate description of spinal kinematics. Understanding the text is not dependent upon following the conventions used here. However, they are helpful for more precise communications and understanding of the biomechanics literature.

The right-handed orthogonal (90°-angle) coordinate system has been recommended for precise orientation about the human body.[61,84] Its orientation in space and its conventions are shown in Figure 2-2.

Motion Segment

The motion segment, the traditional unit of study in spinal kinematics, is constituted by two adjacent vertebrae and their intervening soft tissues. Motion is described in terms relative to the subjacent vertebra (see Appendix:Glossary).

Rotation

A body (any piece of matter) is said to be in rotation when movement is such that all particles along some straight line in the body or a hypothetical extension of it have zero velocity relative to a fixed point. Rotation is a spinning or angular displacement of a body about some axis. The axis may be located outside the rotating body or inside it.

Translation

A body is said to be in translation when movement is such that all particles in the body at a given time have the same direction of motion relative to a fixed point.

Degrees of Freedom

One degree of freedom is motion in which a rigid body may translate back and forth along a straight line or may rotate back and forth about a particular axis. Vertebrae have six degrees of freedom, translation along and rotation about each of three orthogonal axes.

Range of Motion (ROM)

The difference between the two points of physiologic extremes of movement is the range of motion. Translation is expressed in meters or inches and rotation is expressed in degrees. The

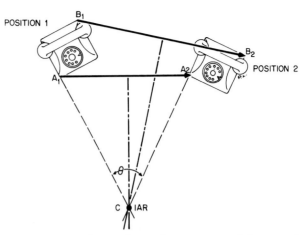

Fig. 2-3. This figure shows the concept and the actual method of determining the instantaneous axis of rotation in *uniplanar* motion. The IAR is determined by the intersection of the perpendicular bisectors of the two lines A_1A_2 and B_1B_2 (the translation vectors of the two points A and B on the telephone). The angle θ formed at the IAR by points A_1, A_2 or B_1, B_2 is the angle of rotation. (White, A. A., III, and Panjabi, M. M.: Spinal kinematics. The Research Status of Spinal Manipulative Therapy. NINCDS Monograph (No. 15). p. 93. Washington, D.C., U.S. Department of Health, Education and Welfare, 1975.)

range of motion can be expressed for each of the six degrees of freedom.

Coupling

Coupling refers to motion in which rotation or translation of a body about or along one axis is consistently associated with simultaneous rotation or translation about another axis.

Pattern of Motion

This is defined by the configuration of a path that the geometric center of the body describes as it moves through its range of motion.

Instantaneous Axes of Rotation (IAR)

At every instant, for a rigid body in plane motion there is a line in the body or a hypothetical extension of this line which does not move. The instantaneous axis of rotation is this line. Plane motion is fully defined by the position of the instantaneous axis of rotation and the magnitude of the rotation about it (Fig. 2-3).[A]

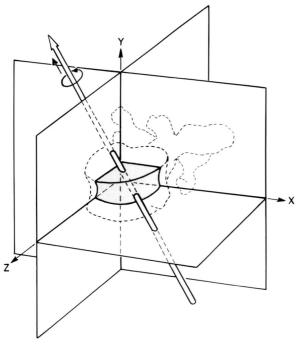

Fig. 2-4. Helical Axis of Motion. The screw motion which fully describes three-dimensional motion is a superimposition of rotation and translation about and along the same axis. Here a vertebra is shown with a hypothetical helical axis. See the Appendix:Glossary for a more detailed explanation.

Helical Axis of Motion (HAM)

The instantaneous motion of a rigid body in three-dimensional space can be analyzed by regarding it as a simple screw motion. The screw motion is a superimposition of rotation and translation about and along the same axis. This axis has the same direction as the resultant of the three rotations about the x, y, and z axes. For a given moving rigid body in space, the location of this axis and the designation of numerical values for rotation and translation constitute a complete, precise, three-dimensional description of the motion (Fig. 2-4). For a more detailed discussion of this concept, consult the Appendix: Glossary.

KINETICS AND MUSCLE ACTIVITY

Kinematics has been defined as that phase of mechanics concerned with the study of move-

Vertebral Muscles and Their Motor Functions

ANTERIOR

Muscles in front flex the spine. If the muscle runs a little obliquely and contracts independently of the corresponding muscle on the opposite side, it rotates and bends the spine laterally, as well as flexing it.

Longus colli*	Obliquus internus
Longus capitis	abdominis*
Rectus capitis anterior	Psoas major†
Rectus capitis lateralis†	Psoas minor†
Obliquus externus	Iliacus
abdominis*	Quadratus lumborum

POSTERIOR

Muscles in back extend the spine. If the muscle runs a little obliquely and contracts independently of the corresponding muscle on the opposite side, it rotates and bends the spine laterally, as well as extending it.

Superficial stratum	*Deep stratum*
Splenius capitis*†	Semispinalis
Splenius cervicis*†	Thoracis*
Erector spinae	Cervicis*
(sacrospinalis)	Capitis*
Iliocostalis*†	Multifidi*
Longissimis*†	Rotatores*
Spinalis*†	Interspinales
	Intertransversarii*

LATERAL

Muscles on the side bend the spine laterally.

Trapezius	Scalenus*
Sternocleidomastoid*	Anterior
Quadratus lumborum	Medial
	Posterior

* Muscles with axial rotation function
† Muscles with lateral bending function

ment of rigid bodies, with no consideration of what has caused the motion. *Kinetics* includes the study of the forces responsible for the motion. The muscles are the primary source of force resulting in motion of the vertebrae. This extremely complex topic is one that has been studied least from the viewpoint of biomechanics. Kinetics of the spine will not be discussed here.

The muscles which may produce motion of the spine include the anterior muscles, which are in front of the vertebrae, the posterior muscles, and the lateral muscles. The anterior muscles include the abdominal muscles and the iliopsoas. They flex the spine. If an anterior muscle runs

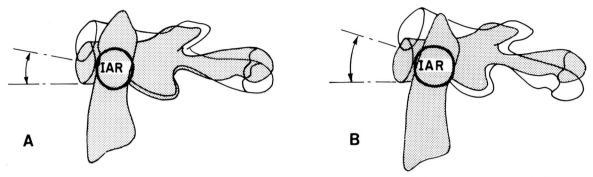

Fig. 2-5. (*A*) Representation of sagittal plane motion of C1 on C2, with the approximate IAR also indicated. Rotation is usually 10 to 11 degrees. (*B*) The anterior curvature of the dens may permit some degree of additional sagittal plane motion in both rotation and translation.

obliquely and contracts independently of the muscle on the opposite side, then it will axially rotate the spine as well as flex it. Similarly, a posterior muscle in the back extends the spine when it contracts. If the muscle runs obliquely and contracts independently of its counterpart on the opposite side, it will axially rotate and bend the spine laterally. If the lateral muscles are on the side and contract, the spine will bend laterally.

THE OCCIPITAL-ATLANTO-AXIAL COMPLEX (Ocp-C1-C2)

The occipital-atlanto-axial joints are the most complex joints of the axial skeleton, both anatomically and kinematically. Although there have been some thorough investigations of this region, there is considerable controversy about some of the basic biomechanical characteristics. In the following presentation, the best available information is analyzed with some discussion of salient questions.

Range of Motion

The representative figures for the ranges of motion for the units of the occipital-atlanto-axial complex are shown in Table 2-1.

Both joints of the complex participate about equally during flexion/extension in total motion in the sagittal plane. The contribution of the C1-C2 joint to sagittal plane rotation has been questioned by Fick, who reported that there is insignificant motion at this joint.[19] Porrier and Charpy reported 11 degrees of movement.[65] Werne showed that upon radiographic study sagittal plane movement is definitely present.[81] An example from his work is shown in Figure 2-5, with an angle of rotation indicated. It was found that the curvature of the dens in the sagittal plane may also allow some additional rotary displacement in that plane.

Some of the curvatures of the dens in the sagittal plane are shown in Figure 4-12 (see Chapter 4), where they are related to a threshold of posterior dislocation of C1 or C2. Subluxations and

Table 2-1. Representative Values of the Range of Rotation of the Occipital-Atlanto-Axial Complex[*]

UNIT OF COMPLEX	TYPE OF MOTION	DEGREES OF MOTION
Occipital-atlantal joint (ocp-C1)	Flexion/Extension ($\pm\theta x$)	13°(Moderate)
	Lateral bending ($\pm\theta z$)	8° (Moderate)
	Axial rotation ($\pm\theta y$)	0° (*Negligible*)
Atlanto-axial joint (C1-C2)	Flexion/Extension ($\pm\theta x$)	10° (Moderate)
	Lateral bending ($\pm\theta z$)	0° (*Negligible*)
	Axial rotation ($\pm\theta y$)	47° (Extensive)

* Based on review of literature and authors' analysis.

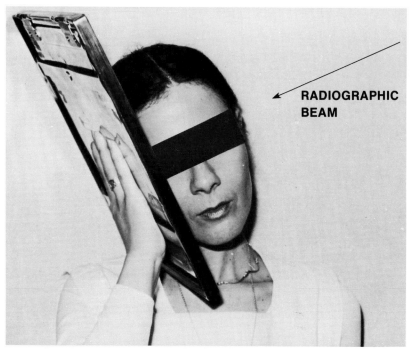

Fig. 2-6. The model is simulating the so-called "cock robin" position that the head may be held in, in a case of rotary subluxation or dislocation of C1 on C2. In order to get a true lateral view of the atlas, the film is placed parallel to the lateral aspect of the skull as shown. The central beam is directed perpendicular to the plane of the cassette. This maneuver makes use of the fact that there is no axial rotation between the skull and C1.

dislocations are often an exaggeration or over-extension of the normal range of motion.

Axial rotation is prevented by the geometric anatomy of the articulation of the ocp-C1 joint, and the two structures move as one unit about the y-axis. The joint surfaces are cup-shaped or arcuate in the sagittal plane, with the arcuate occipital articulation fitting into the cup of C1.

The absence of axial rotation between the occiput and C1 has at least one practical clinical application. In the radiologic evaluation of injury at the ocp-C1-C2 complex, it is important to have a truly lateral view of C1. This can be readily obtained by disregarding the position of the neck and shoulders and placing the film at the lateral side of the skull as shown in Figure 2-6.[73] Because there is no rotation between the skull and C1, this gives a lateral view of C1 unless there is dislocation between the occiput and C1.

There is extensive axial rotation between C1 and C2. A representative figure is 47 degrees.

Studies have shown that 50 per cent of axial rotation in the neck occurs at C1-C2, and that the remainder occurs at the joints of the lower cervical spine. This figure should be regarded only as a rough guideline. In any situation there may be a good deal more or less than 50 per cent of the total axial rotation at the C1-C2 articulation. In our representative normal (Fig. 2-25), the ratio of axial rotation is about 40 to 50 per cent in the upper cervical spine and 50 to 60 per cent in the lower portion. Usually the first 45 degrees of axial rotation takes place at C1-C2, before the lower cervical spine begins to participate.

The extensive amount (47°) of axial (y-axis) rotation at C1-C2 can sometimes cause clinical problems with the vertebral artery. Symptoms of vertigo, nausea, tinnitus, and visual disturbances may occur from occlusion of the vertebral artery associated with axial rotation of the atlas.[6] With axial rotation of the head in one direction on the side away from the direction in which the head

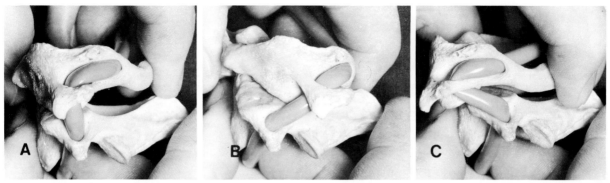

Fig. 2-7. The vertebral artery is represented by a piece of rubber tubing. (*A*) The atlas and axis are in neutral position. (*B*) The atlas is rotated to the left (+θy). (*C*) The atlas is rotated to the right (−θy). There is considerable excursion of the vertebral artery when rotary displacement takes place between the vertebrae. (Fielding, J. W.: J. Bone Joint Surg., 39A:1280, 1957.)

turns, the atlas moves forward in relation to the lateral portion of the axis. The portion of the artery between these two sections is stretched and narrowed. Selecki showed that the contralateral artery was first affected at 30 degrees of rotation and that it became markedly kinked at 45 degrees. Moreover, he observed that with more than 45 degrees of rotation, the contralateral vertebral artery was altered by either kinking or stretching.[72] If the flow in the vertebral artery on the ipsilateral side is compromised, then symptoms may be illicited. This potential problem has been well illustrated by Fielding (Fig. 2-7).[20]

The most detailed and convincing work on the kinematics of this region was done by Werne.[81] His investigations included anatomic dissections as well as anatomic studies of kinematics and radiographic kinematic studies in vitro and in vivo. Most of the information presented here is based upon the studies of Werne. In summary, rotation of the head about the three axes occurs through the occipital-atlanto-axial complex with participation of all three units: the occiput, the atlas, and the axis. Flexion extension (θx) occurs at ocp-C1 as well as at C1-C2. Lateral bending (θz) occurs at the ocp-C1 joint only, and axial rotation (θy) occurs at the C1-C2 joint only. There is negligible rotation at the ocp-C1 joint and negligible lateral bending at C1-C2. These findings are summarized in Table 2-1.

Translatory movements at the occipital-atlanto-axial complex are small. Between the occiput

and C1 there is insignificant translation. At the C1-C2 articulation, sagittal (±z-axis) and horizontal (±x-axis) plane translations are minimal because of the snug fit of the ring of C1 about the dens.

During translation in the mid-sagittal plane, the distance between the anterior portion of the dens and the posterior portion of the ring of C1 is clinically significant. Normal translation is 2 to 3 mm and is used as a guideline to radiologically evaluate the possibility of transverse ligament inadequacy, either from laxity or failure.[37] Jackson carried out radiologic studies of 50 adults and 20 children in which the distance between the posteroinferior margin of the anterior arch of the atlas and the anterior surface of the dens was measured. He found that the distance for adults was constant in full flexion and extension; the maximum was 2.5 cm. For children the maximum was 4.5 cm. Jackson often noted some forward subluxation in children during flexion.[41] This data is important in the diagnosis of rotary subluxations and fixation of C1 and C2 (see Chapter 5.)

Lateral (x-axis) translation of the C1-C2 joint is a highly controversial subject. We believe that there is only an apparent translation, and it is due to axial rotation between C1 and C2. The rotary changes produce a shift in the projection of the lateral masses of C1 in relation to the dens. This has been described by Werne[81] and demonstrated well by Shapiro and colleagues.[73] The rotary displacement pattern and the radiographic

from above

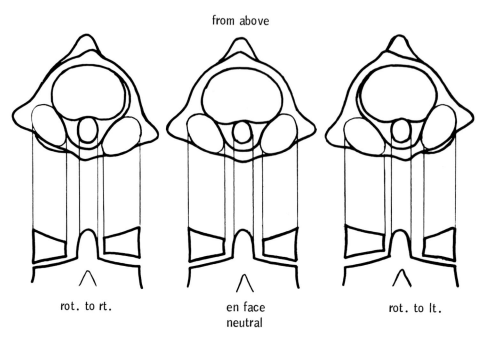

rot. to rt.   en face   rot. to lt.
                       neutral

Fig. 2-8. When C1 rotates to the right ($-\theta y$) on C2, the distance from the dens to the articular mass (lateral mass) of C2 moves forward. The concomitant posterior movement of the right lateral mass of C1 results in an apparent increase in the distance between the right lateral mass and the dens as seen on anteroposterior radiograph. The converse is true for rotation in the opposite direction. (Shapiro, R., Youngberg, A. S., and Rothman, S. L. G.: The differential diagnosis of traumatic lesions of the occipito-atlanto-axial segment. Radiol. Clin. North Am., *11*:505, 1973.)

projection are shown diagrammatically in Figure 2-8. Although Hohl had a different interpretation of this aspect of C1-C2 kinematics, he too made the point that lateral displacement (we believe *apparent* lateral displacement) of up to 4 mm between the dens and the lateral masses as an isolated radiographic finding is *not* indicative of subluxation or dislocation.[37]

Coupling Characteristics

It is generally accepted that there is a strong coupling pattern at the atlanto-axial joint (Fig. 2-9). The axial ($\pm y$ axis) rotation of C1 is associated with vertical ($\pm y$ axis) translation. However, there is some disagreement. The problem goes back at least as far as Henke, who in 1858 described a "double threaded screw" joint, due to the biconvexity of the articulations between C1 and C2.[34] This analysis was criticized by Hultkrantz, who studied sagittal sections of the C1-C2 articulations. He found that some of the surfaces were slightly biconvex, and others were slightly biconcave.[39] It has been observed that although the actual bony configuration may be concave, the configuration of the cartilage is such that the complete articulation has a biconvex design. This design is thought to account for the screw motion. Hultkrantz deduced that the screw movement (y-axis translation) was not characteristic of turning the head but probably only occurred in the extremes of the range of movement. There is more evidence on both sides of this discussion. Hohl has described the coupling of vertical translation of C1 with axial rotation of C1 on C2.[37] His conclusions were based on observations of cineradiographs. Werne's investigations led him to the conclusion that the screw motion depended somewhat on the extent to which the longitudinal axis of the dens correlates with the imaginary longitudinal axis of the body. The more parallel the two are, the more distinctive is the vertical displacement.[81] Figure 2-23 shows the extent to

LEFT ROTATION   **NEUTRAL**   **RIGHT ROTATION**

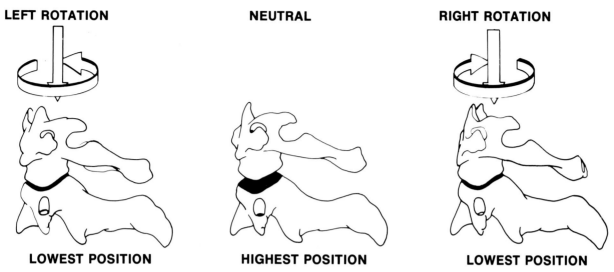

LOWEST POSITION   **HIGHEST POSITION**   **LOWEST POSITION**

Fig. 2-9. Because of the anatomic design of the lateral articulations, C1 is highest in the middle position and lowest with the extremes of axial rotation to the right or the left.

which the parallelism between the vertical axis of the coordinate system and the longitudinal axis of the dens can vary. In the example shown in the Figure 2-23, there is an angle of approximately 45 degrees. One can readily appreciate that the translation along the longitudinal axis of the dens can carry the atlas posteriorly or vertically, depending on the direction in which the dens is pointed.

Instantaneous Axes of Rotation (IAR)

Henke identified IAR for occipital-atlantal motion by determining the centers of the arches formed by the outline of the joints in the sagittal and frontal planes. The transverse axis passed through the centers of the mastoid processes (Fig. 2-10) and the sagittal axis was located at a point 2 to 3 cm above the apex of the dens. Although these points were identified more than a

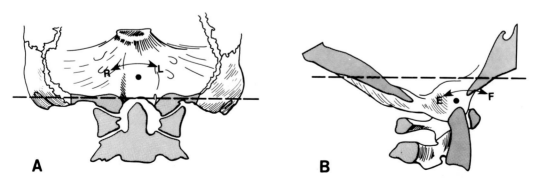

A   **B**

Fig. 2-10. (A) The approximate location of the IAR for the occipital-atlantal joint in the frontal plane is shown here. Lateral bending (R, L) of the occiput on C1 is thought to take place around the indicated dot. The broken line indicates the approximate location of the IAR for the flexion/extension (F, E) motion in the sagittal plane. (B) The converse is shown in the sagittal plane. The broken line localized the IAR for lateral bending and the dot shows the axes for flexion/extension.

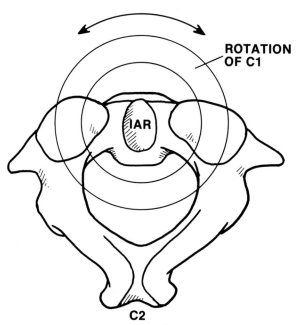

Fig. 2-11. This is a diagrammatic representation of the approximate location of the IAR for axial rotation of C1 on C2. The points are located in the region of the appropriately named *axis*.

century ago, they remain the only approximation of the instantaneous axes of rotation for occipital-atlantal articulation. The method used does not necessarily give accurate results. In order to locate the axes accurately, experimental investigations must be carried out, involving analysis of plane motion in carefully measured, controlled situations. The authors are not aware of such investigations of this region. Since there is no horizontal plane ($\pm\theta$y) rotation at the C1-C2 articulation, an instantaneous axis of rotation for this plan is not considered.

For the atlanto-axial joint the instantaneous axes of rotation can be estimated from the kinematic studies of Werne.[81] Sagittal plane motion shown in Figure 2-5 locates the instantaneous axes of rotation for flexion/extension somewhere in the region of the middle third of the dens. For axial ($\pm\theta$y) rotation, the instantaneous axes of rotation may be assumed to lie in the central portion of the *axis*,[19] a fact which attests to the astuteness of the scholars who named the structure (Fig. 2-11).

Lateral bending (x, y) plane rotation of the atlanto-axial joint is controversial, minimal, negligible, or most probably absent. Thus, given our present knowledge, the question of IAR for this plane is moot.

Functions of Anatomic Elements

At the ocp-C1 articulation, flexion movement is checked by skeletal contact between the anterior margin of the foramen magnum and the tip of the dens. Werne discovered a well developed, previously undescribed bursa which communicated with the joints of the dens. He called it the bursa apicis dentis. Extension is limited by the tectorial membrane (the cephalad continuation of the posterior longitudinal ligament). With flexion of the ocp-C1 joint beyond neutral, the tectorial membrane becomes taut and limits forward flexion at the C1-C2 joint. Similarly, with extension of the ocp-C1 joint, the tectorial membrane again becomes taut and limits extension between C1 and C2.[81] Axial rotation between C1 and C2 is limited by the alar ligaments. Right axial ($-$y-axis) rotation is limited by the left alar ligament. The opposite is true for rotation to the left.

THE LOWER CERVICAL SPINE (C2–C7)

Most of the information presented in this section is based on the work of Lysell.[51] He carried out detailed examinations of the kinematics of fresh autopsy specimens using a precise radiographic technique, which allowed for measurement of three-dimensional motion. The axis, C2, is a transitional vertebra between the occipital-atlanto-axial complex and the lower cervical spine, and therefore it is also discussed here.

Range of Motion

Rotation ranges for the cervical spine are shown in Table 2-2 and Figure 2-25. Most of the motion in flexion/extension is in the central region. The C5–6 interspace is generally considered to have the longest range. There may be some causal relationship between this observation and the incidence of cervical spondylosis at that interspace.[85] For lateral bending and axial rotation, there is a tendency for a smaller range of motion in the more caudal segments. The relationship between disc degeneration and motion was examined by Lysell. The intervertebral disc for each motion segment was cut and graded for degeneration. There was no change in range of motion as a function of disc degeneration.[51] Other investigators have observed that a compensatory increase in motion occurs in cervical spine segments adjacent to interspaces with reduced motion, due either to degeneration or post-traumatic changes.[21,44]

The maximum sagittal plane translation (z-axis) occurring in the lower cervical spine under "physiologic loads" simulating flexion/extension has been measured directly.[83] The representative figure is 2 mm and the maximum was 2.7 mm. The same measurement on a radiograph would vary with the technique employed in taking the film. The authors suggest 3.5 mm as a guide for the upper limits of normal, taking into account radiographic magnification (see p. 192).

Patterns of Motion

As a vertebra goes through its ranges of motion the pattern of motion is determined by a combination of the geometric anatomy of the structures and their physical properties. The positions of a vertebra from full extension to full flexion, for example, have certain similarities throughout the spine, and yet there are some characteristic regional differences and even gradations of differences within regions. Lysell showed clearly that the routes (patterns) were the same for any given vertebra whether it was going from flexion to extension or visa versa.[51] The movement is a combination of translation and rotation. He used what he called the "top angle" to indicate the steepness of the arch that was described by the vertebra while moving from full extension to full flexion.[c] The arches were flat at C2. The steepest was at C6, followed by C7. Those in between were all about the same.

The pattern of motion in the sagittal plane is shown diagrammatically in Figure 2-12. The acuity of the arc was found to decrease in association with disc degeneration; this overall pattern was shown to be a statistically significant variation.[51] The pattern of motion in the sagittal plane involves a strong coupling element.

Table 2-2. Limits and Representative Values of Range of Rotation of the Lower Cervical Spine

INTERSPACE	FLEXION/EXTENSION (x-axis rotation)		LATERAL BENDING (z-axis rotation)		AXIAL ROTATION (y-axis rotation)	
	LIMITS OF RANGES (degrees)	REPRESENTATIVE ANGLE (degrees)	LIMITS OF RANGES (degrees)	REPRESENTATIVE ANGLE (degrees)	LIMITS OF RANGES (degrees)	REPRESENTATIVE ANGLE (degrees)
C2–C3	5–23	8	11–20	10	6–28	9
C3–C4	7–38	13	9–15	11	10–28	11
C4–C5	8–39	12	0–16	11	10–26	12
C5–C6	4–34	17	0–16	8	8–34	10
C6–C7	1–29	16	0–17	7	6–15	9
C7–T1	4–17	9	0–17	4	5–13	8

(White, A. A., III, and Panjabi, M. M.: The basic kinematics of the human spine. Spine, 3:12, 1978.)

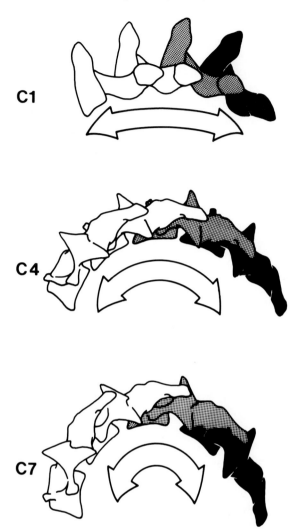

C1

C4

C7

Fig. 2-12. This is a diagrammatic approximation of the relative cephalocaudal variations in radii of curvature of the arches, defined by the cervical vertebrae as they rotate and translate in the sagittal plane. The diagram depicts the patterns of motion of C1, C4, and C7, moving back and forth between full flexion and full extension.

Coupling Characteristics

The coupling patterns in the lower cervical spine are dramatic and clinically important. The coupling is such that with lateral bending the spinous processes go to the convexity of the curve.[51] In lateral bending to the left the spinous processes go to the right, and in lateral bending to the right they go to the left (Fig. 2-13). (In the coordinate system $+\theta z$ is coupled with $-\theta y$ and $-\theta z$ is coupled with $+\theta y$.) This coupling is significant in understanding scoliosis as well as some aspects of spine trauma and its treatment. For example, a dislocation may result when a traumatic force carries a joint beyond its normal range of motion. The coupling phenomenon plays a role in that some ratios of axial rotation and lateral bending may result in a unilateral facet dislocation (see Chapter 4).

The amount of axial rotation that is coupled with lateral bending at various levels of the spine has been studied and described[51]. At the second cervical vertebra, there are 2 degrees of coupled axial rotation for every 3 degrees of lateral bending, a ratio of 2 to 3 or 0.67. At the seventh cervical vertebra, there is 1 degree of coupled axial rotation for every 7.5 degrees of lateral bending, a ratio of 1 to 7.5 or 0.13. Between C2 and C7 there is a gradual cephalocaudal decrease in the amount of axial rotation that is associated with lateral bending. This phenomenon of gradual change in the coupling ratio may be related to a change in the incline of the facet joints. Although this has not been measured and proven, we believe that the angle of incline of the facet joints in the sagittal plane increases cephalocaudally.

Instantaneous Axis of Rotation

The instantaneous axis of rotation for the cervical spine *motion segments* has been placed in a variety of different locations by different research workers. This is partially the result of a lack of consistency among investigators (Fig. 2-14).[D] Suggested locations include the body of subadjacent vertebrae, the center of the vertebral body, the disc, and the nucleus pulposus. An additional theory contends that the instantaneous axis of rotation for C2 lies in the posterior, caudal portion of the subadjacent vertebra, but that there is a progression in which the instantaneous axis of rotation moves anterior and cephlad, such that for C6 it is located at the anterior, cephalad portion of the subadjacent vertebra. Others suggest that there are large numbers of motion centers for

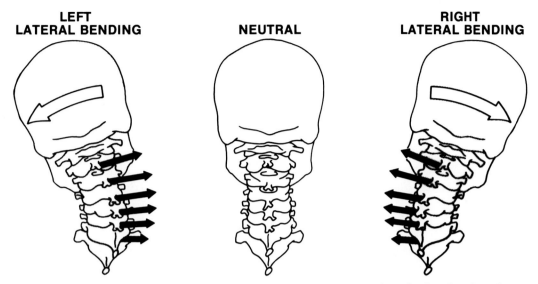

LEFT LATERAL BENDING **NEUTRAL** **RIGHT LATERAL BENDING**

Fig. 2-13. An important, major cervical spine coupling pattern. When the head and neck are bent to the right, the spinous processes go to the left. The converse is also shown. (Expressed in the coordinate system, +z axis rotation is coupled with −y axis rotation, and −z axis rotation is coupled with +y axis rotation.)

each vertebra. The authors are not aware of any investigation designed specifically to locate the instantaneous axis of rotation for cervical spine motion.

Based on personal judgment of observations of patterns of motion, Lysell postulated the locations of the instantaneous axes of rotation in the cervical region.[51] The locations were not determined quantitatively.

For sagittal and horizontal plane motion the instantaneous centers are thought to lie in the anterior portion of the subadjacent vertebra. The more anterior location is suggested by Lysell, who observed very little movement of his anterior measuring point. For lateral bending, they are probably in the region of the question mark shown in Figure 2-15, but this is even more speculative.

Functions of Anatomic Elements

The function of anatomic elements in the cervical spine is discussed in detail in Chapter 5. Investigations comparing the kinematics of a motion segment under "physiologic loads," with and without various elements, show that as long as either all anterior elements or all posterior elements are intact, there is no grossly abnormal motion.[83]

The strength and orientation of the annular fibers, along with the tenacious attachment to the periphery in all regions of the vertebral body and end-plate, contribute to the great resistance of the annulus to horizontal translation. This has an important role in the clinical stability of the spine.

The range of motion of flexion/extension is to some extent dictated by the geometry and stiffness of the disc.[19,45,49,86] For example, in flexion/extension the greater the height of the disc and the smaller the anteroposterior diameter, the greater is the motion. Similarly, if lateral bending is analyzed, the motion would be greater when the disc is higher and its lateral diameter is smaller. In addition, the greater the stiffness of the disc, the smaller is the motion.[E] A mathematical analysis of the dependence of rotatory motion upon properties of the disc is provided in Figure 2-16.

When there is a smaller diameter in the plane

FLEXION   LOADING

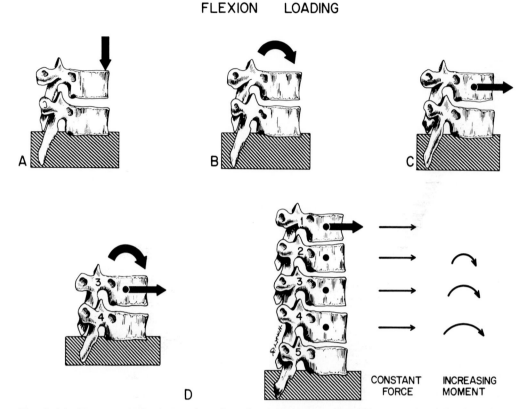

Fig. 2-14   Various methods employed in the in vitro experiments to produce flexion of the spine. Note that when multiple segments are studied simultaneously, there are different moments applied to the motion segments under study.[D] (White, A. A., III, and Panjabi, M. M.: Spinal kinematics. The Research Status of Spinal Manipulative Therapy. NINCDS Monograph (No. 15). p. 93. Washington, D.C., U.S. Department of Health, Education and Welfare, 1975.)

of motion, other things being equal, bony impingement is less likely and more motion is possible. In the cervical spine, where there is the greatest motion, the disc diameters of the sagittal and coronal plane are less than in the thoracic and lumbar regions. In addition to the disc, the stiffness of the other ligaments, especially the yellow ligament, also plays a significant role in the kinematics of the cervical spine.[5]

The uncinate processes, which began to develop at 6 to 9 years of age and are fully developed at 18 years, may be of importance in the patterns of motion in the cervical spine. They are thought to prevent posterior translation and also to limit lateral bending. In addition, the uncinate processes serve as a guiding mechanism to the patterns of flexion/extension.[8,15,24,64]

THE THORACIC SPINE

Range of Motion

The range of sagittal plane rotation (flexion/extension) for the thoracic spine is given in Table 2-3 and Figure 2-25. The median figure is 4 degrees of motion in the upper portion of the thoracic spine and 6 degrees of motion in the middle segments. In the lower portion (T11–12 and T12–L1) there are 12 degrees of motion at each segment. In the frontal plane (lateral bending) there is 6 degrees of motion in the upper thoracic spine, with 8 degrees or 9 degrees in the two lower segments. In the horizontal plane (axial rotation) there is 8 to 9 degrees of motion in the upper half of the thoracic spine and 2 degrees for each interspace of the three lower segments.

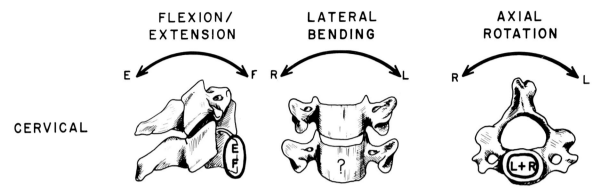

FLEXION/EXTENSION   LATERAL BENDING   AXIAL ROTATION

CERVICAL

Fig. 2-15. The approximate locations of instantaneous axes of rotation in the lower cervical spine. E is the location of IAR in going from a neutral to extended position. F is the location in going from a neutral to a flexed position. L shows the axes in left axial rotation, and R shows them in right axial rotation. The question mark indicates that there are at present no convincing estimates of the IAR for lateral bending in the cervical spinel. (White, A. A., III, and Panjabi, M. M.: Spinal kinematics. The Research Status of Spinal Manipulative Therapy. NINCDS Monograph (No. 15). p. 93. Washington, D.C., U.S. Department of Health, Education and Welfare, 1975.)

Here, the figures for axial rotation coincide nicely with the findings in vivo of Gregersen and Lucas, who studied axial rotation in the thoracic spines of seven medical students by inserting Steinman pins into the spinous processes.[30] They noted an average of 6 degrees of rotation at each level, and when their subjects were walking the maximum amount of rotation was observed at the middle portion of the thoracic spine. Figures for each interspace are given in Table 2-3.

Patterns of Motion

The pattern of motion in the sagittal plane for the thoracic spine is somewhat similar to that in the cervical spine. In describing the patterns of cervical spine motion the T angle, or "top angle," was employed to indicate the acuity of the arch formed by a given point as a vertebra moved in a plane. To evaluate thoracic spine motion in the sagittal and frontal planes, the average curvature

Table 2-3. Limits and Representative Values of Range of Rotation of the Thoracic Spine

| INTERSPACE | FLEXION/EXTENSION | | LATERAL BENDING | | AXIAL ROTATION | |
	LIMITS OF RANGES (degrees)	REPRESENTATIVE ANGLE (degrees)	LIMITS OF RANGES (degrees)	REPRESENTATIVE ANGLE (degrees)	LIMITS OF RANGES (degrees)	REPRESENTATIVE ANGLE (degrees)
T1–T2	3–5	4	5	6	14	9
T2–T3	3–5	4	5–7	6	4–12	8
T3–T4	2–5	4	3–7	6	5–11	8
T4–T5	2–5	4	5–6	6	4–11	8
T5–T6	3–5	4	5–6	6	5–11	8
T6–T7	2–7	5	6	6	4–11	8
T7–T8	3–8	6	3–8	6	4–11	8
T8–T9	3–8	6	4–7	6	6–7	7
T9–T10	3–8	6	4–7	6	3–5	4
T10–T11	4–14	9	3–10	7	2–3	2
T11–T12	6–20	12	4–13	9	2–3	2
T12–L1	6–20	12	5–10	8	2–3	2

(White, A. A., III, and Panjabi, M. M.: The basic kinematics of the human spine. A review of past and current knowledge. Spine, 3:12, 1978.)

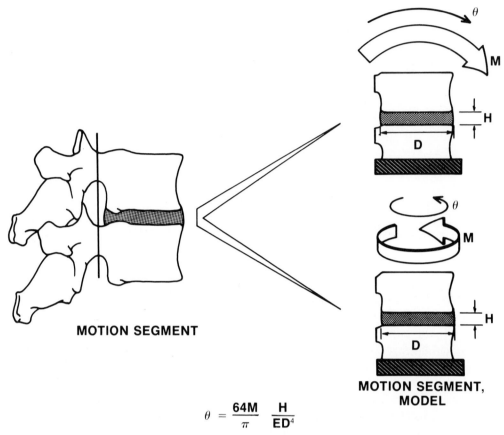

$$\theta = \frac{64M}{\pi} \ \frac{H}{ED^4}$$

Fig. 2-16.   Rotatory motion as a function of the height, diameter, and material of the intervertebral disc.

(the reciprocal of the radius of the arch) is used. In sagittal plane motion (flexion/extension) the average curvature is quite small, indicating a rather flat arch (Fig. 2-17A). There is no pattern of cephalocaudal variation. The average curvature in the frontal plane is also flat, but nevertheless greater, or steeper, than the arches of the sagittal plane (Fig. 2-17B). Also, in the frontal plane there is a cephalocaudal variation. The acuity of the arch tends to increase between T1 and T12.

Coupling Characteristics

There are a number of different coupling patterns, many of which may prove to be of clinical significance in the future. Of most interest at present in both the cervical and thoracic spines is coupling between lateral bending and axial rotation. Considerable interest in the thoracic

spine is due to the significance of normal coupling and abnormal coupling in scoliotic deformities (see Chapter 3).

Coupling has caused considerable literary controversy; not only are there debatable characteristics, but the occurrence of such a phenomenon is sometimes questioned. The historical aspects of this controversy have been reviewed.[82] The disagreement is due to a wide variety of different techniques, as well as the complexity of the motion under analysis.

The pattern of coupling in the thoracic spine is of the type that has been described in the cervical spine. Lateral bending is coupled with axial rotation, such that the spinous processes move toward the convexity of the lateral curvature. The cephalocaudal variation of this coupling pattern within the thoracic spine is of considerable interest. In the upper portion of the thoracic spine, the two motions are strongly coupled, although not as strongly as in the cervical spine. In the middle portion of the thoracic spine, the coupling pattern is by no means as distinct; moreover, it is inconsistent, and in some instances in the middle portion, the spinous processes rotate toward the concavity of the lateral curvature. Also, in the lower portion of the thoracic spine the coupling pattern is not as strong as in the upper portion. These patterns have been documented in detail elsewhere.[F,82]

Actually, a study by Panjabi and colleagues has shown that all of the six degrees of freedom demonstrate coupling patterns.[58]

Instantaneous Axis of Rotation

The shortcomings of current descriptions of the location of the instantaneous axis of rotation have been discussed.[D] The approximate location of these centers for the thoracic spine are represented diagrammatically in Figure 2-18.

Helical Axis of Motion

Although the concept of helical axis of motion in the thoracic spine has been introduced,[82] there have been no studies designed to precisely determine the site and orientation for a representative sample of vertebral motion.

Functions of Anatomic Elements

The functions of various anatomic elements have been studied in thoracic spine kinematics. With regard to the effect of removal of all posterior elements on the mechanics of the thoracic spine, several parameters were studied in individual motion segments.[82] In the movement where extension was simulated, there was a statistically significant increase in extension following removal of the posterior elements. This is due to the fact that the intervertebral joints and the spinous processes limit the amount of extension that occurs in this region. This also supports the description of these structures as load bearing elements. The differences throughout the full range of flexion/extension are shown in Figure 2-19. The increase in rotation also occurred in the horizontal plane (y-axis rotation) upon removal of

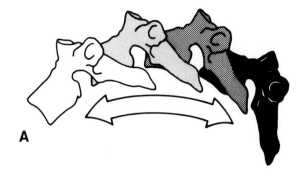

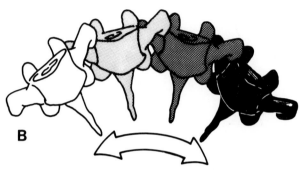

Fig. 2-17. A diagrammatic approximation of the relative variations in the radii of curvature of the arches defined by the thoracic vertebrae as they move in the sagittal and in the frontal planes. The arches described in the pattern of motion for lateral bending (*B*) are more accentuated than those described in flexion/extension (*A*).

the posterior elements. These biomechanical changes were also shown to be statistically significant. Due to the spatial alignment of the facet articulations, bony impingement resisting axial rotation is not believed to occur (Fig. 2-24). The posterior ligaments, primarily the yellow ligaments and also the facet joint capsules, are probably the major structures that resist axial motion. The resistance results from the development of tension in spinal structures. After the posterior elements are removed, the motion is restricted solely by the annulus fibrosis. In a clinical situation, motion is restricted by the annulus fibrosis and the muscles.

The effect of the removal of the posterior elements on the instantaneous axes of rotation has been studied in the three traditional planes of motion. Only a slight shift of the points was

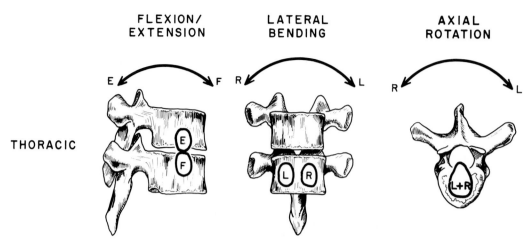

FLEXION/
EXTENSION

LATERAL
BENDING

AXIAL
ROTATION

THORACIC

Fig. 2-18.   The approximate locations of the instantaneous axes of rotation in the thoracic spine. E is the location of the axes going from a neutral to an extended position. F is the location of the axes going from a neutral to a flexed position. L shows the IAR in left lateral bending or left axial rotation, and R shows the axes in right lateral bending or right axial rotation. (White, A. A., III, and Panjabi, M. M.: Spinal kinematics. The Research Status of Spinal Manipulative Therapy. NINCDS Monograph (No. 15). p. 93. Washington, D.C., U.S. Department of Health, Education and Welfare, 1975.)

noted. This observation is of theoretical interest regarding the significance of the spatial alignment of the facet joints with regard to the patterns of motion. If the removal of these joints does not effect the rotation axes, the role of the facet joints in the mechanics of the spine comes

into question. At present, resolution of this question awaits further study.

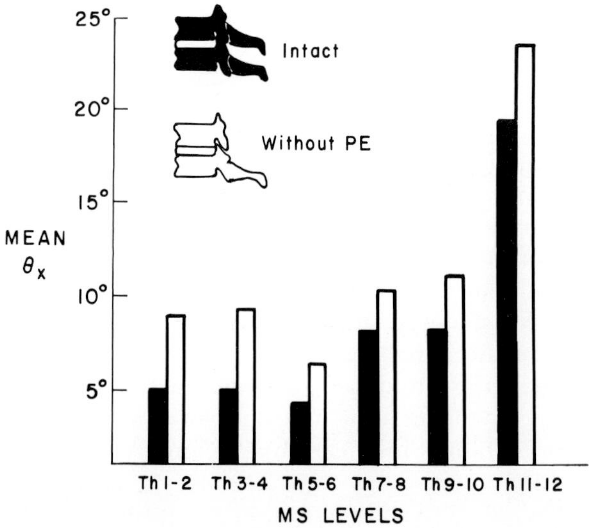

THE LUMBAR SPINE

Range of Motion

The representative rotations in flexion/extension, lateral bending, and axial rotation are shown in Table 2-4 and Figure 2-25. In flexion/extension there is usually a cephalocaudal increase in the range of motion in the lumbar spine. The lumbosacral joint offers more sagittal plane motion than do the other lumbar joints. For lateral bending each level is about the same, except for the lumbosacral joint, which shows a relatively small amount of motion. The situation is the same for axial rotation, except that there is more motion at the lumbosacral joint.[50] It is not unreasonable to speculate that the high incidence of clinically evident disc disease at L4–5 and L5–S1 may be related to mechanics. These two areas bear the highest loads and tend to undergo the most motion.

Coupling Characteristics

There are several coupling patterns that have been observed in the lumbar spine. Rolander

25°

Intact

20°

Without PE

15°

MEAN
θ_x

10°

5°

Th1-2 Th3-4 Th5-6 Th7-8 Th9-10 Th11-12
MS LEVELS

Fig. 2-19.   This is a graphic representation of average total sagittal plane rotation (flexion/extension) at the different thoracic levels, with and without the posterior elements.

Table 2-4. Representative Values of the Range of Rotation of the Lumbar Spine

INTERSPACE	FLEXION/EXTENSION (x-axis rotation)		LATERAL BENDING (z-axis rotation)		AXIAL ROTATION (y-axis rotation)	
	LIMITS OF RANGES (degrees)	REPRESENTA-TIVE ANGLE (degrees)	LIMITS OF RANGES (degrees)	REPRESENTA-TIVE ANGLE (degrees)	LIMITS OF RANGES (degrees)	REPRESENTA-TIVE ANGLE (degrees)
L1–L2	9–16	12	3–8	6	1–3	2
L2–L3	11–18	14	3–9	6	1–3	2
L3–L4	12–18	15	5–10	8	1–3	2
L5–S1	14–21	17	5–7	6	1–3	2
	18–22	20	2–3	3	3–6	5

(White, A. A., III, and Panjabi, M. M.: The basic kinematics of the human spine. A review of past and current knowledge. Spine, 3:12, 1978.)

observed an interesting coupling of y-axes rotation (axial) with +y-axes translation.[70] However, in more detailed experiments, this particular coupling was found to be rather weak.[60]

One of the strongest coupling patterns is that of lateral bending (z-axis rotation) with flexion/extension (x-axis rotation; Fig. 2-20). Moreover, there is also a coupling pattern described by Miles and Sullivan, in which axial rotation is combined with lateral bending, such that the spinous processes point in the same direction as the lateral bending.[54] This pattern is the opposite of that in the cervical spine and the upper thoracic spine. Although these coupling patterns comprise fundamental and essential elements in the understanding of lumbar spine kinematics, investigators have not been able to attach any clinical significance to them.

Instantaneous Axes of Rotation (IAR)

The rotation axes for the sagittal plane of the lumbar spine have been described in several reports. Calve and Galland in 1930 suggested that the center of the intervertebral disc is the site of the axes for flexion/extension.[7] Rolander showed that when flexion is simulated starting from a neutral position, the axes are located in the region of the anterior portion of the disc,[70] as shown in Figure 2-21. Reichmann and colleagues reported that the instantaneous axes of rotation is occasionally in the region of the disc, but in the majority of situations it is outside the disc and a considerable distance from it. In lateral bending, frontal plane rotation, the axes fall in the region of the right side of the disc with left lateral bend-

ing, and in the region of the left side of the disc with right lateral bending (Figure 2-21).

For axial (y-axis) rotation, the instantaneous axes of rotation are located in the region of the posterior nucleus and annulus.[9] A pattern of displacement of the rotation axes was not apparent according to evidence of disc degeneration.

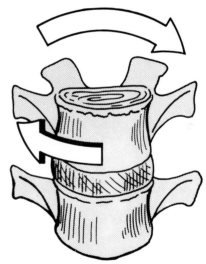

LUMBAR COUPLING

Fig. 2-20. Representation of a coupling pattern in the lumbar spine. Lateral bending (θz) is coupled with axial rotation (θy). Note that this coupling is just the opposite of that shown in the cervical spine in Figure 2-13. In the cervical spine the spinous processes moved toward the convexity of the curve: in the lumbar spine they would move toward the concavity. (Based on Krag, M. H.: Three dimensional flexibility measurements of preloaded human vertebral motion segments. [M. D. Thesis.] Yale University School of Medicine, New Haven, 1975.)

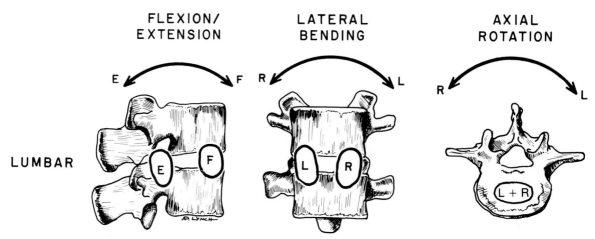

FLEXION/EXTENSION   **LATERAL BENDING**   **AXIAL ROTATION**

LUMBAR

Fig. 2-21. The approximate locations of the instantaneous axes of rotation in the lumbar spine. E is location of the axes going from a neutral to an extended position. F is the location of the axes going from a neutral to a flexed position. L shows the IAR in left lateral bending or left axial rotation, and R shows the axes in right lateral bending or right axial rotation. (White, A. A., III, and Panjabi, M. M.: Spinal kinematics. The Research Status of Spinal Manipulative Therapy. NINCDS Monograph (No. 15). p. 93. Washington, D.C., U.S. Department of Health, Education and Welfare, 1975.)

In the lumbar spine the location of the IAR (or some analogous concept) has received considerable attention. The major thrust of the investigations has been to show differences in the *points* of a diseased lumbar spine as opposed to that of the healthy state, with the rational expectation that this may provide some basic knowledge related or leading to some useful diagnostic tool. The hope is that this type of mechanical observation may provide some insight or understanding concerning the cause of pain or morphologic changes. The other potential value of IAR studies is the possible development of a diagnostic tool that could help identify the source and location of pain.

In both sagittal and frontal plane rotation with a normal disc, the instantaneous axes of rotation were found in a relatively concentrated area.[70] However, in the presence of disc degeneration there was a distinct tendency for the axes to be spread out, as shown in Figure 2-22. Similar observations were made by Pennal and colleagues using radiographic technique in vivo. This general approach of determining "abnormalities" of IAR to diagnose disc degeneration or other diseases is appealing. However, current measuring techniques in vivo involve such variability and measurement error that any real differences between the normal and the pathologic state would be masked.

Although at present there is no distinct, clinically workable use of IAR, there are some speculations which merit discussion. Theoretically, once measuring techniques are developed it should be possible, in addition to disc degeneration, to recognize clinical instability and changes in the physical properties of the ligamentous structures. In addition, the reliable identification of IAR could be of value in predicting the behavior of the spine motor units in response to different injurious vectors (see Chapter 4). Finally, the instantaneous axis of rotation is significant in determining the efficacy of different constructs of spine fusions (see Chapter 8).

Helical Axes of Motion

The authors are not aware of any studies that have been carried out to determine the helical axis of motion for the lumbar spine.

Functions of Anatomic Elements

The lumbar intervertebral joints are thought to be anatomically designed to limit anterior translation and permit considerable sagittal and frontal plane rotation.[46] The intervertebral joints are

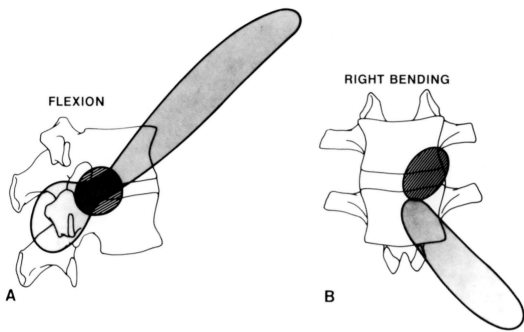

Fig. 2-22. The changes in the location of the instantaneous axes of rotation in lumbar spine motion segment, with and without degenerative disc disease. The axes for the normal discs are shown in the dark areas with longitudinal lines, and those for the degenerated discs are shown in the lighter gray areas. Flexion is represented by *A* and right lateral bending by *B*. Left lateral bending would be represented by a mirror image of *B*. (Based on information from Rolander, S. D.: Motion of the lumbar spine with special reference to the stabilizing effect of posterior fusion [thesis]. Acta Orthop. Scand., *90* [Suppl.], 1966.)

aligned to resist axial rotation. In general, these joints are thought to serve as a guide for the patterns of displacement of the motion segments.[4,56]

COMPARISON OF REGIONAL CHARACTERISTICS AND VARIATIONS

This section includes some generalizations about the characteristic kinematics of the four spinal regions. At the risk of seeming to "second guess" nature and evolution some etiologic considerations about the engineering design of the human spine are discussed.

Anatomic considerations relating to the spine as a whole are important. It is worthwhile to observe, study, and reflect upon regional characteristics and the spatial orientation of the vertebrae in different regions of the spine, especially in relation to clinical biomechanics of the spine.

Much thought and analysis goes into a discussion of the "motion segment." Generally, it is shown with the intervertebral disc parallel to the bottom of the page, and one tends to assume that each motion segment is oriented such that the disc is horizontal. In Figure 2-23, a radiograph in which the subject is standing erect, only a few of the motion segments are parallel or nearly parallel to the horizontal plane. In the normal individual this occurs in the region of C3–4, the middle thoracic region and the middle lumbar region. In other regions, the plane of the intervertebral disc is not parallel to the horizontal plane. Frequent referral to Figure 2-23 may provide valuable spatial orientation for the study of in vivo spine biomechanics.

As the radiographs in Figure 2-23 are studied, it may be useful to review some anatomic factors. In the frontal plane, the spine is straight and symmetrical, with the exception of a slight right

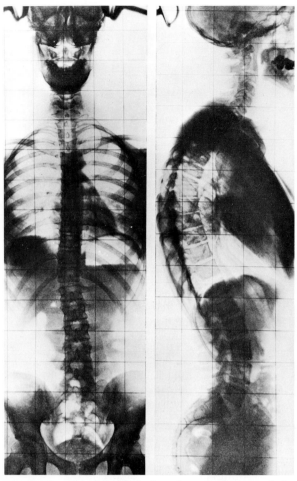

Fig. 2-23. Standing frontal and sagittal view of the entire human spine. This is a valuable picture which is important to study for several reasons: It gives an accurate account of the relative sizes of the vertebrae in different regions of the spine; it shows the spatial relationships of all vertebrae and provides a view of the relative curvatures of different regions in various planes; this picture also allows the viewer to better appreciate the spatial orientation of the facet joints in the standing position; it reminds the viewer that, although motion segments are usually depicted with the disc horizontal, only a few of the motion segments actually have their discs horizontal in a standing position. (Schmorl, G., and Junghanns, H.: The Human Spine in Health and Disease. 2nd English edition. Stuttgart, Georg Thieme Verlag, 1968.)

convex thoracic curve. This may be due to the position of the aorta.[74] Other investigators suggest that it is due to increased use of the right hand.[12,23] The relation of handedness has been supported by the observation of left convex curvature in left-handed individuals.[28]

There are four normal curves in the sagittal plane. They provide increased axial flexibility with stability and augmented shock-absorbing capacity. The curves are convex forward in the cervical and lumbar region, and concave forward in the thoracic and sacral regions. The lumbar curve, quite aesthetically, is slightly more accentuated in the female. The dorsal or the thoracic curve is structural and can be looked upon as the persisting curve of the embryonic axis.[23] This curve is the result of an intravertebral variation in height, the anterior height being less than the posterior height.[29] Its convexity is 20 to 40 degrees. When it exceeds 40 degrees it is considered abnormal.[68] The thoracic curve has been observed to increase with age. Below the age of 40, the female thoracic spine is straighter than that of the male. This difference is not found after 40 years of age, when the dorsal spine of the female becomes as curved as that of the male. The lordosis of the cervical curve is due to the wedge-shaped disc and the greater anterior height of the vertebral body. Note that from C1 to L5 the vertebral bodies increase consistently in volume.[29,74] In the frontal plane the width of the vertebral bodies increases from C2 to L3.[29] In the thoracic spine, the sagittal and frontal diameters are about equal[29] or slightly greater in the saggital plane.[75]

The spatial orientation of the facet joints in the human spine is shown in Figures 2-24 and 1-14. These structures play a significant role in the characteristic regional variations in the kinematics of the human spine.

The representative ranges of motion for all segments in the traditional planes are given in Figure 2-25, which summarizes the basic kinematics and regional variations.

Occipital-Atlanto-Axial Complex

This region contains the most complex, unique, and highly specialized structures. It is the transition zone between the more standard vertebral design and the radically different skull. The three units maintain structural stability and at the same time combine to allow sizable quantities of motion in flexion/extension, lateral bending, and especially axial rotation. In order to protect the vital medullary structures in the area more free space for the spinal cord is present here than anywhere else in the spine (see Fig. 4-10). In addition, an anatomic mechanism for axial rotation has evolved, in which the instantaneous axis of rotation is placed as close as possible to the spinal cord, permitting a large magnitude (47°) of rotation without bony impingement upon the spinal cord. Other than the crucial medullary structures in this area, there is also the unique problem of allowing motion and at the same time achieving and protecting the transport of the vertebral arteries into the calvarium. A large amount of axial rotation is allowed at C1–C2, but there is virtually none between the occiput and C1, where the arteries enter the calvarium. All loads are borne through the occiput and the lateral masses of C1 on to those of C2. These articulations are crucial to structural stability, and without an intervertebral disc both good load bearing and motion are not possible. Consequently, there is very little or no lateral bending at this articulation.

The axis (C2) is also anatomically unique and is certainly a transitional vertebra with its large spinal canal. The axial rotation is much less at C2–3, largely because the yellow ligament that starts at this level is much stiffer and more restricting than the lax atlanto-occipital membrane which lies at the level above. Moreover, the anatomic complex of the dens and the transverse apical and alar ligaments are designed to allow significantly more axial rotation than would be expected of the intervertebral disc and the facet joint.

Lower Cervical Spine (C2–C7)

The second cervical vertebra is also part of the lower cervical spine. In this region stability and mobility must be provided, and at the same time the vital spinal cord and, in most of this region, the vertebral arteries must be protected. There is a good deal flexion/extension and lateral bending in this area. This region has at least one distinct characteristic coupling pattern, in which lateral bending and axial rotation are coupled such that the spinous processes point in the opposite direction to that in which lateral bending takes place. Arkin put forth an interesting hypothesis that

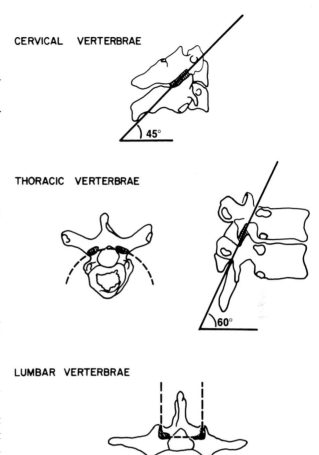

Fig. 2-24. Characteristic facet orientation in the cervical, thoracic and lumbar regions. The spatial alignment of the facet joints determines, to a large extent though not completely, the characteristic kinematics of different regions of the spine.

coupling is due to the mechanics related to soft-tissue tensions.[3] However, the spatial orientation of the facet joints is a more plausible explanation, illustrated in Figure 2-24. Because these joints are oriented at about a 45-degree angle to the vertical, in the sagittal plane the lateral bending results in axial rotation. During lateral bending to the left, as the left facet of the upper vertebra moves down the 45-degree incline to the left, it is also displaced somewhat posteriorly. As the facet on the right moves up the 45-degree incline on the right, it is displaced somewhat anteriorly.

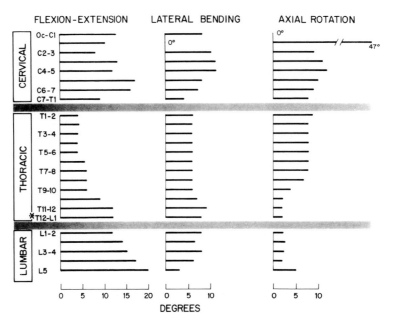

Fig. 2-25 This is a composite of the representative values for rotation at the different levels of the spine in the traditional planes of motion. It is designed to allow a ready comparison of the motion in the various regions of the spine, as well as the different types of movement in each region. The figures for the T12–L1 interspace are derived from interpolations. (White, A. A., III, and Panjabi, M. M.: The basic kinematics of the human spine. A review of past and current knowledge. Spine, 3:12, 1978.)

The total effect is an axial rotation, such that the spinous process points to the right (+y-axis rotation).

Thoracic Spine

The thoracic spine is a transitional region between the relatively more mobile cervical and lumbar regions. It is thought to be designed for rigidity, vital for general, erect bipedal support and protection of the cord as well as the other organs in the thoracic cavity, and to facilitate the mechanical activities of the lungs and rib cage.

First, consider the anatomic and kinematic factors. The upper thoracic spine is similar to the cervical region, and the lower thoracic spine is similar to the lumbar region. The upper thoracic vertebrae are relatively small, similar to those in the cervical region. The spatial orientation of the facet joints is somewhat similar to those of the cervical spine, but the angulation in the sagittal plane is a good deal more (Fig. 2-24). The spatial orientation of the facets in the thoracic spine changes from the upper to the lower region.[13,75]

In a given individual, the spatial orientation of the facet joints may change abruptly to that of the lumbar region anywhere between T9 and T12.[29,69] In the lower thoracic spine the vertebral bodies are larger and the discs are larger.

In regard to kinematic changes, the upper thoracic spine exhibits more axial rotation than the lower thoracic spine. Axial rotation in the cervical spine is ample, but in the lumbar spine there is relatively little (Fig. 2-25). The lower portion of the thoracic spine, unlike the upper portion, is capable of ample flexion/extension, a motion which is sufficient and gradually increasing in the lumbar spine. The coupling characteristic of the cervical spine is clearly present in the upper portion of the thoracic spine. However, it becomes weaker or changes in the middle and lower portion of the thoracic spine.

Lumbar Spine

The most unique characteristic of this area is that it must bear tremendous loads. This is due to the large, superimposed body weight which interacts with additional forces generated by lifting and other activities that involve powerful muscle forces. In addition, the lumbar spine in conjunction with the hips is responsible for the mobility of the trunk. Together these impose formidable mechanical demands on the region, and it is not surprising that the lumbar spine may not always be capable of meeting them.

The anatomic location of the fifth lumbar vertebra and the unique spatial orientation of its facet articulation with the sacrum qualifies it as a transitional vertebra. The ample flexion extension may be attributed to the sizable intervertebral disc, and the ample axial rotation is no doubt associated with the facet joint orientation.

There is an interesting coupling pattern in the lumbar spine, which is the opposite of a salient pattern in the cervical and upper thoracic spine. In the cervical and upper thoracic regions, with lateral bending the spinous processes move toward the convexity of the curve. However, in the lumbar region, the spinous processes move toward the concavity of the curve.

AGE, SEX, AND SPINE KINEMATICS

Many observations have been made with regard to the decreased mobility of the spine associated with aging. It is not clear whether this is an independent variable, having to do with the spontaneous changes in the mechanical properties of the tissues, or whether it is related to changes that occur as a result of inactivity (using spinal mobility less).

Penning states that cervical spine motion decreases with age.[64] Moll and Wright carried out measurements of thoracolumbar spine motion in 237 normals, 119 males and 118 females. Their results showed an increase in spinal mobility between the decades of 15 to 24 and 25 to 34, followed by a progressive decrease with advancing age. They also found an interesting sex difference related to spine kinematics. Male mobility exceeded female mobility in the sagittal plane during flexion/extension, whereas during lateral flexion, the converse was true.[55] These findings may challenge the imagination of even the most prudish sexologist.

Galante noted that after age 35 there was no significant change in the tensile *properties* of the lumbar annulus fibrosis as a function of aging.[25] Tanz, in studies of the lumbar spine, observed a significant motion loss between childhood and adolescence or young adulthood, but he found that the motion loss after age 35 was not significant.[77] This observation is better explained by *intrinsic* tissue changes than by disuse of the full range of motion.

Although the number of women included in his study group was small, Allbrook did not find any sex difference in the range of lumbar spine motion in his study of live subjects. He did, however, note a decreasing range of flexibility with age. This study also showed that there was less movement in the presence of osteophytes at the interspace.[1] Evans and Lissner studied a group of 11 specimens of lumbar spines and pelves and found no apparent relationship between the age of the individuals and the biomechanical properties that effect kinematics.[17]

DISEASE AND SPINE KINEMATICS

One of the primary reasons for studying spine kinematics is to identify and study any changes that may occur in relation to disease.

Reports have suggested that variations in mobility associated with a given interspace is indicative of pathologic changes. A bibliography of these studies is available in the work of Pennal and colleagues.[63]

Increased sagittal plane translation may be an early sign of disc degeneration.[31] Some investigators have not agreed with this observation. Hirsch and Lewin studied the lumbosacral joint and found that disc degeneration did not effect the range of motion of the L5 facet in relation to the sacrum.[35] Rolander showed that there is generally only 1 to 2 mm of translation in the frontal or sagittal axes. These in vitro studies involved direct measurements and observations on the discs. Rolander found no increased translation with degenerative discs.[70]

Mensor and Duvall studied the motion of the lumbosacral joint in 527 consecutive patients in their office. This was done with lateral radiographs in full flexion/extension with the subject sitting. The motion was measured by superimposing the two films and meauring changes in the angle at the lumbosacral junction. The findings were compared with a control group of 94 healthy individuals. Although there is not a statistical analysis, the authors observed that while only 15 per cent of the normal control group showed absence of mobility, 43 per cent of the patients with low back pain from a variety of diseases had no motion of L4 and L5.[53]

Jirout and Tanz have noted that 11 and 20 per cent of normals (individuals without back pain) have restriction of spinal movement at the L4–5 and L5–S1 interspaces, respectively.[42,77] Tanz observed no differences in lumbar motion between normals and those with a history of low back pain. Howes and Isdale reported greater joint mobility in women patients with no specific back pain.[38] However, Sweetman and colleagues found no relationship between sagittal mobility of the lumbosacral spine and past history of low back pain in a study of 500 postmen.[76]

Some hypotheses suggest an increase in motion associated with disease; others propose a decrease. Generally, this type of approach to analysis of disease has not been used, for several reasons. First of all, there is a considerable normal variation. In addition, the measuring techniques in most studies have been cumbersome and of questionable reliability.

A large number of studies have employed a variety of devices, techniques, and methods in an attempt to develop a useful measure of various segments of the spine in order to distinguish between health and disease. None of these appear to be practicable techniques. A description of various methods follows.

In 1924 Cyriax described a torsionometer designed to measure lateral curvature in the lumbodorsal region.[10] Since that time a number of techniques have been proposed. These include a photographic technique,[32] spondylometers,[14,27,33] inclinometers,[79] skin measurements,[52,80] and recently a combined skin and pendulum method.[55] Finally, there is the combined flexirule/hydrogomometer.[2] This device combines two methods and gives a record of the curvature of the lumbar spine, as well as a numerical figure which represents the mobility of the segments measured. None of these seem to have achieved widespread clinical usage. This type of gross measurement of motion has been used to follow patients with ankylosing spondylitis,[33,52] but has not been helpful in evaluating or predicting low back pain.[76]

CLINICAL BIOMECHANICS

A knowledge of basic normal kinematics of the spine is crucial to the understanding of the pathology, clinical interpretation, and treatment of a large majority of spine disorders.

Accurate description and communication of this knowledge requires certain terms, definitions, and conventions.

Because there is no axial rotation between the occiput and C1, it is possible to obtain a truly lateral radiograph of C1 by positioning the film parallel to the lateral aspect of the skull.

There is a large amount (47°) of axial rotation possible at the C1 = C2 articulation. If there is compromise of the flow of the vertebral artery, symptoms of basilar insufficiency may result. Stretching and narrowing of the artery due to axial rotation between C1 and C2 may cause this.

The kinematics of this extremely complex articulation must be carefully studied in order to understand rotary subluxation between C1 and C2. The two key points here are to appreciate that normal axial rotation on an anteroposterior radiograph gives the appearance of abnormal frontal plane motion of C1 in relation to C2, and that true rotary subluxation and dislocation is manifested by an abnormal separation between the dens and the anterior ring of C1 on a true lateral radiograph of C1.

The large amount of motion in the C5–6 area of the cervical spine, especially in the sagittal plane, may be related to the higher incidence of cervical spondylosis there. Studies of the maximum range of sagittal translation ($\pm$z-axis) in the cervical spine are helpful in the interpretation of radiographs for clinical instability. The observed maximum is 2.7 mm. With radiographic magnification, the suggested upper limits of normal are 3.5 mm.

In the cervical spine there is a strong pattern of coupling, such that axial rotation is associated with lateral bending. When bending to the left the spinous processes point to the right. This fact is important in the analysis of mechanisms of injury in the cervical spine.

There is no grossly abnormal motion in the cervical spine under "physiologic loads" as long as either all the anterior elements or all the posterior elements are intact.

The coupling characteristics in the middle and lower portion of the thoracic spine may have some significance in the pathologic biomechanics that lead to scoliosis. In some instances the coupling pattern has an axial rotation associated with lateral bending, which is the same as that seen in the deformity of scoliosis.

In the lumbar region a good deal of attention has been directed to the possibility that in some states either the range of motion or the pattern of distribution of the instantaneous axes of rotation is altered by disease processes. This is not true for the range of motion. Well presented documentation of in vitro changes in the instantaneous axes of rotation associated with disease has not resulted in widespread clinical usage.

Analysis and comparison of the characteristic kinematics in different anatomic regions of the spine is helpful in the analysis and evaluation of spine trauma. The hypermobility of the cervical spine has been implicated in whiplash and related problems. The less mobile thoracic spine, with the abrupt transition between it and the lumbar spine has important mechanical influences in the fracture patterns in these regions with regard to axial rotation and general mobility.

Larger segments of the spine and the entire spine have been studied extensively to determine the effects of age and sex on mobility. There is generally a decrease in motion with advancing age, but there is not a uniformity of opinion concerning this issue.

Except in patients with ankylosing spondylosis, the clinical measurements of mobility of large segments of the spine have not been particularly useful.

NOTES

[A] The problem of determining the instantaneous axis of rotation and the angle of rotation for a certain rigid body undergoing plane motion may be solved by several different methods. A simple graphical method is described here. In Figure 2-3, a telephone is drawn in position 1, and the two translation vectors, A_1A_2 and B_1B_2, are graphed for the two points A and B. Next, the perpendicular bisectors to the two translation vectors are constructed. The intersection of the two bisectors is point C. Lastly, lines A_1C and A_2C are drawn, and the angle between them is called θ.

If the telephone were simply rotated about point C, through an angle equal to θ degrees, the point A_1 is displaced to A_2, and similarly the point B_1 to B_2. Thus, a pure rotation about the point C has displaced the telephone from position 1 to position 2. We call the point C the instantaneous axis of rotation of this body motion, and θ is the angle of rotation.

Since the motion discussed takes place in a plane, and the instantaneous axis of rotation is a line, it has a point of intersection with this plane. This point of intersection is called the center of motion and is synonymous with the instantaneous axis of rotation.

[B] The state of the science of spine kinematics is really in a rather curious situation in regard to the instantaneous axes of rotation and helical axes of motion. The strict concept of IAR is really applicable only to motion that is limited to one plane. We know that vertebral segment motion is rarely uniplanar. Nevertheless, it has been studied that way for several reasons: the anatomic tradition of describing motion in three planes, flexion/extension, lateral bending, and axial rotation; the use of radiography which provides only uniplanar analysis of complex motion; the clinical tradition of thinking of the motion in terms of rotation in three perpendicular planes. Thus, when we speak of IAR, we are generally talking of a complex motion and studying it in a simplified uniplanar view.

On the other hand, the helical axis of motion may be used to precisely describe the three-dimensional movement of one vertebra in relation to its subadjacent fellow. However, at present, this is of virtually no practical importance because the information is not available, nor is the clinical setting such that it would be accepted and utilized at the present time.

[C] Although the top angle is a satisfactory term, the radius of curvature may be a preferable method of indicating and quantitating a curve or arch. Radius of curvature is described in the Appendix:Glossary.

[D] Even studies from which instantaneous axes of rotation have been calculated have varied considerably in principle and technique. Here is a review of some of the salient considerations.

A given instantaneous axis of rotation depends upon the structure as well as the type of loading. In other words, it is not sufficient to say that, for example, vertebra T3 has an instantaneous axis of rotation, with respect to its subadjacent fellow, located 3 mm anteriorly and 23 mm caudal to the anatomic center of its body. Although it is a precise physical location, it is not sufficient. In addition, we must also specify the type of loading, which in itself is an ambiguous term. Let us take for example, flexion loading. Although everyone understands what is meant by flexion (i.e., forward bending), when it comes to simulating this loading in cadaver experiments, different researchers use different types of loading. Figure 2-14 shows some versions of flexion loading. A compressive force placed anteriorly was used by Rolander[70] when he studied the lumbar spine and White,[82] who studied the thoracic spine. Flexion can also be created by applying a moment about a horizontal axis as shown in Figure 2-14. This method was used by Markolf. Figure 2-14 also shows a method in which a horizontal force is applied to the center of the vertebral body and directed forward. This method was used by Panjabi and colleagues.[60] Another type of loading has been used by Lysell[51] and White[85] in experiments where multiple segments are employed with the lowest vertebra fixed. A transverse load is applied to the top vertebra to produce flexion. In this type of loading, all intermediate vertebrae are subjected to varying amounts of load. The top vertebra is loaded through a pure transverse force. All intermediate vertebrae are loaded with a combination of the transverse force, which is the same at all levels, and bending moments, which are increasing in magnitude in a cephalocaudad direction. Since the instantaneous axis of rotation is a function of the type of load applied, it is clear that for the load depicted in Figure 2-14 the instantaneous axis of rotation calculated for each vertebra is going to vary because of the different combinations of force and moment at different levels. This concept applies equally to extension and lateral bending. With these loading considerations in mind, one should be quite circumspect in comparing results when there are such crucial differences in experimental techniques. Studies of the instantaneous axes of rotation in axial rotation have been treated more consistently by various investigators. However, it has been documented that axial rotation and lateral bending are coupled and are part of three-dimensional motion. Therefore, such a motion does not have an instantaneous axis of rotation but, instead, a helical axis of motion.

^E Other things being equal, rotatory motion can be expected to vary directly with the height of the disc, with the disc material, and with the fourth power of the disc diameter, and inversely with its stiffness. In lateral bending the disc height is therefore relatively less important than it was in the case of flexion/extension.

For the moment, disregarding the effect of the posterior elements and representing a motion segment by two rigid bodies connected by a cylindrical disc (Fig. 2-16), the following trends can be projected for the motion as a function of the height, diameter, and material of the disc. According to the simple engineering theory of strength of materials, the rotation θ produced by application of a bending moment M (flexion/extension, and lateral bending) is

$$\theta = \frac{64M}{\pi}\frac{H}{ED^4}$$

where H = the disc height
   D = the diameter
   E = the modulus of elasticity of the disc material
   π = 3.14

This formula represents axial rotation θ produced by the axial moment (torque) M if G replaces E (G = the modulus of shear of the disc material) and 32 replaces 64.

^F If the reader examines the study by White,[82] note that the coordinate system in the experimental investigation is not the same as the system used here.

CLASSIFICATION OF REFERENCES

Anatomy 12, 19, 23, 28, 29, 34, 40, 65, 69
   Occipital-atlanto-axial 39, 81
   Lower cervical 8, 15, 24
   Thoracic 13

Basic biomechanics 3, 16, 49, 57, 71, 75, 85
   Occipital-atlanto-axial 11, 72
   Lower cervical 5, 51
   Thoracic 30, 58, 59, 82
   Lumbar 9, 17, 18, 25, 30, 50, 56, 60, 70
Clinical biomechanics 10, 14, 20, 27, 33, 38, 45, 47, 48, 52, 55, 64, 67, 68, 74, 78
   Occipital-atlanto-axial 36, 37, 73
   Lower cervical 21, 43, 44, 84
   Lumbar 1, 2, 26, 31, 35, 42, 54, 63, 66, 76, 77, 79, 80, 86
Clinical topics 7, 32
   Occipital-atlanto-axial 6, 22, 41, 62
   Lower cervical 85
   Lumbar 4, 46, 53

REFERENCES

1. Allbrook, D.: Movements of the lumbar spinal column. J. Bone Joint Surg., *39B*:339, 1957.
2. Anderson, J. A. D., and Sweetman, B. J.: A combined flexi-rule/hydrogomometer for measurement of lumbar spine and its sagittal movement. Rheum. Rehab., *74:* 173, 1975.
3. Arkin, A. M.: The mechanism of rotation in combination with lateral deviation in the normal spine. J. Bone Joint Surg., *32A*:180, 1950.
4. Armstrong, J. R.: Lumbar Disc Lesions. Edinburgh, E. & S. Livingstone, 1958.
5. Ball, J., and Meijers, K. A. E.: On cervical mobility. Ann. Rheum. Dis., *23*:429, 1964.
6. Barton, J. W., and Margolis, M. T.: Rotational obstruction of the vertebral artery at the atlantoaxial joint. Neuroradiology, *9*:117, 1975.
7. Calve, J., and Galland, M.: Physiologie Pathologique Du Mal De Pott. Rev. Orthop., *1:*5, 1930.
8. Compere, E. L., Tachdjian, M. D., and Kernakan, W. T.: The Luska joints—their anatomy, physiology and pathology. Orthopedics, *1:*159, 1958/59.
9. Cossette, J. W., Farfan, H. F., Robertson, G. H., and Wells, R. V.: The instantaneous center of rotation of the third lumbar intervertebral joint. J. Biomech., *4:*149, 1971. (*An important and well done study of the IAR for axial rotation in this region.*)
10. Cyriax, E. F.: An apparatus for estimating the degree of rotation of the spinal column. Lancet, p. 1024, 1924. (*This work is of historical interest.*)
11. Dankmeijer, J., and Rethmeier, B. J.: Lateral movement in the atlanto-axial joints and its clinical significance. Acta Radiol., *24*:55, 1943. (*An in vivo and in vitro radiographic study of lateral movement only.*)
12. Davis, G. G.: Applied Anatomy. ed. 5. Philadelphia, J. B. Lippincott, 1918.
13. Davis, P. R.: The medial inclination of the human thoracic intervertebral articular facets. J. Anat., *93:*68, 1959.
14. Dunham, W. F.: Ankylosing spondylitis. Measurement of hip and spine movements. Br. J. Physiol. Med., September–October, 1949.
15. Eklin, U.: Die Alterveranderumgen der Halswirbelsaule. Berlin, Springer-Verlag, 1960.
16. Elward, J. F.: Motion in the vertebral column. J. Roentgenol., *42*:91, 1939. (*This work is primarily of historical interest.*)
17. Evans, F. G., and Lissner, M. S.: Biomechanical studies

on the lumbar spine and pelvis. J. Bone Joint Surg., 41A:278, 1959. (*A detailed study of flexibility and motion of multiple groups of motion segments in the lumbar spine.*)

18. Farfan, H. F.: Muscular mechanism of the lumbar spine and the position of power and efficiency. Orthop. Clin. North Am., 6:135, 1975.

19. Fick, R.: Handbuch der Anatomie und Mechanik der Gelenke. Jena, S. Fischer Verlag, 1904, 1911.

20. Fielding, J. W.: Cineroentgenography of the normal cervical spine. J. Bone Joint Surg., 39A:1280, 1957.

21. ———: Normal and selected abnormal motion of the cervical spine from the second cervical vertebra to the seventh cervical vertebra based on cineroentgenography. J. Bone Joint Surg., 46A:1779, 1964. (*Some basic characteristics of cervical spine kinematics demonstrated well and documented in vivo.*)

22. Fielding, J. W., and Hawkins, R. J.: Spine fusion for atlanto-axial instability J. Bone Joint Surg., 58A:400, 1976.

23. Frazier, J. E.: The Anatomy of the Human Skeleton. ed. 4. London, J. & A. Churchill, 1940.

24. Frykholm, R.: Lower cervical vertebrae and intervertebral discs. Surgical anatomy and pathology. Acta Chir. Scand., 101:345, 1951.

25. Galante, J. O.: Tensile properties of the human lumbar annulus fibrosis [thesis]. Acta Orthop. Scand., 100 [Suppl.], 1967.

26. Gianturco, C.: A roentgen analysis of the motion of the lower lumbar vertebrae in normal individuals and in patients with low back pain. Am. J. Roentgenol., 52:261, 1944. (*This work is of historical interest.*)

27. Goff, D., and Rose, G. K.: The use of a modified spondylometer in the treatment of ankylosing spondylitis. Rheumatology, 20:63, 1964.

28. Gray, H.: Anatomy of the Human Body. ed. 23. Lewis, W. H. [ed.]. Philadelphia, Lea & Febiger, 1936.

29. ———: Descriptive and Applied Anatomy, ed. 34, Davies, D. V. [ed.]. London, Longmans, Green & Co., 1967.

30. Gregersen, G. G., and Lucas, D. B.: An in vivo study of the axial rotation of the human thoracolumbar spine. J. Bone Joint Surg., 49A:247, 1967. (*A very important study showing the functional kinematics of the spine.*)

31. Hagelstam, L.: Retroposition of lumbar vertebra. Acta Chir. Scand., 143 [Suppl.], 1949. (*An important study of lumbar spine kinematics.*)

32. Hart, F. D., Robinson, K. C., Allchin, F. B., and Maclagan, N. F.: Ankylosing spondylitis. J. Med., 18:217, 1949.

33. Hart, F. D., Strickland, D., and Cliffe, P.: Measurement of spinal mobility. Ann Rheum. Dis., 33:136, 1974.

34. Henke, W.: Handbuch der Anatomie and Mechanik der Gelenke. Leipszig und Heidelberg, 1863.

35. Hirsch, C., and Lewin, T.: Lumbosacral synovial joints in flexion-extension. Acta Orthop. Scand., 39:303, 1968.

36. Hohl, M.: Normal motion in the upper portion of the cervical spine. J. Bone Joint Surg., 46A:1777, 1964.

37. Hohl, M., and Baker, H. R.: The atlanto-axial joint. J. Bone Joint Surg., 46A:1739, 1964. (*A milestone study which touches upon the crucial clinical kinematic problems of this area.*)

38. Howes, R. G., and Isdale, I. C.: The loose back: an unrecognized syndrome. Rheumatol. Phys. Med., 11:72, 1971.

39. Hultkrantz, J. W.: Zur Meehanik der Kopfbewegungen beim Menschen. Kurgl. Sv. Vet. Akad. Handl. Bd. 49, nr. 8, Stockholm, 1912.

40. Humphrey, G. M.: A Treatise on the Human Skeleton. London, Macmillan, 1958.

41. Jackson, H.: The diagnosis of minimal atlanto-axial subluxation. Br. J. Radiol., 23:672, 1950.

42. Jirout, J.: The normal mobility of the lumbo-sacral spine. Acta Radiol., 47:345, 1957.

43. ———: The mobility of the cervical vertebrae in lateral flexion of the head and neck. Acta Radiol., 13:919, 1972.

44. Jones, M. D.: Cineradiographic studies of the normal cervical spine. Calif. Med., 93:293, 1960.

45. Keller, H. A.: A clinical study of the mobility of the human spine, its extent and its clinical importance. Arch. Surg., 8:627, 1924.

46. Lewin, T.: Osteoarthritis in lumbar synovial joints. A morphological study. Acta Orthop. Scand., 73 [Suppl.], 1964.

47. Loebl, W. Y.: Measurement of spinal posture and range of spinal movement. Ann. Phys. Med., 9:103, 1967.

48. Lovett, R. W.: Lateral Curvature of the Spine and Round Shoulders. Philadelphia, Blakiston & Sons, 1967. (*A classic article describing one of the best early studies of spine kinematics.*)

49. Lucas, D. B., and Bresler, B.: Stability of the ligamentous spine. Biomechanics Laboratory, Univ. Calif., San Francisco and Berkley. Technical Report. Ser. 11, Re. 40, 1961.

50. Lumsden, R. M., and Morris, J. M.: An in vivo study of axial rotation and immobilization at the lumbosacral joint. J. Bone Joint Surg., 50A:1591, 1968. (*One of the major in vivo studies of spine kinematics.*)

51. Lysell, E.: Motion in the cervical spine. Acta Orthop. Scand., 123 [Suppl.], 1969. (*The most exhaustive and carefully done study of the kinematics of the lower cervical spine.*)

52. Macrae, I. F., and Wright, V.: Measurement of back movement. Ann. Rheum. Dis., 28:584, 1969. (*One of the better studies of the movement of large segments of the spine.*)

53. Mensor, M. C., and Duvall, G.: Absence of motion at the fourth and fifth lumbar interspaces in patients with and without low-back pain. J. Bone Joint Surg., 41A:1047, 1959. (*A thorough and well presented analysis of a large amount of clinical and radiological data.*)

54. Miles, M., and Sullivan, W. E.: Lateral bending at the lumbar and lumbosacral joints. Anat. Rec., 139:387, 1961.

55. Moll, J. M. H., and Wright, V.: Normal range of spinal mobility. Ann. Rheum. Dis., 30:381, 1971. (*An excellent study which probably represents the best work in the area of large spine segment mobility per physical examination.*)

56. Nachemson, A.: The influence of spinal movements on the lumbar intradiscal pressure and on the tensile stresses in the annulus fibrosis. Acta Orthop. Scand., 33:183, 1963.

57. Panjabi, M. M., Aversa, J., Conati, F. C., and White, A. A.: Three dimensional motion of the metacarpophalangeal joint: a measuring technique. Orthopaedic Research Society, Vol. 1, January 1976.

58. Panjabi, M. M., Brand, R. A., and White, A. A.: Three dimensional flexibility and stiffness properties of the human thoracic spine. J. Biomech., 9:185, 1976.

59. ———: Mechanical properties of the human thoracic spine as shown by three-dimensional load-displacement curves. J. Bone Joint Surg., 58A:642, 1976.

60. Panjabi, M. M., Krag, M., White, A. A., and Southwick,

W. O.: Effects of preload on load-displacement curves of the lumbar spine. Orthop. Clin. North Am., 8:181, 1977.

61. Panjabi, M. M., White, A. A., and Brand, R. A.: A note on defining body parts configurations. J. Biomech., 7:385, 1974.

62. Paul, L. W., and Moir, W. W.: Non-pathological variations in relationship of the upper cervical vertebrae. Am. J. Roentgenol., 62:519, 1949.

63. Pennal, G. F., Conn., G. S., McDonald, G., Dale, G., and Garside, H.: Motion studies of the lumbar spine. A preliminary report. J. Bone Joint Surg., 54B:442, 1972. (*This article discusses a noteworthy radiological technique that could have some clinical significance.*)

64. Penning, L.: Functional pathology of the cervical spine. Amsterdam, Excerpta Medica, 1968.

65. Poirier, P., and Charpy, A.: Traite d'Anatomie Humaine. 1:74, 1926.

66. Reichmann, S., Berglund, E., and Lundgren, K.: Das Bewegungszentrum in der Lendenwirbelsaule bei Flexion und Extension. Z. Anat. Entwicklungsgesch, 138:283, 1972.

67. Roaf, R.: Rotation movements of the spine with special reference to scoliosis. J. Bone Joint Surg., 40B:312, 1958.

68. ———: Vertebral growth and its mechanical control. J. Bone Joint Surg., 42B:40, 1960.

69. Rockwell, H., Evans, F. G., and Pheasant, H. C.: The comparative morphology of the vertebral spinal column; its form as related to function. J. Morphol., 63:87, 1938.

70. Rolander, S. D.: Motion of the lumbar spine with special reference to the stabilizing effect of posterior fusion [thesis]. Acta Orthop. Scand., 99 [Suppl.], 1966. (*An exhaustive bibliography on the lumbar spine and a very meticulous study of kinetics and kinematics.*)

71. Schulthess, W.: Uber die lehre des zusammenhanges der physiologischen torsion der wirbelsaule mit lateraler biegung und ihre beziehungen zur skoliose unter berucksichtigung der lovettschen experimente. Z. Orthop. Chir., 10:455, 1902.

72. Selecki, B. R.: The effects of rotation of the atlas on the axis: experimental work. Med. J. Aust., 1:1012, 1969.

73. Shapiro, R., Youngberg, A. S., and Rothman, S. L. G.: The differencial diagnosis of traumatic lesions of the occipito-atlanto-axial segment. Radiol. Clin. North Am., 11:505, 1973. (*Highly recommended as the best overview of the clinical radiological problems related to this region.*)

74. Steindler, A.: Kinesiology of the Human Body. Springfield, Ill., Charles C Thomas, 1955.

75. Strasser, H.: Lehrbuch der Muskel und Gelenkmechanik. *Vol. 2.* Berlin, Springer-Verlag, 1913.

76. Sweetman, B. J., Anderson, J. A. D., and Dalton, E. R.: The relationship between little-finger mobility, lumbar mobility, straight-leg raising and low-back pain. Rheum. Rehab., 13:161, 1974.

77. Tanz, S. S.: Motion of the lumbar spine. A roentgenologic study. J. Roentgenol., 69:399, 1953. (*An important and well done radiographic study of the lumbar spine.*)

78. Thomas, D.: A spondylometer: apparatus developed under Dr. R. Harris, Buxton. Physiotherapy, 42:113, 1956.

79. Troup, J. D. G., Hood, C. A., and Chapman, A. E.: Measurements of the sagittal mobility of the lumbar spine and hips. Ann. Phys. Med., 9:308, 1968.

80. Van Adrichem, J. A. M., and Van der Korst, J. K.: Assessment of the flexibility of the lumbar spine. Scand. J. Rheumatol., 2:87, 1973.

81. Werne, S.: Studies in spontaneous atlas dislocation. Acta Orthop. Scand., 23 [Suppl.], 1957. (*A thorough and careful study of the function of the C1-C2 complex, which includes some interesting mechanical models and theoretical concepts. It is the most detailed study of this area.*)

82. White, A. A.: Analysis of the mechanics of the thoracic spine in man [thesis]. Acta Orthop. Scand., 127 [Suppl.], 1969.

83. White, A. A., Johnson, R. M., Panjabi, M. M., and Southwick, W. O.: Biomechanical analysis of clinical stability in the cervical spine. Clin. Orthop., 109:85, 1975.

84. White, A. A., Panjabi, M. M., and Brand, R. A.: A system for defining position and motion of the human body parts. Med. Biol. Eng., 13:261, 1975.

85. White, A. A., Southwick, W. O., DePonte, R. J., Gainor, J. W., and Hardy, R.: Relief of pain by anterior cervical spine fusion for spondylosis. A report of 65 patients. J. Bone Joint Surg., 55A:525, 1973.

86. Wiles, P.: Movements of the lumbar vertebrae during flexion and extension. Proceeding of the Royal Society of Medicine, 28:647, 1935.

3 Practical Biomechanics of Scoliosis

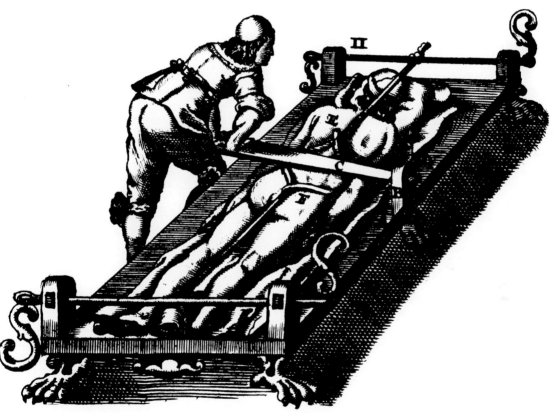

Fig. 3-1. This illustration, taken from Scultetus' The Surgeons Store-House, shows that "biomechanics" has been involved in the correction of spine deformities for several centuries. (Scultetus: The Surgeons Store-House. p. 63, London. Printed for Starken at The Miter on Fleet Street, near Temple Bar, 1674. Courtesy of Yale Medical Library.)

ANATOMIC CONSIDERATIONS

Normal Curves. In the frontal plane the normal spine appears straight and symmetrical, with the exception of a very slight right thoracic curve. This may be due to the position of the aorta.[37]

Other investigators suggest that it is due to increased use of the right hand.[7,13]

The Facets. Humphry pointed out that movements in the spine are possible mainly due to the shape and position of the articulating processes of the diarthrodial joints.[19] It is the orientation and position of these joints in space that influence the mechanics of the spine (see Figs. 1-14, 2-24). This is important to keep in mind when the phenomenon of coupling is considered. In the thoracic spine the superior facet is almost flat and directed backward, a little laterally, and upward. The inferior facet is directed forward, slightly downward, and medially.[16] The orientation of the facets in the thoracic spine may be related to the irregular pattern of coupling found in this region. The significance of this is discussed on page 97.

The Ligaments.   Little is known about the physical properties and activity of the ligaments in scoliosis. Walters and Morris carried out in vitro studies to compare mechanical properties of the interspinous ligaments in subjects with idiopathic scoliosis to those with scoliosis of known cause. No differences were observed.[41]

Nordwall compared mechanical properties of interspinous ligaments and tendons of the erector spinae muscles in patients with idiopathic scoliosis, patients with scoliosis of known cause, and patients with spondylolisthesis only. No significant differences were found.[28]

A good deal has been written concerning the mechanical importance of the ligamenta flava. Rolander credited them with a major role in restricting or dictating the kinematics of normal motion.[35] The following considerations involving the yellow ligaments may have clinical relevance to scoliosis. The yellow ligaments and facets have been shown experimentally to limit the amount of axial rotation in the normal thoracic spine.[44] Also, hemilaminectomy, which releases "check rein" force of yellow ligaments, can result in experimental scoliosis.[26]

NORMAL KINEMATICS

. . . It is as if one undertook, for example, to investigate a railroad accident solely from a study of the wrecked cars. Much could be learned as to the effect and direction of the destructive forces the amount of force expended, and the kind of damage done, but more could be learned and future accidents could be better prevented by a study of the normal running time of the trains, their proper relation to each other at the time of the accident, and by an investigation of the signal system and the routine precautions adopted. (Lovett, *In* The Mechanics of the Normal Spine in Relation to Scoliosis, 1905.)

Lovett termed his study "mechanics." This discussion focuses primarily on the kinematics of the thoracic spine. *Kinematics* is defined in Chapter 2.

Kinematics of the thoracic spine has been studied using two well developed experimental methods. One method analyzed motion segments by applying known forces and measuring displacement with electrical recording devices. This technique provided two-dimensional analysis. Controlled studies were made using this technique to compare the motion with and without the posterior vertebral elements. A detailed account of this experimental method is available in the literature.[44] The other method employed steel balls as markers and analyzed larger segments of the spine. Radiographs were taken of the vertebrae at different points in the characteristic ranges of motion. From this experiment it was possible to calculate precise three-dimensional kinematics of the spine. A detailed explanation of this technique may be found in a thesis by Lysell.[23]

Degrees of Freedom.   This concept, which is basic to the understanding of kinematics, is defined in Chapter 2. A vertebra in motion thus has six degrees of freedom for its movement. It may translate along or rotate about any of the three axes (Fig. 3-2). Until recent years for clinical and experimental purposes the motion has been measured in only two dimensions. The tendency has been to describe this motion in each of the three traditional planes, frontal, sagittal, and horizontal. Most analyses have dealt with only those components of the translation or rotation vectors that lie in one of these planes. This has been done most often with radiologic studies, taking into consideration only the rotary components. Such an analysis betrays an accurate description, as there is almost always an element of translation along with rotation. Moreover, various motions occur in planes other than the traditional anatomic planes. This oversimplification is present in clinical measurements of the relative positions of the vertebrae in scoliosis; the deformity and the measurements are depicted in the single plane of radiographic film.

Coupling. This is applied to motion in which rotation or translation about or along one axis is consistently associated with rotation or translation about or along a second axis. Some interesting questions concerning this phenomenon in the normal and scoliotic spine follow.

In the cervical spine and the upper portion of the thoracic spine, there is a relatively marked and consistent coupling of *axial rotation with lateral bending.* The direction of coupling is such that axial rotation of the vertebral body causes its anterior aspect to point toward the concavity of the lateral bending curve. In other words, the spinous processes point more to the convexity of the physiologic curve.[A] In the middle and also in the lower regions of the thoracic spine, this same pattern is still present and probably predominant. However, in these areas it is not as marked, nor is it consistently present. Furthermore, the direction of the coupled axial rotation in the middle regions is in some cases the reverse of that of the cervical and upper thoracic spine.[B] These observations relate to some possible etiologic mechanisms (see p. 97).

Posterior Elements. Under controlled conditions the mechanics of the motion segments were studied with and without posterior elements.[44] The removal of these structures resulted in significant increases in the amount of axial rotation. The posterior elements set a limit on axial rotation in the normal spine. Most probably, their release allows for considerably more correction of the abnormal axial rotation in the scoliotic spine. The study implies that yellow ligament transection and release of the facet joint capsules, either through osteotomy or soft-tissue release, facilitates derotation in the scoliotic spine. These considerations become more important as techniques are available to apply a moment about the axial (y) axis to correct the abnormal rotation. Such a procedure is not likely to result in instability, since the spine is fused as part of the surgical treatment of scoliosis. It is of interest to note that other investigators using a computer model of the spine showed that surgical ablation of the intervertebral disc (the anterior elements) significantly reduced the resistance of the spine to correc-

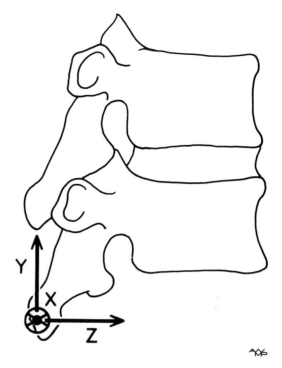

Fig. 3-2. This demonstrates the use of an orthogonal coordinate system on the spinal motion segment in a standard orientation. (White, A. A., III, Panjabi, M. M., and Brand, R. A.: A system for defining position and motion of the human body parts. Medical and Biological Engineering and Computing, p. 261. March, 1975.)

tion.[36a] All of these points are mechanically sound. When or if they should be utilized depends upon surgical judgment and technology.

Helical Axis. A truly three-dimensional analysis involves a description of the motion in terms of the equivalent helical motion of the vertebrae in space. This equivalent helical motion is a superimposition of rotation and translation about and along the same axis, the helical axis of motion. This axis has the same direction as that of the rotation axis (see Fig. 2-4). It is important to include accurate three-dimensional considerations, which allow the relationship of each vertebra to its subadjacent fellow to be precisely defined. Questions regarding scoliotic deformity and correction come to mind. How much displacement is necessary for a normal vertebra to move from its place in a normal curve to its place in a scoliotic curve? And, how much of this displacement is regained after a correction by means of a Milwaukee brace, exercises, or surgery? Since these displacements are three-dimensional, definition in terms of helical motion is advantageous.

BIOMECHANICAL DEFINITION OF SCOLIOSIS

Scoliosis is defined as an appreciable lateral deviation in the normally straight vertical line of the spine. Since the ultimate effect of the disease is an extensive alteration in the mechanical structure of the spine, a biomechanical definition of the disease is necessary: abnormal deformation between and within vertebrae; too much curvature in the frontal plane; too much vertical axis rotation in the wrong direction.

In other words, the relative position of vertebrae in regions of the spinal column is abnormal, and deformation within an individual vertebra is abnormal. There is too much curvature. Instead of a straight spine in the frontal plane (x, y plane) or the subtle, right physiologic curve, there is an exaggerated curvature in the frontal plane. The curves are in the wrong plane. Generous curves in the sagittal plane are normal. (There is normal cervical and lumbar lordosis and thoracic kyphosis.) The axial rotation is in the wrong direction. In scoliosis, there is considerable deformation within a given vertebrae. There may be wide pedicles on one side and a short pedicle on the other. The transverse processes may be asymmetrical in their spacial orientation. The spinous process may be bent and not in the midline. The laminae and the vertebral bodies are asymmetrical (Fig. 3-3).

ETIOLOGIC CONSIDERATIONS

Biomechanical Classification

There is a long list of known causes, conditions, or diseases that are associated with scoliosis. There are several methods of classification. A biomechanical classification is provided here, and may best be appreciated in the following context. The spine remains normal due to the maintenance of a delicate and precarious balance. This balance depends on a precise functional status and dynamic symmetry, the key ele-

ments being the bony structure, the ligaments, the intrinsic neuromuscular mechanics, and, finally, the general balance and symmetry of the body. Scoliosis can result from either gross or subtle disruptions of the delicate balance.

Biomechanical Classification of Scoliosis

Alterations of intrinsic osseous structures
  Abnormalities of material properties of support structure
    Rickets (primary and secondary)
    Osteogenesis imperfecta
    Neurofibromatosis
    Infections or tumors
  Abnormalities of the geometry of the support structure
    Hemivertebrae
    Maldeveloped vertebrae
    Myelomeningocele
    Asymmetrical spina bifida
    Asymmetrical lumbosacral vertebral structure and articulation
    Fractures and dislocations
    Various surgical procedures
  Abnormal regional kinematics
    Congenital unilateral bars
    Partial failures of segmentation
    Asymmetrical sacralization of fifth lumbar vertebra
    Fractures and dislocations
    Surgery
Alterations of intrinsic ligamentous structures
  Marfan's disease
  Mucopolysaccharoidosis
  Myelomeningocele
  Surgery
Alterations in static or dynamic balance
  Neuromuscular static balance
    Polio
    Myelomeningocele
    Syringomyelia
  Neuromuscular dynamic balance
    Cerebral palsy
    Freidreich's ataxia
    Muscular dystrophy
  Postural dynamic balance
    Abnormalities of vestibular apparatus
    Visual disturbances
    Torticollis
    Leg-length discrepancies
  Thoracic static balance
    Rib removal (thoracoplasty); ipsilateral convexity
    Excessive thoracic scarring; contralateral convexity
Congenital scoliosis (deformity intrinsic to body)
  Infantile type
  Sprengel's deformity
  Klippel-Feil syndrome
  Multiple congenital anomalies
Miscellaneous forms of scoliosis
Idiopathic scoliosis

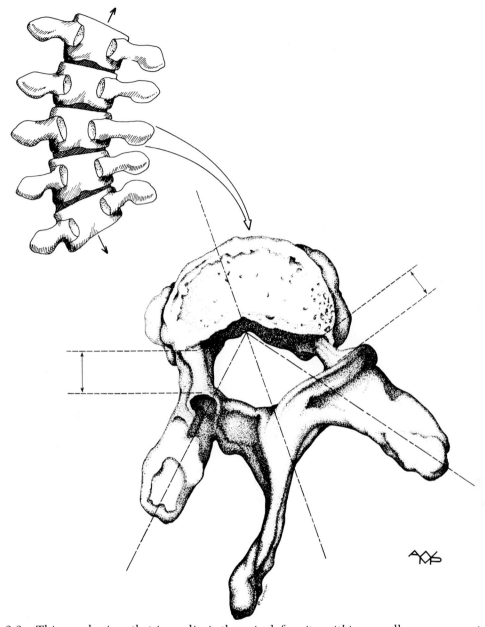

Fig. 3-3. This emphasizes that in scoliosis there is deformity *within* as well as among vertebrae.

The disease entries are not exhaustive for each category. There is also some overlap; a given disease may contribute or be presumed to contribute to the imbalance through more than one mechanism.

Experimental Studies

The cause of 85 to 90 per cent of cases of scoliosis is unknown. Idiopathic scoliosis occurs in an otherwise perfectly healthy child, often associated with a familial history of the disease. Numerous hypothetical, etiologic explanations are offered. From a mechanical point of view, the hypothesis should explain the cause of the abnormal curvatures, the abnormal rotation, and the forces necessary to cause deformation within a vertebra.

One of the major experimental thrusts has

been to establish some imbalance in the neuromuscular and osseous ligamentous structures of the spine in experimental animals, the assumption being that imbalances that result in a scoliotic pattern may be sought as potential etiologic factors in idiopathic scoliosis. This presumes that scoliosis is caused by the weakness or absence of a structure on the convex side of the curve or an overactivity of its antagonist on the concave side. A large number of anatomic elements have been studied in either rabbits or pigs. Table 3-1 is a comprehensive list of various surgical procedures that have produced scoliosis. All operations were unilateral, performed at five levels.

Michelsson listed operations that most consistently induce scoliosis. They were (A) resection of the dorsal ends of the ribs, (B) hemilaminectomy, and (C) transection of the posterior costotransverse ligaments. The factor that is common to both A and B is C. Michelsson suggested that the posterior costotransverse ligaments are crucial in maintaining equilibrium and symmetrical growth in the spine.

When one finds a consistent unilateral alteration resulting in scoliosis, the assumption is that with a growing spine, the initial, functional scoliosis ultimately develops into a structural deformity. This is explained on the basis of what has been traditionally called Heuter Volkman's law. The theory suggests that increased pressure across an epiphyseal growth plate inhibits growth, whereas decreased pressure across the plate tends to accelerate growth. This theory purports that, on the concave side of the curve, the epiphyseal plates have abnormally high pressures that result in decreased growth, whereas on the convex side of the curve the pressures are less, resulting in accelerated growth. These two factors contribute significantly to vertebral asymmetry. Work by Stillwell on monkeys nicely supports this hypothesis.[38]

Two experiments involved the fixation of the spine in a curved position and fixation of the spinous processes of the vertebrae. The first tended to result in occasional scoliosis, and the second resulted in severe scoliosis with lordosis and rotation.

Another etiologic consideration related to mechanics is asymmetrical radiation of the spine,

resulting in curvature due to changes in the epiphyseal growth plates, with either unilateral stimulation or unilateral ablation.

Experimental scoliosis has also been produced by radiologic exposure of the growing spine, induction of lathrysm, oxygen deficiency, unilateral labyrinthine stimulation, and unilateral labyrinthine ablation.[26,32] The very broad variety of experimental variables which have resulted in a "scoliotic" deformity suggests that the maintenance of a normal spine in a growing animal is dependent upon a delicately balanced, easily disrupted equilibrium.

This general experimental approach is questionable, since the goal is to explain idiopathic scoliosis *in man*, an erect, biped organism. The frequency, duration, direction, and magnitude of the loads are significantly different in the pig, dog, rabbit, or mouse. There are obvious differences in the anatomy of the spine in animals. Subtle anatomic factors, such as facet orientation, can significantly alter the mechanics of the spine. Thus, there is yet another limiting factor in the use of animals to study scoliosis in man. Using quadripeds as experimental prototypes is, no doubt, valuable but should be viewed in this perspective.

Etiologic Theories

A review of the salient theories that have a basis in biomechanical principle follows.

Roaf suggests that the basic problem in scoliosis is relative lengthening of the anterior components of the spine compared with the posterior elements.[34] Such a situation in an unyielding anterior musculoskeletal wall of the body results in lateral deviation of the spine and the subsequent development of scoliosis. The theory does not explain why the deviation is so predominantly to the right. Also, there is unconvincing evidence that the muscles of the anterior abdominal wall can not stretch, yield, or accommodate the long anterior elements. Moreover, the muscles are not particularly tense in patients with scoliosis.

MacEwen produced scoliosis experimentally in animals by transection of the dorsal nerve root and suggested that the result may be due to a loss of sensory input.[25] The convexity of the resultant curve was to the side of the disrupted neural

Table 3-1. Michelsson's Experimental Surgical Scolioses*

	RABBITS			PIGS		
OPERATION	NO. OF ANIMALS	FUNCT. SCOLIOSIS	STRUCT. SCOLIOSIS	NO. OF ANIMALS	FUNCT. SCOLIOSIS	STRUCT. SCOLIOSIS
Transection or resection of muscles and/or ligaments						
Transection of the costotransverse ligaments	59	+	±	7	+	+
Transection of the ligaments of the heads of the ribs	38	+	+			
Transection of the ligaments attached to the dorsal ends of the ribs	17	+	+	2	+	+
Transection of the intercostal muscles	9	+	±	3	+	+
Transection of all muscles and ligaments between the transverse processes and between these and the arches in the lumbar spine	8	+	+			
Operations on Nerves						
Transection of the intercostal nerves	13	+	±			
Operations on Bones						
Hemilaninectomy in the thoracic spine	56	+	+	2	±	±
Hemilaminectomy in the thoracic spine	9	+	+			
Transversectomy in the lumbar spine	7	+	±			
Transversectomy in the lumbar spine	2	+	+			
Resection of the heads of the ribs	14	+	+	1	+	+
Provoked epiphysiolysis of the heads of the ribs or transection of the necks of the ribs	16	+	±			
Resection of the dorsal ends of the ribs	125	+	+	25	+	+
Transection of the thoracic wall lateral to the tubercles of the ribs	8	+	+			
Resection of the ribs laterally of their tubercles	25	+	+			

* Modified from Michelsson, J.: The development of spinal deformity in experimental scoliosis. Acta Orthop. Scand., *81* [Suppl.], 1965.
+ Scoliosis usually resulted.
± Persistent structural scoliosis sometimes resulted.

sensory elements. Alexander, Bunch, and Ebbesson showed with histologic staining techniques and examination of the anterior nerve cells that the ablation of the dorsal sensory roots also caused an associated motor root impairment.[2]

A theory proposed by White is as follows. The observation that occasional coupling of axial rotations of the vertebrae causes the anterior aspect to point toward the convexity of the lateral curve in normal bending in the middle portion of the thoracic spine must be considered. It is generally acknowledged that scoliosis frequently starts in this mid-thoracic area. There is already a physiologic, slight, right thoracic curve in this region. If some precarious balance of the normal thoracic motion should be disturbed, vertebrae in the physiologic, right thoracic curve might somehow rotate too much into the convexity of the curve (Fig. 3-4). Such an occurrence could set off a chain of events which lead to asymmetrical loads on the epiphyseal plates, muscle, and ligamentous imbalance, with ultimate progression to scoliosis. The precipitating condition may be an abnormal or malaligned facet, a discrete traumatic episode, a chemical hormonal change, extreme handedness of the individual, or any number of other possible embarrassments that upset the delicate balance. The crucial variable may be whether or not the thoracic vertebrae of the normal curve rotate toward the concavity or the convexity of the lateral curve.[45]

The relation of handedness to scoliosis has been supported by the observation of the left convex curvature in left-handed individuals.[15] It is tempting to speculate about the great proportion of right thoracic curves in idiopathic scoliosis. Do left-handed individuals with scoliosis tend to have left thoracic curve deformities? McCarver and colleagues reviewed left thoracic and related curve patterns.[24] Of 14 patients with left thoracic curves, ten were right-handed, only two were left-handed, and two were ambidextrous. One left-handed patient and one of the two ambidextrous patients had infantile idiopathic scoliosis.* This data does not support a hypothesis suggesting some association of left thoracic deformity with left-handedness.

Another possible neurologic basis for the etiology of scoliosis has been proposed. This is based on epidemiologic studies carried out by Yamada and colleagues. These investigators found that of 100 patients with scoliosis, 99 had abnormal equilibrium. This malfunction progressed with the severity of the scoliotic curve. At full growth, the findings gradually diminished and disappeared. The dysfunction was noted in the proprioceptive and optic reflex systems.[47] This

observation shows an association, but not necessarily a cause. Observers in the United States have not discerned any such changes in patients with scoliosis.

Loynes carefully reviewed 241 patients who had thoracoplasty and removal of three to ten ribs. A convex scoliotic curve to the side of the operation developed in 99 per cent of these patients. Scoliosis tended to progress with time.[22]

Ponsetti suggested that a shift in the position of the nucleus pulposus toward the convex side of the curve might be the cause of scoliosis. The normal physiologic shift of the nucleus pulposus is toward the concavity of the curve.

Occasionally a patient is seen who has a single or a double curve over a tilted, or asymmetrical or malformed fifth lumbar vertebrae. The situation can also exist with pelvic obliquity. Such asymmetry may result in a moment about the z-axis which would tilt the entire spine off to one side. In order to keep the center of gravity over the sacrum, a physiologic curve develops in the lumbar spine. With time, the unbalanced forces acting on the epiphyses lead to structural changes. If compensation is then needed above the lumbar curve, and the epiphyses are young enough to respond, a similar process may occur in the thoracic curve. That is, an initially compensatory function curve may become structural (Fig. 3-5).

BIOMECHANICAL CONSIDERATIONS INVOLVED IN TREATMENT

The mechanics of treatment attempt to return the spine to a normal configuration. There are basically two types of deformation that must be corrected. The first is called the functional curve. This is an abnormal curvature that is always present, except when some force is applied to correct it, such as active muscular strain by the patient. The patient may also bend toward the convexity of the functional curve. This curve is maintained by less rigid ligaments, muscles, and gravitational forces.

In contrast to the functional curve is the structural curve, which is more rigid and cannot be

---

* Personal communication, D. Levine.

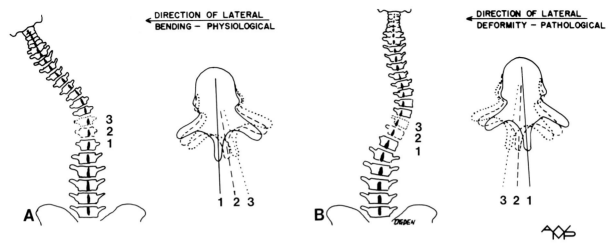

Fig. 3-4. Axial rotation into the normal (physiologic) lateral curve (A) and the scoliotic curve (B) is represented. (A) The normal curve generally shows axial rotation of the anterior portion of the vertebra into the concavity of the physiologic curve. However, *sometimes* the normal curve may rotate into the convexity. (B) In the scoliotic spine, the associated axial rotation is *always* into the convexity of the lateral curve. (White, A. A., III: Kinematics of the normal spine as related to scoliosis. J. Biomech., 4:405, 1971.)

corrected by active muscle forces. This curve usually consists of deformation within vertebrae; there is wedging and distortion of the osseous structure, and the ligamentous components of the curve are stiff. Either curve may have some component of rotation.

The correcting loads may be applied through a variety of different techniques. The loads vary in frequency, amplitude, duration, and mode of application. Basic engineering principals are involved in the correction of scoliosis.

Creep and Relaxation

Creep is an important concept in the treatment of scoliosis. The phenomenon is due to the viscoelastic properties of the muscles, ligaments, and bones. *Creep* is the deformation that follows the initial loading of a material and that occurs as a function of time without further increase in load. When a force is applied to correct a spinal deformity, and the force continues to work after the initial correction, the subsequent correction that occurs over a period of time as a result of the same load is due to creep (Fig. 3-6). When a load is applied to a viscoelastic material and the deformation remains constant, the observed subsequent decrease in load with time is *relaxation*. There are a number of clinical examples

of the use of either creep or relaxation: the use of halo femoral traction (creep); the pause of several minutes between distraction increments with a Harrington rod (relaxation); and reoperation 10 to 14 days following implantation of a rod in order to gain additional distraction (relaxation).

In an experimental study, a Harrington rod with a pressure transducer was constructed with the ability to reflect axial loading. With the use of a wireless telemetry system, it was possible to obtain information about axial forces on the rod associated with different activities. Nachemson and Elfstrom found that the distraction force is decreased 20 to 45 per cent in the first hour following surgery.[27]

Comparison of Axial and Transverse Load for Scoliosis Correction

True simulation of the scoliotic spine mathematically requires a complex, three-dimensional model. However, there is some merit in studying the behavior of the spine by highly simplified models in order to test a basic concept. A simplified model is employed here in order to study the comparative efficiency of different types and combinations of loads applied to a scoliotic spine for correction. The scoliotic spine is modeled by three components: two rigid links AC and BC,

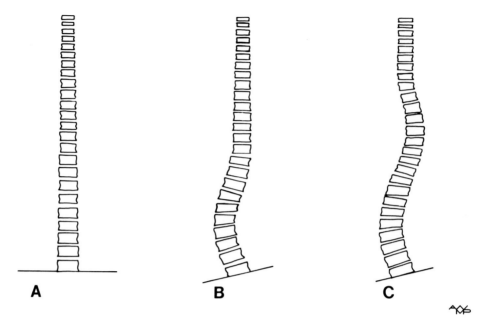

Fig. 3-5.   (*A*) A normal balanced spine. (*B*) "Tilt" or asymmetry in lumbosacral area, with a functional or structural lumbar curve. (*C*) A superimposed functional and structural thoracic curve.

connected by way of a torsional spring C (Fig. 3-7). The components lie and move in the frontal plane. The links are oriented to simulate spine deformity in θ degrees as measured by the Cobb's method. The static behavior of this model is studied under three separate loading conditions, axial force, transverse force, and a combination of axial and transverse forces.

The principle of axial loading in correcting a scoliotic spine is used frequently. Examples include skeletal traction, the Milwaukee brace, and Harrington rod. Figure 3-8A shows the spine being stretched by the axial force. A three-component model for this loading is shown in Figure 3-8B. An axial force is applied at the two ends of the spine segment, represented by points A and B in the model, to elongate and straighten the spine. The mechanism of angular correction by elongation is not due to tensile stresses in the spine, but rather to the bending moments (stresses) created at the various disc spaces. It is these bending moments which correct the angular deformity.

In contrast to axial loading, transverse loading

has not been utilized as extensively. In the Milwaukee brace and on the Risser table, use of the lateral pad applies transverse loading. Figure 3-9 shows the spine being subjected to lateral loads. A three-component model for this load type is shown in Figure 3-9B. The lateral force is applied at C and reactive forces half its size, are taken up at points A and B. The angular correction is again obtained by creating corrective bending moments at the disc spaces. Simple expressions for the bending moments produced at the disc space, represented by point C in Figure 3-9B, for axial and transverse loads separately, may be derived.

Studying Figure 3-8A in a little more detail, one notices that the corrective bending moment at the apex of the curve is the axial force F multiplied by its perpendicular distance D to the apex of the curve. It is easily seen that the greater the deformity, the greater is the distance D. In other words, the correctional ability of the force *increases* with the severity of the deformity.

A similar situation occurs when the spine is subjected to transverse loading. Figure 3-9A shows that the corrective bending moment at the apex of the curve equals half of the force at the apex (the other half works on the other half of the spine) multiplied by D, the perpendicular distance to the apex of the curve. In contrast to the axial force the corrective bending moment for the lateral force *decreases* as the deformity of the spine increases.

From this discussion it becomes apparent that the combination of axial and transverse loads is most beneficial for all situations. In other words, the axial component provides most of the corrective bending moment when deformity is severe, and the transverse component takes over the correcting function when deformity is mild. The load situation for the combined case may look like Figure 3-10. This fits well with the findings of Schultz and Hirsch which were based on computer generated models of the human spine. They found that with the mild curves axial loading with the distraction rods provided relatively very little incremental correction and required relatively large forces.[36a] Using equal loads at the three loading points, the two end forces will have to be tilted 30 degrees towards the center force for the equilibrium of the spine. These arguments are supported by engineering analysis of the simple models shown in Figures 3-8 through 3-10.[c]

Comparison of the efficiency of the three loading types can be made on the basis of the corrective bending moment produced at the disc space. The greater the bending moment, the greater is the angular correction obtained. Figure 3-11 shows the comparative results in graphical form. The diagram shows, on the horizontal axis, the angular deformity θ in degrees as measured by Cobb's method and, on the vertical axis, a factor M/FL which represents the amount of corrective bending moment obtained at the apex of the curve due to any of the three load types. If F and L have the same values in the three methods (a given scoliotic spine is loaded to the same load level), then M/FL represents the *relative* corrective moment.

Comparing the graphs of the axial load to the transverse load it can be seen that these two curves cross at about where the angle θ is 53 de-

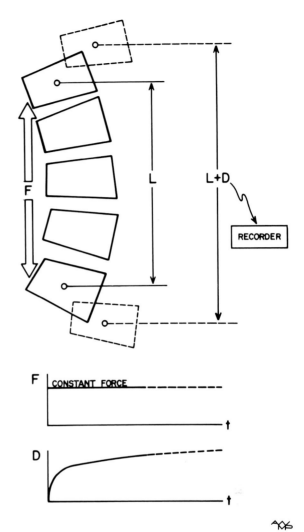

Fig. 3-6. Creep in scoliosis. F is a constant force applied with axial traction. The original length of the scoliotic segment L corrects and increases to L + D as a function of time. D is the deformation or change in the length of the curved segment of spine.

grees. Therefore, based on the analysis of this theoretical model, axial loading is more beneficial for severely deformed scoliotic spines, while transverse loading is ideal for correcting milder curves. However, when all three graphs are compared, it becomes clear that the combined load is the most efficient load type for all degrees of deformity.

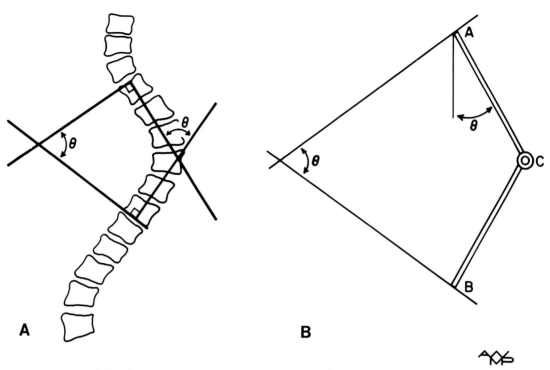

Fig. 3-7. A model to study the correction efficiency of axial and lateral forces. (*A*) Scoliotic spine curvature as measured by the Cobb's method. The angle θ in degrees is the measure of the deformity. (*B*) A highly simplified mathematical model of the scoliotic spine is made up of two rigid links AC and BC connected at C by way of a torsional spring.

Use of the three graphs in Figure 3-11 determines the most efficient treatment for a given patient. Suppose there are two patients whose curves measure 30 and 70 degrees respectively, by Cobb's method. Assuming that all three load types are feasible and available for treatment, the problem is to choose the most efficient. Plotting the value of $\theta = 30$ degrees on the horizontal axis, for the patient with mild deformity (Fig. 3-11), one can read off the vertical axis the three values of the quantity M/FL provided by the axial, transverse, and combined load types. These are 0.26, 0.48 and 0.71, respectively. Considering the M/FL value provided by the axial load as 100 per cent, then the corresponding values for the other two load types are 185 per cent and 273 per cent. Thus, for this patient, transverse load is more efficient than the axial load, while the combined load is the best. Similarly, one can plot and read off the values for the patient with

severe deformity, 70 degrees. From Figure 3-11 the M/FL values are 0.57, 0.41, and 0.91, respectively. Again counting on the percentage basis and considering the M/FL value provided by the axial load type as 100 per cent, the values are 72 per cent and 160 per cent, respectively for the transverse and the combined loadings. Thus, for the patient with severe deformity, the axial load is more efficient than the transverse load, but again the combined load is superior. Based on these theoretical considerations, patients with severe deformity should be treated by axial loading in the beginning, and as the deformity decreases the loading should be changed to the transverse type, assuming that axial and the transverse loading cannot be combined and applied simultaneously.

Connock and Armstrong have made an innovative contribution in the development of the apparatus which allows for the direct application of

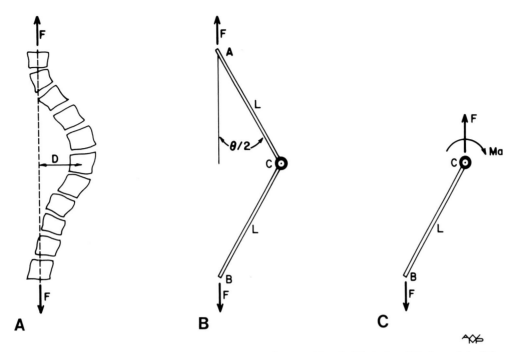

Fig. 3-8.   Axial load. (*A*) The scoliotic spine under axial load. (*B*) A simplified model of the spine being subjected to axial distraction force F. (*C*) Free body diagram of the model link BC and the joint C.

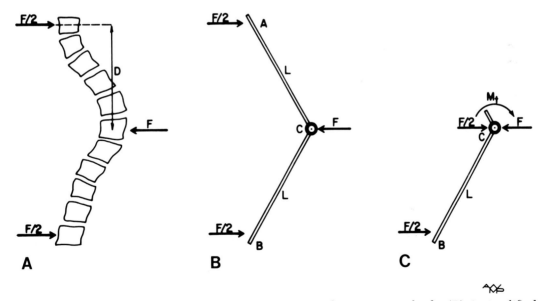

Fig. 3-9.   Transverse loads. (*A*) The scoliotic spine under transverse loads. (*B*) A simplified model of spine being subjected to three-point transverse forces. (*C*) Free body diagram of the model link in BC and the joint C.

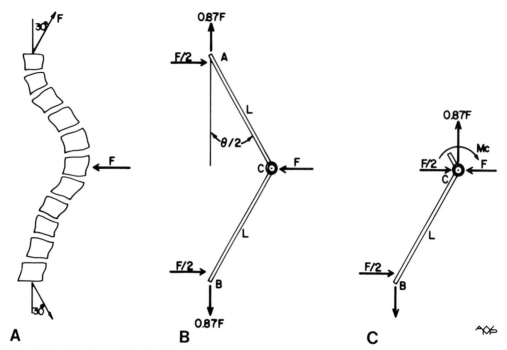

Fig. 3-10. Combined loads. (A) The scoliotic spine under combined axial and lateral loads. (B) A simplified spine model being subjected to combined loading. (C) Free body diagram of the model link BC and the joint C.

transverse loading to scoliotic vertebrae. The principle of the technique is shown in Figure 3-12A,B. By applying tension between the rod and metal devices attached to the posterior element, a transverse load TL is applied.[6] There is an advantage, however, in applying the transverse load at a different point (Fig. 3-12C). This tends to correct the abnormal axial rotation of the scoliotic vertebra. The element of abnormal frontal plane curvature is nearly corrected with the current treatment armamentarium. Application of transverse loads to a point to *correct* the axial rotation is being developed.

MECHANICS OF DIFFERENT TREATMENT METHODS

Exercises

It is questionable whether or not exercises alone significantly correct scoliosis. However, theoretically a vigorous and thoroughly super-

vised exercise program may reeducate patient and muscles so as to correct a functional curve. The muscle forces that can be applied are of relatively low amplitude and frequency, and the duration of application is limited. Most probably, exercises should not be relied upon to hold or correct a curve when they are used alone. Some of the traditional exercises to treat scoliosis are shown in Figure 3-13.

It is interesting to speculate why exercises alone have not been found beneficial in the treatment of scoliosis. Muscular forces are rarely working at a significant mechanical advantage for correction of the scoliotic spine. Certainly, the erector spinae muscles are not able to function at the most efficient mechanical advantage. The other factor, which is perhaps more important, is the need for prolonged force application in order to take advantage of the viscoelastic creep. It is difficult to maintain voluntary muscle contraction and apply forces to the spine for a time long enough for the resisting viscoelastic structures to yield. These two factors limit the capacity of pure exercises in achieving correction. Most surgeons do not consider exercise alone to be of significant value in the treatment of scoliosis. However, vigorous and well organized exercise programs are still offered with enthusiasm by some surgeons. If there is careful periodic observation of the curve, then no harm is done.

Electrodes powered by intermittent cyclical currents are being implanted in the erector spinae muscles on the convex side of the curve to stimulate muscle contraction. A totally implantable unit with its own power supply has been developed. Transcutaneous stimulation of muscles is also being used in humans to correct scoliosis. Preliminary reports indicate that this may prove beneficial in some cases.[3]

The Milwaukee Brace

The Milwaukee brace is advantageous in the treatment of scoliosis: Active exercise is performed while in the brace; a *normal mold* is constructed into which the deformed patient is fit; and corrective forces are applied to a growing spine. The brace applies corrective forces to the spine for 23.5 hours each day. The spine is being supported, splinted, and stretched constantly between the throat and occipital mold on one end and the pelvic girdle on the other. Additional forces are applied through corrective pads attached to the uprights of the brace and the axillary sling. The brace takes advantage of growth potential, so that it has the possibility of correcting structural deformity. Active correctional forces are being applied to the spine by the patient both consciously (the active exercise program) and unconsciously (occasional moving away from the pads, the axillary sling, and the throat mold and occipital piece). The amplitude of the active forces is limited by the patient's muscle strength and the mechanical advantage. The passive correctional forces are limited by the stiffness of the tissue transmitters (ribs, muscle, skin, fat), biological tolerances (pain threshold, organic functions), and the psychosocial tolerances of the patient (see page 348).

A special exercise program is a crucial aspect of the use of the Milwaukee brace. Exercises in

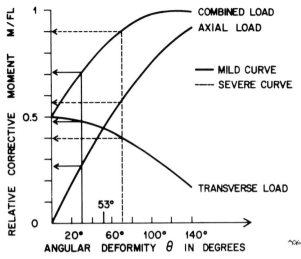

Fig. 3-11. A graphic representation of "relative corrective moment M/FL" as a function of spine deformity in degrees (Cobb's method) for the three loading types. According to the theoretical model studied here, we note the following: The combined load is the most efficient for any degree of deformity; the axial load efficiency increases with the angular deformity; and the transverse load efficiency decreases with angular deformity. The deformity angle of 53 degrees is a break even point for the axial and transverse loads. Examples of two theoretical patients with mild (30°) and severe (70°) curves are shown.

breathing and pelvic alignment are an important adjunct. These combat lumbar lordosis, enhance the active correctional forces of the patient's own intrinsic muscle groups, and stimulate normal activity in the brace. When the brace is constructed, it must be "made straight." That is, it must not yield or be fit in any degree to the deformity as it exists. The basic brace should thus be made on a level pelvic support, with the uprights erect and perpendicular to the horizontal plane of the pelvis. In other words, the deformed body must go into a straight, normal, dynamic mold. It follows from the concept of dynamic molding that growth potential should remain in order to have the best functional or working brace. It is important to hold the correction once it is achieved until maturity and, finally, to wean the patient gradually.

The Milwaukee brace has been valuable as a holding device both pre- and postoperatively.

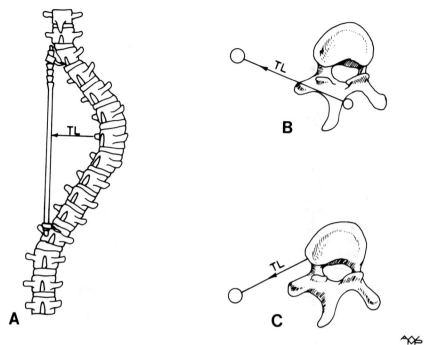

Fig. 3-12. A comparison of the effects of two types of transverse loading (TL) on the axial rotation of a scoliotic vertebra. (A) Both types of transverse loading correct the lateral curvature. (B) Transverse loading tends to increase the abnormal θy rotation. (C) Transverse loading tends to increase the abnormal rotation.

It is known for its success in the complete and final correction of a number of patients with scoliosis, without any surgical intervention. (However, it must be kept in mind that following completion of treatment some patients can progress as much as 1 to 2 degrees yearly, up to age 25 or 29.[25a])

Nachemson and Elfstrom implanted telemetrized Harrington rods in patients with idiopathic scoliosis and obtained data about the effects of several pertinent factors upon forces exerted upon the rods.[27] Much of this information is of clinical importance. Questions such as how much a scoliosis patient may be allowed to move and how different reclining positions influence the forces in the Harrington rod have been subject to discussion. Figure 3-14 shows the axial force in the distraction rod with the patient lying in three different positions. It is interesting to note that although the axial force increased in both the side lying positions, the increase was smaller when the patient was lying on the side away from the convexity of the curvature. This is due to the fact that the spine is loaded like a two-point supported beam, in its middle by the weight of the trunk. The two points of support are the pelvis and shoulder girdles. This particular pattern produces tensile loads on the side of the spine next to the bed and compressive loads on the side away from the bed. Therefore, the measured loads on the telemeterized rod and the laminae are greater with the patient lying on the convex side of the curve. Based on this information, it is probably worthwhile to avoid allowing patients to lie on the convex side of their curve during the first 2 weeks after rod implantation.

When forces on the rod with a Risser cast, a Milwaukee brace, and no support were compared, Nachemson and Elfstrom found the brace to be superior in terms of reducing the axial forces on the rod (Fig. 3-15). They also showed that when different parts of the brace are re-

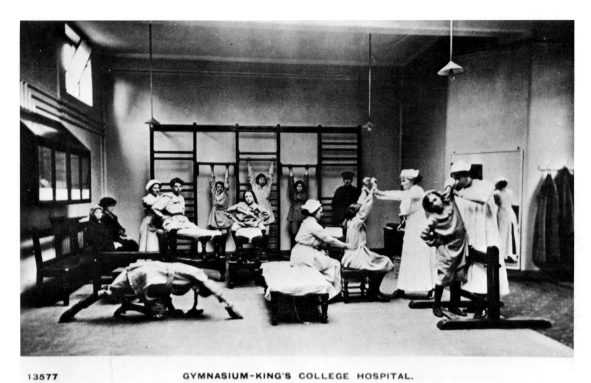

13577   GYMNASIUM-KING'S COLLEGE HOSPITAL.

Fig. 3-13. Some of the typical exercises and activities for correction of scoliosis. The principles of axial traction and transverse loading and the direct application of bending moments are all well demonstrated in this historic photo. Despite the sometimes soundly based mechanics, the evidence does not justify the assumption that exercise alone can either correct or prevent progression of deformity. (Courtesy of King's College Hospital, London, with the assistance of Mr. R. Q. Crellin.)

moved, the axial forces increase.[27] When the patient coughs or vomits coming out of anesthesia, the forces are increased tremendously, and the patient may fracture the lamina and have the rod pull out. A smooth recovery period from anesthesia is therefore crucial to the use of the Harrington rods. In lifting the patient from the bed to the frame, the forces were also noted to increase significantly. There is argument about whether or not a Milwaukee brace should be kept on when the patient is recumbent. If one lies down and takes off a Milwaukee brace, there is an increase in the axial force upon the Harrington rod. Therefore, the Milwaukee brace does diminish the load even in a supine position.

Galante and associates carried out an investigation using a strain gauge device under the occipital and mandibular pads of Milwaukee braces.

They found that if the axillary pad or the sling was removed, there was increased axial loading. This implies that a loss of correction results in increased load on the brace. The Milwaukee brace provides both active and passive correction, as shown by this experiment. The removal of the lateral forces from the axillary pad or the thoracic pad caused increased axial loading; therefore, these pads were presumably applying corrective loads to the spine. The patient is corrected passively. Further, Galante and colleagues found that when a patient moves away from the thoracic pad, which actively corrects the lateral curve and axial rotation, there is also passive stretching of the spine. This experiment showed that the average force on the brace in a standing position was 19 N (4.25 lbf). However, if the patient pulled away from the thoracic pad, the aver-

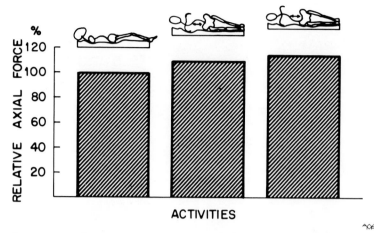

Fig. 3-14. The relative axial force in the telemeterized Harrington rod in the patient lying in bed supine, on the concave side of the curve, and on the convex side of the curve. The force in a patient lying supine has been assigned a value of 100 per cent. (Based on data from Nachemson, A., and Elfstrom, G.: Intravital wireless telemetry of axial forces in Harrington distraction rods in patients with idiopathic scoliosis. J. Bone Joint Surg., 53A:445, 1971.)

age force increased to 63 N (14 lbf), slightly greater than three times as much. This shows that the brace gives passive distraction when the patient moves away from the pads.[14]

Localizer Casts

With this treatment, which is generally used before and after surgery, the patient is placed on a special table where traction and localizer pads for lateral and rotary loads are applied. Correction is achieved and the patient is wrapped in a rigid, well molded, plaster jacket, and the correction forces are released. The goal is to hold the patient in the corrected position. The forces are constant; they may be reapplied as often as is practical to replace the cast. The cast may be left on for 2 to 4 months. Weight loss and compression of tissue results in diminution of the forces.

Traction

There are a variety of methods that may be employed. Head halter and/or ankle pelvic straps can be used. Greater forces can be applied for longer periods of time using skeletal traction. Halo traction is combined with the pelvic hoop or

the more common femoral pins. The halo-hoop has been shown to be valuable in the treatment of a variety of different types of scoliosis. It is especially valuable for straightening out the usually recalcitrant pelvic obliquity. The distractive forces of this apparatus can be measured by placing dynamometers in the four uprights. This is desirable wherever feasible. DeWald and associates showed that forces of 360 to 400 N (80–90 lbf) were readily tolerated by patients. Kyphotic deformities may also be corrected by the apparatus. Any neurologic signs were reversible by reducing the traction. The investigators also proved by objective in vivo monitoring that one of the four uprights may be removed for surgery without loss of correction.[10]

There are certain advantages of preoperative traction in the treatment of severe scoliosis. There is the maximum opportunity to benefit from gradual correction, which takes advantage of the creep phenomenon. This minimizes the possibility of spinal cord damage through correction that is too rapid. Moreover, the patient is awake and any neurologic change can be readily recognized. This minimizes the need for intra-operative maneuvers, such as monitoring spinal responses and awakening the patient during the procedure to check for motor or sensory function. Since the resisting structures are significantly corrected preoperatively, the final force on the Harrington rod is presumed to be diminished. This should reduce the possibility of failure of the thoracic lamina and "pull out" of the rod. Another advantage of preoperative traction is found in the correction of double curves with different stiffnesses. Radiographs taken during full traction give an excellent idea of the relative final correction for each curve that is compatible with good balance.

Recent studies have shown, however, that axial traction is probably not advantageous in patients under 20 years of age with idiopathic curves with a Cobb angle of less than 90 degrees.[27a] Our preceding considerations remain applicable, however, in treating severe scoliosis deformities in other circumstances.

Harrington Instrumentation

Here the forces are applied directly to the two end vertebrae of the curve. These distraction forces are applied manually and maintained by a locking mechanism in the rod. However, they are not measured. The forces are applied in small increments. Their amplitude is limited by the strength of the bony structure to which the rod is attached. The limiting factor is the lamina of the thoracic vertebrae, which may fail if the distraction rod has a force of 370 N (83.3 lbf).[42] The force may be applied indefinitely. The use of this rod is always in conjunction with a spinal arthrodesis of the involved vertebrae. The surgeon can take some advantage of relaxation by waiting at least 5 minutes between the last three increments of force applied to the distraction rod. The corrective value of the last notches on the rod is low, and the forces involved are high.[36a]

Waugh conducted studies on the biomechanics

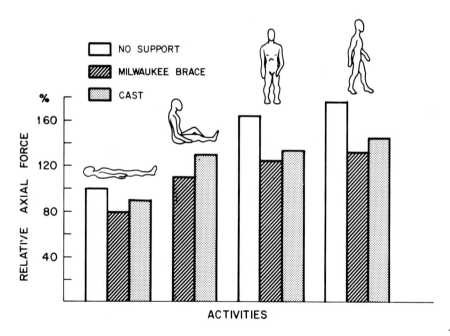

Fig. 3-15. Relative axial force in the telemeterized Harrington rod in patients wearing no external support, a Milwaukee brace, and a Risser cast. The force in a patient with no support and lying supine has been assigned a value of 100 per cent. The bar graphs show patients under these three conditions performing different activities. (Based on data from Nachemson, A., and Elfstrom, G.: Intravital wireless telemetry of axial forces in Harrington distraction rods in patients with idiopathic scoliosis. J. Bone Joint Surg., 53A:445, 1971.)

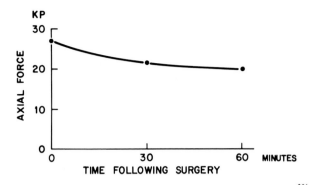

Fig. 3-16.   Axial force in kiloponds (kp) in the Harrington rod in a patient immediately following surgery. Immediate relaxation of force with time is shown. 1 kp = 9.81 N = 2.21 lbf. (Based on data from Nachemson, A., and Elfstrom, G.: Intravital wireless telemetry of axial forces in Harrington distraction rods in patients with idiopathic scoliosis. J. Bone Joint Surg., 53A: 445, 1971.)

and technique of the Harrington rod. He found that there is considerable stress concentration of the hook in the upper lamina, which is the weak point of the system. The tolerance limit was found to be equal to a force of about 200 to 300 N (43.9–65.8 lbf). These studies showed that in flexible curves, 200 to 300 N (43.9–65.8 lbf) of force was adequate for 60 to 70-per cent correction. Over 300 N (65.8 lbf), the rod is likely to pull out. Waugh suggested that for greater contact area between the hook and the lamina, a different hook design should be used.[42] He has subsequently experimented with the use of methylmethacrylate to reduce stress concentration by increasing the contact area. He also suggested that the steps on the Harrington rod be placed closer together, since the increment of one additional step augments the force on the rod from 200 N (43.9 lbf) to above the crucial 300 N (65.8 lbf) load. If the steps are not as great, the force may range from 200 to 280 N (43.9–61.4 lbf), gaining more correction and still remaining within the range of the tolerance of the lamina.

Axial Forces.   Since we know that the limiting factor in the amount of corrective force that may be applied to the scoliotic spine with the distraction rod is the load-bearing tolerance of the thoracic lamina, in vivo measurements of axial loads on the Harrington rod become quite important.

The experiments of Nachemson and Elfstrom generated some relevant data on this subject.[27] Forces during operation and immediately after surgery are shown in Figure 3-16. On the ordinate is the force in kiloponds, and on the abscissa is the time in minutes after operation. One sees that there is a marked decrease in the axial force with time due to the viscoelastic properties of the ligaments (relaxation). Within the first hour the average axial force had fallen to 78 per cent of the original value. Therefore, distraction is best applied with some time lapse between application. The use of the outrigger distraction in surgery, with occasional small increments of axial load, can expand the time range over which the maximal axial load is applied. Thus, greater correction may be obtained by the same load.

It is important to handle the patients carefully. Lifting and turning the patient in bed produces a great increase in the axial force. Some of the highest forces are produced with coughing. If bucking and coughing is a factor in patients awakening from anesthesia, large forces can be created. One strong cough or buck can tear the upper hook from the thoracic lamina. The importance of a smooth, early recovery phase from anesthesia cannot be overemphasized.

Compression Rod.   This is a corrective device that is used on the convex side of the curve. The rod is in tension and thus applies two colinear compressive forces to the spine. The change in the positions of the vertebra between the ends of the rod is dependent upon the bending moments produced at the centers of rotation for the vertebrae. If the centers of rotation are between the rod and the concavity of the curve, these vertebra tend to be corrected. However, if the centers are between the rod and the convexity of the curve, the bending moments produced may tend to exaggerate the deformity.

The total corrective effect depends upon the balance between the two, upon the distribution of the centers of rotation of the vertebral bodies with respect to the direction of the compressive forces. In general, the corrective effect is small and may even be negative. Waugh attached a compression rod to the convex side of a scoliotic curve after applying a distraction rod to the other side. There was a 9.8 N (2.2 lbf) reduction of the axial forces with the compression rod in place.[42] It does not appear that this small difference contributes significantly to correction.

A modification of the compression rod principle is the spring used by Gruca.[17] An extension spring is used with the hooks attached to the pedicles and its length lying over the convex side of the spine. It applies compressive forces at the hook-pedicle junctions and, radially, inward forces to the bodies of the vertebrae encompassed by the spring. Here again the corrective bending moments are rather small. The situation can be greatly improved if wedge resection of the discs is performed to shift the centers of rotations to the side of the colinear compressive forces that produce the corrective bending moments.

Dwyer's Method

The Dwyer technique is another surgical procedure for the correction of scoliosis.[11] The technique is especially valuable where there is a large anterior curvature (lordosis) or where there is absence of the posterior anatomic structures, as with meningomyelocele. The biomechanical principle of Dwyer's method is shown in Figure 3-17. Compressive forces are applied to the spine on the convex side of the curve at each segmental level. This consists of removing the discs and inserting screws into the vertebral bodies on the convex aspect. A braided wire is passed through holes in the screw heads. By applying tension to the wire, corrective bending moments are created at the intervertebral spaces. The magnitude of the force is limited only by the fixation of the cable holes to the vertebrae and is reported to be in the range of 450 N (101 lbf) of tensile force in the braided wire. The correction is maintained by swaging all screw heads onto the wire. Looking at one motion segment, the corrective bending moment provided at each disc space is the tension in the wire multiplied by the length of the lever arm to the instantaneous center of the motion segment. Since the length of the lever arm is small, a large amount of tension is required in the wires to produce a significant correction. Thus, the spine is subjected to a very large force for a given bending moment. To understand what these forces do to the epiphyseal plates, it is necessary to look at the two vertebrae. In Figure

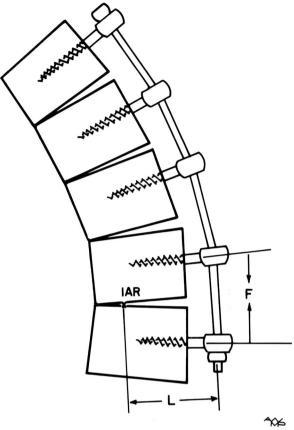

Fig. 3-17. The biomechanical principle of the Dwyer technique is to apply compressive forces on the convex side of the curve. The force F is created by applying tension to the wire on the convex side. The correction is produced by the bending moment F × L.

3-17 the two vertebrae are shown with the instantaneous axis of rotation when a pair of axial forces are applied at the screw heads. With the application of these forces, motion takes place. From the definition of instantaneous axis of rotation, this motion is a rotation about the instantaneous axis of rotation. Figure 3-17 shows that such a rotation brings the portions of the vertebrae anterior to the instantaneous axis of rotation closer together, while those portions posterior are pulled apart. Thus, the epiphysis is put under compression on the convex side, and in tension on the concave side. By way of Heuter Volkmann's law, this may be beneficial in the same manner as medially placed staples are effective in the correction of a valgus deformity.

Anterior Epiphysiodesis

Anterior unilateral epiphysiodesis on the convex side of the curve in a growing child has also been employed by Tylman as a form of treatment in scoliosis.[39] The rationale here is that if growth can be arrested on the convex side of the curve, then the concave side can continue to grow, balance the asymmetry, and achieve correction. Tylman also employs posterior arthrodesis on the convex side. Timing and analysis of potential growth to the untreated areas are crucial and difficult to estimate.

CONCLUSIONS

Scoliosis probably constitutes one of the most challenging and complex clinical problems in the field of orthopaedic biomechanics. In some elusive and insidious manner, biological and mechanical factors combine to produce a disease process which can develop into a major cosmetic deformity and, ultimately, ill health due to cardio-respiratory changes.

This chapter has sought to bring together the important biological and mechanical considerations which constitute a current understanding of scoliosis.

CLINICAL BIOMECHANICS

Removal of posterior elements allows increased axial rotation in the thoracic spine.

Biomechanical theories suggest that removal of the disc may also improve correction potential.

Three-dimensional analysis of scoliosis is crucial to a comprehensive understanding of the disease.

The surgeon may take advantage of the creep and relaxation characteristics of the tissues, primarily by allowing ample time to pass between application of various correctional forces.

The surgeon may take advantage of the analysis of the relative value of axial, transverse, and combined loading in the correction of scoliosis. Theoretically, axial loading is more efficient for severe curves and moderate curves and transverse loading is more efficient for less severe curves. *Combined* loading is always more effective than either type alone.

Certain factors are important in using the Milwaukee brace. Evidence suggests that the brace is as effective as a cast in reducing axial forces adjacent to a scoliotic curve. Removal of axillary supports and thoracic pads increases the axial forces and thus reduces the effectiveness of the brace. The brace continues to resist axial loads in the spine when the wearer is recumbent. Thus, the brace should also be worn when the patient is in this position.

The major practical considerations regarding the use of Harrington instrumentation are as follows: The distraction force that may be applied with the Harrington rod is determined by the tolerance of the thoracic lamina; 295 N (65.8 lbf) is the upper limit of this force; coughing or bucking during the stages of recovery from anesthesia can apply dangerously high forces to the Harrington rod; greater surface contact of hook to lamina and smaller increments between notches on the rod increase the tolerance limits of the mechanism; compression rods on the convex side have little or no correctional value.

The Dwyer technique is a biomechanically sound and effective technique, which has an additional advantage of applying asymmetrical loads to the epiphyseal plate.

NOTES

[A] Using the coordinate system, when axial rotation is coupled with lateral bending, a negative θz is associated with a positive θy.

[B] In the middle and lower regions of the thoracic spine, a negative θz is associated with a negative θy.

[C] Figure 3-8C is a free-body diagram of the link BC and the spring C under axial load. The equilibrium condition for the link BC gives the expression for the bending moment M_a at the junction C:

$$M_a = FL \operatorname{Sin} (\theta/2) \qquad (1)$$

where F is the maximum safe load applied to the vertebra in the axial direction, L is the link length, and θ is the angular deformity. Equation (1) shows that, for given values of F and L, the bending moment M_a varies as a sine function of angle $(\theta/2)$. A free-body diagram for the transverse loading is shown in Figure 3-9C. Again, the equilibrium condition at the junction C gives the expression for the bending moment:

$$M_t = \frac{FL}{2} \operatorname{Cos} (\theta/2) \qquad (2)$$

Here F is the transverse force applied to the middle of the curve and F/2 are the reactive forces. In this case, for given values of F and L, the bending moment M_t is proportional to half of the cosine of angle $(\theta/2)$. One may take this analysis a step further and study the effect of combining axial and transverse loads. Such a combined situation is shown in Figure 3-10. Using equal loads at all three loading points, A, B, and C, the axial components of forces at A and B are 0.87F, while the horizontal components are F/2. (The end force vectors are tilted 30° towards the center force.) From the free-body diagram, Figure 3-10C, and the equilibrium conditions for the link BC, we can write the expression for the bending moment at C caused by the combined loading. This is

$$M_c = FL \sin (30° + \theta/2) \qquad (3)$$

CLASSIFICATION OF REFERENCES

Anatomy 7, 13, 15, 16, 19, 28, 41
Kinematics 9, 21, 23, 35, 37, 45
Etiological considerations 2, 12, 18, 22, 24, 25, 26, 32, 33, 34, 40, 45, 47
Treatment 3, 5, 6, 10, 11, 14, 17, 25a, 27, 27a, 36a, 39, 42
Advanced reading 29, 30, 31, 36, 43, 46

REFERENCES

1. Akerblom, B.: Standing and sitting posture [thesis]. Stockholm, A/B Nordiska Bokhandelns, 1948.
2. Alexander, M. A., Bunch, W. H., and Ebbesson, S. O. E.: Can experimental dorsal rhizotomy produce scoliosis? J. Bone Joint Surg., 54A: 1509, 1973.
3. Bobechko, W. P.: Scoliosis spinal pacemakers. J. Bone Joint Surg., 56A:442, 1974.
4. Braus, H.: Anatomie des Menschen, Band I: Bewegungsapparat. Berlin, Springer-Verlag, 1921.
5. Cobb, J. R.: Spine arthrodesis in the treatment of scoliosis. Bull. Hosp. Joint Dis., 19:187, 1958. (*The best description of the technique for an orthopaedic operation that the authors are aware of.*)
6. Connock, S. H. G. and Armstrong, G. W. D.: A transverse loading system applied to a modified Harrington instrumentation. J. Bone Joint Surg., 53A:194, 1971.
7. Davis, G. G.: Applied Anatomy. ed. 5. Philadelphia, J. B. Lippincott, 1918.
8. Davis, P.: The medial inclination of the human thoracic intervertebral articular facets. J. Anat., 93:68, 1959.
9. Davis, P., Troup, J., and Burnard, J.: Movements of the thoracic and lumbar spine when lifting: a chronocyclophotographic study. J. Anat., 99:15, 1965.
10. DeWald, R. L., Mukahy, T. M., and Schultz, A. B.: Force measurement studies with the halo-hoop apparatus in scoliosis. Orthop. Rev., 2:17, 1973.
11. Dwyer, A., Newton, N., and Sherwood, A.: An anterior approach to scoliosis. A preliminary report. Clin. Orthop., 62:192, 1969. (*An innovative surgical technique for the treatment of scoliosis.*)
12. Farkas, A.: Mechanism of scoliosis in experimental lathyrism. Bull. Hosp. Joint Dis. 19:260, 1958.
13. Frazier, J.: The Anatomy of the Human Skeleton. ed. 4. London, J. & A. Churchill, 1940.
14. Galante, J., Schultz, A., and DeWald, R.: Forces acting in the Milwaukee brace on patients undergoing treatment for idiopathic scoliosis. J. Bone Joint Surg., 52A:498, 1970. (*Some clinically useful information.*)
15. Gray, H.: Anatomy of the Human Body. ed. 23. Lewis, W. H. [ed.]. Philadelphia, Lea & Febiger, 1936.
16. ——— Descriptive and Applied Anatomy. ed. 34. Davis, D. V. [ed.]. London, Longmans, Green & Co., 1967.
17. Gruca, A.: Protocol of the 41st congress of Italian Orthopaedics and Traumalogy. Bologna, Italy, 1956.
18. Heuter, C.: Anatomische studien an den extremitaten gelenken neugeborener und erwachsener. Virchow's Arch. Path. Anat., 25:575, 1862.
19. Humphry, G.: A Treatise on the Human Skeleton. London, MacMillan, 1858.
20. Junghanns, H.: Die zwischenwirbelscheiben im roentgenbild. Fortschr. Röntgenstr., 43:275, 1931.
21. Lovett, R.: The mechanism of the normal spine and its relation to scoliosis. Boston Medical Surgical Journal, 153:349, 1905. (*An old classic.*)
22. Loynes, R.: Scoliosis after thoracoplasty. J. Bone Joint Surg., 54B:484, 1972.
23. Lysell, E.: Motion in the cervical spine [thesis]. Acta Orthop. Scand., Suppl. 123 [Suppl.], 1969. (*Valuable experimental concept and an excellent study of the kinematics of the lower cervical spine.*)
24. McCarver, C., Levine, D., and Veliskakis, K.: Left thoracic and related curve patterns in idiopathic scoliosis. J. Bone Joint Surg., 53A:196, 1971.
25. MacEwen, G. D.: Experimental scoliosis. In Proceedings of a Second Symposium on Scoliosis: Causation. Zorab, P. A. [ed.] Edinburgh, E. & S. Livingstone, 1968.
25a. Mellencamp, D. D., Blount, W. D., and Anderson, A. J.: Milwaukee brace treatment of idiopathic scoliosis. Clin. Orthop., 126:47, 1977.
26. Michelsson, J.: The development of spinal deformity in experimental scoliosis. Acta Orthop. Scand., 81 [Suppl.], 1965. (*An excellent review of animal experiments related to scoliosis.*)
27. Nachemson, A., and Elfstrom, G.: Intravital wireless telemetry of axial forces in Harrington distraction rods in patients with idiopathic scoliosis. J. Bone Joint Surg., 53A:445, 1971. (*A classic in vivo study with valuable clinical information.*)
27a. Nachemson, A., and Nordwall, A.: Effectiveness of the operative cotrel traction for correction of idiopathic scoliosis. J. Bone Joint Surg., 59A:504, 1977.
28. Nordwall, A.: Mchanical properties of tendinous structures in patients with idiopathic scoliosis. J Bone Joint Surg., 56A:443, 1974.
29. Olsen, G. A.: New Development in the Correction of Scoliosis. Proceedings of Workshop on Bio-engineering Approaches to the Problems of the Spine. Sponsored by the Surgery Study Section Division of Research Grants, National Institute of Health, Bethesda, Md., 1970.
30. Panjabi, M. M.: Three-dimensional mathematical model of the human spine structure. J. Biomech., 6:671, 1973. (*Construction and uses of a mathematical model in spine problems.*)
31. Panjabi, M. M., and White, A. A.: A mathematical approach for three-dimensional analysis of the mechanics of the spine. J. Biomech., 4:3, 1971. (*Three-dimensional*

motion analysis including the effect of experimental errors.)

32. Ponsetti, I. V.: Experimental scoliosis. Bull. Hosp. Joint Dis., *19*:216, 1958.

33. Ponsetti, I., Pedrini, V., and Dohrman, S.: Biomechanical analysis of intervertebral discs in idiopathic scoliosis. J. Bone Joint Surg., *56A*, 1973.

34. Roaf, R.: The basic anatomy of scoliosis. J. Bone Joint Surg., *48B*:786, 1966. (*An interesting and important theory.*)

35. Rolander, S.: Motion of the lumbar spine with special reference to stabilizing effect of posterior fusion [thesis]. Acta Orthop. Scand., *90* [Suppl.], 1966. (*A monumental bibliography on basic and applied scientific aspects of the human spine.*)

36. Schultz, A. B., Larocca, H., Galante, J. A., and Andriacchi, T. P.: A study of geometrical relationships in scoliotic spines. J. Biomech., *5*:409, 1972. (*An attempt at simulating scoliosis by a simple mathematical model.*)

36a. Schultz, A. B., and Hirsch, C.: Mechanical analysis techniques for improved correction of idiopathic scoliosis. Clin. Orthop., *100*:66, 1974.

37. Steindler, A.: Kinesiology of the Human Body. Springfield, Ill., Charles C Thomas, 1955.

38. Stillwell, D. L.: Structural deformities of vertebrae.: bone adaption and modeling in experimental scoliosis and kyphosis. J. Bone and Joint Surg., *44A*:611, 1962.

39. Tylman, D.: Anterior epiphysiodesis and posterior spinal fusion in the treatment of scoliosis. American Digest of Foreign Orthopaedic Literature, Fourth Quarter. p. 203, 1972.

40. Volkmann, R.: Chirurgische erfahrungen ueber knochenverbiegungen und knochen wachstum. Arch. Path. Anat., *24*:512, 1862.

41. Walters, R., and Morris, J.: An in vitro study of normal and scoliotic interspinous ligaments. J. Biomech., *6*:343, 1973.

42. Waugh, T.: Intravital Measurements During Instrument Correction of Idiopathic Scoliosis. Gothenburg, Sweden, Tryckeri Ab Litotup, 1966.

43. Weiss, E. B.: Quantitation of Curvature and Torsion in X-rays of the Spine. Proceeding of Workshop on Bioengineering Approaches to Problems of the Spine. Sponsored by the Surgery Study Sections Division of Research Grants, National Institute of Health, Bethesda, Md., 1970. (*Some important biomechanical considerations involving the Harrington rod.*)

44. White, A. A.: Analysis of the mechanics of the thoracic spine in man. An experimental study on autopsy specimens. [thesis]. Acta Orthop. Scan., *127* [Suppl.], 1969. (*Recommended to those with special interest in biomechanics of the thoracic spine.*)

45. —— Kinematics of the normal spine as related to scoliosis. J. Biomech. *4*:405, 1971.

46. White, A. A., Panjabi, M. M., and Brand, R.: A system for defining position and motion of human body parts. J. Med. Biol. Eng., *261*:261, 1975. (*Basic ideas concerning position and motion of irregular bodies (vertebrae) in space are presented.*)

47. Yamada, K., et al.: A neurological approach to the etiology and treatment of scoliosis. J. Bone Joint Surg., *53A*:197, 1971.

4 Practical Biomechanics of Spine Trauma

You have to hang Mr. A. He is 5 ft., 10½ in. in height, and weighs 12 st., 2 lbs., 6 oz., 1 dwt. His neck from the sternocleidomastoid to the sterno-hyoid measures 6¾ in. The neck is strong and 17 in. in diameter. Calculate to three places of decimals the drop necessary to hang this man thoroughly, without risk of giving pain to on-lookers. Also give the diameter and quality of the rope you would employ, in terms of pounds "avoirdupois of strain."

Charles Duff: *A Handbook on Hanging*, London, 1938

Upon completion of this chapter, the reader is not expected to calculate the answer to this question to more than one decimal place.

The serious emphasis of this chapter is the practical biomechanics of spine injuries. A good deal is known about the mechanism of injury in spine trauma. However, there are also a number of assumptions that lead to copious conclusions in the analysis of spine trauma. It is not uncommon for physicians to look for 2 to 3 seconds at a lateral radiograph of the cervical spine and then to embark upon detailed deliberations about the directions and magnitudes of the forces responsible for the observed injuries. In many of these situations the "learned dissertations" constitute inappropriate, unfounded speculations. Given the current thrust in the direction of a more scientific engineering study of clinical phenomenon, this type of speculation is no longer valid. However, such an analysis cannot yet be replaced by precise, valid scientific data. The current state of knowledge lies somewhere between gross speculation and precise science. This chapter seeks to go beyond glib explanations based on speculation and imprecise understanding of mechanics. It offers a framework for a more sound analysis.

GENERAL CLINICAL CONSIDERATIONS

In the discussion of the suggested treatment of spine injuries, the authors assume that the fundamentals of emergency treatment and basic care of the patient with an injured spinal cord are being carried out. These include the usual attention to the air way and treatment of hemorrhage and shock. We assume that adequate fluid replacement is initiated, and the splinting of injured parts is carried out whenever necessary. The patient should be treated with due consideration of early drainage of the bladder and careful monitoring of vital signs and neurologic status, along with the recording of a medical history and physical examination. Initial care should also include radiologic evaluation, baseline laboratory studies, and the indicated consultations. Collaboration among orthopaedist, neurosurgeon, and radiologist can be invaluable in piecing together the possible mechanism of injury and evaluating the damage imposed to important, stabilizing, anatomic structures (see Chapter 5).

MECHANISM OF INJURY

The mechanism of injury is of major importance in the complete understanding of spine trauma. An analysis of injury mechanisms is beneficial and practical and can be helpful in choosing the technique of reduction and management of certain injuries. A recognition of the resultant injury as opposed to the mechanism of injury is also important. There are "families" of injuries that result from identical or similar mechanisms of injury. With a thorough understanding of the biomechanics involved, the association of certain injuries may come to be expected.

To build a system for evaluating injury mechanisms, it is necessary to challenge, if not destroy, some of the current "ways of thinking," which may create difficulties with terminology. Physicians speak of flexion injuries, extension injuries, rotation injuries, lateral bending injuries, and compression injuries. Studies of kinematics and analysis of forces in the motion segment have shown that these types of traditional descriptions of patterns of motion in the spine are no longer adequate to completely explain spine mechanics and injury mechanisms. The traditional concept of flexion or extension is not one simple motion, but involves two types of motion, such as translation as well as rotation in the sagittal plane. Depending upon the force vector, markedly different patterns of motion as well as vertebral deformation may be produced. Another case in point is lateral bending, which involves rotations about the horizontal and vertical axes, respectively, as well as translation perpendicular to the sagittal plane. In other words, lateral bending may cause any combination of transverse shear in the horizontal plane, rotational shear about the vertical axis, and tensile and compressive stresses in the vertebral bodies. Therefore, to assume that a mechanism of injury involves only lateral bending is an oversimplification. In order to develop a system for describing mechanisms of injury, the analysis may be carried out with the motion segment as the analytical unit. The load-displacement and failure patterns may then be analyzed and described in that context.

Any of the six degrees of freedom of a motion segment can carry with it an associated force or bending moment (torque). Kinematics explains that the coupling patterns are inherent to the motion segments in most regions of the spine (see

Chapter 2). Orientations in three-dimensional space of different motion segments at the time of injury modify these coupling patterns.

Crucial to an analysis of the forces involved is an understanding of the instantaneous axis of rotation. This axis dictates the pattern of deformation that occurs in the motion segment as a function of its relationship to the force applied. For example, a vertical force applied anterior to the IAR causes flexion. The same force applied posteriorly to the IAR produces extension. Therefore, in analyzing the mechanism of injury, the motion segment or motion segments involved must be evaluated, considering the six possible degrees of freedom and the various IAR due to application of different force vectors.

After taking into consideration the varying degrees of freedom of movement of the vertebra, it is then important to analyze some of the characteristics of the forces and moments that may be applied. Generally, in civilian injuries, forces come in at some slightly inclined angle, off one of the three orthogonal axes, x, y, or z. As a result of clinical habit, patterns, and reality, the large majority of analyses have been involved with sagittal plane motion, with the injuring force vector presumed to be somewhere in the sagittal plane. In other words, vertical compression and flexion/extension mechanisms tend to predominate in the injuries physicians observe. In airplane ejection injuries, there is nearly vertical force, with minimal eccentricity close to the y-axis in the sagittal plane. Even here, the various regions of the spine are subjected to flexion, compression, or extension due to varying curvature of the spine. Civilian flexion/extension injuries include whiplash, bilateral facet dislocations, and hangman's fractures.

The forces vary tremendously in the rate of application and magnitude. Due to the difference in stiffness and energy-absorbing capacities of the ligamentous structures and the bone, it is theoretically possible that the failure point of the bone-ligament complex of the motion segment may vary as a function of the magnitude, direction, and rate of application of these forces. This factor may explain some of the discrepancies and disagreements in the literature concerning whether the bone or the ligamentous structure fails first. An example in point is the controversy of the fracture of the dens versus the rupture of the transverse ligament of the dens. Although there have been no experiments to test this in the spine, it may be that the rate of application of the load determines whether the ligament or the bone fails first. The work of Noyes and colleagues shows that such a phenomenon is operative elsewhere in the body.[87] There is another possibility to be considered. For a given individual, one structure may be stronger than the other. There is adequate basis to assume that there is a broad variation in the strength of the dens, given the numerous congenital variations in the ossification centers and the complex lines of potential weakness due to failure of normal maturation and fusing together of these centers. These considerations exemplify the complications that may be involved in an analysis of the mechanism of injury.

An understanding of normal kinematics in the various regions of the spine is essential. For example, the amount of rotation that is permitted about the y-axis (in the horizontal plane) in the cervical spine is significantly greater than that observed in the lumbar spine. The alignments of the facets in the lumbar region does not allow much rotation about the y-axis. When the normal range of rotation about the y-axis is forcefully exceeded, there is fracture or disruption of the lumbar facets and/or posterior elements.

The spine has certain characteristics that predispose different areas to injury. The classic example is the thoracolumbar area. Predisposition to injury here is thought to be due largely to the stress concentration imposed by the abrupt increase of the stiffness from the thoracic to the lumbar spine. This is due to a rather abrupt change of the alignment of the facet joints, from the thoracic type of orientation to that of the lumbar, which involves a rotation of the facet joint planes by almost 90 degrees about the y-axis (see p. 40; Chap. 2). Most studies of injury have shown this region to be the most frequent site of spine fractures. However, Griffith and colleagues have published an article which describes the changing patterns of fractures in the dorsal and lumbar spines. They noted that there were two peaks of incidence of injury. The highest was in the mid-portion of the thoracic spine, the second being at the thoracolumbar junction.[52] The authors can only offer a theoretical explanation for this area of high incidence. Since it is a relatively stiff area, it is less able to absorb energy before failure. Moreover, because of its location, large bending moments are readily exerted.

RESEARCH DATA

There have been a number of experimental studies designed to evaluate the mechanics of spinal injuries. Studies on the application of forces to the spine have been reviewed in Chapter 1. Here, some of the salient experiments and findings regarding spine trauma are discussed.

Roaf applied static loads to fresh frozen autopsy motion segments, using an experimental apparatus that applied compressive loads.[106] He recognized that this was not the most characteristic rate of application of loading found in injuries of the spine. The method was thought to be justified by the fact that on a few occasions, a more rapidly acting force was applied, and the same pattern of failure in the motion segment was observed. There are no values given for either of the rates of application. This basic work provides some reasonable guidelines to the sequence of events that may be involved in the compressive loading of vertebrae in trauma. There is the initial deformation. The disc is relatively less compressible than the vertebra when tested in a normal motion segment. Therefore, there is bulging of the vertebral end-plate. The process continues to subsequent failure of the end-plate, which is probably the first structure to fracture. As deformation proceeds there is a fracture of the cortical shell and compression of the cancellous bone. This study did not demonstrate the phenomenon suggested by Armstrong, which involves pressing of the nucleus material on the annulus, causing a localized protrusion.[6] However, in the older specimens where the nucleus was no longer fluid, Roaf recognized that there was asymmetrical compression and sometimes pressure transmitted to the annulus, resulting in either tearing of the annulus or general collapse of the vertebra due to the buckling at the sides. This study also included experiments in which the resistance of the annulus with and without the presence of a fluid nucleus pulposus was compared. After denucleation (the removal of the nucleus pulposus), compressive loading produced typical annulus prolapses of the type seen in operations involving disc protrusions. Roaf suggested that this may have considerable medicolegal significance, since a vertebral endplate fracture with extrusion of the nucleus into the vertebral body and loss of disc turgor may result in the subsequent development of typical annulus herniation.

There were other fundamental facts related to spine trauma that came out of this work. Roaf indicated that he was not able to produce a "hyperflexion injury" of a normal intact spinal unit because vertebral body crush always occurred prior to the rupture of the posterior ligaments. Similarly, he recognized it was not possible to rupture the anterior longitudinal ligament in the cervical spine by pure hyperextension force prior to producing crushed fractures of the neural arch. He noted that the ligamentous structures, while significantly resistant to compression and tensile loading of the motion segment, were quite vulnerable to rotation. He also noted that the disc was subject to injury due to the horizontal shear forces produced by the rotation. Thus, when there are extensive ligamentous ruptures, clinically the possibility of rotation (moments about the y-axis) should be strongly considered in an analysis of the mechanism of injury.

Farfan and colleagues carried out experiments which led them to the hypothesis that the annulus does not tend to fail with compressive loading, but rather with shear loading.[40] This is no reason, however, to assume that compression and shear, as well as bending, may not be contributing factors. In this same study it was observed that, with compressive loading of the motion segments, blood was squeezed out of the cancellous bone of the vertebral body. This phenomenon led to the rather appealing hypothesis that the fluid component of the blood in the spongy elastic vertebral body serves as a shock-absorbing mechanism. Such a mechanism is assumed to

work only at high rates of deformations, which is generally the situation in clinical spine trauma.

The study of Gosch and colleagues provides some interesting information about spine trauma. This investigation examined the effects of impact loading applied to the heads of monkeys. The animals were anesthetized, placed on a track, and accelerated into a fixed metal barrier. A transducer load cell mounted on the impact block measured the energy delivered to the head at the time of impact. High speed cinematography was used to analyze the movement following the impact. Lateral radiographs of the spine were taken after the injury, and specially prepared mid-sagittal cuts of the frozen vertebral column were made in order to study spinal cord compression by displaced bone fragments. The experimental design included three groups of animals. The magnitude of the force was varied in each of the three groups. In addition, the three groups were distinguished by loading the necks at the time of trauma in flexion, in extension, and under vertical compression (−y-axis). The investigators found that in addition to flexion or hyperextension, it was necessary to induce an axial rotation to the spine (y-axis rotation) in order to produce dislocation.[48] This of course corroborates the observations by Roaf and is especially significant because it employs living animals and more clinically realistic impact loading. Gosch and colleagues emphasized that the anterior and posterior compressive forces, especially those occurring in hyperextension, produced the greatest damage to the central portion of the spinal cord.

They also indicated that the muscle tone at the time of impact had a profound effect on the threshold of forces required to produce cord damage. Muscle tone was necessary to produce the cord injury. This is compatible with and somewhat supportive of the often stated assumption that, all other things being equal, the more relaxed individual (an infant or drunk) is less likely to be injured in a situation involving physical trauma.[A] A qualifying point should be added here. The assumption holds unless the magnitude of the traumatizing forces is low enough to be checked by the intrinsic splinting power of the subject's muscles.

There are a number of other research studies

related to spine trauma. The biomechanics of trauma to the spine is based upon studies of mathematical modeling, studies of anatomic specimens, studies of animals in vivo, studies of man in vivo, and clinical observations.

SOME COGENT STUDIES OF SPINAL CORD TRAUMA

This section presents some basic information about the pathoanatomic changes that occur in the spinal cord following trauma. Most of the points presented here have been selected from a comprehensive review by Dohrmann.[28] The studies are organized according to three basic questions: What happens to the spinal cord following mechanical impact, and when does it happen? What, if anything, can be done to therapeutically alter the sequence of events?

Pathoanatomic Changes

A number of investigators have reported posttraumatic alterations in nerve cells and myelinated fibers and demonstrated hemorrhage within the gray matter, which is generally followed by edematous changes in the white matter.[137-141] The amount of hemorrhage was grossly related to the magnitude of the contusing forces. Dohrmann's electron microscopic studies revealed that the hemorrhages in the spinal cord contusion were probably related to tears in the walls of the muscular venules that are located in the gray matter.[30] Turnbull noted that the central vessels in the spinal cord are oriented so as to be stretched and compressed by a posteroanterior force.[135] This implies a greater vulnerability of the cord to forces in the sagittal plane of the z-axis. In other words, abnormal anterior or posterior translation of the vertebrae is more likely to cause damage to these vessels and therefore the spinal cord.

Temporal Considerations

It has been shown that when the intrinsic vessels of the spinal cord of the cat are injured to the point of paraplegia, the perfusion of the gray matter is reduced as early as 15 minutes after experimental trauma, and after one hour the flow is virtually nonexistent.[29-32] However, it is injury to the major sensory and motor tracts, located in the white matter, that is responsible for the devastating functional loss following contusion of the spinal cord. After trauma, the perfusion of the white matter decreases and begins to stabilize by approximately 1 hour, but returns within 24 hours after injury (transitory traumatic paraplegia), or continues to decrease (permanent traumatic paraplegia).[30] This decrease in blood flow patterns in the white matter is due to vasospasm and is probably secondary to the posttraumatic subarachnoid hemorrhage.[29]

Investigators have observed a centrifugal progression of edema in feline spinal cords during the first 8 hours following trauma.[50,138] At 1 hour following contusion, edema primarily involved the gray matter. At 4 hours, it had progressed to the immediately adjacent white matter. By 8 hours, the entire contused spinal cord had become edematous. As expected, there is a correlation between the magnitude of the force applied to the spinal cord and the associated damage.

Magnitude of Trauma and Degree of Damage

Allen in 1911, first quantitated experimental trauma applied to the spinal cord. He found that by dropping a 30-g mass approximately 10 cm perpendicularly onto the thoracic spinal cord of dogs, temporary paraplegia was produced.[B] If the impact was increased by dropping the 30-g mass from a height of 14 cm, the dogs were rendered permanently paraplegic. Intramedullary hemorrhage and edema were the changes noted within 4 hours following impact. In a recent paper, correlation has been established, at least in cats, between the magnitude of trauma (as measured by impulse) and the resulting spinal cord lesion.[B,29a] Another method of quantitating spinal cord trauma is to place a small hydraulic balloon in the epidural space and apply measured compressive forces. These studies were done by Tarlov and colleagues, who observed degeneration at the level of the balloon and also extension of pathology in both directions away from the site, commensurate with the amount of pressure applied.[128-130] This observation is significant because it probably explains the frequently observed clinical finding of spinal cord damage a variable distance from the location of the recognized trauma.

The observation of coalition or extension of damaged areas of the spinal cord has other clinical significance. Dohrmann and colleagues showed experimentally in monkeys that a "transitory traumatic paraplegia," which appeared to be complete, could resolve spontaneously in 1 to 2 weeks after injury.[29] This was the case provided that bleeding was local, central, and did not coalesce to form a large hemorrhage involving the entire gray matter. This implies that recovery is at least partially dependent on the size and extent of the damage caused by the initial trauma and also fits with the generally good prognosis in the clinical central spinal cord syndrome. In some instances, recovery may be related to collateral circulation. Kamiya carried out studies in which he experimentally compressed the anterior region of the cervical spinal cord in dogs. Through his studies he was able to recognize a fair amount of compensatory circulation between the anterior spinal artery, the central arteries, and the longitudinal anastomotic vessels near the central canal.[68]

Effects of Treatment

What, if anything, can be done to prevent the pathologic changes associated with spinal cord trauma? Richardson and Nakamura applied local compression that produced intramedullary edema but no hemorrhage.[105] Interestingly, these investigators were apparently able to reverse all of the electron microscopic alterations associated with the low grade trauma with a combination of local hypothermia and steroids. White and colleagues reported that local hypothermia beginning 6 to 8 hours after the contusion did not significantly alter the pathologic changes in spinal cord morphology.[150] Albin and colleagues contused spinal cords and then applied local hypothermia. They observed that if the hypothermia was instituted within 4 hours of contusion, the animals regained most of their sensory and motor function. However, if this was not initiated until 8 hours following contusion, then there was a failure to demonstrate recovery.[1] Other studies demonstrating recovery included those by Ducker and Hamit, who were able to demonstrate

recovery using either local hypothermia or steroids within the first 3 hours following injury.[33]

Hartzog and colleagues and Kelly and colleagues, following contusion on the spinal cords of experimental animals, were able to demonstrate functional recovery with the use of hyperbaric oxygen.[56,73]

Black and Markowitz observed that steroids enhanced functional recovery, while incision of the dura mater had deleterious effects in monkeys with contused spinal cords. They also noted that recovery rates were the same for monkeys decompressed with a one- or a three-level laminectomy.[12]

In general, most studies evaluating various treatments in experimental spinal cord contusion have utilized small control (untreated) groups. In a group of over 100 unrelated animals with spinal cord contusions, the lesions produced were found to be more clinically variable than initially believed. This suggests that some of the "improvements" observed with various treatments may not have been caused by the treatments. Therefore, to make definite conclusions apropos of treatment efficacy, large control groups are necessary.*

Osterholm and colleagues described an increase in intramedullary norepinephrine after trauma. Excessive accumulation of norepinephrine and hemorrhage into the gray matter of contused spinal cords was prevented for up to 6 hours by administering alpha-methyl tyrosine within 15 minutes after the experimental trauma.[89,90] However, other investigators have not been able to confirm this reported increase in norepinephrine.[26,33,57,84,103]

In order for these factors to demonstrate any effect in the experimental situation, they must be operative soon after the injury. It is rarely possible in the clinical situation to achieve this. Nevertheless, based on these and other experimental studies, clinical practices continue to include the use of a number of such variables, so far with inconclusive results.

Summary of Spinal Cord Trauma

The major points regarding spinal cord trauma are as follows. The primary pathoanatomic

---

* Personal communication, G. J. Dohrmann.

changes are hemorrhage and edema. The severity is related to the magnitude of the injuring force, or more precisely the energy, the momentum, and the impulse. The hemorrhage is usually in the central gray matter. The source of the hemorrhage is probably small tears in the walls of the muscular venules. Initially, the lesion is more central and then moves peripherally where it involves the white matter and causes most of the clinical damage. There are sometimes associated areas of hemorrhage rostrad and caudad to the site of impact. Steroids, local hypothermia, hyperbaric oxygen, and other agents to some degree have been shown in experimental animals to diminish or eliminate the hemorrhage and/or associated neurologic deficit. The modalities must, however, be applied as soon as possible, at least within the first 4 hours after injury. Neither laminectomy nor any of the other experimental treatments have had any degree of success in the clinical situation.

A SYSTEMATIC APPROACH TO ANALYSIS OF MECHANISM OF INJURY AND CLASSIFICATION OF SPINE TRAUMA

The problem of accurately analyzing mechanisms of injury in clinical spine trauma is a formidable one. In any given situation, for a mechanism of injury to be identified, a systematic analysis must be carried out. With thorough analysis of cumulative cases, accuracy and understanding is improved. In this section it is suggested that the thorough evaluation of a case of spine trauma, to determine mechanism of injury, include analysis in the following categories: detailed clinical history, detailed physical examination, application of research data, and biomechanical interpretation of radiographs.

Clinical History

The information here is often very unreliable for a variety of reasons. There may be amnesia, with no information or with confabulation. Often, in the excitement of the mishap, there is failure to observe, or there may be inaccurate observation. Sometimes, the history is quite definitive, as

in seat ejection injury or hangman's fracture. Injuries occur in unfortunate individuals on both sides of the law. Sometimes, especially in athletic injuries, the history is vivid and accurate to the smallest detail and can be confirmed and reexamined on slow motion film. The clinical history includes information that can be obtained from police records, direct examination, and photography of the accident site. Careful observations of skid marks and associated property damage in conjunction with expert consultation may generate useful and accurate information. On-site examination or photographic study of vehicles involved in an accident can provide clues or hard data. In a diving injury, where possible, a site visit can often contribute significantly to piecing together the complete analysis. One should gather as much relevant data as possible and weigh it according to circumstances, sources, and internal consistency.

Physical Examination

Bruises, lacerations, and associated fractures about the face and head can be helpful in determining the possible direction of force vectors. However, impact trauma may occur on *rebound* and a particular laceration may not be indicative of the direction of the force that caused the injury to the spine. Associated fractures in other areas of the spine, as well as in the long bones, may be helpful in determining the magnitude and direction of vectors involved in the injury.

Application of Research Data

There are basically three types of research information that may be usefully applied, clinical, experimental, and mathematical. There are a number of series of cases in the literature in which the mechanism of injury is reasonably well-defined and the pattern of failure of the spine is well documented. Examples include the hangman's fracture, seat ejection fractures, seat belt fractures, and some compression fractures of the thoracic and lumbar spine. A number of experimental studies have subjected animals and cadavers to various types of trauma in controlled situations. The injuries were studied anatomically and through movies, cineradiography, and radiography. This data can be reasonably extrapolated and applied to clinical situations in a manner that provides additional analytical insight and some standard with which to check "deduced" mechanisms of injury.

Biomechanical Interpretation of Radiographs

Here the clinician analyzes the radiographs, taking into consideration the information from the history and physical examination. In addition, the radiographs are interpreted in the context of current biomechanical knowledge and principles. Some guidelines for the biomechanical interpretation of radiographs of the spine after trauma follow. These are not absolute rules, but acceptable maxims based on current knowledge.

Guidelines for Biomechanical Interpretation of Radiographs

Bone tends to fail first along lines of tensile stress, then it may fail as a result of either shear or compression. Presumably it is best designed to withstand compressive loads.

One may assume that in the cervical spine, the anterosuperior or the anteroinferior triangle of bone, seen frequently on lateral radiographs, is pulled off by the peripheral annulus fibrosus fibers. Thus, the triangular portion of the vertebral body (actually the anterosuperior rim) may be pulled off in an extension type of injury, where the triangular fragment stays with the annular fibers, which remain attached to the intact vertebra, and the fractured vertebra is pulled away by the tensile loads. However, it is also possible in a flexion injury for compressive loading to result in high shear stresses, causing failure along approximately the same lines in which tensile failure would occur (Fig. 4-1).

In compression of a motion segment, the vertebral body endplate generally fails first.

Wedging of the configuration of vertebral bodies occurs as a result of compression from eccentric forces.

In the normal anatomy of the motion segment, with most loading vectors, the bone tends to fail before the ligamentous structures. There are exceptions.

Where there is wide separation between the anterior and posterior elements, indicating ligamentous rupture, most probably a significant element in the mechanism of injury is axial rotation (torque about the y-axis).

Narrowing between vertebral bodies at a given interspace where there is other evidence of trauma is suggestive of failure of the annulus or its attachment, implicating a mechanism involving shear or tensile loading.

There is an important variable that is time dependent and must be taken into consideration. In any injury to a complex structure such as the spine, there are a number of changes that occur between the onset and completion of the injury. The structures change in geometric and physical prop-

---

erties, and the force vectors of injury change in direction and magnitude. As a consequence, the clinician is faced not with just the analysis of one isolated injury, occurring instantaneously at one structure, but also with a series of rapidly changing injury mechanisms occurring at a series of rapidly changing structures. Current analyses need not seek this level of complexity. However, the oversimplification involved in the use of a static two-dimensional representation of a complicated series of dynamic, three-dimensional events should be kept in mind.

The radiographic evidence is interpreted and analyzed along with available information from the clinical history, physical examination, and research data. A major injuring vector (MIV) is determined. This is challenged by the evaluator, to see that there is internal consistency and that the information from all four categories corresponds. Rarely will everything fit perfectly, but the extent to which this or some other systematic approach is applied determines the accuracy of analysis and the level of understanding.

Designation and Analysis of Injury Using MIV

In 1972 Roaf suggested an international classification for spinal injuries.[108] Here, an independently determined system, similar to the one suggested by Roaf, is used. The coordinate system has a different orientation and has been submitted for consideration as an international standard.[93,148] Concluding that an injury is merely the result of flexion or extension is not an adequate analysis of the forces acting on the motion segment. The text is written so that the reader who does not, so to speak, get down to the xyz of it can progress smoothly without the classification. However, the reader is encouraged to consider the system, since its use is a step toward a biomechanical understanding of the spine.[c]

The system is as follows. Dislocations are described cephalocaudally; the more cranial unit is described as dislocated in relation to its normally positioned subjacent fellow. Examples include occipital-atlantal, atlanto-axial, C5 on C6, T8 on T9, and L3 on L4. The dislocations are described as posterior, anterior, lateral, or rotary. Occasionally the coordinate system is used in parentheses to indicate the displacement. The anteroposterior radiographs are viewed and de-

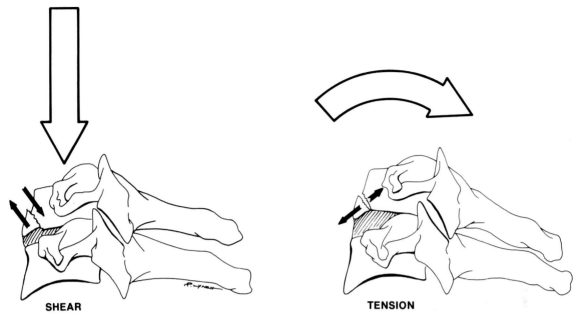

SHEAR   **TENSION**

Fig. 4-1. A triangular fragment of bone at the anteroinferior portion of the vertebral body may result from either shear or tensile failure. In compressive loading there are shear stresses along a line about 45 degrees to the force vector. In extension loading, the same region of bone is subjected to tensile stresses.

scribed as though the examiner is behind the patient, looking at the back of the radiograph. The examiner's right is the patient's right. Open mouth views of the dens are viewed with the examiner and patient face to face.

The term *major injuring vector (MIV)* is used to describe the mechanism of injury. Any given injury results from a complex series of forces and moments applied to the body in a variety of different ways. Ultimately the loads are transmitted to the motion segment in the region of the spine where the injury takes place. The most important complex of forces that causes the injury may be summarized and represented by the vector MIV. The coordinate system and a three-dimensional diagram to show the most representative orientation in space are used. The diagrammatic spatial orientation is occasionally supplemented by designating where the MIV is pointing in the coordinate system. No attempt has been made to estimate or indicate vector magnitude. Where certain bending motions are of particular importance they have been indicated on the diagram.[D]

REVIEW OF SOME SPECIFIC CERVICAL SPINE INJURIES

Occipital-Atlantal Dislocation

This rare and often fatal injury usually consists of an abnormal anterior displacement of the skull in relation to the atlas (Fig. 4-2).

Mechanism of Injury. The mechanisms in these injuries are speculative. Presumably there is a major force vector of high magnitude, along the +z axis. The skull is translated anteriorly in relation to the atlas. Mainly, this causes a shear type of loading at the atlanto-occipital joint, rupturing the articular capsule and causing the dislocation.

Discussion. In this injury, the central nervous system is usually damaged or transected at the medulla oblongata or at the spinal medullary junction. The injury usually causes death and may not be recognized at autopsy unless specifically looked for with flexion/extension radiographs. Alken and colleagues studied 146 accident fatalities and found that 21 per cent had

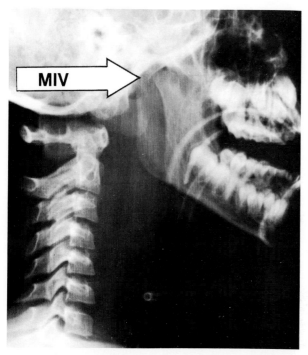

Fig. 4-2. A radiograph of a 9-year-old girl who sustained an occipital-alantal dislocation when hit by an automobile. The MIV is a large magnitude force vector, directed mainly in the positive direction along the z-axis (anterior translation in the sagittal plane). There is also an increased space between the spinous processes of C1 and C2 suggestive of disruption of the posterior ligaments and/or a fractured odontoid. The patient died shortly after this injury, which is usually fatal. (Courtesy of Teaching Library, Department of Diagnostic Radiology, Yale University School of Medicine.)

demonstrable neck injuries. Most of these injuries involved ocp–C1 or C1–C2.[2a]

There is one reported case of a patient who survived with an occipital-atlantal dislocation.[44] This involved a 41-year-old male who suffered an automobile accident. There was a lateral displacement of the occiput in relation to the atlas. The MIV was oriented along the x-axis. The injury was treated with a small amount of traction in a cervical brace for 5 months. Following this, the patient had a sensation of precariously balancing his head on his neck and had a clicking sound on moving his head. He was treated with a posterior cranio-cervical fusion.

It should be mentioned that occipital-atlantal dislocation has been reported in patients who have not suffered trauma.[38,80,143]

Suggested Treatment. Because of the precarious stability and the danger of fatality with minor injury, it is recommended that these injuries be treated with fusion from the occiput to C2 following 2 to 3 weeks of moderate skeletal traction of 3 to 4 kg (6–9 lb) weight.[H]

Fractures of the Posterior Arch of C1

Such a fracture occurs just behind the lateral masses, where the ring is grooved by the vertebral artery (Fig. 4-3).

Mechanism of Injury. Fractures of the ring of the first cervical vertebra are thought to occur primarily as a result of vertical compression on the posterior aspect of the arch of C1.[120] There may also be some acute rotation of the skull counterclockwise about the x-axis (some element of extension). In addition, the lateral masses of C2 may serve as a fulcrum at the site of injury. The anterior arch of C1 is locked, buttressed, or fixed by these lateral masses, while the posterior ring is displaced in the caudad (−y) direction. This results in a tensile failure of the bone on the cephalad surface of the ring, where these fractures generally appear to start. This is compatible with the presumed mechanism of injury and the generally accepted maxim that bone fails in tension. The cephalad surface of the ring is in tension in this injury mechanism. This is the weakest point of the ring because it is thinnest and has the lowest area moment of inertia against the type of loading involved. This is due to grooving at the site bilaterally, where the vertebral artery courses from its osseous vertebral canal across the ring of C1 and into the foramen magnum.

Since this fracture is sometimes seen along with the so-called hangman's fracture, presumably the two injuries have similar mechanisms (Fig. 4-4). In both situations, some element of extension is involved. However, in this fracture the major associated force is compression, whereas in the other injury bending is a significant factor.

Discussion. The symptoms associated with this injury are headaches, suboccipital pain, or nonspecific pain associated with stiffness. The

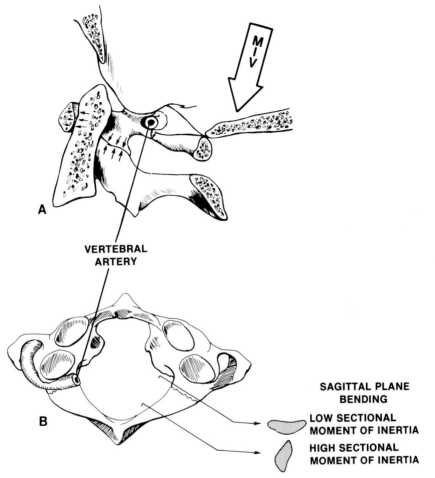

VERTEBRAL ARTERY

SAGITTAL PLANE BENDING

LOW SECTIONAL MOMENT OF INERTIA

HIGH SECTIONAL MOMENT OF INERTIA

Fig. 4-3. This diagram demonstrates how biomechanical and anatomic factors work together to result in a typical fracture of the posterior arch of C1. (A) A mid-sagittal section of the occipital-atlanto-axial complex shows a possible mechanism of injury, one which causes fracture of the ring of C1. A force causing extension (−x-axis rotation) results in fixation of the anterior ring of C1 against the dens, and fixation bilaterally at the articular condyles between the ring of C1 and C2. With this fixation, it is possible for the impingement of the occiput against the posterior ring of C1 to cause a bending moment about the ring of C1, as shown. Note the position of the vertebral artery, at which point the ring of C1 is grooved and weakened. (B) The top view of the ring of C1 shows the vertebral artery on the left in the region of the fracture. On the right side the sectional moment of inertia against bending in the sagittal plane is much smaller where the fracture occurs than it is in the more posterior area, where the resistance to bending in that plane is much greater. The areas are shown by the cross-sections at these two points. In addition to the considerations of the effects of the sectional moment of inertia on the location of the fracture site, there is another factor. Forces are applied at the tip of the ring of C1 by the occiput; thus, the maximum bending moment is also at the site where the fracture occurs.

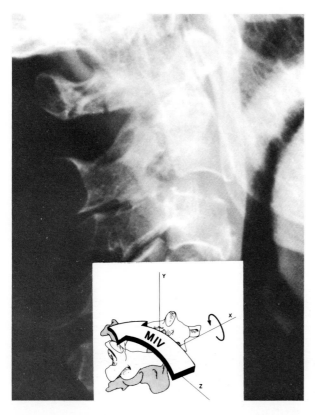

Fig. 4-4. A radiograph of an elderly woman who fell down a flight of stairs and sustained a fracture of the posterior ring of C1 and a traumatic spondylolisthesis. This exemplifies the association of the fracture of the ring of C1 with traumatic spondylolisthesis. The ring of C1 is thought to be bent such that the convexity points caudad. Note that the fracture appears to begin on the caudad side of the ring. The MIV is a negative bending moment in the sagittal plane about the x-axis, shown diagrammatically in the inset. This injury is interesting to contrast with the one shown in Figure 4-3 where the fracture starts on the cephalad side of the ring. In this fracture, there is a traumatic spondylolisthesis and failure of the annulus anteriorly. Note the abnormal separation between the bodies of C2 and C3. As a result of these two injuries, C1 is *not* fixed by impinging against a stable C2, as in Figure 4-3. Consequently, it rotates and impinges on the posterior elements of C2, creating a bending moment in the same plane but in an opposite direction. Thus, the fracture starts at the caudad portion of the ring. Such a fracture of the ring of C1 should alert the clinician to the probability of disruption of the anterior elements of C2.

diagnosis can be readily made by a lateral radiograph of this area.

In rare instances the vertebral artery may be involved, which may cause symptoms of basilar insufficiency. In the classic review by Jefferson in 1920,[66] he referred to two patients who had vertebral artery involvement, mentioned by Delorme in 1893.[27] In the review by Sherk and Nicholson, arteriovenous fistula involving the vertebral artery was discussed as a complication of this injury.[120] Arteriography should be considered in cases where there is a question of vascular involvement.

Suggested treatment. When these fractures are not displaced or only moderately displaced and not comminuted, they may be presumed to be stable. This should be confirmed with flexion/extension films, taken with caution after local symptoms subside, provided there is no neurologic injury. These injuries may be treated for 3 months with an orthosis that offers intermediate control of the cervical spine, a cervical appliance

that has, in addition, shoulder and thoracic support. Orthotic devices are discussed in Chapter 7.

If the fracture is thought to be unstable, the patient should be treated with traction for 2 to 3 weeks, followed by either a Minerva cast, halo plaster fixation, or a fusion of occiput to C2. The choice is made according to the individual surgeon's evaluation of the specific patient, since none of the three offers a distinct advantage. This is a stable injury in most instances and therefore does not require any such vigorous treatment.

Comminuted Fracture of the Ring of C1

This so-called Jefferson fracture is classically described as a four-part fracture of the ring of the atlas.

Mechanism of Injury. The mechanism was first described in 1920. The fracture is a result of compression, usually due to a direct blow on the vertex of the head. The spatial orientation of the occipital condyles are such that when they are driven axially in the caudad direction they act as a wedge, causing a bursting effect and separating the ring of the atlas, usually into four parts. This is shown in Figure 4-5. The mechanism of this injury is not unlike that of a simple fracture of the ring of C1. There are two differences. The MIV in

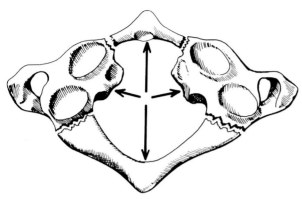

Fig. 4-5. This is the classical fracture described by Jefferson. Separation of the ring of C1 into four fragments is shown at the usual sites of failure.

transmitted through the skull to the anterior ring of C1, transmits the force to the dens, causing a shear failure as shown in Figure 4-7. This fracture can also occur in flexion or anterior translation injuries (+z-axis), in which an intact transverse ligament is strong enough to transmit enough force to fracture the dens.

Discussion. The dens may be thought of as a large stake with a horseshoe around it (Figure 4-8). The open end of the horseshoe has stretched across it a firmly attached strong bridal strap. The horseshoe is analogous to the anterior osseous ring of the atlas. The powerful transverse ligament of the atlas may be thought of as the bridal

the Jefferson fracture has a greater magnitude, and it is more in line with the y-axis.

Discussion. The salient radiologic characteristic of this fracture is bilateral displacement of the articular facet of the ring of C1, seen on an open mouth view with the head in a neutral position (Fig. 4-6).

Suggested Treatment. In the large majority of cases, this is a stable injury without neurologic involvement and may be treated by protective immobilization with a cervical orthosis of intermediate control. If there is gross lateral displacement of the lateral joints, their position may be improved by traction. In the less common situations where instability can be demonstrated, fusion of occiput to C1 should be considered and employed if necessary. The construct of choice is shown in Chapter 7.

Fractured Dens (Odontoid)

These fractures are grouped into three categories, those occurring in the dens, in the juncture of the dens and the body of C2, and at the base of the dens in the body of C2.

Mechanism of Injury. Fractures of the dens have apparently been associated with several mechanisms. Such fractures are seen in association with the hangman's fracture and presumably may be due to hyperextension forces, with the anterior ring of C1 transmitting the energy and causing the failure of the dens. A more direct force vector from anterior to posterior (−z-axis),

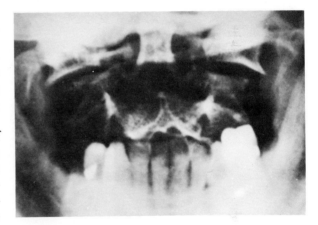

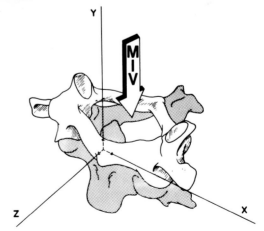

Fig. 4-6. A radiograph of a 47-year-old male with a Jefferson fracture. Note the wide separation of the lateral masses on the open mouth view of the dens. The MIV is shown on the inset. The orientation is not always exactly parallel with the vertical (y) axis.

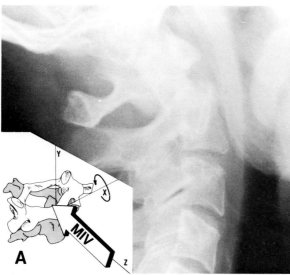

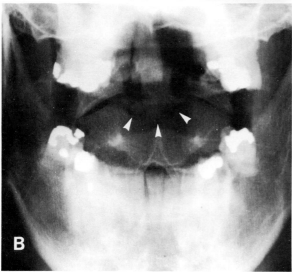

Fig. 4-7. Radiographs of a 33-year-old man who was struck in the front of the head with a heavy weight. He sustained a Type III fracture of the dens, which is most likely to heal. With the posterior dislocation and a history of a blow to the front of the head, we assume an MIV as shown. The vector is primarily in the horizontal plane parallel to the z-axis. The blow produces shear as well as a bending moment (hyperextension) of C1, as shown by impinging of the spinous process of C1 on C2. In comparison, there is relatively more shear here and relatively more torque than in Figure 4-4, traumatic spondylolisthesis and fracture of the ring of C1. Note that in Part *B* a tooth gives the appearance of a laterally displaced high odontoid fracture. The true fracture, documented on laminagrams, is indicated by the three small arrows. (Courtesy of Teaching Library, Department of Diagnostic Radiology, Yale University School of Medicine.)

strap. With powerful posterior translation resulting from large forces, the rigid horseshoe fractures the stake. With translation of sufficient force in the opposite direction, one of three forms of injury may occur: The well attached strong bridal strap may remain intact, and the stake becomes fractured; the bridal strap may rupture, and the stake remains intact (if there is sufficient displacement in this situation, cord damage occurs through the posterior ring of C1, which is not shown in the diagram); or the bridal strap may avulse at its attachment to the horseshoe. When avulsion occurs, a small fragment of bone between the dens and the lateral mass is sometimes visible radiographically on the open mouth view. Avulsion of the transverse ligament may permit displacement and cord injury. The determination of the occurrence of each of the three injuries in any given situation depends upon the physical properties of the involved structures, and the rate of application of the MIV, as well as other factors.

Suggested Treatment. Current knowledge suggests that treatment of the undisplaced dens fracture is based on a classification into three types.[4] Type I is an oblique fracture through the upper portion of the odontoid process. Type II is a fracture at the junction of the dens with the vertebral body of the second cervical vertebra. Type III is really a fracture through the body of the atlas at the base of the dens. Type I is common and benign. Treatment with a cervical orthosis of minimum or intermediate control is satisfactory. Even failure of union should not be a problem, as the fracture is too far above the level of the transverse ligament to cause any loss of stability.

Type II fractures are probably the most difficult to treat, are dangerous, and controversial. In this type, the rate of failure of union is 38 per cent, which is as high in undisplaced as in displaced dens. One alternative is to treat initially with immobilization for 4 months, followed by flexion/extension radiographs. Then, if union and stability are not present, fusion can be carried out.[109] The alternative approach is to proceed with elective fusion of Type II fractures in adults who are not undue surgical risks. There are other considerations here also. With surgery, at least 10 to 15 per cent of neck rotation is lost.[4] This figure may be higher, since normally about 50 per cent

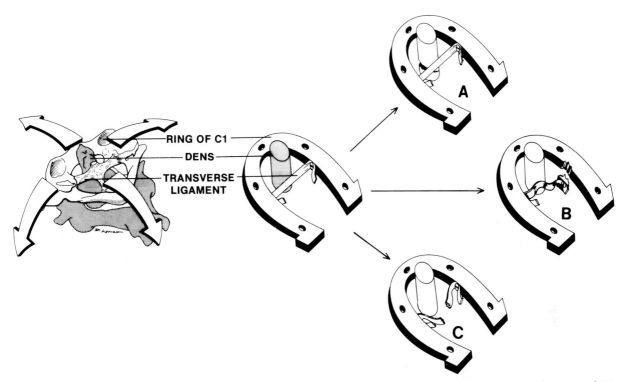

Fig. 4-8. Representation of the relationship between the dens and the transverse ligament in the ring of C1. A stake represents the dens, a horseshoe represents the bony ring of C1, and a bridal strap represents the transverse ligament. With various types of loading on these structures, three basic kinds of injury can occur. (*A*) There can be a fracture of the dens (a failure of the stake) with displacement in any direction. This may be due to impingement of the horseshoe against the stake, or impingement by the bridal strap. (*B*) There can also be a failure of the attachment of the stake or transverse ligament to the horseshoe. When this occurs, it is sometimes possible on the open mouth view of the dens to see a small fragment of bone lying between the odontoid and the lateral mass. (*C*) This shows the simple failure of the transverse ligament (bridal strap).

of axial rotation in the neck is at C1–2. On the other hand, a good deal of inconvenience and time and monetary loss may result when there is residual instability following conservative treatment. If the patient recovers without surgery, then of course there is no exposure to the unique and usual surgical risks involved. It is probably advantageous to present the pros and cons of surgery to the patient. The authors recommend the Brook's technique (see Chapter 8).[53]

Type III fractures (Fig. 4-7) may be expected to heal satisfactorily with conservative treatment, which consists of 10 to 14 days of traction, followed by a cervical orthosis that offers the most effective control for an additional 18 to 20 weeks. The healing rate is over 90 per cent,[4] but stability should be demonstrated by flexion/extension radiographs.

Traction is applied primarily to anchor the head and thereby splint for soft-tissue healing. It is not a particularly effective mechanism for reducing a deplaced dens fracture. This is because the anatomy of the region is such that there are few anatomic structures to transmit the necessary corrective forces to the odontoid for proper reduction and alignment. When there is no neurologic deficit and fusion has been elected, complete anatomic reduction of the dens fracture is not necessary.

Traumatic Atlanto-Axial Dislocations and Subluxation

These are a group of conditions in which trauma results in an abnormal relationship between the ring of C1 and the ring of C2. There may be either an anterior or posterior abnormal displacement of C1 on C2, or there may be a rotary subluxation of C1 on C2. These are discussed in detail in Chapter 5.

Mechanism of Injury. Obviously, the mechanism of injury in the three situations is not the same. For the anterior dislocation, the MIV is primarily along the +z-axis, causing an abnormal anterior translation and the dislocation. This is associated with a significant amount of flexion ($+\theta x$ rotation). The equilibrium between the magnitude of the MIV and the "strength" of the bone is such that in addition to a fractured dens, there is also enough force to cause a displacement. The MIV is oriented similar to that of the undisplaced dens fractures, and in addition consists of a force of sufficient magnitude to cause displacement as well as fracture.

When the fracture dislocation is posterior, the same analysis applies, except for a change in the direction of the MIV. The resultant translation and rotations are in the opposite directions. Two very unusual posterior dislocations of C1 on C2 have been described, in which the dens is spared and the ring of C1 is carried up over the tip of the dens.[55,96] An example is shown in Figure 4-9. In both of these case reports there was no significant fracture of the odontoid. There was a small fragment of bone anterior to the second cervical vertebra in one of the cases. The MIV in these injuries probably had a significant −y-axis component, in order to raise the ring of C1 up over the dens. Thus, the MIV is presumed to have been primarily in the sagittal plane, acting at the *origin* of the coordinates and directed 30 to 40 degrees between the −z-axis and the positive y-axis (Fig. 4-9).

The rotary subluxation of this joint presumably occurs when the force vector is not directly along the z-axis but is off center enough to create a torque about the y-axis and cause rotary dislocation or subluxation.

Discussion. In considering the clinical biomechanics of the atlanto-axial complex, what are the normal relationships at the ring of C1, and how are they maintained? What kinds of forces and structural failures are necessary to disrupt this relationship? What is necessary to reestablish and maintain the normal relationship?

A basic understanding of the functional anat-omy at the ring of C1 is crucial to any study of atlanto-axial pathology. Three anatomic perspectives of the ring of C1 are shown in Figure 4-10.

The normal relationships at the ring of C1 are maintained by a complex of the normal intact structures. The spatial relationship of the cord and the dens at the ring of C1 has been popularized as Steele's rule of thirds.[124] The anteroposterior diameter of the ring of C1 is approximately 3 cm. This space is allocated such that there is about 1 cm for the dens, 1 cm for the cord, and 1 cm of free space. In a detailed study by Wolf and colleagues, the spinal canal at the level of the atlas, in 200 subjects, was found to have a sagittal diameter ranging from 16 mm to 33 mm.[156] Carella carried out measurements in this area and found the sagittal diameter of the ring of the atlas to be consistently greater than that of the axis, sometimes by only a few millimeters. However, more significantly perhaps, was the observation that in patients who experienced hypoplasia or failure of fusion of the components of the ring of the atlas, there was a significant reduction in the sagittal diameter.[116] This should be kept in mind when making clinical judgments concerning patients who have congenital irregularities of the atlas. Relative allocation of space into three equal parts presumably remains the same throughout that range of variation of sagittal diameter. However, proper radiologic studies to evaluate the absolute and relative magnitudes of the dens, the spinal medulla, and the free space can be employed if required.

A review of some of the basic anatomic considerations may be helpful. Detailed discussions of the functional anatomy of this region are available and can be reviewed in the work of Martel and Werne.[80,145] The important relationship of the three anatomic perspectives of the ring of C1 (Fig. 4-10) on radiographic analysis has been summarized in the work of Shapiro and colleagues.[119] In the adult, the distance between the anterior arch of the atlas and the dens in flexion or a neutral position should not exceed 2–3 mm. In the child, this distance can be up to 3–4 mm. When these distances are exceeded, there is either rupture or laxity of the supporting ligaments, primarily the transverse ligament, and secondarily the alar, apical, and the capsular liga-

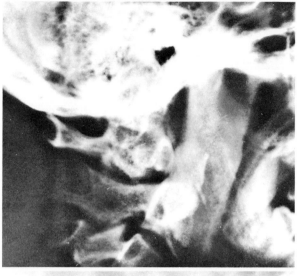

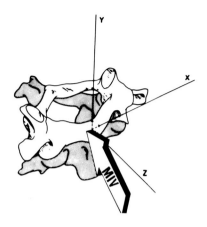

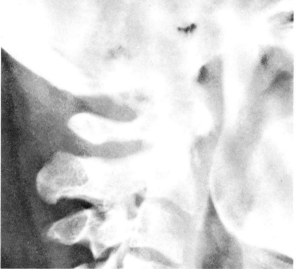

Fig. 4-9. Radiographs of a 34-year-old man involved in a motorcycle accident. The patient sustained a posterior dislocation of the atlas on the axis. The patient had a 4 × 4-cm abrasion over the left parietal region. The fracture was reduced by manual traction and manipulation applied through Vinke tongs without anesthesia. Note the small splinter of bone at the anterior base of the dens that can be seen in both the pre- and post-reduction films. The MIV is shown in the inset and is primarily a vector orientated in the y, z plane, making approximately a 30-degree angle with the positive y-axis. In order to force the anterior ring of C1 up to the tip of the dens and then posterior to it, a posteriorly directed extension injury must have occured. (Radiographs from Patzakis, M. J., et al.: Posterior dislocation of the atlas on the axis: a case report. J. Bone Joint Surg., 56A:1260, 1974.)

ments of the atlanto-axial joint. The other mechanism through which these special relationships may be disrupted is of course through a displaced fracture of the dens.

It has generally been accepted that significant traumatic displacement occurs only with fracture of the dens. Transverse ligament rupture has been thought to occur only secondary to other disease processes, or it is considered to be a spontaneous rupture.[145] In the past, it was believed that with loading which causes anterior translation (+z-axis), the bone generally fails

rather than the ligament, unless there is some active disease process involving the ligament or its bony attachment. However, recent experimental studies have shown that traumatic rupture of the transverse ligament in horizontal loading (+z-axis translation) can occur in the absence of odontoid fractures (Fig. 4-11).[41] The experimental work is supported by several case reports.

It is possible that traumatic rupture of the transverse ligament in patients with multiple trauma causes sudden death and is not recognized at autopsy; the cause of death is assigned

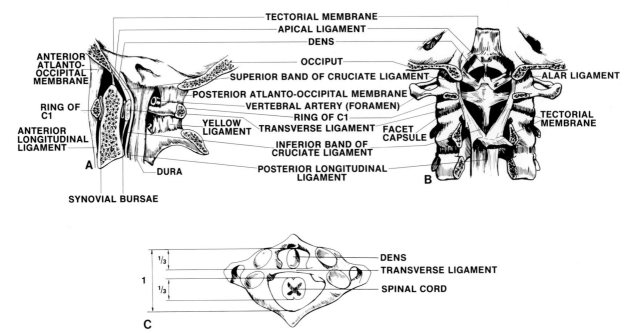

Fig. 4-10. Three anatomic perspectives at the ring of C1, including the functional anatomy of this region relevant to the biomechanics of spine trauma. (*A*) In the lateral view, note the bursa between the ring of C1 and the dens anteriorly, and the transverse ligament and dens posteriorly. There is also a bursa between the transverse ligament and the tectorial membrane. These bursae contain synovial tissue. They may be involved in abnormal displacements related to inflammatory processes resulting from either erosion of the dens or laxity or weakening of the transverse ligament. The apical ligament is seen in this view. It is one of the accessory ligaments of the occipital-atlanto-axial complex which, in conjunction with the alar ligaments, can offer some resistance to horizontal displacement after rupture of the transverse ligament. (*B*) This view shows the tectorial membrane folded down and up, with the superior portion of the cruciate ligament transected to view the apical and the alar ligaments, along with the tip of the dens. The posterior longitudinal ligament is a well developed structure which offers considerable stability to this area. Partial stability is offered by the apical and alar ligaments. (*C*) This view emphasizes Steele's rule of thirds. It shows the perspective of the upper view of the ring of C1 along with the odontoid and the spinal cord. One-third of the total anteroposterior diameter is constituted by the dens, one-third by the spinal cord, and one-third by free space.

to one or more of the other more readily recognized injuries. This assumption is well supported by the work of Alker and colleagues, who found that a large number of the 21 per cent fatal cervical spine injuries involved the C1-C2 articulation.[2a] These considerations raise pertinent and difficult questions in this already complex area of spine trauma.

Another possible mechanism of displacement of the ring of C1 is reported by Patzakis and colleagues.[96] If the odontoid is not fractured, and the transverse ligament is not ruptured, then displacement can occur by raising the ring of the horseshoe and bridal strap up over the stake (tip of the dens). Following this it either relocates by

falling back down anteriorly or it dislocates by falling posteriorly. Obviously, this displacement can be resisted or facilitated by the size and/or shape of the dens. Figure 4-12 readily shows that some dentes are more likely to allow the ring of C1 to ride up and over the tip of the odontoid. This may be caused by a force great enough to overcome the tensile forces imposed by the anterior longitudinal ligament. Figure 4-12 further shows that other anatomic characteristics can play a role in determining the type of injuries that result from a particular spatial orientation of a force vector.

Probably the most common atlanto-axial dislocation occurs with fracture dislocation of the

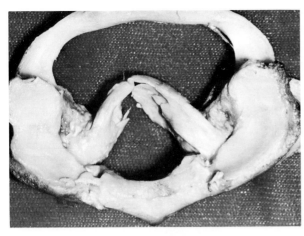

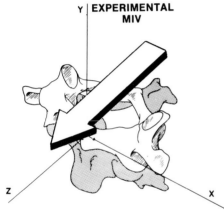

Y | EXPERIMENTAL
MIV

Z   X

Fig. 4-11. A photograph of experimental rupture of the transverse ligament. In cadaver studies this pattern of failure was observed in the absence of fracture. The experimental MIV is shown. This shows that it is mechanically possible to have transverse ligament failure and a C1-C2 dislocation without a fractured dens. (Fielding, J. W., Cochran, G. V. B., Lawsing, J. F., and Hohl, M.: Tears of the transverse ligament of the atlas, a clinical biomechanical study. J. Bone Joint Surg., 56A: 1683, 1974.)

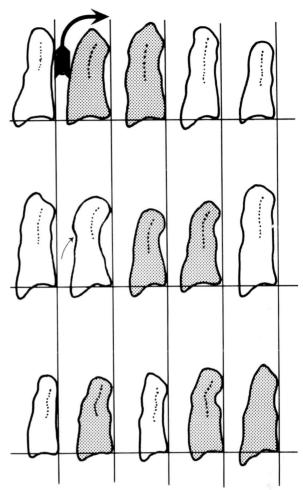

Fig. 4-12. The outlines of lateral radiograph of the dentes. Note the gentle posterior curves; those with dark shading appear more likely to allow the ring of C1 to slide up over the top of the dens and off posteriorly. This is indicated by the large arrow. The dens with the small arrow was not shaded, even though it has a considerable posterior curve. This is because of the little anatomic notch, indicated by the small arrow, which tends to prevent posterior dislocation. (Modified from Werne, S.: Studies in spontaneous atlas dislocation. Acta Orthop. Scand., Suppl. 23:35, 1957).

dens. Elliot and Sachs were among the first to focus on the problem in this perspective. They carried out a clinical and anatomic analysis in conjunction with a case presentation, a fascinating saga of a Russian carpenter who lived and worked for 32 years with an anterior atlanto-axial fracture dislocation. The patient experienced five subsequent injuries following his original fracture dislocation. On several occasions he recovered from formidable neurologic deficits of paralysis and sensory loss. He finally succumbed to

an injury which involved an irreversible neurologic deficit. Examination showed the encroachment of the spinal cord through a "tonsillotome" mechanism (Fig. 4-13). The posterior ring of C1 serves as the fixation fulcrum. Elliot and Sachs observed the relatively large space for the spinal cord at this level and suggested that this

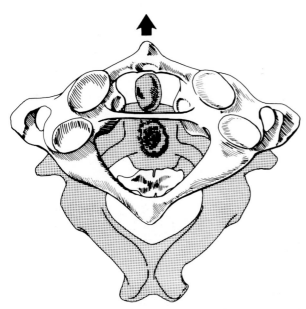

Fig. 4-13. Guillotine mechanism. This is a top view of the ring of C1 and C2. It demonstrates trauma in the upper portion of the cord through what may be called a "guillotine" mechanism. With this, various anatomic structures allow a displacement of the ring of C1 in relation to the ring of C2 to occur following a grossly displaced dens fracture. A relative horizontal translation of the ring of C1 on C2 applies shear forces of large magnitude to the cord. This is somewhat analogous to the mechanism by which a guillotine operates.

was probably the reason that the patient was able to live and work as long as he did.[135]

In discussing the atlanto-axial subluxation, it is important to mention the clinical significance of occipital pain due to the irritation of the sensory nerve at the occipital nerve which emerges between C1 and C2. This nerve may be irritated as a result of the abnormal displacement between the two vertebrae.

Suggested Treatment. The mechanical goal in the treatment of these patients is to reestablish, as much as possible, the normal anatomic relationships at the level of the ring of C1 and maintain them. The suggested treatment of traumatic C1–C2 subluxations and dislocations is reduction by skeletal traction, followed by fusion of C1 to C2. When there is no neurologic deficit, probably perfect anatomic reduction is not that important, in view of Steel's rule of thirds. Thus, if reduction

is not readily achieved, it need not be vigorously pursued. A solid fusion is the most important factor. The most compelling argument for fusion is that it is good insurance. There is evidence that a significant portion of atlanto-axial injuries can result in prolonged neurologic sequela and death if not stabilized by fusion. Some physicians have suggested nonsurgical treatment,[23] and others, fusion, if osteosynthesis is not achieved with conservative therapy.[43,94,109] Most have advocated some type of fusion.[2,4,25,35,58]

Deciding which levels to fuse and how to fuse them is open for discussion. If the ring of C1 is not fractured and is intact, a posterior fusion of C1–C2 is completely adequate to stabilize the joint. Including either the occiput or C3 further restricts the already compromized motion and is not necessary for stability. When there is a compromise of the ring of C1, the occiput should be fused to C2. The Brooks type of posterior fusion works well and has certain biomechanical advantages.[53] These are described in Chapter 8.

Most probably, some of the failures reported with fusion of C1–C2 are related to the choice and the execution of the surgical technique employed. Removal of the ring of C1 is rarely necessary as even a partial reduction, and adequate stabilization is usually sufficient to decompress and protect the cord.

Conservative treatment with prolonged immobilization, using either Minerva casts or fixation, has been recommended. Although the reported results in most cases have been satisfactory, the potential risk of depending on healed ligaments to maintain stability in this vital situation does not seem to be warranted.

"Spontaneous" Atlanto-Axial Dislocations

Abnormal displacement of the ring of C1 occurs either without trauma or with quite trivial trauma. These lesions have been given a long list of names which include torticollis nasopharyngien, malum suboccipitale rheumaticum, spontaneous hyperemic dislocation of the atlas, dislocation nontraumatique, distensionsluxation, maladie de Grisel, and nontraumatic subluxation. In the group of "spontaneous" atlanto-axial dislocations, a broad variety of other conditions are included, in which there may be abnormal displacement with little or no trauma. Figure 4-14 shows a spontaneous anterior subluxation of the atlas secondary to rheumatoid arthritis.

Mechanisms of Injury. There are a variety of different situations that predispose an individual to this injury. They are listed below. The final, common factor is that normal or only slightly greater than normal forces acting in the region cannot be tolerated by the anatomic structures and abnormal displacement occurs. The transverse ligament of the atlas is the most commonly involved "weak link." Presumably, it stretches, ruptures, or pulls out from its osseous attachment, allowing the displacement.

Discussion. An old, unrecognized, forgotton, or unsuccessfully treated injury can cause an apparent "spontaneous" atlanto-axial subluxation. Griswold and Southwick pointed out that a review of the literature showed an overall rate of failure of union for fractured dens of 20 to 40 per cent.[53] Although this is not generally considered to be a cause, when the diagnosis of "spontaneous" atlanto-axial subluxation is suggested, the patient should be questioned carefully, and when there is a history of injury, old radiographs should be reviewed.

Suggested Treatment. The subluxation should be reduced with appropriate traction and associated infection treated. Stabilization by posterior arthrodesis of C1–C2 is then carried out.

Conditions Associated With "Spontaneous" Atlanto-Axial Dislocations

Primary synovitis
    Rheumatoid arthritis
    Ankylosing spondylitis
    Psoriatic arthritis
Regional infections (viral, bacterial, spyrochetal,
    granulomatous)
    Nasal
    Oropharangeal
    Cervical
Primary or metastatic neoplasms
Congenital anomalies of the dens
Congenital laxity of the ligaments
    Down's syndrome
Poliomyelitis*
Previous, forgotten and/or undiagnosed traumatic injuries

---

* In 1934 Coutts described true subluxation of atlas in a patient with unilateral polio of the stabilizing muscles.

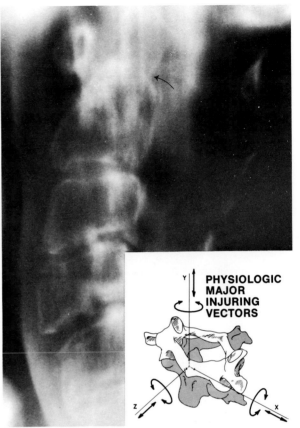

Fig. 4-14. Laminogram of an elderly man with severe rheumatoid arthritis. There is an abnormal separation between the dens and the anterior ring of C1. The MIV consists of the normal complex of physiologic forces acting on the weakened structures. The transverse ligament is lax; moreover, there has been some erosion of the posterior portion of the dens (note the bursa in Fig. 4-10), which allows for even more of an abnormal anterior (+z-axis) translation. (Courtesy of Teaching Library, Section of Neuroradiology, Yale University School of Medicine.)

Rotary Subluxation of C1,C2

In this entity there is a fixed abnormal rotation between C1 and C2. C1 is rotated about the y-axis in relation to C2 and is fixed in that position.

Mechanism of Injury. Presumably, the mechanism of this injury is acute axial rotation, resulting in disruption of the articular capsules of the joints articulating with the lateral masses. The MIV is a torque about the longitudinal axis. The injury can occur in the absence of fracture and is not generally associated with neurologic deficit.

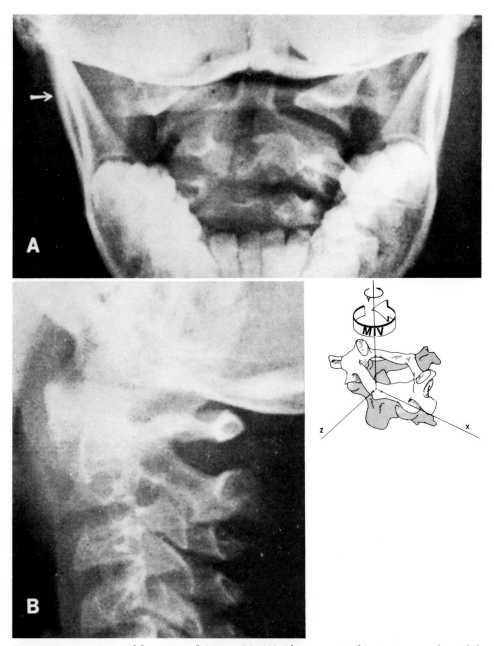

Fig. 4-15. A rotary subluxation of C1 on C2. (*A*) The arrow indicates an overlap of the lateral mass of C1 in relation to the articular facet of C2. This overlap occurs as a result of lateral as well as anterior displacement. (*B*) On the lateral view, one can see an abnormal displacement between the anterior portion of the dens and the posterior portion of the anterior ring of C1. The MIV for this type of injury is primarily a moment about the y-axis, as shown in the inset. (Radiographs from Garber, J. N.: Abnormalities of the atlas and the axis: vertebral, congenital and traumatic. J. Bone Joint Surg., *46A:*1782, 1964.)

Discussion. The diagnosis of this lesion can be elusive. Many patients may be seen with the head rotated to one side and tilted away from the side toward which it is rotated. This has been referred to "as a bird with his head cocked, *listening* for a worm." Based on the fact that the bird's eyes are at the sides of its head and are among its most precise sensory organs, and the assumption being that worms make little noise, the authors suggest that maybe the bird is *looking* rather than listening. In any case, a patient with head held in this position may have a C1,C2 rotary subluxation or spasmodic torticollis. The differential diagnosis of this entity constitutes a sizable list which includes psychiatric disease.

The key to the diagnosis of this condition is radiologic. Several articles have been written suggesting complex radiologic analysis, with one or two open mouth views to make the diagnosis.[63,64,119,142] Actually, this is unduly complicated and the normal anatomic variants make those evaluations difficult to interpret.* There are two radiologic signs that strongly suggest the diagnosis. One is unilateral superimposition of the lateral mass of C1 on one of the articular facets of C2, seen on the open mouth view. The other is anatomic anterior displacement (greater than 2 mm in an adult, greater than 3 mm in a child[119]) of the ring of C1 in relation to the dens, seen on a lateral film. Both of these findings are demonstrated in Figure 4-15.

Suggested Treatment. Reduction should be attempted with adequate axial traction. The evaluation and management of these injuries are discussed in detail in Chapter 5.

Vertical Subluxation of the Axis

Vertical subluxation of the axis can occur as a secondary process in rheumatoid arthritis. Figure 4-16 is an example of vertical subluxation with rheumatoid arthritis. This y-axis translation is due to the repeated gravitational loading on the lateral articular masses of C1 and C2. These weakened structures allow for the vertical cephalad (−y) displacement of the dens into the foramen magnum. Displacement can occur as a result of other

---

* Personal communication, R. Shapiro.

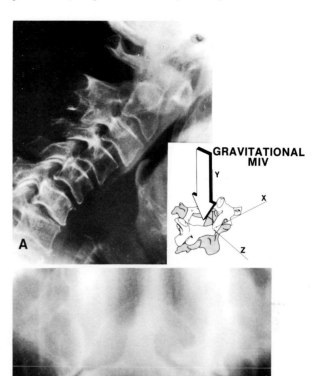

Fig. 4-16. Radiographs of an elderly male with severe rheumatoid arthritis. (A) Vertical subluxation of the axis. This is best described as a vertical (−y-axis) subluxation of the occiput. The dens is at the level of the occipital bone and just at the mouth of the foramen magnum. There is anterior subluxation of C1 on C2 and spontaneous fusion of the lateral masses of C2 and C3. (B) Lateral displacement of the dens and asymmetrical erosion of the lateral mass of C1. The vertical subluxation is largely due to the inadequate supporting structure of the lateral masses. The MIV is primarily the vertical component of the gravitational forces of the head, acting over a long period of time on the weakened bone. (Courtesy of Teaching Library, Section of Neuroradiology, Yale University School of Medicine.)

diseases including tuberculosis, Paget's disease,[86] and osteogenesis imperfecta.[104] It should be noted that there is not a consistent correlation between neurologic status and radiographic evidence of destruction and displacement.[126]

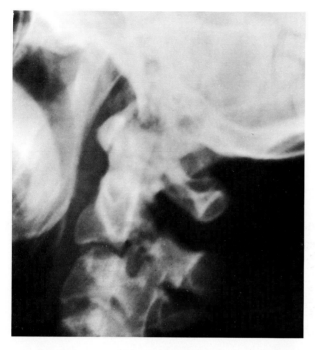

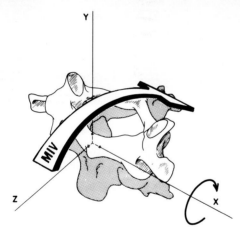

Fig. 4-17. Radiograph of an adult male who sustained in a motorcycle accident a fracture of the parietal bone and a hyperextension injury which resulted in a traumatic spondylolisthesis of C2. The separation of the posterior elements from the anterior elements are well demonstrated in this particular lateral view. The MIV is shown. A major factor is a negative torque about the x-axis. The vector creating the torque may be oriented so that it points more in the +y-axis, as in judicial hanging, or it may tend to point more in the direction of the −z-axis, as in the case of an automobile accident. (Courtesy of Teaching Library, Department of Diagnostic Radiology, Yale University School of Medicine.)

Treatment of these patients is highly individualized. When neurologic symptoms cannot be arrested or treated by conservative measures, such as rest, traction, and orthotic support, then surgery is indicated. Fusion of the posterior occiput to C3 is suggested. A construct designed to resist vertical (−y-axis) forces should be employed. For post-fusion fixation, a halo apparatus is best able to protect the neural elements while the graft matures.

Traumatic Spondylolisthesis of the Axis or "Hangman's Fracture"

There is a very important biomechanical consideration related to the phenomenon of judicial hanging. A considerable amount of information has been generated which relates radiographs and autopsy findings to a known mechanism of injury in a living human being. When the clinician observes similar failure patterns in different patients, a similar mechanism can be presumed to have been operative.

The hangman's fracture is a fracture of the second cervical vertebra which separates the anterior from the posterior elements of the vertebra. An example is shown in Figure 4-17. Thus, the fracture occurs in the anterior most portion of the lateral masses, or into the pedicle area of the vertebra. This fracture may be associated with fractures of other spinous processes or fractures involving the vertebral body of C3. There may be no associated neurologic findings, or there may be symptoms ranging from nerve root irritation to complete flaccid paralysis. There are several works that thoroughly describe this injury.[15a,37,79,115,153,157]

Mechanism of Injury. In judicial hanging with the submental knot, a number of observers have confirmed the lesion commonly known as hangman's fracture. In association with the fracture of the area between the two articular facets of C2, there are several other injuries. There may be complete disruption of the annulus fibrosus, with a dislocation of C2 on C3. Similar injuries are seen in automobile and diving accidents. Certainly, with the submental position of the rope, it is possible to document an extension-distraction type of injury in judicial hanging. The moment exerted on the dens and body of C2 may also create tensile forces on the intervertebral disc and sometimes result in an associated failure of that structure, with the possibility of large displacement between the anterior elements. Cornish observed disruption of the annulus in specimens that he studied.[22] The posterior ligamentous structures are thought to remain intact as they are compressed. Figure 4-18 gives a diagrammatic representation of the hangman's fracture.

There are some interesting anatomic considerations that are relevant here. The transverse foramen for the vertebral artery is in the region of the pedicle (isthmus) of C2.[22] Because of this foramen and the configuration of the neural arch, the structure of C2 in this region has a relatively low area moment of inertia to bending in the sagittal plane. This may be a factor in determining the site of failure. In addition, there is another structural consideration. The occipito-atlanto-axial complex has other characteristics which indicate failure at the pedicle (isthmus). The large extension force creates a bending

moment on the dens, so that it rotates in the sagittal plane about the −x-axis (Fig. 4-19). This bending moment is balanced by two forces. The tensile force produced in the anterior longitudinal ligament, the disc, and the posterior longitudinal ligament on one side, and a compressive joint reaction force between the facet joints of C2 and C3 on the other side. These two equal and opposite forces create the balancing bending moment. The effect of all of these loads is to produce maximum bending moment in the region of the pars interarticularis. As the cross-section of the bone is small, this site is the weakest and thus most susceptible to fracture during the type of load that results in a hangman's fracture.[E]

Discussion. Traumatic spondylolisthesis is an appropriate name for this fracture, since the defect occurs in the posterior elements as a result of trauma. The romantic and emotionally charged appellation of hangman's fractures will no doubt continue, despite the fact that this form of execution is less popular and it is really the "hangee" rather than the "hanger" who sustains the injury. In view of broadening equal occupational oppor-

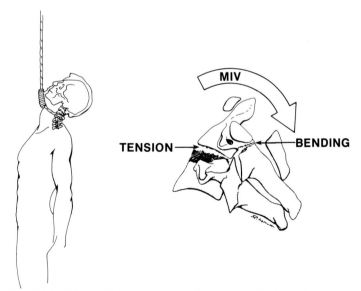

Fig. 4-18. The judicial hangman's fracture. With the submental knot there is a negative torque created about the x-axis. There is failure in the posterior osseous elements and separation anteriorly at the annulus fibrosus. The pattern of this injury varies with the relative magnitude of the component of the vector in the +y direction as well as the −z direction.

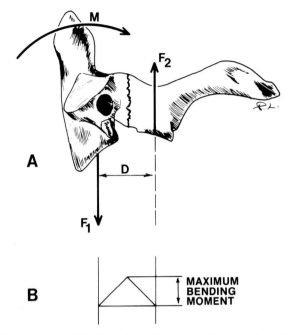

Fig. 4-19. (A) Vertebra C2 is acted upon by the bending moment M, applied by the anterior ring of C1, and a couple of equal, parallel, and opposite forces, F_1 and F_2, applied by C3. The bending moment and the couple balance each other. (B) The bending moment distribution along the pedicles is represented by the triangular bending moment diagram, which shows that in the middle of the pedicle, there is maximum bending moment.

tunities for women, perhaps it should be called the "hanged person" fracture.

The use of this name and the presumably similar mechanism in auto accidents and other injuries has been questioned by some physicians. They point out that many individuals who sustain this injury are not infrequently without even transient neurologic symptoms. The difference is explained by the magnitude and *direction* of the MIV and the duration of load application in the judicial victim, who must "hang by the neck until dead." With the prolonged duration of the load, viscoelastic instability becomes operative, and the critical failure load of the soft tissues is reached, causing separation of vertebra and neurologic death. Should this somehow fail to happen, strangulation assures demise.

These injuries, when secondary to diving or auto accidents, are often without neurologic symptoms. Perhaps this occurs because spondy-

lolisthesis creates a loose neural arch that can further accommodate the cord in an area where it normally has more than ample space.[97]

Actually, there are a large family of injuries which have in common a fracture in the region of the pedicle (isthmus) of C2. The complex of injuries that occurs depends on the specific force vectors involved, the magnitude, direction, point of application, and the duration of application. In addition, the position of the structures of the spine at the time of impact and the individual mechanical properties of the structures in that particular patient all determine the particular injury, the elements destroyed, and the amount of displacement. When one observes a traumatic spondylolisthesis of C2, $-\theta x$ bending moment is the major component of the injuring forces. Therefore when this type of fracture is found, we know from judicial hanging that the most likely mechanism of injury is extension.

In auto accidents, where the extension may be due to the forehead hitting the steering wheel or a slanted windshield, a vertical axial component of compression may be involved, along with the rotary bending moment (Fig. 4-20). Rogers has noted considerable crushing of the third cervical vertebra in addition to the C2 fracture.[110] He also noted other injuries that did not fit neatly with a simple extension mechanism. One of his patients had facet fractures between C7 and T1, which strongly suggests a compressive force. In judicial hanging there is a bending moment creating extension with *tensile* forces on the cervical spine, where as in the auto accident there is a similar bending moment but with *compressive* forces on the cervical spine.[153]

Suggested Treatment. It is obvious that not all hangman's fractures should be treated in the same manner. The treatment actually depends on what, if any, associated injuries are present. Although the posterior ligaments are generally intact, they make no contribution to stability because of the defect of the pedicle. Clinical experience has shown that the defect usually heals with effective protection and immobilization.[15a] However, if, in addition, there is a defect of all the anterior ligaments, then the level is most probably unstable and should be treated with an anterior fusion, such as a Bailey-Badgley trough

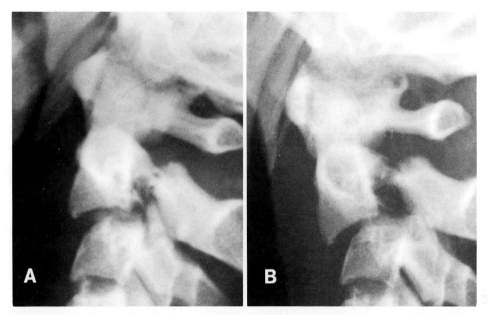

Fig. 4-20. Radiographs of a young male who sustained a traumatic spondylolisthesis in an automobile accident. (A) Fracture dislocation without traction. (B) The instability of the lesion and the effect of 3 lb of axial traction. In this situation the annular and longitudinal ligament fibers between C2 and C3 were obviously destroyed in the injury. It is assumed that the MIV has a significant +y-axis component. In addition to the major y- and −x-axis torque, there is a tensile or shear load applied to the annulus. This does not always occur in such an injury. Note that the posterior elements of C2 had been pulled anteriorly, which was, no doubt, injurious to the cord. This patient died soon after admission to the hospital. (Courtesy of Teaching Library, Section of Neuroradiology, Yale University School of Medicine.)

graft, and well protected by effective immobilization until there is radiographic evidence of osteosynthesis.

Some surgeons vigorously advise against traction.[22] This is because of the large distractions that may occur (Figs. 4-20, 4-21). Such distractions document that the annulus fibrosus and other anterior elements have been disrupted and that the situation is unstable. Carefully monitored axial traction with close observation may be used to safely illicit this information (see Chapter 5). Traction of 30 to 40 N (7–9 lbf) may be used prior to surgery or orthotic immobilization to improve reduction, relieve muscle spasm, and rest the tissues.

Of course, the use of seat belts with shoulder harnesses would greatly reduce this injury in auto accidents. Also, staying on the right side of the road and the law is of considerable help.

Cervical Compression Fractures

This group includes several fractures. They all have to do with vertebral body failure and include simple compression fractures, vertical compression fractures, and communited or "tear drop" fracture dislocations.

Mechanism of Injury. These lesions are thought to be flexion injuries.[151] A major component of the force vector is exerted along the y-axis in the negative direction and primarily in the region of the anterior elements. The type of fracture that results is a function of the magnitude, the spatial orientation, and location with respect to the spine of the force vector on one side versus the physical properties of the various anatomic structures of the vertebra on the other side.

A simple compression fracture with minimal deformation suggests a lower magnitude of force directed toward the midline and axially onto the

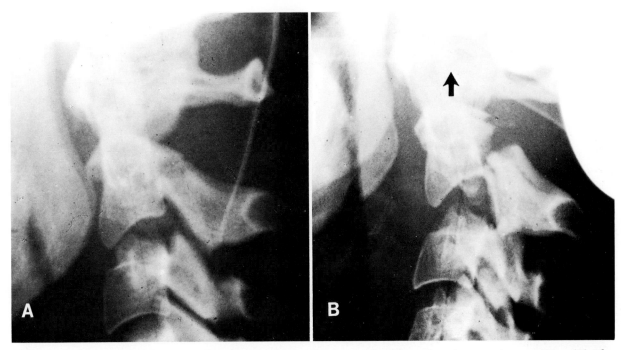

Fig. 4-21.   Radiographs of an adult in an automobile accident. (A) The patient in a resting position. (B) The patient after the application of 8 kg of axial traction. The separation of the anterior elements is drammatically demonstrated. Note that there is little change in the relationships of the posterior elements. The implication is that the ligamentous structures are intact posteriorly. They were not ruptured by tensile loading at the time of injury, as were the anterior elements. This fits with the presumed mechanism of injury; the posterior elements were under compression at the time of failure. (Courtesy of Dr. Mason Hohl, Beverly Hills, Calif.)

vertebral body. A vertical compression fracture with central depression probably has a similar mechanism, with a force of greater magnitude. In addition the annulus fibrosus acts as a wedge, which is driven through the end-plate into the vertebral body.

Finally, there is the communited cervical vertebral body fracture, often referred to as the "tear drop" fracture dislocation. Presumably, this is due to a vertical force vector of high magnitude, which causes an explosive failure with a variable amount of cord compression. There is usually significant cord damage, which may be caused by posterior vertebral fragments being driven into the spinal canal.

Discussion.   The simple compression fracture is generally straight forward, but can sometimes be difficult to distinguish from the normal slight wedging that appears in lateral radiographs of the cervical spine in young individuals. Usually, significantly more or less relative wedging of one

particular vertebra, along with the pattern of the entire clinical picture, leads to a correct diagnosis. The vertical compression fracture without neurologic deficit is not significantly different from the simple compression fracture.

The "tear drop" fracture is of interest for several reasons. First of all, consider the appelatory semantics. Most would agree that the term is catchy, poetic, and popular. The accord probably ends here. There are different theories explaining how the name was chosen and to precisely what it refers. Is it the radiograph, the mechanism, the clinical picture, or the prognosis? Rand and Crandall elected to classify "tear drop" fractures as hyperextension injuries, based on the triangular shape of the fragment of bone often seen at the anteroinferior border of the involved vertebra.[102] Penning suggests that the name comes from the shape of the anteroinferior wedge of bone that is sometimes seen in these injuries.[98] It has also been proposed that the name was given by Schneider because of the sadness resulting from the associated neurologic damage. Perhaps a quote from the article by Schneider and Kehn may be helpful:[114]

This lesion is characterized by crushing of one vertebral body by the vertebral body superior to it in such a manner that the anterior part of the involved centrum is not only compressed, but often is completely broken away from its major portion. In most of these cases, this fragment has resembled a drop of water dripping from the vertebral body and it has been associated with dire circumstances so frequently that the terms "tear drop" and "acute flexion" fracture dislocation of the cervical spine seemed to describe the lesion and to suggest the mechanism of injury [(see Fig. 4-1)].

This particular group of fractures is of interest in yet another aspect. The picture of the residual deformation of an injury is what is seen on the initial radiograph. In other words, a given motion segment or fragment may displace a certain amount at the time of injury, but on the initial radiograph, only the residual displacement is seen, which may be a good deal less than the initial displacement. There may be no residual displacement, leaving a normal alignment and causing perplexity concerning the presence of neurologic deficit. There is sometimes a residual subluxation at the level involved or an obvious residual fragment of vertebral body remaining in the region of the spinal canal. In some instances, however, radiographs show little or no infringement on the canal by a posterior fragment. The fragment presumably has been repositioned due to the restraining forces around the expulsion, which push the fragments back into the region where they came from. This type of deformation of the vertebra at right angles to the MIV is an example of Poisson's effect. The original volume of space occupied by the vertebral body may now be relatively less as a result of impaction from the compressive forces. Figure 4-22 is offered as a diagrammatic explanation of these ideas.

A clinical example is provided which demonstrates several of the factors that have been discussed (Fig. 4-23). This injury was sustained by a college football player following a head-on tackle. The patient was rendered quadraplegic at the level of C5. The lateral laminogram (Fig. 4-23B) shows very minimal posterior displacement of the body of C5. This is a small residual

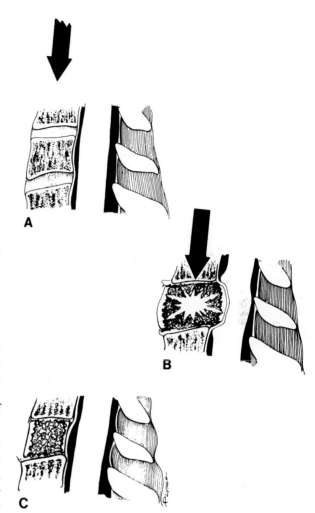

Fig. 4-22. Representation of the presumed dynamics involved in both the compression or the "tear drop" fracture with cord damage. (*A*) A primary vertical force or a flexion moment occurs. (*B*) There is an expulsion of the vertebral body, with deformation of the posterior shell of the vertebra, which pushes back and causes spinal cord impingement. (*C*) When the force is removed, the recoil phenomenon in tissues locally and through the body may leave only a very modest displacement of the vertebrae into the spinal canal, as shown in Figures 4-23 and 4-24, or no residual displacement in the canal, as shown here. The spinal cord injury may be severe, even though there is no residual impingement.

displacement. However, Figure 4-23A shows a complete block at the C5–C6 level, and the clinical picture was that of major spinal cord injury. Note the increased density, the decreased height,

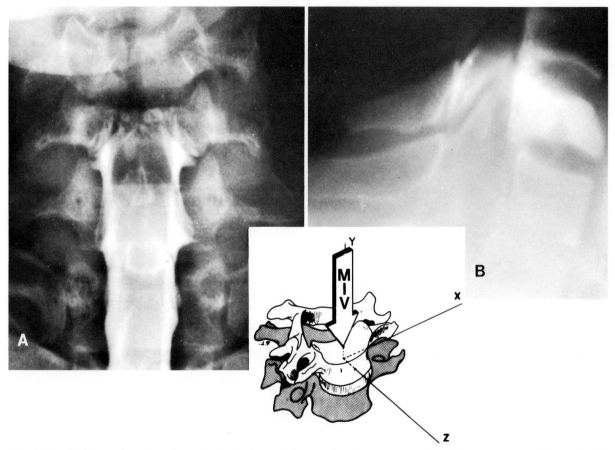

Fig. 4-23. Radiographs of a college football player following head-on, spear tackle. The patient was immediately tetraplegic following the injury. (*A*) Moderate compression of the body of C5, with complete block on myelogram. (*B*) A laminogram which shows increased density and slight increase in radiodensity of C5 secondary to compression. There is also a vertical fracture and some posterior displacement of the body of that vertebra. This injury is thought to exemplify the diagram of Figure 4-22. The MIV is primarily a high magnitude force, exerted along the y-axis in the negative direction. (Courtesy of Teaching Library, Section of Neuroradiology, Yale University School of Medicine.)

and the vertical fracture line involving the body of C5. These are all findings related to the compression injury, with the MIV oriented in the sagittal plane in the direction of the −y-axis.

Another clinical example is provided in Figure 4-24A, which reiterates these points, but, more importantly, it demonstrates the more classic "tear drop" configuration of fragmentation. This is seen best at the anterior inferior portion of C4. There is compression of the vertebral body and minimal posterior displacement. This patient sustained a diving injury and was quadriplegic at the C3–C4 level. The distinct block and a larger

residual displacement is seen in Figure 4-24B, a cysternal myelogram.

Before discussing treatment, the characteristic neurologic picture that accompanies this fracture should be described. The classic findings indicative of *anterior spinal syndrome* are usually present in the typical "tear drop" fracture dislocation. There is immediate complete paralysis and cutaneous sensory loss below the level of the lesion; however, there is bilateral sparing of vibratory and position sense. The neurologic patterns associated with some of the different patterns of spine trauma are discussed in more detail on page 163.

Suggested Treatment. The patient should be evaluated to determine the presence or absence of clinical instability. The simple anterior compression fractures without neurologic deficit can be managed by bed rest in the acute phase, followed by a minimal or a cervical orthosis of intermediate control for 3 to 6 weeks, depending on the clinical conditions. The communited compression fracture, without any suggestion of instability or neurologic deficit, may be treated in a similar manner. These latter injuries, however, are more likely to require additional bed rest with traction and an orthosis of intermediate control for a longer period of time.

It should be noted that in some cases of this injury, presumably when the posterior longitudinal ligament remains intact, axial traction completely reduces the posteriorly displaced fragments. Thus, skeletal traction of an appropriate magnitude is recommended as the first step in the treatment of this injury. Axial traction should always be applied incrementally and checked by lateral radiographs in order to recognize problems of overpull or a positive stretch test. In some patients, when the reduction is satisfactory there is no clinical instability and other aspects of the clinical picture are good, treatment may consist of 1 week of traction, followed by another 5 to 6

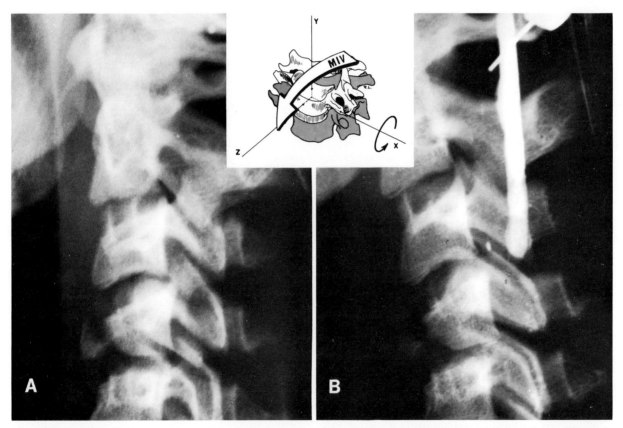

Fig. 4-24. Radiographs of a classical example of the "tear drop" fracture. The patient was tetraplegic following a diving injury. (*A*) The triangular fragment off the anteroinferior body of C4. Compression is also seen here, as well as displacement of the posterior portion of the vertebral shell into the spinal canal. (*B*) The complete block at that level as a result of the injury. The MIV is shown. Because of the significant wedging of C4, C5, and C6, some +x-axis torque is hypothesized. Note also that in both *A* and *B* there is slight separation of the posterior vertebral elements at C4–C5. This is due to tensile loadings associated with the +x-axis torque. The triangular portion of bone ("tear drop") off the portion of the body of C4 is an example of shear failure shown in Figure 4-1. (Courtesy of Teaching Library, Department of Diagnostic Radiology, Yale University School of Medicine.)

weeks in a cervical orthosis of intermediate control.

In the "tear drop" fracture dislocation, the emphasis has been on early laminectomy with dentate ligament transection, followed either immediately or in 2 to 3 weeks by spine fusion. This was recommended by Schneider, on the basis that this was of benefit to the cord in both the immediate and advanced stage of the disease.[112,114] The anterior cord compression is presumed to be related to fragments of bone or disc material displaced into the canal, traumatizing the cord and/or compromising the anterior spinal artery. It is not possible to clearly distinguish those instances in which the findings are due to damage caused by transient compression from those caused by a dislodged fragment of tissue. Moreover, it is reasoned that the injury to the disc and the dislocation have set up conditions for subsequent anterior cord irritation as a result of degenerative processes. Thus, the recommendations are made even when the traditional indications, such as progressing neurologic deficit and a positive jugular vein compression test, are not present.

Although the surgery of decompression remains controversial in this particular situation, it probably has a place. While we have been less enthusiastic about the cord recovery generated, we too advocate decompression. However, in our view it should be by way of an anterior corporectomy and fusion. The site of the spinal cord embarrassment is presumably anterior, not posterior. There may be recovery of an additional root, and in addition the traumatized cervical spine, stabilized by fusion, prevents cervical kyphosis and may allow for better overall nursing care and patient rehabilitation. Therefore, we have decompressed and reconstructed the spine as shown in Chapter 8.

Lateral Bending Injuries of the Cervical Spine

There are injuries to the cervical spine that result in unilateral wedging or fracture of the vertebra, with or without neurologic deficit.

Mechanism of Injury. The major injuring vector in this injury causes a significant degree of rotation about the z-axis. The vector, as seen in the coronal plane (y,x), generally is somewhere between the y-axis and the x-axis. Thus, the head is forced to tilt either to the left or the right. Due to physiologic coupling, there is a component of axial rotation ($\pm\theta y$) involved. As in the case of bending, there is compression on one side (the concave side) and tension on the opposite side (the convex side) of the neutral axis. Consequently, the injury involves wedging of the vertebral body and possible unilateral facet dislocation or fracture of the lateral masses on one side with ligamentous sprains, and ruptures on the opposite side. The forces that create these injuries are readily generated in motorcycle, automobile, and football injuries. During such an automobile injury, the person is thought to be hit from the side by some object when thrown from one side of the vehicle to the other. In the football injury, the mishap occurs in the process of tackling or blocking.

Discussion. The lateral bending football injury has been well documented by Chrisman.[19] Radiographically, the injury may suggest tearing of the intertransverse ligaments and/or an acute angulation in the frontal plane. The radiograph may also show asymmetry of the interspace at the site of injury. These structural changes are often associated with either chronic or prolonged asymmetrical neurologic deficits. Given the mechanism of injury, it is readily apparent that it may be frequently associated with a type of avulsion of the brachial plexus on the convex side of the bending deformation at the time of injury. Neurologic deficits have ranged in severity from a rapidly resolving (15 seconds to several minutes or hours) pain, parasthesis, and paralysis, to a complete, unresolving tetraplegia as in a football player reported by Roaf.[107] Chrisman noted in these patients a limitation of lateral flexion to the involved side in addition to the neurologic deficit.

It is interesting to speculate on the observation that players with a short "bull neck" and players with a long, supple neck are less frequently injured than those in the medium range. It fits with a biomechanical evaluation that the long supple neck may bend over a longer radius of curvature, and thus less bending stress is produced. On the other hand, the short, bulky "bull neck" is stronger, and the short length offers a shorter moment arm and results in less of a bending moment, which causes less damage.

Suggested Treatment. In severe types of injury, similar to those described by Roaf, it is important to bear in mind that treatment with longitudinal traction may amplify the deformity and displacement of the vertebra. In severe injuries, the patient benefits from a cervical orthosis of intermediate control.

Chrisman noticed an increase in these injuries in college football players when their equipment was changed from the high type of shoulder pads to the lower, professional type of shoulder pads. The lower pads allowed a greater range of lateral bending of the cervical spine and therefore did not protect the spine against this type of motion when the high magnitude forces involved in competitive football were applied. Consequently, prevention of these types of injuries is accessible through the use of the high type of shoulder pads or use of a heavily padded horseshoe-shaped cervical collar.

Unilateral Facet Dislocations With and Without Fractures

These injuries involve an abnormal relationship between the articular facets on one side, at the involved level. The caudad articular surface of the superior vertebra is fixed too far anterior to the cephlad articular facet of the inferior vertebra. This may or may not be associated with a fracture of the superior articular facet or lamina. A portion of a ruptured articular capsule may or may not be interposed. This injury is usually associated with rupture of the posterior ligaments, a variable amount of anterior displacement ($+z$-axis translation), and axial rotation ($\pm\theta y$). The annulus fibrosus may be damaged to a variable degree. The anatomic changes with this injury are well described by Beatson.[11]

Mechanism of Injury. An appreciation of this injury is intimately linked with an understanding of the normal kinematics of the cervical spine. A unilateral facet dislocation is caused by an exaggeration of the normal kinematics of the spine. Physiologic lateral bending is coupled with axial rotation, such that the spinous processes tend to move toward the convexity of the physiologic curve (see Fig. 2-13). When this is exaggerated in trauma, the facet on one side goes too far caudad, and the one on the opposite side goes too far cephalad and dislocates (Fig. 4-25). An example of this type of dislocation without fracture is shown in Figure 4-26.

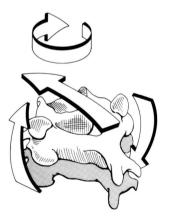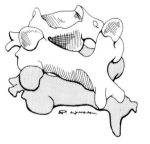

Fig. 4-25. The mechanism of injury in a unilateral facet dislocation. Basically, this injury results from an exaggeration of the normal coupling of axial rotation and lateral bending. If a significant vertical compression ($-y$-axis) component is added, then there may be a *fracture* of the *left facet*. If there is flexion and lateral bending, as shown here, but with a severe torque in the *opposite* direction ($+\theta y$), then there may be a fracture of the right facet.

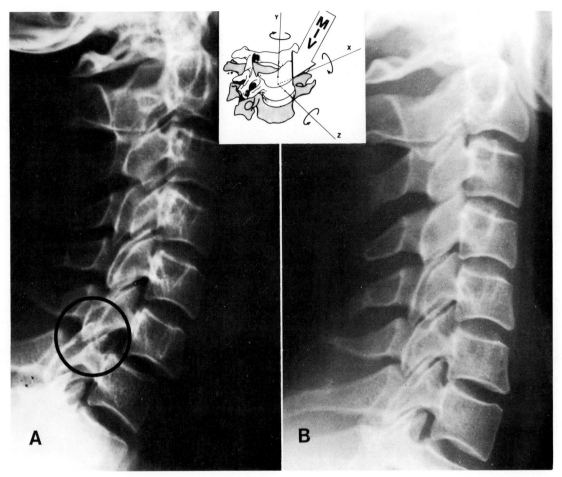

Fig. 4-26.   Radiographs of unilateral left facet dislocation. (A) The dislocation prior to reduction. There is an abnormal anterior translation of C6 on C7. Note the "interdigitation sign." The peaks of the lateral masses seen on this lateral view are not in their normal, shingled relationship, but there is an interdigitation of peaks shown in the circle. This is not always as readily seen, but when present at the same level where there is a moderate abnormal anterior translation, the findings are diagnostic of unilateral facet dislocation. Essentially, this injury is an exaggeration of physiologic flexion, lateral bending, and axial rotation. (B) The reduced state and the normal "shingling relationship" that the lateral masses exhibit on the lateral radiograph. (Courtesy of Teaching Library, Department of Diagnostic Radiology, Yale University School of Medicine.)

In unilateral facet dislocation where there is a fracture, a different mechanism is involved. Figure 4-27 shows an example of such a fracture.

Mechanism of Injury.   When there is a fracture along with dislocation, a large joint reactive force has been created at the fractured facet articulation. There is an impingement of the surfaces that results in failure through the base of the more cephalad facet, which sometimes goes into the lamina. This can develop in one of two ways.

There is either a significant element of axial compression involved with rotation and lateral bending, or there is an *unphysiologic* association of axial rotation with lateral bending. In the example presented in Figure 4-25, a unilateral facet fracture dislocation on the left can occur, with either a large component of axial compression or unphysiologic bending to the left.

Discussion.   The relationships of the mechanisms of injury involving facet dislocations and

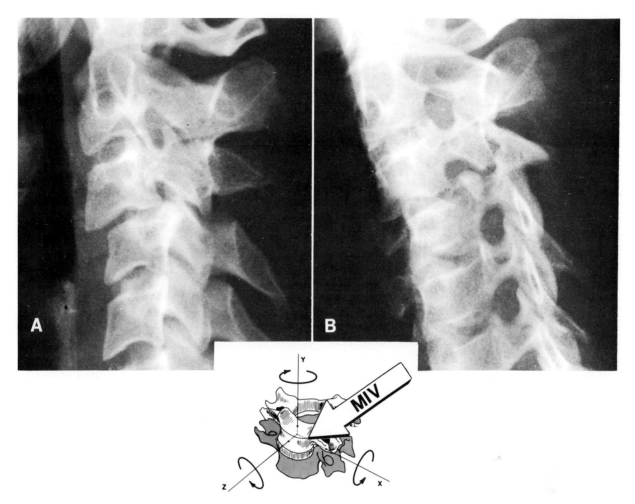

Fig. 4-27. Radiographs of young male who sustained a unilateral fracture dislocation of the left facet. (*A*) The anterior subluxation, which includes a significant element of rotation. (*B*) This oblique view shows the fracture of the caudad portion of the left articular facet, which actually involved a small portion of the lamina. This was observed at the time of surgical exploration. The MIV for this injury has caused flexion, compression, and axial rotation. (There is respective +x-axis rotation, −y-axis compression force, and −y-axis torque.) The mechanism here is similar to that shown in Figure 4-25, but here there is a greater compressive force. The compressive force accounts for fracture of the facet (fracture dislocation) rather than pure unilateral facet dislocation.

fracture dislocations result in an intriguing biomechanical analysis. The importance of a knowledge of normal kinematics in the clinical biomechanics of the spine has been pointed out. The relationship between physiologic and unphysiologic coupling patterns and unilateral facet dislocations and fracture dislocations provides a neat example for such a biomechanical analysis. Table 4-1 shows the relationships between abnormal forces causing certain movements and the

injuries to be expected. It is also of interest to note that the reason these combination of injuries are found in the lower cervical spine is due to the special orientation of the facet joints. Their 45-degree angle is just right to permit either dislocation or fracture dislocation depending upon the factors previously discussed. Table 4-1 does not include considerations of the effects of axial compressive loads on these patterns of injury. The axial compression load (−y-axis) increases

Table 4-1. Hypothesized Mechanisms of Unilateral Facet Dislocations and Fracture Dislocations in the Cervical Spine

		$+\theta z$ RIGHT LATERAL BENDING	$-\theta z$ LEFT LATERAL BENDING
$+\theta y$	Head turns to left	Unphysiologic coupling ↓ Right facet fracture dislocation	Physiologic coupling ↓ Right facet dislocation
$-\theta y$	Head turns to right	Physiologic coupling ↓ Left facet dislocation	Unphysiologic coupling ↓ Left facet fracture dislocation

the probability of a facet fracture in all the patterns but more so in the situations where there is unphysiologic coupling.

These injuries may be readily diagnosed on a routine lateral radiograph when there is abnormal sagittal plane rotation, abnormal anterior translation, and the "interdigitation sign" as seen in Figure 4-26A. Sometimes, however, the injury can be difficult to recognize and is only seen on oblique views, pillar views, or laminograms.

In the pure, isolated, unilateral facet dislocation, there is usually no neurologic deficit. the spine is clinically stable but painful. When there is associated disruption of the annulus fibrosus and fracture involving the facet joints, neurologic complication may also be present.

Suggested Treatment. The treatment may well be divided into pure unilateral facet dislocation and dislocation with variable amounts of associated injuries.

In situations where there is no evidence of neurologic involvement or fracture, and there is little residual displacement, much of the ligamentous complex of the motion segment may be presumed to be intact. It is possible with considerable difficulty to reduce this dislocation and treat the patient with an orthosis of minimum or intermediate control, with a satisfactory result. There may be a late sequela of degenerative arthritis, but it can be managed as indicated.

The safe effective reduction of such an injury constitutes a challenging and interesting problem in the clinical biomechanics of the spine. Skull traction is employed in the treatment of this problem; Vinke tongs are preferable. These are thought to be the most useful because the site and mechanism of fixation to the skull allows for the application of very large loads without the tongs being pulled out. When there is an isolated dislocation, the ligaments effectively assist the muscles in holding the dislocated facet in the overlapped position. Considerable axial (+y-axis) displacement is required to permit the dislocated facet to snap back into place. When the reduction is successful, it often occurs with an audible pop and an immediate dramatic reduction in pain.

When the tongs are in place an initial weight of 7 to 10 kg (15–22 lb) is applied, and lateral radiographs are taken. The surgeon looks carefully for abnormal axial separation between vertebral bodies, indicating disruption of the annulus and a much more severe injury. If this is not present, weights are then added in increments of 4 to 5 kg (9–11 lb), up to 28 kg (61 lb). After each increment of weight, radiographs are taken, and 1 to 2 hours should pass before the next increment, to take full advantage of creep. The patient may need some analgesics and sedation, with encouragement and a positive attitude on the part of the physician. Usually, before the maximum load is reached, the reduction is visible on the radiograph or heard by the patient. If there is still no reduction in the 28- to 29-kg range (61–64 lb), the following procedure should be tried before abandoning closed reduction. With the traction reduced to 20 to 23 kg (45–50 lb), the head is gently flexed laterally away from the dislocated side approximately 60 degrees and rotated toward the dislocated side approximately 60 degrees. (First there is z-axis rotation followed by y-axis rotation. To reduce a left facet dislocation, a $+\theta z$ should be followed by a $+\theta y$; to reduce a right facet dislocation, a $-\theta z$ should be followed by a $-\theta y$.) While the head is still held in this position, 50 per cent of the traction is removed to allow the facet to slip back into place. If subsequent radiographs show persistent dislocation, open reduction is required. These maneuvers are based on an analysis of the kinematics of the spine and the presumed mechanism of injury.

At the time of open reduction, a portion of the cephalad articular process of the facet of the inferior vertebra on the side of the dislocation is removed. Due to the mechanical and anatomical disruption, as a result of injury and treatment, as well as the opportunity presented by the open reduction, fusion is advisable. A posterior wiring and fusion of the two involved vertebrae is sufficient. For unilateral facet dislocations that have posterior element fractures and are clinically unstable by other criteria, open reduction, internal fixation, and fusion are also suggested.

Bilateral Facet Dislocation

This injury involves the caudad articular facets on both sides of the superior vertebra being displaced anterior to the cephalad articular facets of the inferior vertebra. These injuries are generally associated with considerable disruption of the ligamentous structures of the motion segment.[11]

Mechanism of Injury.   In order for the facets to ride up, as they do in this injury, and displace superiorly (+y-axis) and anteriorly (+z-axis), there has to be considerable tensile loading on the posterior elements. This is most likely due to a flexion injury, involving little compression. The forces involved are probably of considerable magnitude. The MIV is presumed to be a flexion bending moment very close to the sagittal plane, as shown in Figure 4-28. Any significant asymmetrical application tends to result in lateral bending and axial rotation and unilateral rather than bilateral dislocation (Figure 4-25).

Discussion.   These injuries are readily diagnosed and usually the criteria of instability are suggested by a systematic evaluation of clinical stability in the cervical spine (see Chapter 5).

Suggested Treatment.   Regardless of neurologic status, the overall rehabilitation and comfort of the patient may be facilitated by internal stabilization. This decision is best made on an individual patient basis. In instances where there is partial neurologic loss and potential for considerable activity, reduction followed by internal fixation and fusion is more likely to be helpful. A definitive recommendation of treatment of these injuries awaits further objective study.

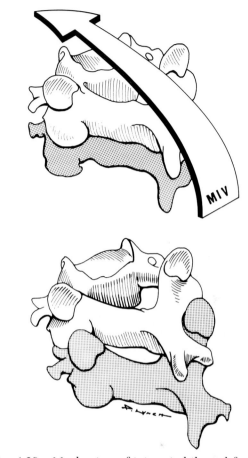

Fig. 4-28.   Mechanism of injury in bilateral facet dislocation. There is a major anterior displacement (+z-axis), with a significant element of force in the vertical direction (+y-axis). The MIV is as shown in the figure as a torque (about the +x-axis).

Gross Dislocations and Fracture Dislocations of the Lower Cervical Spine

This grouping includes a large variety of injuries below the level of C2.

Mechanism of Injury.   Gross dislocations and fracture dislocations of the lower cervical spine occur as a result of forces of large magnitude. Although there are a variety of possible injuries, each is discussed separately to distinguish it from the less severe but similar afflictions. The large majority of these injuries tend to occur in the sagittal plane. The MIV is either a large bending moment exerted about the x-axis, causing movement in the positive direction (+z) and resulting in a flexion injury, or the bending moment is in the negative direction ($-\theta x$), resulting in an extension injury. The major injuring vector is thought to be a moment, since the hypothesized mechanisms consist of a tensile failure of the intervertebral disc. The annular fibers are presumably ruptured or are more likely torn from the vertebral end-plate. These fibers are probably the most effective of the structures that resist translation in the sagittal and coronal planes. In order for gross dislocations to occur, the mechanical integrity of the disc must be destroyed, along with the anterior and posterior longitudina ligaments and the posterior elements.

Discussion. Figure 4-29 is presented as rep-

resentative case for the analysis of mechanism of injury. Gross dislocations and fractures are usually catastrophic; however, occasionally they can be amazingly benign with respect to cord damage. An instantaneous auto-decompression results in gross displacement of the posterior elements, allowing the cord to go free and unscatched by any portion of its osseous canal. In Figure 4-29, the patient fell approximately 6 m (18 ft) and struck his face, sustaining the injury shown. The force vector has two components, a horizontal force directed posteriorly ($-z$-axis) and a vertical force ($-y$-axis). The horizontal force, because of its distance from the site of injury, produces an MIV that has a large bending moment about the

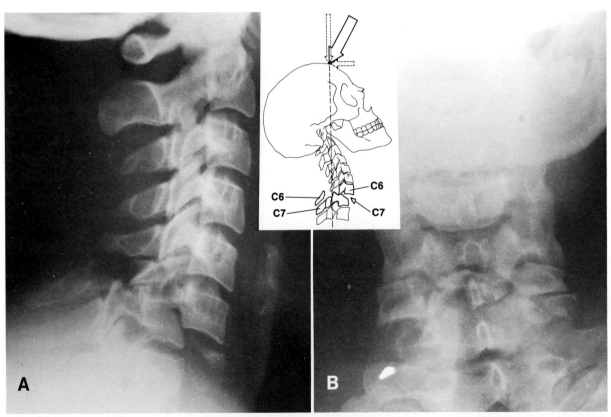

Fig. 4-29. Radiographs of a 38-year-old male who fell and struck his face. There is an anterior dislocation of C6 on C7. There is fracture and wide separation of the laminae and spinous process of C6. The MIV is primarily a negative torque about the x-axis, created by the posteriorly directed horizontal force, with a significant $-y$-axis force vector, as indicated by the compression of the lateral masses of C6, shown in *B*. Note the triangular fragment of bone in *A*. This is probably a shear failure due to the vertical compression force. The fragment probably remains attached to the annulus, which is still attached to the inferior body of C6. (Courtesy of Teaching Library, Department of Diagnostic Radiology, Yale University School of Medicine.)

−x-axis. In all probability the disc, including the upper cartilaginous end-plate of C7, translated forward with the body of C6. Note the triangular configuration of bone located beneath the antero-inferior corner of the body of C6. This is the anterosuperior rim pulled off the body of C7 by the peripheral, circumferential annular fibers, which are firmly affixed to the bone through Sharpey's fibers. The vertical compressive force accounts for compression of the lateral mass, the fracture of the pedicles, the laminae, and the base of the spinous process of C6. On the antero-posterior view, it can be seen that the lateral masses are not symmetrically compressed, indicating that the MIV is not acting purely in the sagittal plane. However, there is some component of the force acting around the z-axis (some element of lateral bending). Apparently, the trauma to the face was not purely in the midline, but slightly to one side, creating this component. Finally, there is little or no disruption of the relationship between the spinous processes of C6 and C7. This fits with an extension mechanism.

Suggested Treatment.

These severe fracture dislocations with or without neurologic deficit are probably best treated with reduction using skeletal tong traction followed by fixation and fusion. The traction is gradually applied in increments of 40 to 50 N (9–11 lbf) with radiographs and clinical neurologic monitoring. Fusion may be carried out through an anterior or posterior approach, depending upon the nature and character of structural damage and any site of decompression. Postoperative fixation can include internal wiring or plating, with or without halo fixation, which is determined by the stability required.

Whiplash

Although it has been suggested that this term be abandoned, such a project may not be desirable or feasible, as it is thoroughly descriptive and well entrenched. However, when one attempts to define the term, this suggestion seems worth considering.

The term whiplash applies to a complex and variable set of clinical circumstances. There is usually a history of a minor or moderately severe rear end collision. The patient presents with some combination of a large variety of symptoms, the only common factor being neck pain. Radiographs of the cervical spine are generally normal, except for the possible loss of physiologic cervical lordosis. There is enough literature on whiplash to fill an entire book of this size. Selected information on the topic and an overview of the current state of confusion are presented here.

Mechanism of Injury.

The exact mechanism of injury is not certain, although it is generally considered to involve hyperextension. There is too much rotation about the x-axis in the negative direction ($-\theta x$). The inertia of the head tends to hold it in a resting position following the sudden acceleration of the remainder of the body. The forward pull applied by the trunk to the lower portion of the head produces a moment and a rotation of the head in the negative direction around the x-axis, causing extension of the cervical spine. The injury can also result from a phenomenon in which the head undergoes positive rotation around the x-axis due to sudden deceleration of the body, followed by a negative rotation around the x-axis as a result of recoil.

Discussion of Experimental Studies.

Macnab simulated whiplash employing monkeys as experimental subjects. He dropped the animals from varying heights and they were suddenly decelerated, with the head left unsupported and free to move. The gravitational forces were varied by altering the height from which the animals were dropped. The anatomic lesions created were studied. The damage ranged from minor tears in the sternocleidomastoids to partial avulsions of the longus colli muscle. There were retropharangeal hematomas and damage to the sympathetic nerves. Hemorrhages in the muscle layers of the esophagus were also noted. The most frequent and reproducable lesions were ruptures of the anterior longitudinal ligament and separation of the annulus fibrosus from the associated vertebra.[76]

Work by Patrick showed that if hyperextension or hyperflexion in either direction ($\pm\theta x$) describes a certain critical angle, then damage in the area presumably results.[95]

A discussion of whiplash injuries must include the associated head injuries. With the usual type of whiplash injury (an acceleration of the body leaving the head and neck to its own inertia) often there are associated contusions of the brain. These come from essentially two sources. The first is a contrecoup phenomenon, in which there is movement of the skull, causing subsequent trauma to the cortex and cerebellum. There are also occasional injuries at the base of the brain due to the sudden angular acceleration of the skull. In addition to these injuries, an external blow to the skull may occur when the patient's body is thrown forward into some structure in the automobile. Thus, there is the possibility of brain injury due to sudden rotation of the head, as well as impact forces transmitted by the skull. Torres and Shapiro, Pruce, and Wickstrom and colleagues have reported significant electroencephalographic abnormalities in patients following whiplash injuries.[101,134,152] In some instances these findings have been similar to those observed in other types of closed head injuries. There is no doubt that some of these intracranial lesions may account for, or at least contribute to, some of the bizarre local symptoms, as well as some of the psychoneurotic problems that are often associated with this disease complex. Such information deserves due consideration in maintaining a humane, professional attitude toward patients with this injury.

It is interesting to estimate the magnitude of collision impact necessary to result in a concussion. Ommaya and Hirch studied this problem using scaling techniques and extrapolating from data obtained in experiments on chimpanzees and monkeys. The results indicated that a head rotation acceleration of about 1,800 rad/s² would result in a 50-per cent probability of cerebral concussion.

An angular acceleration of the head of 1,800 rad/s² (100,000 deg/s²) is reached when a car is hit from behind, producing 5 g* horizontal acceleration of the car.[88] This acceleration of 5 g is equal to attaining a speed of approximately 18 km/h from standstill within 0.1 second. In other words, if a car is hit from behind causing it to move at a speed of 18 km/h (10.8 mph) within 0.1 second, there is a 50-per cent probability of cerebral contusion for the occupants.

A considerable amount of work has been done on various experimental studies and mathemat-

ical modeling of the phenomena involved in whiplash injuries.[81] In the bibliography, some of the salient mathematical and experimental studies on this topic are included.

There are several ways to explore the mechanism of injury. Anthropometric dummies that have been instrumented to provide data on complete motion of various body parts may be used. Mathematical models may simulate the occupant-car system; this method has the advantage of great flexibility. In addition, animals can be used in real life experiments. Unfortunately, the anatomy is much different from the human.

Figure 4-30A shows the experimental results obtained by Severey and colleagues when they simulated the whiplash injury mechanism by using well instrumented anthropometric dummies and human volunteers (at slow speeds) during controlled experimental collisions.[118] Typically, a 13-km/h (8 mph) rear end collision produced a 2 g acceleration of the vehicle and a 5 g acceleration of the head after a lapse of about 0.25 second.[118] This magnification of the acceleration for the head and the resulting forces are the result of the unrestrained head.

Motion of the head following collision is documented in Figure 4-30B. A typical curve of head rotation versus time is shown. The head first goes into flexion and then into extension within 0.2 second. The maximum injuring forces, however, occur in extension and are found mainly in the region of C6 and C7. The results were obtained by McKenzie and Williams in computer simulation of whiplash using a mathematical model.[75] The question of whether or not the head goes directly into extension or is preceded by some flexion, as depicted above, is debatable.[16,45] Although most evidence may suggest that the major injuries are due to hyperextension, it is important for the clinician to bear in mind that there may also be a significant flexion component involved in the mechanism.

Motion of the head and the loads causing injury to the spine are dependent upon the seatback stiffness. This important effect is shown in Figure 4-30C. The two curves represent horizonatal acceleration of the head, responsible for shear loads in the neck, versus time after collision. The stiffer seatback produces less accelera-

---

* g is the acceleration due to earth's gravity, typically 9.81 m/s² (32.2 ft/s²).

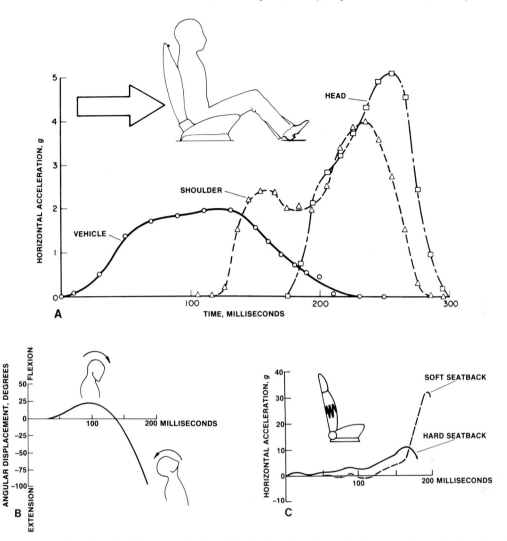

Fig. 4-30. (A) Note that the shoulder and the head lag behind as the vehicle is accelerated when hit, but they catch up and within 0.3 seconds they reach accelerations 2 to 2.5 times the maximum vehicle acceleration. (Based on results from Severy, D. M., Mathewson, J. H., and Bechtol, C. D.: Controlled automobile related engineering and mechanical phenomena. Medical aspects of traffic accidents. Proceedings of Montreal Conference, p. 152, 1955.) (B) The head first goes into flexion and then into hyperextension within the first 0.2 seconds. (C) The horizontal acceleration of the head for two different stiffnesses of the seat-back. The harder seatback has a lower acceleration and therefore is associated with less injurious loading. (B and C based on results from McKenzie, J. A., and Williams, J. F.: The dynamic behaviour of the head and cervical spine during whiplash. J. Biomech., 4:477, 1971.)

tion and therefore less shear stresses. Similar results were obtained for the angular acceleration of the head, indicating that less bending stresses occur in the neck with a stiffer seat. Obviously with regard to whiplash injury, the harder seat is safer.

A study of Figure 4-31 demonstrates three basic safety factors related to whiplash injuries. First there is the headrest, which limits the possible amount of extension that is allowed in the case of rear end collision. Headrests should be at least as high as the level of the ears, which approximates

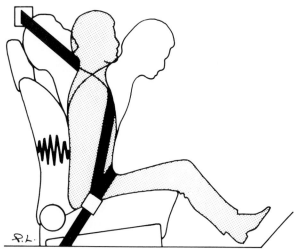

Fig. 4-31. Representation of the headrest, the shoulder strap, and seatback stiffness, three factors related to the extent of injury in whiplash.

Clinical Findings Following Whiplash Injury

Narrowing of one or more intervertebral discs upon radio-graphic examination

Chip fractures or compression damage of vertebral bodies

Compression fractures

Tear of facet joint ligaments shown by subluxation on radio-graph

Hyperalgesia over the cervical dorsal area

Pain, loss of motion, and involuntary muscle spasm in the neck and upper part of the dorsal region

Electromyographic evidence of motor nerve involvement

Sensory pain of a cervical, dermatomic distribution

Disturbance of cervical postural reflex

Blurred vision

(Adapted from Billig, H. E.: Traumatic neck, head, eye syndrome. Journal of the International College of Surgeons, *20*:558, 1953.)

the center of gravity of the skull. Unfortunately, in many designs they are below the center of gravity, in which case they serve as a fulcrum and accentuate injury. Secondly, there is the restraining capacity of the shoulder strap. By restraining the motion of the chest, there is a decrease in the amounts of inertial forces exerted on the cervical spine. Finally, there is the spring, which represents the stiffness of the seatback. The stiffer the spring, the safer the seat.

Discussion of Clinical, Psychiatric, and Medicolegal Considerations. The extensive attention that this group of injuries has received in the medical literature is partially due to the fact that the symptoms associated with it are much broader and less specific than in other neck injuries. Consequently, there is an abundance of medicolegal, psychiatric studies, and dissertations on the topic.

Typically, an individual is involved in a rear end automobile accident. Either immediately following this, or after several symptom-free days, the patient develops some part of a broad symptom complex. There may be associated frontal or occipital headaches, numbness or weakness in one or both upper limbs, as well as vertigo or tinnitus. There may also be dysphagia and blurring of vision or nystagmus. Several clinicians have noted the most common findings to be neck pain with muscle spasm, limited motion, and loss or reversal of the normal cervical lordosis. The

above list gives another clinician's view of the findings that may result from a whiplash injury.[13] Gay and Abbot offer a comprehensive review of the major clinical presentation of this problem and the management of this disease.[45]

There has been much speculation about the possible influence of psychiatric factors and monetary compensation on the severity of the patient's symptoms. Gotten pointed out that there is a dramatic difference in the time lost from work *before* and *after* settlement. He reviewed the work record of a group of 100 patients with whiplash injuries. Prior to settlement, 41 per cent of the patients lost 3 months or more from work. Following settlement, only 7 per cent of the patients had lost that same amount of time. He noted that a number of the symptoms were of psychological origin and were refractory to treatment. Moreover, the symptoms usually resolved following settlement of the litigation. His hypothesis stated that the illness was used as a means of implementing psychological adjustments which had been postponed or unfulfilled because of financial difficulties.[49]

In contrast, there is the work of MacNab, who purports that these patients are not simply a group of hysterical, neurotic, or dishonest people. He notes that the symptoms are much more frequent in patients who have had hyperextension injury as opposed to flexion or lateral neck injury. He reasons that this strong predilection to extension injuries would not exist if it were based simply on psychiatric and compensation factors. He noted further that some of the concomitant injuries, such as broken ankles and other limb injuries, generally heal without prolonged refractory histories. Finally, he points out that if compensation and litigation are major factors, one would not expect 45 per cent of the patients (as he found in his sample) to continue to have symptoms for 2 years or more after settlement.[76]

A similar study that does not accept the "psychoneurotic litigation" origin of whiplash symptoms is that of Schutt and Dohan. These investigators reviewed a large series of women with neck injuries due to automobile accidents. They noted that there was no association between delay of onset of symptoms and persistence of symptoms and litigation. From this observation they rejected the hypothesis that, after a symptom-free interval, patients develop symptoms as a result of "coaching," to build a case for litigation. Moreover, they found that symptoms persisted for approximately the same amount of time in the same percentage of individuals in two groups of patients, those involved with litigation and those with no litigation pending.[117] It is very difficult to know what role psychological and sociological factors play in whiplash injuries.

Hohl reviewed 146 patients and was able to identify certain clinical characteristics in the early, post-injury stages that were associated with a poor prognosis. These characteristics, which had a statistically significant correlation, are as follows:

Clinical Factors Associated With Poor Prognosis Following Soft-Tissue Injuries of the Neck

Numbness and/or pain in an upper extremity
Radiographic visualization of sharp reversal of cervical lordosis
Restricted motion at one interspece (flexion/extension radiographs)
Need of cervical collar for more than 12 weeks
Need of home traction
Need to resume physical therapy more than once due to symptom exacerbation

(Adapted from Hohl, M.: Soft-tissue injuries of the neck in automobile accidents—factors influencing prognosis. J. Bone Joint Surg., 56A: 1675, 1974.)

Discussion of Radiologic Considerations. Wagner and Abel carried out clinical and experimental studies which led them to the conclusion that the whiplash phenomenon may include occult injuries. With specialized radiographic

---

Radiographic Studies*

Anterior view of cervical spine
Open mouth view of the dens
Lateral view of cervical spine, with chin relaxed and in maximum flexion
Lateral view in maximum extension
Right and left oblique view of 45°

* Adapted from Zatzkin, H. R., and Kveton, F. W.: Evaluation of the cervical spine in whiplash injuries. Radiology, 75:557, 1960.

---

techniques they identified several lesions: interarticular isthmus fractures, with or without lamina fractures; fractured transverse process of C1; rotary subluxation of C1 with respect to the occiput and the axis; and Luschka joint fractures. This work suggests that some patients thought to have normal radiographs following a whiplash injury may well have some of the above injuries, which are occult on routine radiographs.[141]

Zatzkin and Kveton compared radiologic findings in 50 patients with whiplash injury with 35 normal adults. The radiographs taken and the relative frequency of "abnormal" findings in the two groups are included in the list above and in Table 4-2, respectively.[158] A radiograph should not be called abnormal unless several of the findings in Table 4-2 are present.

Suggested Treatment. Treatment of these injuries involves support for the neck during the

---

Table 4-2. Abnormal Findings in Whiplash Victims and Their Relative Frequency Compared with Normals*

RADIOGRAPHIC FINDINGS IN ORDER OF IMPORTANCE	FREQUENCY RATIO	
	WHIPLASH PATIENTS	NORMALS
Marked decrease in ability to flex cervical spine	10	1
Marked straightening of normal curve	5	1
Scoliosis curvature in coronal (y, x) plane	5	1
Reversal of cervical lordosis	3	1
Slight to marked inability to extend cervical spine	2	1
Wedging or narrowing of one or more intervertebral discs	2	1
Encroachment on one or more intervertebral foramina	2	1

* Adapted from Zatzkin, H. R., and Kveton, F. W.: Evaluation of the cervical spine in whiplash injuries. Radiology, 75:557, 1960.

phases of severe muscle spasms and stiffness. This can be achieved with a cervical orthosis of intermediate control. Various modalities of physical therapy have also been employed. The primary consideration, however, seems to be time, which allows the soft-tissue lesions to heal. The patient may be symptomatic for 2 or 3 days, months, or years. Certainly, appropriate analgesics are also useful and some physicians may choose to use some of the so-called muscle relaxants, although these have not been proven to be advantageous. Traction has also been suggested in the treatment of these patients.

When symptoms persist for 3 months or more the physician may want to perform an anterior cervical spine fusion at a moderately suspicious level.[125] If the usual indications for the procedure are present, then it is reasonable to go ahead with it. However, a mere history of whiplash should not alter the usual conservative indications for anterior cervical spine fusion.[149] In the broad spectrum of spine problems, this is one of the most difficult syndromes to manage, and considerable supplementary objective information is required to solve this problem.

Careful examination, understanding, accurate, empathetic communications, and reassurance carry even more than their usual importance in the care of patients with whiplash injuries.

In the prevention of this injury, the most important consideration is that a proper head rest be available. This prevents the excursion of the neck to a degree of hyperextension that might be injurious to the intrinsic structures of the spine. It has been noted by Wickstrom and colleagues that some of the headrests in current auto models are not high enough and may actually serve as a fulcrum accentuating rather than preventing the injury (Fig. 4-31).[152] Moreover, the work of Patrick demonstrated that when it is possible to anticipate an injury, a potential victim can protect himself by clasping the hands together and placing them behind the head, and falling in this same position across the seat of the car. This maneuver makes use of the upper limbs and the adjacent seat to protect against hyperextension of the neck.[95]

Other preventive methods include designing a seat back with some type of attenuating mechanisms that would absorb some of the forces and diminish the initial acceleration of the body in relation to the head and neck. A damping mechanisms included in the shoulder and lap restraint system may also be helpful. Patrick suggested that a primary consideration in seat design for protection against this injury is to limit the extension angle of the neck to below 80 degrees and preferably below 60 degrees. Meanwhile, observant motorists can protect themselves by paying attention to the vehicles that approach from behind.

Hyperextension Injuries Beyond Whiplash

This group of injuries is said to comprise 50 per cent of serious cervical spine injuries, and they may be associated with significant cord or root damage. They may have an associated posterior element fracture and/or fracture of the anterior inferior tip of the dislocated vertebra.

Mechanism of Injury. Hyperextension injuries differ from the usual whiplash in clinical appearance and prognosis. It is tempting to hypothesize that in the hyperextension injury, the amount of rotation is greater than in whiplash. This may be true but is unproven. In contrast to the mechanism of hangman's fracture, the major forces are applied lower in the cervical spine. This may be due to the instantaneous axes of rotation created by the location of major force vectors. Another factor is the relative ability of the vertebra in the two regions, in any given patient, to resist the applied loads. In other words, major injuring vectors that are very similar in two patients may produce different injuries. There is enough variation in the mechanics of the complex structure of the human spine, so that an extension injury could cause a hangman's fracture in one patient and a hyperextension injury involving C5–C6 in another.

Taylor, in an article on the mechanisms of injury to the spinal cord in the absence of damage to the vertebral column, proposed the following. There are hyperextension injuries in which there is considerable extension of the spine without any temporary dislocation. However, the damage to the cord is a result of impingement of the forward bulging of the ligamentum flavum. This hypothesis is supported by five cadaver studies, in which there was hyperextension of the spine and observable impressions on the posterior

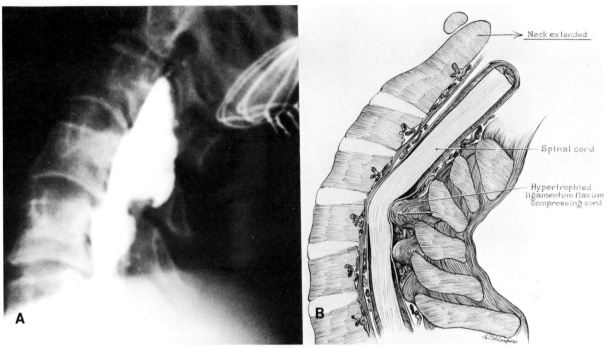

Fig. 4-32. (*A*) Myelogram shows significant encroachment upon the spinal canal by an extradural structure in a patient who has Brooks' C1–2 fusion. This encroachment is due to the enfolding of the yellow ligament. (*B*) The situation diagrammatically. Such findings are sometimes associated with symptoms. (Johnson, R. M., Crelin, E. S., White, A. A., and Panjabi, M. M.: Some new observations on the functional anatomy of the lower cervical spine, Clin. Orthop., *111:*192, 1975.)

portion of the cord at the level of the interlamellar spaces. It was noted in these studies that the thecal space for the cord was narrowed as much as 30 per cent. Figure 4-32 is supportive of this interesting hypothesis.[67] However, in cadaver spines, in which these experimental tests were carried out, the ligamenta flava have probably lost some of their elasticity. When normal elasticity is present, these ligaments shorten with hyperextension and thus do not normally impinge upon the spinal cord.

Forsythe suggested a mechanism of injury in which hyperextension is associated with shear loading that develops at the site of dislocation. The injury results in rupture of the anterior longitudinal ligament, separation of the intervertebral disc at the vertebral end-plate, separation of the posterior longitudinal ligament from the vertebral body and fracture or dislocation of the facets. The overall residual deformation may sometimes have a normal or near normal appearance. The residual lesion might show only slight *anterior*

subluxation of the involved vertebra, a fracture, or no changes on routine radiographic examinations.[42] These considerations may contribute to the confusion over whether encroachment during hyperextension that is due solely to the yellow ligament, without fracture and/or dislocation, can result in cord damage.

In a more recent publication, Marar submitted some new considerations on this subject. His study reviewed 45 patients with severe hyperextension injuries and noted the primary soft-tissue failure shown in Figure 4-33A. In addition, he studied four patients who died from their injuries. Careful autopsy evaluation was carried out, and a rather dramatic observation emerged from the investigation. In each of the four autopsy studies, a complete transverse fracture was found in the vertebral body at the level of the inferior portion of the pedicles (Fig. 4-33B). The cord had been compressed between the upper portion of the fractured vertebra and the lamina of the subadjacent vertebra. Spontaneous reduction had

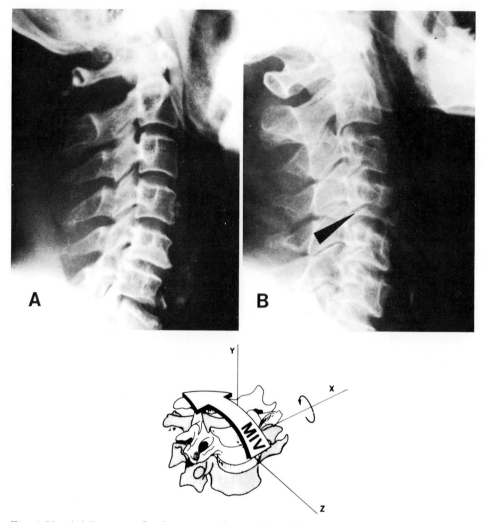

Fig. 4-33. (A) Posterior displacement of C6 and C7 following a hyperextension injury. The patient had an incomplete tetraplegia. The triangular fragment from the anterio-inferior lip of the body of C6 results in tensile failure of the bone, which has remained attached to the annulus through Sharpey's fibers and not the delicate anterior longi-tudinal ligament. The remainder of the separation has occurred at the cartilaginous end-plate, where the attachment is less secure. (B) This fascinating radiograph shows a transverse fracture of the body of C4 below the level of the pedicle. There is backward subluxation of the upper fragment. These findings suggests the presence of large shear forces. There was an incomplete tetraplegia. This fracture most likely would be missed on a routine radiograph should it spontaneously reduce, from either elastic recoil or moving the patient. The MIV for both injuries is shown in the inset. The major factor is a torque of high magnitude about the x-axis in the negative direction. (Radiographs from Marar, B. C.: The pattern of neurological damage as an aid to the diagnosis of the mechanism in cervical-spine injuries, J. Bone Joint Surg., 56A: 1648, 1974.)

taken place and the fracture could not be visualized on routine radiographs.[78] The failure in these hyperextension injuries can occur either through the osseous structures as shown in this study, through the annulus fibers, or more likely at the attachment of the annulus to the vertebral end-plate. Here, then, are additional patterns of failure that have the same basic MIV as that of hyperextension injuries of the cervical spine and may be associated with significant neurologic deficit. The strain rate at which trauma occurs may be the determining factor in whether the tendon or the bone fails under tensile loading. The work of Noyes on failure patterns of the anterior longitudinal ligament of the knee of monkeys showed that tensile loading may either rupture the tendon or avulse a fragment of bone, depending on the strain rate at which the structure was loaded. In other words, the same MIV can cause different types of anatomic damage, depending on the rate of deformation or rate of loadings. Specific mechanical properties of individual structures also play a role in such determinations.[87]

Discussion   Forsythe and Marar emphasized that this unstable hyperextension injury may spontaneously reduce and have a normal radiographic appearance.[42,78] The stretch test (Chapter 5) may be helpful in the diagnosis of an occult transverse fracture of the vertebral body or an undisplaced failure at the disc end-plate interphase.

The mechanism of cord lesion in many of these injuries is probably due to the "pincher phenomenon" described by Taylor and Penning.[98,131] There is a significant compromise of the anteroposterior diameter of the spinal cord between the posteroinferior lip of the vertebra above and the anterior superior portion of the subadjacent lamina. The threshold for cord damage through this "pincher phenomenon" is greatly accentuated when there are either osteophytes or yellow ligament encroachment present at the level of the translatory displacement. This is shown in the radiograph in Figure 4-34. A summary of the various pathoanatomic conditions that can traumatize the spinal cord through abnormal translation in extension injuries is presented in Figure 4-35. The yellow ligament, the osteophytes and, the pincher effect are the three

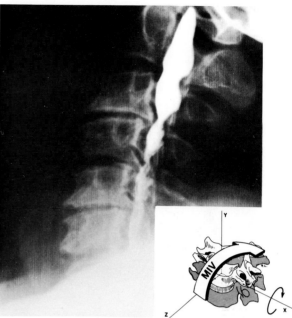

Fig. 4-34.   Radiograph of a 50-year-old male with cervical spondylosis who suddenly became paraplegic following a moderate fall off of a curb due to intoxication. The patient struck his head and extended his neck at the time of the fall. The cord damage here is due to the encroachment of the spinal cord at the C4–5 level by midline osteophytes anteriorly, and invaginated ligamentum flavum posteriorly, both shown by the partial block on myelogram. A radiologic estimate of the true sagittal anteroposterior diameter of the spinal canal in this patient is only 6 mm at the C4–5 level. This is an example of minor or possibly even a physiologic motion causing damage when the margin of safety and space for the cord has been significantly reduced. (Courtesy of Teaching Library, Section of Neuroradiology, Yale University School of Medicine.)

main considerations. If any combination of these three factors is operative, the injury to the cord for a given displacement is certain to be greater.

Suggested Treatment.   Carefully monitored axial traction should be used to treat these injuries. Posterior fusion with wiring and bone grafting has been recommended.[42] If the posterior longitudinal ligament is intact and there is good spontaneous reduction, the injury may be stable. The clinician cannot always be sure of the condition of the posterior longitudinal ligament. Thus, in order to avoid the catastrophy of initial or subsequent neurologic damage, it is suggested that these injuries be systematically evaluated for

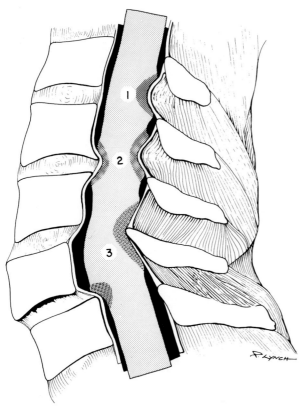

Fig. 4-35. Anatomic factors which may compromise the space for the spinal cord and cause neurologic problems. (*1*) Encroachment by the yellow ligament. (*2*) Encroachment by the midline osteophyte anteriorly and the yellow ligament posteriorly. (*3*) The "pincher phenomenon." This can occur from anterior translation of the vertebra, as shown. It can also occur from posterior translation of that same vertebra, in which case the spinal cord is damaged by the posteroinferior edge of the vertebral body and the superior edge of the subjacent lamina (see Fig. 8-4). These effects of these factors are summative, and any combination of the three may occur at the same level. They either lower the threshold at which trauma can cause neurologic damage, or they cause such damage.

clinical stability; the unstable cases should be treated by posterior fusion, followed by an orthosis of intermediate control.

If there are no posterior elements fractured, a posterior approach is the procedure of choice. This is because posterior wiring to an intact vertebra above and below the level of the ligamentous or the boney injury will provide some degree of immediate stability. In the case of pos-

terior element fractures or ligamentous disruption with this injury, the anterior approach may leave the patient unstable both anteriorly and posteriorly in the immediate prolonged postoperative period.[123b] However, this may be compensated for by halo fixation. If the surgeon can be sure of intact posterior elements, both anterior and posterior fusion are nearly equally suitable. However, satisfactory *immediate* internal postoperative stability may be achieved with posterior fusion and wiring.

Central Spinal Cord (Medulla) Syndrome

In individuals with cervical spondylosis, hyperextension injuries of the cervical spine without fracture or dislocation sometimes produce a pattern of neurologic defects known as the central spinal cord syndrome. The syndrome classically consists of motor deficit in the upper limbs and a segmental level of impaired sensation. Because the fibers in the spinothalamic tract conveying pain and thermal sensation are located posterolaterally and the touch fibers are grouped anteromedially a dissociated sensory loss of pain and temperature sensation may occur depending on the size of the central lesion. In other words, sensation to pain and temperature is lost but sensation to touch remains. If the central lesion involves more of the surrounding white matter, various long tract signs and bladder dysfunction may be noted.

Mechanisms of Injury. Taylor studied the effect of hyperextension of the neck on the distribution of pantopaque between C3 and C7 in normal cervical spines. He found a decrease in the anteroposterior diameter of the canal of up to 30 per cent. Presumably this is due to the invagination of the yellow ligament. If, in addition to the space encroachment by the yellow ligament, there is also a transverse osteophyte protruding posteriorly, obviously considerable damage to the spinal cord may occur. Figure 4-35 shows how a combination of these factors can result in a compromise of the anteroposterior diameter of the cord and subsequent damage.

Schneider and colleagues constructed a crude model of the cord out of foam rubber and drew on it the cross-sectional anatomy, covered it with rubber to represent the meninges, and compressed it in what would be the sagittal diameter of the cord. This study suggests that in addition to compressive forces, there are associated longitudinal tensile forces which cause damage proximal and distal to the site of compression.[F] This may partially explain the axial progression of neurologic damage cephalad and cuadad to the site of maximum compression.[113] The primitive biomechanical model does not take into consideration the role of the anterior spinal artery or the differential susceptibility of the various cord elements to the different strains they must encounter in anteroposterior compressive loading. These general findings are supported by a recent work of Dohrmann and Panjabi on experimental spinal cord trauma in cats. They found the traumatic lesion to spread axially in both directions from the site of impact. The spread is related to the magnitude of trauma or more precisely to the impulse of the transverse impact.[B,29a]

Discussion. Rand and Crandall have suggested several possible neuropathologic sequences that may result from the mechanical changes described above:

A small local area of hematomyelia with associated edema and swelling in the central portion of the cord may develop.

There may be central local recess of the gray matter which occurs secondary to hemorrhage. This is somewhat analogous to the experimentally produced lesions by Wagner and colleagues through direct impact loading of the exposed spinal cords of cats.[138]

There may occur simple central concussion with surrounding edema.

There may be infarction with central softening secondary to compression or damage of the anterior spinal artery.[102]

There are a number of possible mechanisms which may produce the final neuropathology once the external forces are generated. Some of the major investigations on this subject have been reviewed on page 119.

It should be noted that a midline posterior osteophyte alone may compromise the cord enough to cause damage even without discrete trauma. Murone emphasized the importance of the role of the initial normal sagittal diameter of the cervical spinal canal, as related to the development of myelopathy. In his study of Japanese males with cervical spondylosis, he found that those who developed myelopathy had initial sagittal diameters that were less than normal, and those without myelopathy had saggital diameters greater than normal.[83] Thus, cord injury can also occur gradually or as a result of a mild or severe flexion injury. A crucial variable in either situation is the initial sagittal diameter of the cervical canal for the particular patient.

The injuries may not have obvious associated fractures, and this may be difficult to diagnose radiographically. There are several characteristics that may help piece together the complete clinical picture. One obvious finding is cervical degenerative disease with one or more transverse bars (osteophytes).

An avulsion fracture of an anterior osteophyte may be present, suggesting a hyperextension injury. The old, reliable sign of retropharyngeal soft-tissue swelling or hemorrhage may be manifested. Other clues include any clinical consideration in the history suggestive of an extension injury and the presence of bruises or lacerations of the forehead or face.

Table 4-3 is presented here but in fact it is relevant to the entire section on cervical spine trauma. Marar presented a classification of neurologic injury patterns in cervical spine trauma and attempted to correlate them to specific injury mechanisms. Table 4-3 comes from this study. The classifications and correlations are not sharply delineated. However, the approach is novel and interesting, and the analysis constitutes a noteworthy endeavor to impose some order to an extremely complicated and difficult clinical area. To a large degree, progress in this area can be measured by the extent to which it is possible to collect, analyze, and interpret observations. Physicians can then more clearly develop, define, and delineate the entities in Table 4-3, placing them in precise, functional categories. A good deal is still to be learned.

Figure 4-36 is provided as a summary and review of the pathoanatomical considerations important in the understanding of the anterior spinal cord syndrome and the central spinal cord syndrome.

Table 4-3. Associations of Gross Neurological Patterns and Broad Injury Mechanisms in the Cervical Spine

	NEUROLOGIC DAMAGE	INJURY
Group I	Total motor and sensory loss to all four limbs. Total transection of cord. No recovery occurred.	Burst fracture or bilateral facet dislocation, flexion injury.
Group II	Motor loss of varying degrees, either in all four extremities or in the upper limbs only. Sometimes there was segmental or patchy transient sensory loss associated. (*Central spinal cord damage*)	Hyperextension injuries.
Group III	Complete motor loss in the extremities, with hypoesthesia and hypalgesia up to the level of the lesion. No loss of position and vibratory sense. (*Anterior spinal cord damage*)	Vertical compression, bursting injury, "tear drop" fracture dislocation; possibly some associated flexion or extension.
Group IV	Motor power in all four limbs or the upper extremities alone with no sensory loss.	Unilateral facet dislocation, fractured arch of atlas and a variety of injuries.
Group V	Brown-Séquard syndrome.	Unilateral facet dislocation or a burst fracture.

(Marar, B. C.: The pattern of neurological damage as an aid to the diagnosis of the mechanism in cervical-spine injuries. J. Bone Joint Surg., 56A:1648, 1974.)

Suggested Treatment. Several investigators, Bailey and Rand and Crandall, have emphasized that surgical intervention is not indicated for the central spinal cord syndrome.[19,102] Schneider suggested that it is probably contraindicated.[113] Thus, the diagnostic considerations leading to recognition is important. Surgery contributes nothing. The emphasis has been to protect the cord and to attempt to reduce edema. The patient should be systematically evaluated for the presence of clinical stability. If there is no stability, then after 3 to 4 weeks in traction, when the neurologic picture is stable, the patient may progress to a cervical brace of intermediate control. The patient may be freed of all immobilization by 12 weeks post-injury.

Clay Shoveler's Fracture

These injuries consist of fractures of one or more of the spinous processes in the lower cervical or upper dorsal spine. They occur in individuals who have been working at some form of shoveling or similar activity. Many of the patients have been undernourished, unhealthy, out of condition, or unaccustomed to heavy labor. The classic example is that of an unhealthy or unconditioned worker who has had symptoms of pain between the shoulders for several days or weeks when he lifts a shovel full of clay. Some of the clay sticks to the shovel, and there may be the sound of a crack, followed by severe pain in the back between the shoulders. Lateral radiographs show the fracture of one or more spinous processes (Fig. 4-37).

Mechanism of Injury. Presumably, injury is due to forces transmitted to the spinous processes from the shoulder girdle by the muscles attached to them.

The trapezius, rhomboid, and the posterior serratus muscles originate in the spinous processes. The fracture can be one, sudden, staccato type of force, or it may be a fatigue type of phenomenon. Many, if not most of such fractures, occur as a result of a fatigue mechanism. Support for this is suggested by the fact that it frequently occurs in the uninitiated shoveler and is associated with a repetitive activity, usually preceded by symptoms in the lower cervical or upper dorsal spine for a period of time prior to the actual fracture.

The major vector of force of these muscles in relation to the spine is horizontal ($\pm$x-axis; Fig. 4-38). Their function during shoveling is to firmly support the shoulder girdle in relation to the spine and the thoracic cage. This allows for the most efficient transmission of force from the trunk by way of the shoulder girdle and arms to the shovel. Repeated forces are transmitted from the

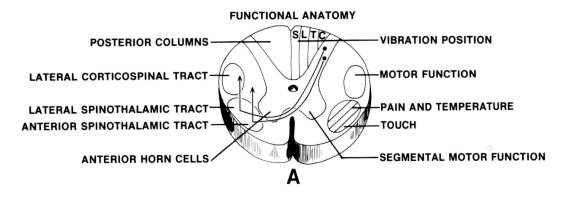

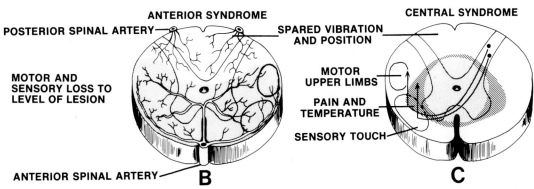

Fig. 4-36. The pathoanatomic considerations in spinal cord trauma. (A) A cross-section of the cervical portion of the cord. On the left, the important anatomic structures are labeled. On the right, their functions are indicated (S, L, T, C: sacral, lumbar, thoracic, cervical). (B) The *anterior spinal cord syndrome.* The arterial supply is shown in this diagram. The anterior spinal artery supplies the shaded area which includes the corticospinal tracts, the anterior horn cells, and the spinothalamic tracts. The posterior columns supplied by the posterior spinal arteries are not involved. Therefore, the resulting clinical neurologic picture is one of preservation of vibratory and position sense, with complete motor and sensory loss (pain, temperature, and touch) up to the level of the lesion. (C) The *central spinal cord syndrome.* The hemorrhage and edema located centrally involves the anterior horn cells, and the segmental sensory fibers with sparring of the more peripheral structures. This gives a clinical picture of motor defect in the upper limbs with a segmental sensory loss. Depending upon the degree and progression of the lesion, there may be paralytic involvement in the upper and lower limbs, with more involvement of the upper limbs. This is thought to be due to the lamination of the corticospinal tracts in which the cervical tracts are more centrally located. In addition, there may be more involvement of the lateral than of the anterior spinothalamic tracts, resulting in loss of pain and temperature sensation with preservation of touch. The two types of shading demonstrate the many variable patterns that are possible.

shovel through arms, shoulders, and the muscles to the spinous processes. These bony structures, due to the state of health or lack of biomechanical adaptation from previous loadings, may not be able to withstand the forces. Although individual loads may be within the load bearing tolerance of the bone, repeated loads result in a type of fatigue failure.

Discussion. There are some additional biomechanical concepts that are related to this injury. One of the theories of injury suggested, in a report by Hall, is the possibility of failure due to pull through the ligamentum nuchae and the supraspinous ligaments.[54] This is not likely in view of the rather delicate, almost nonexistent nature of the ligamenta nuchae in the human and

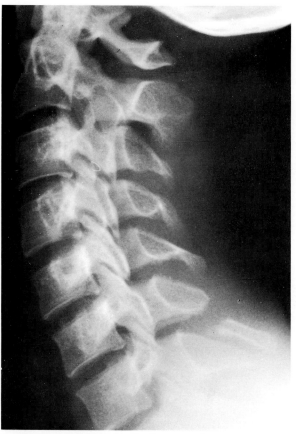

Fig. 4-37. Radiograph of a fracture of spinous process of C6, characteristic of the "clay shoveler's" fracture. The MIV may be a bending moment applied to the spinous processes in the horizontal (x, z) plane. The failure occurs either as an isolated episode or, more likely, through a fatigue type of mechanism. (Courtesy of Teaching Library, Department of Diagnostic Radiology, Yale University School of Medicine.)

the rather thin interspinous and supraspinous ligaments in the cervical and thoracic spine.[67,147] There are other interesting anatomic facts that relate to the mechanics of this injury. The sectional moment of inertia per area of the spinous process is greater against bending in the sagittal (y, z) plane than in the horizontal (x, z) plane. The site of the fracture within the spinous process occurs at the smallest cross-sectional area of that structure (Fig. 4-38). The observation that most of the fractures are at C7, followed by C6,[5] may well be related to the length of the spinous processes, since C7 and C6 have the longest process.

The fractures probably occur at these sites because the longer processes allow for the application of a greater bending moment.

A clay shoveler's fracture is also recognized in whiplash injury. The mechanism is supported through experimental studies. Gershon-Cohen and colleagues carried out some crude experiments on cadavers, in which acute forces simulating hyperextension and hyperflexion were found to be associated with avulsion injuries of the spinous processes. These investigators suggested that the ligamenta nuchae and the intraspinous ligaments may be responsible.[46]

Suggested Treatment. Hall, based on his experience with 13 patients, suggested *early* removal of the fractured fragment.[54] Jones and Annan were in favor of conservative treatment.[5,144] This consisted basically of analgesics and rest, followed by gradual rehabilitation and rebuilding of muscle strength back to the level of the pre-injury performance. Neck movements, flexion/extension in particular, are very painful, especially in the early convalescent phase. Presumably, this is due to motion transmitted to the fracture site through the normal muscolotendenous attachments. A cervical orthosis of intermediate control with a thoracic attachment may be of considerable value for the first 3 to 4 weeks, followed by active exercise.

REVIEW OF SOME SPECIFIC THORACIC AND LUMBAR SPINE INJURIES

Vertebral End-Plate Fractures

There are three types: (A) those that involve the central portion of the end-plate; (B) those that are quite peripheral in the end-plate and involve the cylindrical cortical shells; and (C) fractures that produce transverse fissures extending across the entire end-plate.[99] In some instances there may be extensive disruption, with displacement of the annulus fibrosus and cartilaginous end-plate into the cancellous bone of the vertebral body. In Figure 4-39 the upper end-plate of L3 is fractured but cannot be seen on regular radiograph or on the tomograms. The L2 vertebra

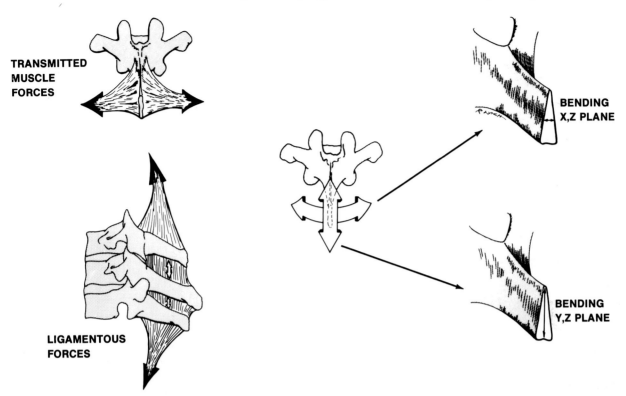

Fig. 4-38. Representation of the mechanism of spinous process fracture in clay shoveler's injury. Large forces are transmitted to the spinous processes through the origin of the muscles that stabilize the shoulder. Relatively smaller forces are transmitted through the interspinous ligaments in flexion and extension of the spine. The spinous process is constructed such that there is a much smaller sectional (area) moment of inertia to resist bending in the x, z plane than there is in the y, z plane. Thus the most likely mechanism of failure is through muscle forces transmitted to the spinous processes causing bending in the x, z plane. There is an additional biomechanical factor operative here (see p. 164).

shows an end-plate fracture of Type (B) described above.

Mechanism of Injury. In the experimental situation, with a gradually applied vertical load there is bulging of the annular fibers and vertical displacement of an intact vertebral end-plate. When the stress on the end-plate exceeds the maximum allowable stress, failure occurs. If the forces continue, the initial crack propagates in different directions and eventually fragments. As this happens, a nonfragmented cartilaginous end-plate and the annular fibers are displaced into the cancellous bone area. Vertebral end-plate fractures are due to vertical compression loads, primarily on the vertebral body. The particular configuration depends on the magnitude and direction of the injuring vector and the mechanical

characteristics of the existing anatomy in the particular vertebra and individual. It has been shown that the load bearing capacity varies with age. A group of vertebrae loaded in individuals over 60 failed at an average load of 4200 N (950 lbf) whereas those under 40 sustained loads of up to 7600 N (1710 lbf).[99]

Discussion. These fractures frequently go undiagnosed. Laminograms show a minimally displaced vertebral end-plate fracture which is not observed on routine radiographs. However, even this technique is unlikely to show an undisplaced fracture, unless healing has progressed with some visible callous formation. The authors make the following recommendation. When diagnosis is important for legal or medical reasons, patients with injuries presumed to result from vertical

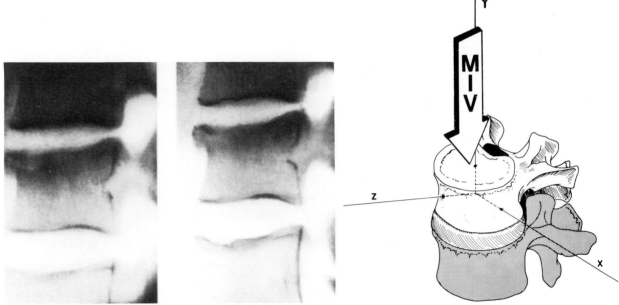

Fig. 4-39.   Laminograms showing two vertebral end-plate fractures. The middle vertebral body L2 shows a fracture of its upper end-plate involving the cortical shell. The vertebra beneath it shows a fracture of the neutral portion of the end-plate. This was not apparent on the plane radiograph nor on the adjacent laminograms, 0.5 cm away. These fractures frequently go undiagnosed. The MIV is shown on the inset as a force of moderate or severe magnitude along the −y-axis. (Radiographs from Perey, O.: Fracture of the vertebral end-plate in the lumbar spine—an experimental biomechanical investigation. Acta Orthop. Scand., 25 [Suppl.], 1957.)

compression loads should have post-injury laminograms, followed by subsequent studies in 3 to 4 weeks.

Rolander has observed that even in normal nontraumatic lumbar spine mechanics, there can be deformation or even fracture of the vertebral end-plate.[111] Perey found in experimental compressive loading of lumbar motion segments that end-plate fractures were relatively more frequent than compression fractures.[99] We submit that in vertical loading, the end-plate is most probably the first osseous structure to fail.

Suggested Treatment.   The treatment is aimed at the relief of symptoms. Bed rest with analgesics is employed until the acute symptoms subside and the patient is able to ambulate. An appropriate spinal orthosis of minimum or intermediate control may be employed in the convalescent period if the symptoms so indicate.

Ejection Seat Injuries

Compression fractures and vertebral end-plate fractures of the spine often occur when pilots must be catapulted from aircraft in dangerous situations.

Mechanism of Injury.   The mechanism of this injury is due to the tremendous force which is applied to the spine in the sitting position as a result of acceleration of the seat up and out of the aircraft. The determination of injury and the extent of the same depends upon a number of variables. Some of the important variables are as follows: the magnitude of the acceleration and its rise time; the stiffness and damping quality of the base of the seat; the design of the seat; the spacial orientation of the vertebral column (that is flexed, extended, or straight, the latter being the most desirable); the training and the readiness of the pilot.

Discussion.   As these injuries are intimately associated with modern technological martial arts, a good deal of investigation has gone into their prevention. It has been suggested that the seat back contour should be designed to maintain, as closely as possible, a normal vertebral alignment, while others consider a straight spine to be the most desirable. Ideally, head flexion should not be induced at the time of ejection. The recommended trunk-thigh angle is 135 degrees. It has also been suggested that a rocket propelled ejection system might be safer, since there would be less *impact* at the time of the initial acceleration. The usual mechanism is to impart acceleration to the seated pilot through the explosion of gunpowder charges. Laurel and Nachemson reported that accelerations up to 20 g acting on the long axis of the spine could be safely tolerated provided that the rate of increase of acceleration does not exceed 300 g per second.[72] In the report by Chubb and colleagues, it was indicated that sitting in the erect position with hips and head firmly against the seat was the most significant factor in prevention of compression fractures.

The middle portion of the thoracic spine was found to be the most frequently involved in the report by Hirsch and Nachemson. Generally, these compression fractures did not cause neurologic disorders. The pilots were able to return to active service as early as 2 months following injury.[59]

Treatment. These fractures may be treated according to the usual guidelines for the management of compression fractures (outlined below).

Compression Fractures

These fractures occur most frequently in the lower thoracic and upper lumbar regions. Generally they show varied amounts of wedging of the vertebral bodies. Such fractures may be associated with an end-plate failure, which may go unnoticed in the presence of the more obvious wedging and communition.

Mechanism of Injury. This fracture is most probably caused by a vertical force exerted either as an axially directed vector ($\pm$y-axis), or by a moment about the x-axis, or a combination of the two. These concepts are demonstrated diagrammatically in Figure 4-40. The effect of these loads on the middle vertebrae is shown. The dot represents the assumed position of the axis of rotation at this level. Therefore, when an axially directed compressive force is applied directly in line with the axis of rotation, the result is a direct compression of the vertebra with end-plate fractures. However, when the compressive force is anterior to the axis of rotation, the vertebra in question is subjected to a compressive force and a bending moment. This causes wedging of the vertebra, as shown in Figure 4-41.

Discussion. It has been pointed out that in pure vertical loading of the vertebral motion segment the posterior elements bear a significant portion of the load. Thus, one would expect to see fractures or disruptions of the posterior elements associated with vertebral body fractures in those compression fractures where vertical loading is the main component. Ewing and colleagues have shown that the fracture threshold can be raised from 10 to 18 g in embalmed human cadavers by moderately hyperextending the vertebral column.[39] This points out the role of the facets in resisting compressive loads (see Chapter 1) and leads to the recommendation that in the presence of a predominantly vertical compression fracture, one should make a careful radiologic evaluation of the posterior elements, where additional fractures are likely to be found.

Most vertebral body comminutions come from some combination of vertical forces and bending moments. The end-plate fracture is a result of relatively pure vertical loading, and a fracture with extensive compression and anterior wedging, as shown in Figure 4-41, is a combination of both types of loading with high magnitude.

McSweeney has noted several cases in which he has observed cervicodorsal injuries associated with sternal fracture dislocation.* There have been wedge compression fractures that were sometimes not readily recognized because of their location in the low cervical or very high thoracic areas. We suggest that these injuries have a large bending moment involved, and the point of application of the force is well anterior to the central axis. There is a large vertical compressive force anterior and in the region of the manubrio-sternal joint. There is wedging due to the anterior forces and fractures of the spinous processes due to the large tensile forces exerted posteriorly (Fig. 4-42). The processes in the lower cervical and upper thoracic spine are long, and thus large bending moments are applied to them. There is an important clinical point to be learned here. In the presence of a manubrio-sternal dislocation, the physician should look

---

* Personal communication, Mr. T. McSweeney.

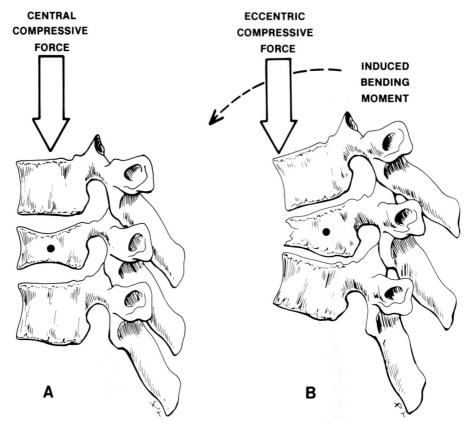

CENTRAL COMPRESSIVE FORCE

ECCENTRIC COMPRESSIVE FORCE

INDUCED BENDING MOMENT

A

B

Fig. 4-40. Different configurations of fractures produced by compression. (*A*) A centrally located axial compressive force close to the neutral axis (represented by the black dot) produces biconcave deformities of the end-plates. (*B*) An eccentrically located force away from the neutral axis results in a greater bending moment and produces a compressive fracture of the body, with characteristic wedging.

carefully for injuries of the cervicodorsal junction, and the converse is also true.

Plaue pointed out that much of the experimental work on the failure of vertebra in compression has not adequately emphasized the sequence of events after the initial failure. In an experimental study of autopsy material he noted that vertebra, after compression fracture, maintain 60 to 70 per cent of their original load bearing capacity. Moreover, vertebrae compressed to one-half the original height began to approach their *original* load bearing capacity.[100] This is presumably due to an increase of load bearing as a result of a "new," impacted vertebra. Thus, consideration should be given the complex and controversial question of the post-fracture management of these patients. If this phenomenon is operational in the clinically compressed vertebra, then it may well be the case that any observed additional angulation of the spine that occurs during the treatment is due to longitudinal strain of the posterior soft tissues as a result of tensile loads applied rather than of further compression of the fractured vertebra (Fig. 4-43). Narrowing of intervertebral discs in the kyphotic curve and excessive fragmentation of the vertebral body may also be contributing factors in the progression of deformity.

Suggested Treatment. The treatment of these injuries is a controversial subject, and the guidelines are not well delineated. The patients should be systematically evaluated for clinical instability. Severe pain and slow healing has been reported in unreduced fractures. Certainly the presence of an unsightly gibbus is not desirable. In fractures with unsightly deformity, treatment with reduction and a hyperextension cast is desirable. Other fractures may be treated with bed rest, exercises, and careful follow-up with radiographs.

Patients with mild compression loss of one-third or less of presumed original height of one or more vertebrae can be treated with active exercise and mobilization after a period of bed rest to allow acute symptoms to subside. Based on the work of Plaue,[100] this should be satisfactory. Patients with more than this degree of compression are probably best treated with reduction and application of a well molded plaster jacket. Even though there is considerable disagreement in the literature, Westerborn and Olsson have shown that in some wedged compression fractures, it is possible to reposition the vertebral body and regain a large portion of its original height and maintain the improvement for 5 years following reduction.[146] The duration of immobilization should be 3 to 6 months, depending on the severity of the injury. We recommend mobilizing these patients sooner under careful observation for evidence of progression of deformity.

Lateral Wedge Fractures

Such fractures are virtually the same as the compression fracture, except that the component force vector is such that there is asymmetrical collapse of the vertebra about the sagittal plane. Thus, there is wedging in the frontal (y,x) plane.

Mechanism of Injury. The injuries occur, as in the cervical spine, with a force which causes severe lateral bending ($\pm\theta z$), associated with some flexion. There may be unilateral injury of the articular facet, the pedicle, or the lamina on the concave side, and fractures of the transverse processes on the convex side (Fig. 4-44). Fractures of the transverse process are due to tension in the intertransverse ligaments. The bone has failed in tension at a lower threshold than the ligamentous structures, therefore, instead of rupture of the intertransverse ligaments, the transverse processes have fractured.

Discussion. Nicoll found these fractures to be

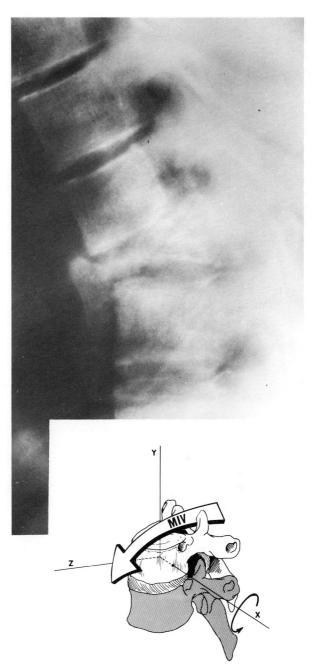

Fig. 4-41. Radiograph of a severe compression fracture of D7, which resulted in paraplegia with a complete block, shown with a myelogram. The MIV shown is vertical load, due largely to torques about the x-axis. This is evidenced by the anterior wedging. Also, there is considerable vertical loading which has resulted in the central compression. (Courtesy of Teaching Library, Department of Diagnostic Radiology, Yale University School of Medicine.)

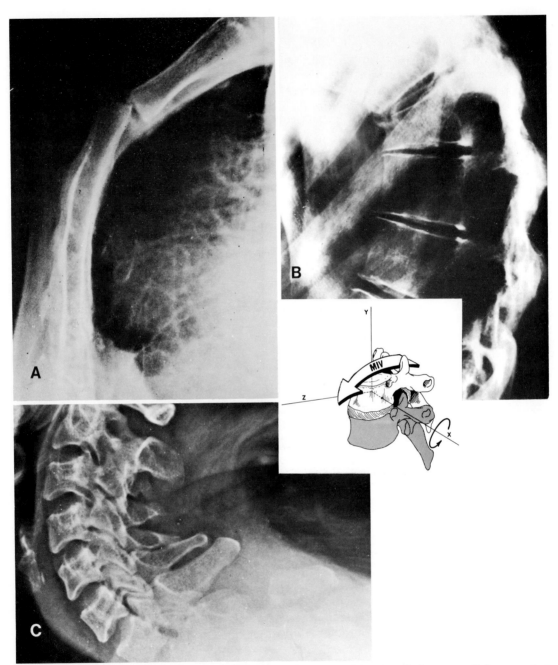

Fig. 4-42. Lateral radiograph of the sternum. (*A*) There is a fracture dislocation of the manubriosternal joint. The patient also had a pneumothorax associated with a fracture of the second rib. (*B*) Lateral radiograph of the dorsolumbar spine shows wedge compression fractures of the fifth and sixth thoracic vertebrae, resulting in a 90-degree kyphosis. This is due to a large +x-axis bending moment. (*C*) A view of the cervicodorsal junction shows that the spinous processes of the three upper thoracic vertebrae have been completely avulsed. This is due to tensile loading associated with the MIV. Cervical lordosis is exaggerated due to the thoracic kyphosis. (Radiographs courtesy of Mr. T. McSweeney, The Robert Jones & Agnes Hunt Orthopaedic Hospital, Oswestry, U.K.)

clinically different from anterior wedge compression fractures in both treatment and outcome. In his overall series he reports complete recovery in 40 per cent of the anterior wedge compression fractures, but in only 21 per cent of the lateral wedge fractures. He indicated several important clinical points about this type of fracture. The residual pain in lateral wedge fractures is greater. This may be related to the relative amount of soft-tissue damage in the two types of fracture. Sometimes there is iliopsoas injury, which may be accompanied by significant retroperitoneal hemorrhage and a clinical picture of an "acute abdomen." Two patients in Nicoll's series had a laparotomy with negative findings before injury to the vertebral complex was diagnosed.[85]

Suggested Treatment. The guidelines suggested for treatment of anterior wedge compression fractures are recommended for lateral wedge fractures also.

Gross Fracture Dislocations of the Thoracic and Lumbar Spine

This group of injuries is separated from end-plate fractures, compression fractures, lateral wedge fractures, and posterior element fractures. Any combination can occur in association with a dislocation. There are distinguishing mechanical characteristics, such as causative factors, damage incurred, and treatment. This section discusses trauma of the thoracic and lumbar spine that involves dislocation and possible neurologic involvement of the cord or the cauda equina.

Mechanism of Injury. The intrinsic anatomic structure of the spine in these regions is quite stable, thus large forces are required to cause fractures and dislocations. The strength and stability of this area is related to several biomechanical factors. As a result of the size of the disc and the vertebra in this region, there is a large component of direct, osseous, annular fiber attachment to the periphery of the end-plate. In this region, the anterior and posterior longitudinal ligaments are strong and well developed.[133] The posterior elements include rigid osseous stability through the spatial orientation of the facet joints, along with strong posterior ligamentous structures. These factors apply more to the lumbar spine than to the thoracic spine.

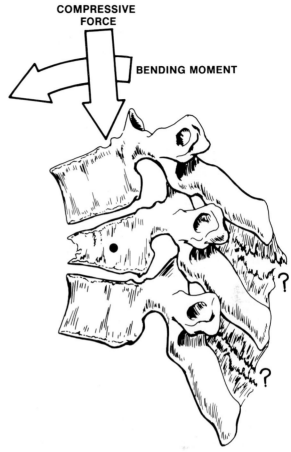

Fig. 4-43. Following a fracture from any combination of compression and bending moment, the tendency for subsequent clinical angulation and kyphosis deformity depends largely on what happened to the posterior elements at the time of injury. If they are intact, the ability of the compressed vertebral body to withstand the loads most probably is great enough so that there will not be extensive clinical progression. On the other hand, if the posterior ligaments have been damaged, then the possibility of clinical progression of deformity or instability is significantly greater. A highly fragmented vertebral body fracture may also be likely to allow progressive kyphosis.

However, the thoracic spine has a significant stabilizing influence through the attachment and inertia of the rib cage. Since there is so much natural stability in these regions, fracture dislocations generally are associated with very high forces, such as falls from considerable heights, auto accidents, heavy weights falling on the back, or "cave-in" injuries of the type sustained by coal

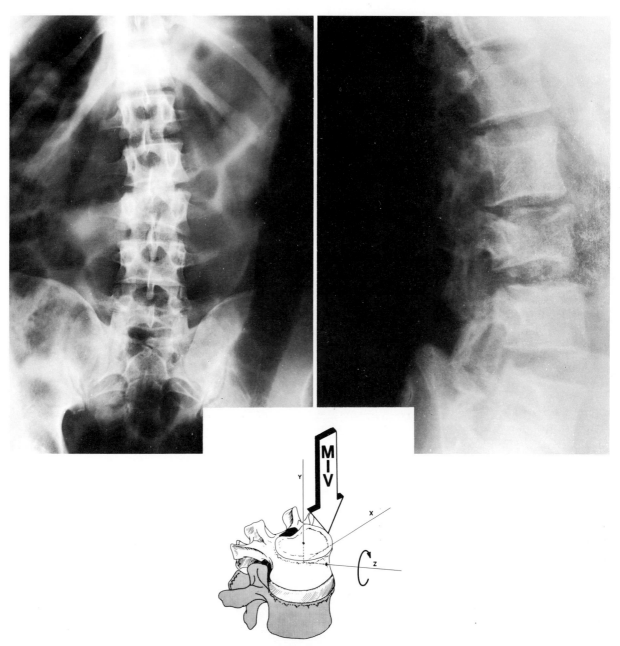

Fig. 4-44. Radiographs of a patient who sustained a high magnitude lateral wedge injury. There is asymmetrical compression of the left side of the third lumbar vertebra. There is slight compression of the pedicle and articular facet, indicating compressive loading. The right transverse process of L3 is fractured due to tensile loading on the opposite side. These factors show that the spine has been subjected to a left ($-z$-axis) bending moment in the coronal plane. Just to the right of the base of the spinous process of L3, there is a displaced fracture of the lamina. This may be a shear fracture; in a beam subjected to bending, there is maximum shear stress around the neutral axis. The radiograph on the right (the lateral view) shows the vertebral end-plate compression fractures.

miners. Pure flexion is usually not enough to rupture the posterior ligaments and facet complexes. In order to disrupt these structures and cause dislocation, an element of shear loading is usually necessary in addition to the large normal loads that are required. Thus, the fracture dislocations in these regions generally involve a major element of axial rotation, flexion, and some primary or coupled lateral bending. An example is presented in Figure 4-45.

Discussion.   Most of the injuries occur in or near the thoracolumbar junction.[52] This may be related to a phenomenon of stress concentration due to several mechanical differences in the two regions. There is generally less motion in the thoracic spine,[147] and the stiffness coefficient is less than in the lumbar spine[91,92] for most of the motion patterns. The attachment of the ribs in the region probably contributes to the stiffness and certainly adds to its inertia. Finally, the patterns of movement are different in the two areas. There is a rather abrupt change in the physiologic range of axial rotation ($\pm\theta y$). This change occurs at the level where the facet joint orientation of the thoracic spine changes to the facet joint orientation of the lumbar spine (see Chapter 2). The anatomic level of that rather abrupt change varies among individuals, from T9 to L1. These anatomic facts are no doubt contributing factors to the tendency for a higher incidence of fracture at these levels.

Suggested Treatment.   The problem of the treatment of these fractures is complex, complicated, controversial, and confusing. It is not reasonable to generalize extensively because each fracture has its unique complex of clinical considerations and because recommendations and experience in the literature abound with contradictory observations, methods, and results. Here we present what we believe to be the basic questions involved, along with the essence of some of the major relevant works on the topic. Finally, our own approach to the problem is offered.

What is the validity of the statement by Watson-Jones, "perfect recovery is possible only if perfect reduction is insisted upon . . ."?[144] What is the relationship between the anatomic and functional results? Does a plaster jacket do more harm than good? Should the plaster jacket, if used, be applied with the spine in a neutral or a hyperextended position? How does one distinguish the stable from the unstable fracture? Should the unstable fracture be treated in plaster, with an orthosis, with an anterior fusion, or with a posterior fusion? Does fusion prevent progression of deformity or neurologic deficit?

Bohler, Davis, Watson-Jones, and Key and Conwell support the view that *anatomic reduction* is important in the management of these fractures.[14,24,25,144,71] On the other side of this controversy, Leidholdt and colleagues, in a retrospective study of 204 patients with fracture dislocations and paraplegia, noted that sagittal plane deformities of 30 degrees or more did not have a significant deleterious affect on either function or pain. Moreover, these investigators found no evidence that these major deformities caused any further deterioration of neurologic function where incomplete neurologic lesions were present.[73] Nicoll and Westerborn and Olsson have not emphasized the anatomic reduction, but rather the importance of determining stability and treating the patient according to that determination.[85,146] Nicoll considered early ambulation, exercises, and activity to be crucial in the successful rehabilitation of his patients. Westerborn and Olsson treated some with hyperextension and plaster jackets, but in other instances, they elected posterior fusion.

The topic of clinical stability is dealt with in detail in Chapter 5. Most writers agree that when there is neurologic involvement, there is usually instability. Nicoll considered a stable fracture to be one in which the interspinous ligaments, the facet joint complex, and the vertebral discs are intact. He suggested that unstable fracture dislocations should be treated in a plaster cast, with the spine in neutral position.[85] Westerborn and Olsson treated some in hyperextension plaster jackets and others with posterior fusion.[146] Holdsworth suggests reduction and anterior or posterior fusion. In instances where the site of the fracture dislocation is through the anterior and posterior elements of the bony structure of the vertebra, he suggests conservative treatment of this most unstable injury. This recommendation was based on his expectation that stability is achieved with healing through osseous unions.[61]

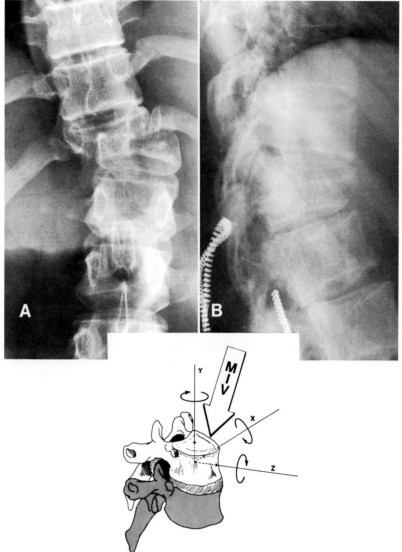

Fig. 4-45. Radiographs show a displaced fracture through the body and posterior elements of D12 sustained by a young woman in an automobile accident. (A) Malalignment of the spinous processes above and below the fracture site indicate abnormal axial rotation in the negative direction about the y-axis. There are fractures of both transverse processes of L1 as well as the right transverse process of L2. The thoracic spine above the fracture is tilted to the left (−z-axis rotation). (B) This lateral view shows compression of the anterior portion of the vertebra, with the thoracic spine tilted forward (+x-axis rotation). Fracture of the pedicle is also shown here. The MIV is shown in the inset. There is an element of torque about all three axes (−y-axis, −z-axis, and +x-axis). There was a high magnitude of force with a significant element of torsional shear involved at the fracture site. This type of complex mechanism of injury is best explained in the helical axis of motion, a concept which is more complicated than the MIV and awaits a better understanding of the biomechanics of spine trauma. (Courtesy of Teaching Library, Department of Diagnostic Radiology, Yale University School of Medicine.)

Rules and guidelines about the treatment of these injuries are limited both by the clinical uniqueness of each injury and by the present state of knowledge. The following approach is our synthesis of current information, with anticipation of more definitive information in the future. We suggest that the guidelines for the evaluation and treatment of clinical instabilities presented in Chapter 5 be followed. When there is a fracture dislocation with no neurologic involvement, one reasonable attempt at closed reduction with skeletal traction should be made. If this is successful, an appropriate orthosis of maximum control for the region involved is applied. The vigorous orthotic treatment is to avoid redislocation. If the closed reduction is not successful, an appropriate orthosis with intermediate control is applied. The orthosis, in either case, is worn for 6 weeks with the patient in bed. During the next 6 weeks, the patient is ambulated with the device. Following this, activities continue without the orthosis and progress toward normality. Flexion/extension radiographs and clinical follow-up are used to monitor the progress. If disabling pain, neurologic symptoms, or abnormal motion should occur, then an appropriate fusion should be considered.

For protection of residual and recoverable neurologic function, fusion is generally required in the unstable fracture dislocations. Generally some simple posterior technique suffices, except in cases where there is marked kyphosis or following extensive laminectomies. In these instances or in cases where anterior decompression is indicated, the anterior approach and interbody fusion is considered. Kelly and Whitesides and others have advised osseous stabilization of these injuries for better overall rehabilitation.[70]

Isolated Posterior Element (Neural Arch) Fractures

These fractures include any and all fractures posterior to the posterior longitudinal ligaments.

Mechanism of Injury. Such fractures are thought to occur with a flexion and axial rotation type of injury. It is also probable that vertical loading with the spine in extension can cause fractures of the posterior elements. When there is a large torque applied to the spine, with a spatial orientation of the lumbar vertebra, there may be damage in this region. This is because the facets in the lumbar region are aligned primarily in the sagittal plane, and significant y-axis torques will fracture them.[G] Axial (θy) rotation of a lumbar motion segment of greater than 3 degrees can cause either intra-articular damage or posterior element fracture (see Chapter 2).[125a]

Discussion. These fractures are frequently overlooked; thus, careful examination and good radiographic techniques are required to make the diagnosis. They may also be associated with fractures of the transverse processes. This should alert the physician to look more carefully at the posterior elements at or near the level of a transverse process fracture.

Suggested Treatment. It has been suggested that above L4 the injuries may be treated functionally.[85] Patients are given bed rest until acute symptoms subside, then mobilized in a spinal orthosis of minimal control for 6 to 8 weeks. Following this, they may gradually resume normal activity as tolerated.

When there is a lesion at the fourth or fifth lumbar level, the treatment depends on the presence or absence of spondylolisthesis. If there is clinical instability, then spine fusion to the normal adjacent vertebra above and below should be carried out. If there is no evidence of instability, then functional treatment of 6 weeks bed rest, followed by gradual mobilization in an orthosis of intermediate control should suffice. In some situations intractable chronic back pain may develop. This should be treated with bilateral posterior lateral fusion, uniting the normal vertebrae cephalad and caudad to the spondylolisthesis.

Lap Belt Injuries

This type of fracture was first described in 1948 by Chance, purposefully.[18] These injuries occur in the region of the upper lumbar spine. They may be purely ligamentous or they may consist of fractures or fracture dislocations of various elements of the spinal column. Sometimes only the facet complexes are involved in the injury. Ordinarily, there is a varied amount of associated vertebral compression fracture. Often there is a residual deformation from the MIV, resulting in a deformity which shows extensive separation of the posterior elements of the spine, with widening of the intervertebral foramen seen on lateral radiographs. On some occasions, the failure may occur entirely through osseous material, resulting in an almost perfect slice through the bony structures of the vertebrae (through the spinous processes, transverse processes, pedicles, and the body of the vertebra).[7]

Mechanism of Injury. The mechanism of this injury is one of rapid deceleration of the passenger, in which the patient is virtually wrapped around the seat belt, causing hyperflexion centered in the upper middle portion of the lumbar spine. Due to the instantaneous axis of rotation imposed by the seat belt in this particular situation, there is relatively little vertebral compression. As a result, the entire structure of the vertebral column is subject to relative amounts of tensile loading. This hypothesis is well described and convincingly supported in the comprehensive report by Smith and Kaufer.[121]

Discussion. This particular pattern of injury offers some provocative questions for discussion, especially in view of the limitations of looking at a radiograph and describing the mechanisms involved in injury. In a sizable series of patients reported by Smith and Kaufer, the mechanism of injury was reasonably well documented. Although the exact magnitude and direction of forces involved were not known, the basic clinical situation was quite similar. Nevertheless, the investigators recognized a wide variety of different patterns of failure in the vertebral motion segment. This spectrum included a purely osseous injury with all of the ligaments apparently intact. In this situation, as shown in Figure 4-46, the fracture went through the spinous process, the transverse process, and the pedicle, almost as a slice. With this same mechanism, however, there were two injuries in which there was absolutely no osseous failure. Instead, the entire ligamentous structure failed, including all the posterior ligaments, the facet capsules, and the annulus fibrosis. Between these two extremes, there were varying patterns of facet fractures, avulsions, and moderate amounts of vertebral compression fractures.[121]

At this point it is tempting to present a *law* of mechanism of injury. *Similar force patterns do not necessarily produce identical failure patterns.* In addition, it is tempting to reject any laws which categorically state that in some particular injury ligaments will fail before bone or that the converse will occur. There are two important variables that lead to a number of exceptions to any such law. One has to do with *individual* biological differences, and the other has to do with subtle but significant *mechanical* differences. In other words, if the exact mechanical situation is applied to a given motion segment in two different individuals, the thresholds for failure of tendon versus bone in the two individuals may be different. On the other hand, if similar load vectors are applied to a given motion segment in two identical twins, except that the strain rate is varied in one of the twins, ligament may fail before bone, or conversely, bone may fail before the ligament. This is supported by an investigation which showed that there is a differential in the threshold of ligament versus bone failure in tensile loading, depending on the rate of deformation.[87] From these considerations it is readily apparent that clinically similar mechanisms of injury can result in significantly different patterns of damage to the motion segments.

We are in accord with various investigators who believe that the presence of lap belt injuries should not be interpreted as a condemnation of seat belts. With 35 per cent fewer major and fatal accidents associated with the use of this safety device, we think that the advantages outweigh the disadvantages. The evidence suggests that the risk of lap belt injury be thought of as a necessary liability, which is especially high when the belt is not properly worn.[51,121]

The belt should not be worn across the abdomen or up above the rim of the pelvis. For correct use of the belt, it is to be strapped across the lower portion of the pelvis at the hip joints. The ideal placement is directly over the anterior capsule of the hip joint. In this situation, the torque is applied closer to the hip joints, which have a greater degree of mobility and intrinsic osseous ligamentous stability than is present in the lumbar spine. Also, the proper use of shoulder straps in conjunction with the lap belt virtually eliminates the possibility of this injury by preventing

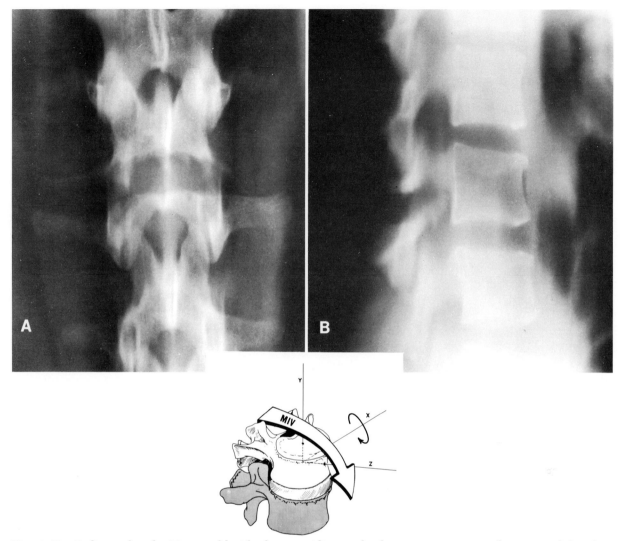

Fig. 4-46. Radiographs of a 16-year-old girl who was riding in the front passenger seat of an automobile when it suddenly decelerated as a result of an impact with a telephone pole. (*A*) Lateral laminogram shows moderate compression fracture of the most anterior portion of the bodies of L3 and L4, with a horizontal fracture through the posterior elements of L3. (*B*) An anteroposterior view of the fractures of the posterior elements. Note how the clean horizontal slice cuts through the spinous process, the lamina, the pedicle, and actually the right transverse process. The MIV is a positive torque about the x-axis. There is compressive loading anterior to the axis of rotation and tensile loading posterior to it. In this particular case, the axis of rotation is somewhere in the central portion of L3. (Radiographs courtesy of Dr. E. M. Rhodes, New Haven, Conn.)

rotation of the thorax about the lap portion of the seat belt.

Suggested Treatment. Treatment should be based on a careful evaluation of clinical stability. In most instances with severe injuries, at least all the posterior elements are destroyed and internal fixation and fusion is the treatment of choice.

Chance reported lap belt fractures with failure through the osseous tissues. He emphasized that good results could be achieved by treatment in hyperextension.[18]

In the management of these patients, physicians should be suspicious of associated intra-abdominal or retroperitoneal hemorrhage.

Sacral and Coccygeal Fractures

These fractures are generally associated with high magnitudes of force. Pelvic fractures can be serious injuries for this reason and also due to the frequent complication of excessive hemorrhage. The pelvis is an osseous ring, and rarely is there a fracture at only one segment, without an associated fracture or dislocation elsewhere in the ring. Vertical fractures of the ala of the sacrum may be overlooked on radiographs. Often, an associated fracture of the pubis ilium or ischium will serve as a "tip-off" for a more careful examination of the sacrum. The sacrum may show only an irregularity of the trabecular pattern or a break in the smooth arch of the bone of one or more of the sacral foramina. The failure seems to occur more frequently through the bone of the sacrum than at the sacroiliac syndesmosis. Injuries to the pelvic rim are shown in Figure 4-47.

The mechanism of injury in these fractures involves very high loads and usually a direct blow to the pelvic ring. In addition, a fracture may occur by transmission to the pelvis through the

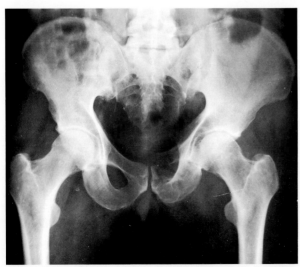

Fig. 4-47. A 52-year-old male with fracture dislocation of sacrum and fracture of pelvis. The pubic fracture is more obvious and should always alert the clinician to the probability of a fracture elsewhere in the pelvic ring. The MIV in these types of injury is always of very high magnitude. (Courtesy of Teaching Library, Department of Diagnostic Radiology, Yale University School of Medicine.)

axially loaded femur. Here, too, the loads involved are of a high magnitude.

Coccygeal fractures can also be difficult to diagnose. The normal anatomic variation in this area makes it almost impossible to make a diagnosis solely on the basis of the angulation at the sacro-coccygeal joint. These injuries occur as a result of a direct blow or a fall on the "tail bone." Coccydynia is notoriously difficult to treat, and often has a significant functional component with or without demonstrable organic disease.

Post-traumatic coccydynia in the presence of a demonstrable fracture is treated with bed rest during the acute phase of 5 to 7 days. Following this the patient may be allowed activities as tolerated and a large sponge donut for sitting. Symptoms which persist after 6 or 8 weeks may fall in the category of chronic functional problems.

REVIEW OF SPECIAL INJURIES TO THE SPINE

Spinal Injuries in Athletics

Spinal injuries in sports constitute only about 3 per cent of all athletic injuries. However, it is thought that 50 to 75 per cent of the fatal injuries involve the head and neck, and cervical spine trauma accounts for about 25 per cent of those injuries.[74] Practically any sport may be involved. A partial list includes the more well known associations, football, soccer, lacrosse, rugby, baseball, judo, skiing, riding in snowmobiles, tobogganing, jumping on trampolines, and diving.

Football, a sport that is frequently filmed and carefully studied, has been analyzed frequently with respect to injury mechanisms. The lateral flexion injury of football has been well documented. Schneider and colleagues and Melvin and colleagues have pointed up the role of the face guard in cervical spine football injuries.[82,116] The lever arm created by the face guard attached to the helmet, which has an excellent grip on the head, supplemented by a snug chin strap, has the potential to apply tremendous torques to the cervical spine. The mechanism can involve either flexion or extension ($\pm\theta x$). Face mask designs that create a smaller moment lever due to the shorter arm (extending only 2.5 cm beyond the tip of the nose) are helpful in diminishing the force applied to the spine in the case of a mishap.

Other spine injuries in football result from the tremendous energy involved in the deceleration of large masses (players of 100–150 kg) colliding with each other (as with spear tackling and blocking) or with the earth. Sometimes, these forces exceed the nonfailure energy absorption capacity of the spine and related structures and result in spine failure. Prevention of these injuries can be minimized by good conditioning to take full advantage of biomechanical adaptation and to decrease the probability of failure; good training to teach players the habit of protecting themselves by splinting their muscles for over two seconds after the stop-action whistle; and the elimination of spear tackling and some of the plays in which players are highly prone to injury. The best example of the latter is the "kick off." The role of the trunk muscles in contributing to the support of the spine has been discussed in Chapter 6, and they certainly should be strengthened along with the cervical muscles, which have the possibility of offering considerable splinting protection.

Stauffer and Fox presented 14 patients with quadraplegia as a result of football injuries. All but one of the injuries occurred in teenagers who were either scrimmaging or playing a game. Eleven of the 14 injuries were compatible with a flexed position of the neck at the time of impact. Also, eleven of the injuries occurred in a defensive back involved in openfield tackling.[123a]

A flexion injury producing a "tear drop" fracture is not uncommon. Many such injuries occur as a result of spear tackling or diving into unfamiliar waters. Others are due to faulty diving techniques. This fracture and its mechanism is discussed on page 141.

Snowmobile and tobogganing accidents usually cause fractures in the lumbar spine. The most common is a type of compression fracture due to sudden vertical loading secondary to hitting a bump. In snowmobiles, these could be dampened to some extent by the seat construction. The toboggan rider can generate a considerable dampening effect through his own joints by riding on his knees and shins, with knees and hips flexed.

Spondylolisthesis

In spondylolisthesis there is a defect in the pars interarticularis, which is associated with anterior translation of the involved vertebra in relation to the subadjacent one.

Mechanism of Injury. The mechanism is unknown. However, a feasible theory suggests that it is due to a fatigue fracture superimposed on a hereditary defect or predisposition.

Discussion. An excellent analysis of etiological factors has been described by Wiltse.[154,155] The possible causes are listed below.

Some Hypothesized Mechanisms of Development of Spondylolisthesis

Separate ossification centers (The lateral masses, which normally have one ossification center, have two which fail to fuse.)

A fracture which occurs at the time of birth

An ordinary fracture of that region

A stress or fatigue fracture

Displacement secondary to increased lumbar lordosis

Displacement secondary to a pinching mechanism of superior and inferior articular processes

Weakness of regional ligamentous and facial support structures

Asceptic necrosis of the pars interarticularis

Dysplasia of the pars interarticularis

The theory that seems to have survived best at present is that of fatigue fracture. This is based primarily on a number of observations, including radiographic documentation of an intact pars prior to vigorous athletic activity and/or discrete trauma, followed by radiologic evidence of spondylolisthesis.[21,155]

There are several factors, however, about the overall clinical picture that are not entirely compatible with the hypothesis of fatigue fracture. There is a significant difference in the incidence of the lesion across genetic barriers. Certain families have a documented predisposition. The disease is thought to have an incidence of 1.95 per cent in American Blacks, 5.8 per cent in American Whites, and about 60 per cent in American Eskimos. Usually fatigue fractures occur *after* the age of 6.5 years. Yet, this is when a precipitous increase in spondylolisthesis is observed. The radiographic changes are not typical of fatigue fractures elsewhere. The clinical history in patients with these lesions is not one of unaccustomed repetitive loading, as in the "military trainee" or the newly initiated "jogger" who sustains a fatigue fracture. Possibly, these differences are due to a different configuration of loading involved in the lumbar segment, resulting in a clinical picture which is atypical of the fatigue fracture. A definitive etiology remains to be proven.

Suggested Treatment. In young individuals, 21 years of age or less, plaster immobilization in a body jacket from the nipples down to the knee, on one side for 3 to 4 months, should allow for healing. In order to rest the lumbosacral joint, it is necessary to include one thigh (see Chapter 7). In adults, and in situations where conservative treatment does not eliminate symptoms, bilateral posterolateral spine fusion to a normal vertebra, above and below the deficit, is indicated. In cases where there is nerve root irritation, removal of the posterior elements of the involved vertebra, as described by Gill,[47] is desirable. We believe that, except for unusual circumstances, this procedure should be done in conjunction with a spine fusion to provide clinical stability and prevent further anterior translation of the body of the involved vertebra.

Pathologic Fractures

When there are alterations in the quality or the quantity of the supporting structures of the vertebra, fracture can occur with loads far below those required to damage the normal vertebra. The location of the abnormality within the vertebra and the orientation of the damaging vector determines the type of fracture that occurs. The details of the mechanical effects of structural loss in osteoporosis is discussed in Chapter 1. Boukhris and Becker have studied the association of vertebral fractures and osteoporosis and have reported the incidence of these fractures with sex and race groups.[15]

Fractures in Ankylosing Spondylitis

The emphasis here is that the morbidity and mortality associated with cervical spines effected with ankylosing spondylitis or rheumatoid arthritis is much greater. Barnes, Janda and colleagues, Vicas, and Hollin reported differences in the clinical picture of trauma in the presence of ankylosing spondylitis. These investigators noted a poor overall prognosis; there was a higher incidence of spinal cord injury and it was more severe and complicated. Even in cases where there was fracture without neurologic deficit, the mortality was greater.[10,62,65,136]

The difference is largely due to the tremendous loss of flexibility of the spine with ankylosing spondylitis. Nature has carefully evolved the highly specialized construct of the normal spine, which is designed for considerable energy absorption through its flexibility. The more rigid spine of ankylosing spondylitis does not have this capacity and therefore fails after the absorption of much less energy. Consequently, it may fragment more and also exert more force onto the cord after fracture. Because of the rigidity of the spine on both sides of the fracture, the probability of large displacements and initial or additional spinal cord trauma is quite significant. Thus, we agree with Janda and colleagues[65] in recommending halo fixation. Immobilization for 5 to 6 months is suggested before carefully controlled flexion and extension studies are conducted to check healing.

Fracture Dislocations in Children

Any discussion of spine injuries in children should include a statement about interpretation of lateral cervical spine radiographs. In children under 10 years of age, there normally may occur at the C2–3 or C3–4 levels as much as 3 to 4 mm of anterior (+z-axis) translation. This should not be diagnosed as a dislocation or subluxation without other distinct clinical evidence.

Spinal injuries and fracture dislocations in children are traditionally thought to be relatively rare. A recent report by Aufdemaur suggests the possibility that their reputation for rarity may in part be due to failure of recognition. He reported on 12 cases of spinal injury in patients from 0 to 18 years. In all these patients, the fracture occurred through the epiphyseal plate. The upper plate was involved twice as frequently as the lower one. The fractures occurred in the growth zone, in either the columnar region or the zone of provisional calcification. These injuries were difficult to see on radiographs. This work has pointed up the fact that epiphyseal injuries occur in vertebra in much the same manner as in the rest of the growing skeleton. Those regions of the epiphysis seem least able to resist loads in tension, under compression, or during shear, because they have the least interstitial support structure and the greatest amount of cell protoplasm.[7]

CLINICAL BIOMECHANICS

Our precise understanding of the mechanisms of injury in spine trauma is a good deal less developed than the usual casual deliberations imply.

The importance of careful handling and splinting is crucial in the immediate and intermediate care of patients with injury to the spine.

Some basic understanding of the normal kinematics of the spine is crucial to a meaningful analysis and interpretation of injuries and their mechanisms.

An understanding of the regional variations in the ranges of motion and the stiffness properties of the spine is fundamental to an understanding of mechanisms of injury. The cervical spine is probably the most flexible and has the widest range of mobility. The thoracic spine is the least flexible and has the smallest range of motion. The lumbar spine lies somewhere in between in respect to these parameters.

Horizontal shear forces are *probably* the most efficient mechanisms for disrupting ligamentous connections between vertebra.

In vertical compression loading, the vertebral end-plate fails first.

When high magnitudes of force are applied to the spine, relaxed muscles seem to be associated with less cord injury than do tense or actively contracting muscles.

The anatomic and clinical damage in spinal cord trauma is not based on an all-or-none threshold of force. It is related to the magnitude of the trauma in a variety of complex ways.

Hemorrhage and edema appear to be the major pathoanatomic result of trauma to the spinal cord.

The clinical history in evaluating the mechanism of injury of spinal trauma is valuable only after it has been carefully checked and collaborated with other evidence.

A variety of bruises and lacerations can occur on rebound impact or during other associated trauma. These should not be confused with the effects of the major injuring force that has caused the spine trauma and which is under evaluation. Therefore, in analyzing the mechanism of injury, these signs are to be weighed and checked along with other information.

The anterosuperior or anteroinferior triangle of bone that is frequently seen on lateral radiographs of the injured cervical spine may represent failure of that bone in either shear or tension. This means that such an injury may occur as a result of compressive or tensile loading.

The site of failure of a number of cervical spine injuries is largely dependent upon the anatomic structures of the bone involved. Fractures of the ring of C1 generally occur in the region the ring is grooved by the vertebral artery. Here the structure is weaker and less resistant to certain bendings loads. Also, in rare instances, the vertebral artery may be involved at the site, causing symptoms of vascular insufficiency.

Odontoid (dens) fractures must be carefully evaluated and their treatment individualized. There are clear-cut instances in which they need not be fused. However, the mechanics of and the risks involved are such that it is advisable to fuse when there is doubt about adequate stability. In injuries that result in an abnormal relationship between C1 and C2, careful biomechanical evaluation is crucial. While the authors do not recommend fusing all of such injuries, if after a systematic analysis there is significant doubt, surgical stabilization is suggested.

Evaluation of persistent post-traumatic torticollis should include careful radiographic analysis of the C1, C2 relationship.

The so-called hangman's fracture (traumatic spondylolithesis) is of considerable biomechanical interest. It provides an opportunity for understanding the group of related injuries that can occur as a result of the forces involved in the process of judicial hanging. This group includes the following injuries: odontoid fractures, fractures of the ring of C1, traumatic spondylolithesis of C2, and others.

An important consideration in the management of a patient with traumatic spondylolithesis is the recognition of the possible association with failure of the anterior longitudinal ligament and the attachment of the annulus fibrosus between the bodies of C2 and C3. The defect may not show up on routine radiographs, but may become evident catastraphically if too much axial traction is applied. Therefore, traction should be applied in increments and monitored by lateral radiographs and neurologic evaluations. These precautions will avoid the undesirable displacement that can occur.

The "tear drop" compression fracture causes trauma to the cord through the impact of the expanding posterior shell of the vertebra. The shell may or may not remain displaced in the spinal canal at the time of radiographic examination. If there is residual displacement of fragments, one can take advantage of an intact posterior longitudinal ligament and carefully monitored axial traction to displace fragments from the canal back to their proper location.

In persistent unilateral facet dislocations without fracture, an understanding of the mechanics of the injury and the kinematics of the cervical spine can be helpful in reduction of cases that are resistent to simple axial traction. The basis of the manipulation is explained and it involves the following: With the head under about 28 kg (63 lb) of traction weight (maximum traction), a carefully controlled bending of the head laterally away from the dislocated side to 60 degrees is followed by an axial rotation of the head toward the dislocated side of about 60 degrees. Finally, with the head held in this position, 50 per cent of the traction is carefully removed. This should achieve reduction.

Despite the frequently present psychiatric and medicolegal factors involved in whiplash, there is clearly good biomechanical and anatomic evidence for considering such injuries to be bonafide organic diseases.

The patterns of failure in severe hyperextension injuries beyond whiplash may include unrec-

ognized tensile failure either through the osseous mass of the vertebral body or at the attachment of the annulus fibrosus. The residual deformation after recoil may result in a spontaneous reduction, which can make recognition on routine radiographs impossible.

Vertebral end-plate fractures can easily go unrecognized. Lateral laminograms are helpful when the diagnosis is not evident.

With manubrio-sternal dislocations, wedge fractures of the cervicodorsal region, and the converse, should be suspected.

In determining the probability of progressive kyphosis following a compression fracture, the clinician should bear in mind that the compacted compressed vertebra may have 60 to 70 per cent or more of its original pre-injury ability to withstand vertebral compressive loads. Therefore, physiologic loads should be tolerated without additional deformity from further vertebral wedging and compression. The clinician must take into consideration the status of the posterior ligaments. If they are intact, then protected ambulation should be adequate to prevent subsequent deformity in most situations.

It is suggested by a number of authorities that in severe unstable fracture dislocations of the thoracic and thoracolumbar spine, protection of any residual cord and nerve root function, as well as the general post-trauma care and rehabilitation of the patient, is greatly facilitated by secure internal stabilization.

If the seat belt were worn properly across the hip joints and in conjunction with a shoulder harness, seat belt injuries would be nonexistent. However, in our opinion, even an improperly worn seat belt is better than no seat belt at all.

Fractures of the spines with ankylosing spondylitis carry high mortality and morbidity and thus are best treated with halo type fixation.

NOTES

[A] The authors are not aware of any epidemiologic documentation of less injury among relaxed individuals. The role of muscle forces before, during, and after spine trauma is not well understood. It appears that there may be some protection for the athlete through splinting when trauma can be anticipated. The work of Soechting and Paslay showed that the reaction time required for the motorist to voluntarily splint his muscles virtually eliminates the possibility of any voluntary muscle activity active at the time of injury.[123] These investigators observed that in a typical automobile, moving at a speed of 10 kmph (6 mph), the head will hit a dashboard, 38 cm (15 in) away from the head, in about 0.15 seconds. The muscles reaction time being the same order of magnitude, it is not possible for the muscles to contribute any protection when collision happens at higher speeds. The critical unit of 10 kmph (6 mph) obviously eliminates the large majority of auto accidents. On the other side of this issue we have the evidence of Gosch and colleagues who showed clearly that cervical spine injuries were less severe in anesthetized than in awake monkeys subjected to trauma.[48] It may be that normal muscle tone rather than splinting is the crucial factor. The important question of the effects of muscle forces in spine trauma needs and merits considerable study.

It has been possible to carry out such an investigation, and the salient findings are presented.

[B] When trauma is created by impacting a given mass M in kg (lb) from a height h in m (ft), there may be different mechanical parameters which are relevant to the trauma of the spinal cord. There are at least three that are readily discernible: the energy of the falling mass due to its height, the momentum of the mass due to its velocity, and the impulse that the mass delivers to the spinal cord. As can be seen from the equations below, these quantities are distinctly different.

$$\text{Energy} = mgh$$
$$\text{Momentum} = m\,v_1 = m\sqrt{2gh}$$
$$\text{Impulse} = m\,(v_2 - v_1)$$

Where g is gravitational acceleration = 9.81 m/s² (32 ft/s²)
v_1 is the velocity of the mass at the time of impact in m/s (ft/s)
v_2 is the velocity of the mass on rebound in m/s (ft/s)

In a recent paper, correlation between Impulse, as defined above, and the traumatic spinal cord lesion produced has been shown.[29a]

[C] In analyzing injury, the more traditional terms are maintained; however, in addition, our classification is used whenever the knowledge is adequate. The standard uses of the coordinate system has been described in Chapter 2. Nevertheless, a partial review is provided here. The traditional anatomic planes are shown in Figure 2-2. These designations assume the anatomical position.

Planes
y, z—sagittal plane
y, x—frontal plane
z, x—horizontal plane
Directions
+ x translation—toward the patient's left
− x translation—toward the patient's right
+ y translation—cephalad or up
− y translation—caudad or down
+ z translation—forward
− z translation—backward
Rotation
+ θx—clockwise about x-axis, as in flexion
− θx—counterclockwise about x-axis, as in extension
+ θy—clockwise rotation about y-axis, as in axial rotation to the left
− θy—counterclockwise rotation about y-axis, as in axial rotation to the right
+ θz—clockwise rotation about z-axis, as in right lateral bending
− θz—counterclockwise rotation about z axis, as in left lateral bending

[D] A more detailed look at the concept of the major injuring vector involves considering the vector to consist of the forces and moments acting on the vertebra in question. Because the traumatic force is seldom directly applied to the spine, there is always a bending moment and/or a torque at the site of injury, along with the original force. The moment or torque is the result of the lever arm between the force and vertebra. As an example, take the case of a man hit from the front on the center of the forehead. If the force is in the sagittal plane, then the MIV present at the vertebra consists of a force, which is exactly equal and parallel to the original force on the head, and a bending moment, equal in magnitude to the force times the shortest (perpendicular) distance from the vertebra to the line of action of the force on the head. Now if the person were not hit exactly in the center of the head or if the force were not in the sagittal plane, then in addition to the force and the bending moment there would also be a torque about the y-axis of the vertebra. To complicate the problem even more, the resulting moments and torques at a vertebra at the time of injury are dependent upon the spatial relationship between the original force and the instantaneous position of the vertebra in space. The MIV presented in the various diagrams for a given injury is the most dominant force and/or moment vector *at the vertebra* responsible for causing the injury, according to the best biomechanical analysis of the injury causing mechanism.

[E] In hangman's fracture the major injury vector is a bending moment acting on C2 by means of the dens and the anterior ligamentous structure. Let this moment be M, as shown in Figure 4-19A. The free-body analysis technique involves isolating C2. Let us assume that the contribution from C1 onto C2 is a bending moment M and the contribution from C3 onto C1 is a pair of forces F_1 and F_2 as shown. Because the vetebra C2 must be in moment equilibrium, the two forces must be equal, opposite, and parallel. The magnitude of these forces is given by the equation

$$F_1 = F_2 = \frac{M}{D},$$

where D is the distance perpendicular to the forces. Force F_1 is a tensile force contributed by anterior ligamentous structures between C2–C3 and force F_2 is a compressive facet joint reaction. The bending moment diagram for this loading situation is shown in Figure 4-19B. The bending moment is maximum in the middle of the two forces. Anatomically this is also the section with the lowest moment of inertia. The probability of fracture at this section with this kind of loading is therefore quite high. If the force F_1 is not parallel to the axis of the disc C2–C3, then this disc will have, in addition to the tensile force, shear forces. Similarly, if F_2 is not perpendicular to the facet joint surfaces shear forces will be present at the joint, thus causing stress in the facet capsular ligaments.

[F] The study of Schneider and colleagues is another example in which Poisson's ratio is operative. A compressive load across the cord produces tensile strains in the axial direction.

[G] One of the very few motion patterns in which the lumbar spine is stiffer than the thoracic spine is that of axial rotation. In axial rotation the stiffness coefficient of the lumbar spine is about two times that of the thoracic spine.[92] Thus the risk of fracture is greater than the risk of dislocation in the lumbar region when there is an axial (y-axis) torque.

ᴴ Traction is a force; the unit of measure is newtons (pound-force). However, it is generally applied by hanging weights that are specified by their mass in kilograms (pounds). Thus, a 1-kg weight applies 9.8 N (2.2 lbf) of traction. Similarly, a 1-lb weight applies about 4.5 N (1 lbf) of traction.

CLASSIFICATION OF REFERENCES

Basic biomechanics 11, 39, 40, 41, 48, 75, 81, 86, 87, 88, 91, 92, 93, 99, 100, 106, 108, 111, 123, 133, 145, 147, 148, 152

Basic neuropathology 1, 3, 8, 12, 28, 29, 29a, 30, 31, 32, 33, 50, 56, 57, 69, 84, 89, 90, 103, 105, 128, 129, 130, 132, 135, 137, 138, 139, 140, 141, 150

Clinical topics

    Occipital-atlanto-axial-complex 2, 2a, 4, 15a, 17, 23, 35, 36, 38, 41, 43, 44, 53, 55, 58, 63, 64, 66, 80, 94, 96, 109, 111a, 119, 120, 124, 126, 142, 143, 145

    Traumatic spondylolisthesis (hangman's fracture) 15a, 22, 34, 37, 79, 115, 153, 157

    Lower cervical spine fractures 9, 10, 11, 42, 65, 67, 77, 95, 97, 98, 107, 110, 123b, 131, 151, 152

    Whiplash injuries 13, 45, 46, 49, 60, 75, 76, 81, 88, 101, 117, 132, 134, 152, 158

    Central spinal cord syndrome 102, 113

    Clay shoveller's fracture, 5, 54

    Thoracic spine injuries 52, 61, 70, 73, 85, 146

    Lumbar spine injuries 6, 40, 51, 52, 61, 70, 73, 85, 99, 111, 122, 146

    Seat ejection fractures 20, 59, 72

    Lap belt injuries 18, 51, 121, 122

    Spinal injuries in athletes 19, 74, 82, 116

    Spondylolisthesis 154, 155

REFERENCES

1. Albin, M. S., White, R. J., Acosta-Rua, G.: Study of functional recovery produced by delayed localized cooling after spinal cord injury in primates. J. Neurosurg., *29:* 113, 1968.

2. Alexander, E., Forsyth, H. F., Davis, C. H., and Nashold, B. S.: Dislocation of the atlas on the axis. The value of early fusion of C₁, C₂, and C₃. J. Neurosurg., *15:*353, 1958.

2a. Alker, G. J., et al.: Post mortem radiology of head and neck injuries in fatal traffic accidents. J. Neuroradiol., *114:*611, 1975. (*An important and revealing article on upper cervical spine trauma and the number of fatal injuries that are not recognized by routine autopsy.*)

3. Allen, A. R.: Surgery of experimental lesion of spinal cord equivalent to crush injury of fracture dislocation of spinal column: a preliminary report. J.A.M. A., *57:* 878, 1911.

4. Anderson, L. D., and D'Alonzo, R. T.: Fractures of the odontoid process of the axis. J. Bone Joint Surg., *56A:* 1663, 1974. (*Probably the best article available on the classification and management of odontoid fractures.*)

5. Annan, J. H.: Shoveler's fracture. Lancet, *1:*174, 1945.

6. Armstrong, J. R.: Lumbar disc lesions. Edinburgh, E.&S. Livingstone, 1952.

7. Aufdermaur, M.: Spinal injuries in juveniles, necropsy findings in twelve cases. J. Bone Joint Surg., *56B:*513, 1974.

8. Bailey, P.: Traumatic hemorrhages into the spinal cord. Med. Rec., *57:*573, 1900.

9. Bailey, R. W.: Observations of cervical intervertebral-disc lesions in fractures and dislocations. J. Bone Joint Surg., *45A:*461, 1963. (*One of the most informative publications on cervical spine trauma.*)

10. Barnes, R.: Paraplegia in cervical spine injuries. Proc. R. Soc. Med., *54:*365, 1961.

11. Beatson, T. R.: Fractures and dislocations of the cervical spine. J. Bone Joint Surg., *45B:*21, 1963. (*One of the best works on the problem of unilateral and bilateral facet dislocations.*)

12. Black, P., and Markowitz, R. S.: Experimental spinal cord injury in monkeys: comparison of steroids and local hypothermia. Surg. Forum, *22:*409, 1971.

13. Billig, H. E.: Traumatic neck, head, eye syndrome. Journal of the International College of Surgeons, *20:*558, 1953.

14. Bohler, L.: The Treatment of Fractures. 4th English ed. Bristol, John Wright & Sons, 1935.

15. Boukhris, R., and Becker, K. L.: The inter-relationship between vertebral fractures and osteoporosis. Clin. Orthop., *90:*209, 1973.

15a. Brasher, H. R., Venters, G. C., and Preston, E. T.: Fractures of the neural arch of the axis. A report of twenty-nine cases. J. Bone Joint Surg., *57A:*879, 1975.

16. Calliet, R.: Neck and Arm Pain. Oxford, Blackwell Scientific Publications, 1964.

17. Carella, A.: Variations of the sagittal diameter of the atlas and axis in cases of slight anomaly of the atlas. Neuroradiology, *5:*195, 1973.

18. Chance, G. Q.: Note on a type of flexion fracture of the spine. Br. J. Radiol., *21:*452, 1948.

19. Chrisman, O. D., Snook, G. A., Stanitis, J. M., and Keedy, V. A.: Lateral-flexion neck injuries in athletic competition. J.A.M.A., *192:*613, 1965. (*Worthwhile reading for one interested in the care of the athlete.*)

20. Chubb, R., et al.: Compression fractures of the spine during USAF ejections. Aerosp. Med., *36:*968, 1965.

21. Collard, M., and Brasseur, P.: Rontgenologischer nachweis des traumatischen ursprungs einer sondylolyse. Fortschr. Röntgenstr., *117/6:*647, 1972.

22. Cornish, B. L.: Traumatic spondylolisthesis of the axis. J. Bone Joint Surg., *50B:*31, 1968. (*A thorough and comprehensive clinical review of this injury.*)

23. Coutts, M. B.: Atlanto-epistropheal subluxations. Arch. Surg., *29:*297, 1934. (*A thorough anatomical and pathophysiological clinical review.*)

24. Davis, A. G.: Fractures of the spine. J. Bone Joint Surg., *11:*133, 1929.

25. ———: Tensile strength of the anterior longitudinal ligament in relation to treatment of 132 crush fractures of the spine. J. Bone Joint Surg., *20:*429, 1938.

26. De la Torre, J. C., et al.: Monoamine changes in experimental head and spinal cord trauma: failure to confirm previous observations. Surg. Neurol., *2:*5, 1974.

27. Delorme: Traité de Chirurgie de Guerre, *1:*868. Paris, 1893.

28. Dohrmann, G. J.: Experimental cord trauma—a historical review. Arch. Neurol., *27:*468, 1972. (*An excellent comprehensive review article up to 1972.*)

29. Dohrmann, G. J., and Allen, W. E., III: Microcirculation of traumatized spinal cord: a correlation of microan-

giography and blood flow patterns in transitory and permanent paraplegia. J. Trauma, 15:1003, 1975.

29a. Dohrmann, G. J., and Panjabi, M. M.: "Standardized" spinal cord trauma: biomechanical parameters and lesion volume. Surg. Neurolog., 6:263, 1976.

30. Dohrmann, G. J., Wagner, F. C., Jr., and Bucy, P. C.: The microvasculature in transitory traumatic paraplegia: an electron microscopic study in the monkey. J. Neurosurg., 35:263, 1971.

31. Dohrmann, G. J., and Wick, K. M.: Demonstration of the microvasculature of the spinal cord by an intravenous injection of the flourescent dye, thioflavine S. Stain Technol., 46:321, 1971.

32. Dohrmann, G. J., Wick, K. M., and Bucy, P. C.: Spinal cord blood flow patterns in experimental traumatic paraplegia. J. Neurosurg., 38:52, 1973.

33. Ducker, T. B., and Hamit, H. F.: Experimental treatments of acute spinal cord injury. J. Neurosurg., 30:693, 1969.

34. Duff, C.: A Handbook on Hanging. The Bodley Head, London, 1938.

35. Dunbar, H. S., and Bronson, R. S.: Chronic atlanto-axial dislocations with late neurologic manifestations. Surg. Gynecol. Obstet., 113:757, 1961.

36. Elliott, G. R., and Sachs, E.: Observations on fracture of the odontoid process of the axis with intermittent pressure paralysis. Ann. Surg., 56:876, 1912. (*A beautifully presented classic case that will satisfy the scholarly appetite. The saga of a hard working man who recovered many times from profound neurologic deficit is followed by an astute analysis of the autopsy findings.*)

37. Elliott, J. M., Rogers, L. F., Wissinger, J. P., and Lee, J. F.: The hangman's fracture. Fractures of the neural arch of the axis. Radiology, 104:303, 1972.

38. Englander, O.: Non-traumatic occipito-atlanto-axial dislocation. Contribution to the radiology of the atlas. Br. J. Radiol., 15:341, 1942.

39. Ewing, C. L., et al.: Structural consideration of the human vertebral column under $+G_z$ impact acceleration. J. Aircraft, 9:84, 1972.

40. Farfan, H. F., Cossette, J. W., Robertson, H. G., Wells, R. V., and Kraus, H.: The effects of torsion on the lumbar intervertebral joints; the role of torsion in the production of disc regeneration. J. Bone Joint Surg., 52A:468, 1970.

41. Fielding, J. W., Cochran, G. V. B., Lawsing, J. F., and Hohl, M.: Tears of the transverse ligament of the atlas, a clinical biomechanical study. J. Bone Joint Surg., 56A:1683, 1974.

42. Forsythe, H. F.: Extension injuries of the cervical spine. J. Bone Joint Surg., 46A:1792, 1964.

43. Fried, L. C.: Atlanto-axial fracture dislocations. Failure of posterior C1 to C2 fusion. J. Bone Joint Surg., 55B:490, 1973.

44. Gabrielsen, T. O., and Maxwell, J. A.: Traumatic atlanto-occipito dislocation: with case report of patient who survived. Am. J. of Roentgenol. Radium Ther. Nucl. Med., 97:624, 1966.

45. Gay, J. R., and Abbott, K. H.: Common whiplash injuries of the neck. J.A.M.A., 152:1698, 1953. (*A good comprehensive review of the salient clinical considerations.*)

46. Gershon-Cohen, J., Budin, E., and Glauser, F.: Whiplash fractures of cervicodorsal spinous processes; Resemblance to shoveler's fracture. J.A.M.A., 155:560, 1954.

47. Gill, G. G., Manning, J. G., and White, H. L.: Surgical treatment of spondylolisthesis without spine fusion. J. Bone Joint Surg., 37A:493, 1955.

48. Gosch, H. H., Gooding, E., and Schneider, R. C.: An experimental study of cervical spine and cord injuries. J. Trauma, 12:570, 1972. (*One of the most important and informative studies on the biomechanics of spine trauma.*)

49. Gotten, N.: Survey of 100 cases of whiplash injuries after settlement of litigation. J.A.M.A., 162:865, 1956.

50. Green, B. A., and Wagner, F. C., Jr.: Evolution of edema in the acutely injured spinal cord: a fluorescence microscopic study. Surg. Neurol., 1:98, 1973.

51. Greenbaum, E., Harris, L., Halloran, X.: Flexion fracture of the lumbar spine due to lap-type seat belts. Calif. Med., 113:74, 1970.

52. Griffith, H. B., Cleave, J. R. W., and Taylor, R. G.: Changing patterns of fracture in the dorsal and lumbar spine. Br. Med. J., 1:891, 1966.

53. Griswold, D. M., and Southwick, W. O.: Lesions of the atlanto-axial complex and their management [thesis]. Section of Orthopaedic Surgery, Yale University School of Medicine, New Haven, 1972.

54. Hall, R. D.: Clay-shoveler's fracture, J. Bone Joint Surg., 12:63, 1940. (*Recommended as one of the best papers on this particular topic.*)

55. Harolson, R. H., III, and Boyd, H. B.: Posterior dislocation of the atlas on the axis without fracture. Report of a case. J. Bone Joint Surg., 51A:561, 1969.

56. Hartzog, J. T., Fisher, R. G., and Snow, C.: Spinal cord trauma: effect of hyperbaric oxygen therapy. Proc. Spinal Cord Inj. Conf., 17:70, 1969.

57. Hedeman, L. S., Shellenberger, M. K., and Gordon, J. H.: Studies in experimental spinal cord trauma. Part I: alterations in catecholamine levels. J. Neurosurg., 40:37, 1974.

58. Hentzer, L., and Schalimtzek, M.: Fractures and subluxation of the atlas and axis. Acta Orthop. Scand., 42:251, 1971.

59. Hirsch, C., and Nachemson, A.: Clinical observations on the spines in ejected pilots. Aerospace Med., 34:629, 1963.

60. Hohl, M.: Soft-tissue injuries of the neck in automobile accidents—factors influencing prognosis. J. Bone Joint Surg., 56A:1675, 1974.

61. Holdsworth, F. W.: Fractures, dislocations and fracture-dislocations of the spine. J. Bone Joint Surg., 45B:6, 1963.

62. Hollin, S. A., Gross, S. W., and Levin, P.: Fracture of the cervical spine in patients with rheumatoid spondylitis. Am. Surg., 31:532, 1965.

63. Jacobson, G., and Alder, D. C.: An evaluation of lateral atlanto-axial displacement in injuries of the cervical spine. Radiology, 61:355, 1953.

64. ————: Examination of the atlanto-axial joint following injury: with particular emphasis on rotational subluxation. Am. J. Roentgenol. Radium Ther. Nucl. Med., 76:1081, 1956.

65. Janda, W. E., Kelly, P. J., Rhoton, A. L., and Layton, D. D.: Fracture-dislocation of the cervical part of the spinal column in patients with ankylosing spondylitis. Mayo Clin. Proc., 43:714, 1968.

66. Jefferson, G.: Fracture of the atlas vertebra, report of four cases and a review of those previously recorded. Br. J. Surg., 7:407, 1920.

67. Johnson, R. M., Crelin, E. S., White, A. A., and Panjabi, M. M.: Some new observations on the functional anatomy of the lower cervical spine. Clin. Orthop., *111*:192, 1975.

68. Kamiya, T.: Experimental study on anterior spinal cord compression with special emphasis on vascular disturbance. Nagoya J. Med. Sci., *31*:171, 1967.

69. Kelly, D. L., Jr., et al.: Effects of hyperbaric oxygenation and tissue oxygen studies in experimental paraplegia. J. Neurosurg., *36*:425, 1972.

70. Kelly, R. P., and Whitesides, T. E.: Treatment of lumbodorsal fracture-dislocations. Ann. Surg., *167*:705, 1968.

71. Key, J. A., and Conwell, H. E.: The Management of Fractures, Dislocations and Sprains. ed. 4. St. Louis, C. V. Mosby, 1946.

72. Laurell, L., and Nachemson, A.: Some factors influencing spinal injuries in seat ejected pilots. Ind. Med. Surg., *32*:27, 1963.

73. Leidholdt, J. D., et al.: Evaluation of late spinal deformities with fracture dislocations of the dorsal and lumbar spine in paraplegias. Paraplegia, *7*:16, 1969.

74. Leidholdt, J. D.: Spinal injuries in sports. Surg. Clin. North Am., *43*:351, 1963.

75. McKenzie, J. A., and Williams, J. F.: The dynamic behavior of the head and cervical spine during "whiplash." J. Biomech., *4*:477, 1971.

76. Macnab, I.: Acceleration injuries of the cervical spine. J. Bone Joint Surg., *46A*:1797, 1964.

77. Marar, B. C.: The pattern of neurological damage as an aid to the diagnosis of the mechanism in cervical-spine injuries. J. Bone Joint Surg., *56A*:1648, 1974. (*An important and interesting analysis, although not completely convincing.*)

78. ———: Hyperextension injuries of the cervical spine. The pathogenesis of damage to the spinal cord. J. Bone Joint Surg., *56A*:1655, 1974. (*A good review and an up to date analysis of the topic.*)

79. Marshall, J. J.: Judicial executions. Br. Med. J., *2*:779, 1888.

80. Martel, W.: Occipito-atlanto-axial joints in rheumatoid arthritis and ankylosing spondylitis. Am. J. Roentgenol. Rad. Ther. Nucl. Med., *86*:223, 1961.

81. Martinez, J. L., and Garcia, D. J.: A model for whiplash. J. Biomech., *1*:23, 1968.

82. Melvin, W. J. S., Dunlop, H. W., Hetherington, F. R., and Kerr, J. W.: The role of the faceguard in the production of flexion injuries to the cervical spine in football. Can. Med. Assoc. J., *93*:1110, 1965.

83. Murone, I.: The importance of the sagittal diameters of the cervical spinal canal in relation to spondylosis and myelopathy. J. Bone Joint Surg., *56B*:30, 1974.

84. Naftchi, N. E., et al.: Biogenic amine concentrations in traumatized spinal cords of cats: effect of drug therapy. J. Neurosurg., *40*:52, 1974.

85. Nicoll, E. A.: Fractures of the dorso-lumbar spine. J. Bone Joint Surg., *31B*:376, 1949.

86. Nonne, M.: Kompression des Halsmarks durch eine chronisch entstandere Luxation zwischen Atlas and Epistropheus sowie swischer Schadelbasis und Atlas. Arch. Psychiat. Nervenkr., *74*:264, 1925.

87. Noyes, R. R., DeLucas, J. L., and Torvik, P. J.: Biomechanics of anterior cruciate ligament failure: an analysis of strain-rate sensitivity and mechanisms of failure in primates. J. Bone Joint Surg., *56A*:236, 1974.

88. Ommaya, A. K., and Hirsch, A. E.: Tolerances for cerebral concussion from head impact and whiplash in primates. J. Biomech., *4*:13, 1971.

89. Osterholm, J. L., and Mathews, G. J.: Altered norepinephrine metabolism following experimental spinal cord injury: I. Relationship to hemorrhagic necrosis and post-wounding neurological deficits. J. Neurosurg., *36*:386, 1972.

90. ———: Altered norephinephrine metabolism following experimental spinal cord injury: II. Protection against traumatic spinal cord hemorrhagic necrosis by norepinephrine synthesis blockade with alpha methyl tyrosine. J. Neurosurg., *36*:395, 1972.

91. Panjabi, M. M., Brand, R. M., and White, A. A.: Three-dimensional flexibility and stiffness properties of the human thoracic spine. J. Biomech., *9*:185, 1976.

92. Panjabi, M. M., Krag, M., and White, A. A.: Effects of preload on load displacement curves of the lumbar spine. Orthop. Clin. North Am., *8*:181, 1977.

93. Panjabi, M. M., White, A. A., and Brand, R. A.: A note on defining body parts configurations. J. Biomech., *7*:385, 1974.

94. Paradis, G. R., and Janes, J. M.: Post traumatic atlanto-axial instability: the fate of the odontoid process fracture in 46 cases. J. Trauma, *13*:359, 1973.

95. Patrick, L. M.: Studies on hyperextension and hyperflexion injuries in volunteers and human cadavers. *In* Gardjian, E., and Thomas, E. [ed.]: Neckache and Backache. Springfield, Charles C Thomas, 1969.

96. Patzakis, M. J., et al.: Posterior dislocation of the atlas on the axis: a case report. J. Bone Joint Surg., *56A*:1260, 1974.

97. Payne, E. E., and Spillane, J. D.: The cervical spine. Brain, *80*:571, 1957.

98. Penning, L.: Functional Pathology of the Cervical Spine. Amsterdam, Excerpta Medica, 1968.

99. Perey, O.: Fracture of the vertebral end-plate in the lumbar spine—an experimental biomechanical investigation. Acta Orthop. Scan., 25 [Suppl.], 1957. (*A thorough, informative, well illustrated analysis of the mechanical, radiological, and anatomic aspects of the subject.*)

100. Plaue, R.: Die mechanik des wirbelkompressionsbruchs [The mechanics of compression fractures of the spine]. Zentralbl. Chir., *98*:761, 1973.

101. Pruce, A.: Whiplash injury: what's new? South. Med. J., *57*:332, 1964.

102. Rand, R. W., and Crandall, P. H.: Central spinal cord syndrome in hyperextension injuries of the cervical spine. J. Bone Joint Surg., *44A*:1415, 1962.

103. Rawe, S. E., et al.: Norepinephrine levels in experimental spinal cord trauma. Presented at the meeting of the American Association of Neurological Surgeons, St. Louis, April, 1974.

104. Ray, B. S.: Platybasia with involvement of the central nervous system. Ann. Surg., *116*:231, 1942.

105. Richardson, H. D., and Nakamura, S.: An electron microscopic study of spinal cord edema and the effect of treatment with steroids, mannitol and hypothermia. Proc. Spinal Cord Inj. Conf., *18*:10, 1971.

106. Roaf, R.: A study of the mechanics of spinal injuries. J. Bone Joint Surg., *42B*:810, 1960.

107. ———: Lateral flexion injuries of the cervical spine. J. Bone Joint Surg., *45B*:36, 1963.

108. ———: International classification of spinal injuries. Paraplegia, *10*:78, 1972. (*An important basic approach to the analysis and classification of spine trauma.*)

109. Roberts, A., and Wickstrom, J.: Prognosis of odontoid fractures. J. Bone Joint Surg., *54A*:1353, 1972.

110. Rogers, W. A.: Fractures and dislocations of the cervical spine. J. Bone Joint Surg., *39A*:341, 1957.

111. Rolander, S. D., and Blair, W. E.: Deformation and fracture of the lumbar vertebral end plate. Orthop. Clin. North Am., *6*:75, 1975.

111a. Schatzker, J., Rorabeck, C. H., and Waddell, J. P.: Nonunion of the odontoid process, an experimental investigation. Clin. Orthop., *108*:127, 1975.

112. Schneider, R. C.: The syndrome of acute anterior spinal cord injury. J. Neurosurg., *12*:95, 1955.

113. Schneider, R. C., Cherry, G., and Pantek, H.: The syndrome of acute central cervical spinal cord injury. J. Neurosurg., *11*:546, 1954.

114. Schneider, R. C., and Kahn, E. A.: Chronic neurological sequellae of acute trauma to the spine and spinal cord. J. Bone Joint Surg., *38A*:985, 1956.

115. Schneider, R. C., Livingston, K. E., Cave, A. J. E., and Hamilton, G.: "Hangman's fracture" of the cervical spine. J. Neurosurg., *22*:141, 1965. (*An excellent overview of this injury.*)

116. Schneider, R. C., Reifel, E., Crisler, H. D., and Oosterbaan, B. G.: Serious and fatal football injuries involving the head and spinal cord. J.A.M.A., *177*:362, 1961.

117. Schutt, C. H., and Dohan, F. C.: Neck injuries to women in auto accidents. A metropolitan plague. J.A.M.A., *206*:2689, 1968.

118. Severy, D. M., Mathewson, J. H., and Bechtol, C. O.: Controlled automobile related engineering and medical phenomena. Medical aspects of traffic accidents. Proceedings of Montreal Conference, p. 152, 1955.

119. Shapiro, R., Youngberg, A. S., and Rothman, S. L. G.: The differential diagnosis of traumatic lesions of the occipito-atlanto-axial segment. Radiol. Clin. North Am., *11*:505, 1973. (*A highly recommended excellent clinical radiological review of this complex region.*)

120. Sherk, H., and Nicholson, J.: Fractures of the atlas. J. Bone Joint Surg., *52A*:1017, 1970.

121. Smith, W. S., and Kaufer, H.: A new pattern of spine injury associated with lap-type seat belts: a preliminary report. Univ. Mich. Med. Center J., *33*:99, 1966.

122. ———: Patterns and mechanism of lumbar injuries associated with lap seat belts. J. Bone Joint Surg., *51A*:239, 1969.

123. Soechting, J. F., and Paslay, P. R.: A model for the human spine during impact including musculature influence. J. Biomech., *6*:195, 1973.

123a. Stauffer, E. S., and Fox, J. M.: Traumatic quadraplegia secondary to football accidents. Meeting of the Cervical Spine Research Society, Toronto, November 1975.

123b. Stauffer, E. S., and Kelly, E. G.: Fracture dislocation and recurrent deformity following treatment by anterior interbody fusion. J. Bone Joint Surg., *59A*:45, 1977.

124. Steele, H. H.: Anatomical and mechanical considerations of the atlanto-axial articulation. J. Bone Joint Surg., *50A*:1481, 1968.

125. Strain, R. E.: Cervical discography and electromyography in the diagnosis of lacerated or torn cervical disc. J. Fla. Med. Assoc., *49*:734, 1963.

125a. Sullivan, J. D., and Farfan, J. F.: The crumpled neural arch. Orthop. Clin. North Am., *6*:199, 1975.

126. Swinson, D. R., Hamilton, E. B. D., Mathews, J. A., and Yates, D. A. H.: Vertical subluxation of the axis in rheumatoid arthritis. Ann. Rheum. Dis., *31*:359, 1972.

127. Tarlov, I. M.: Spinal cord compression studies: III. Time limits for recovery after gradual compression in dogs. Arch. Neurol. Psychiat., *71*:588, 1954.

128. ———: Spinal Cord Compression: Mechanism of Paralysis and Treatment. Springfield, Charles C Thomas, 1957.

129. Tarlov, I. M., and Klinger, H.: Spinal cord compression studies: II. Time limits for recovery after acute compression in dogs. Arch. Neurol. Psychiat., *71*:271, 1954.

130. Tarlov, I. M., Klinger, H., and Vitale, S.: Spinal cord compression studies: I. Experimental techniques to produce acute and gradual compression. Arch. Neurol. Psychiat., *70*:813, 1953.

131. Taylor, A. R., and Blackwood, W.: Paraplegia in hyperextension cervical injuries with normal radiographic appearances. J. Bone Joint Surg., *30B*:245, 1948.

132. Taylor, A. R.: The mechanism of injury to the spinal cord in the neck without damage to the vertebral column. J. Bone Joint Surg., *33B*:543, 1951. (*A classic article which is focal to basic clinical knowledge of spine trauma.*)

133. Tkaczuk, H.: Tensile properties of human lumbar longitudinal ligaments [thesis]. Acta Orthop. Scand., *115* [Suppl.], 1968.

134. Torres, F., and Shapiro, S. K.: Electroencephalograms in whiplash injury: a comparison of electroencephalographic abnormalities with those present in closed head injuries. Arch. Neurol., *5*:40, 1961.

135. Turnbull, I. M.: Microvasculature of the human spinal cord. J. Neurosurg., *35*:141, 1971.

136. Vicas, E. B.: Fractures de la colonne cervicale ankylosee par la maladie de Marie Strumpell. Union Med. Can., *101*:1818, 1972.

137. Wagner, F. C., Jr., and Dohrmann, G. J.: Alterations in nerve cells and myelinated fibers in spinal cord injury. Surg. Neurol., *3*:125, 1975.

138. Wagner, F. C., Jr., Dohrmann, G. J., and Bucy, P. C.: Early alterations in spinal cord morphology following experimental trauma. Fed. Proc., *29*:289, 1970.

139. ———: Histopathology of transitory traumatic paraplegia in the monkey. J. Neurosurg., *35*:272, 1971.

140. Wagner, F. C., Jr., Green, B. A., Bucy, P. C.: Spinal cord edema associated with paraplegia. Proc. Spinal Cord Inj. Conf., *18*:9, 1971.

141. Wagner, R. F., and Abel, M. S.: Small-element lesion of the cervical spine due to trauma. Clin. Orthop., *16*:235, 1960.

142. Wartzman, G., and Dewar, F. P.: Rotary fixation of the atlanto axial joint: rotational atlantoaxial subluxation radiology, *90*:479, 1968.

143. Washington, E. R.: Non-traumatic atlanto-occipital and atlanto-axial dislocation: case report. J. Bone Joint Surg., *41A*:341, 1959.

144. Watson-Jones, R.: Fractures and Joint Injuries. ed. 3. Two Volumes. Edinburgh, E. & S. Livingstone, 1943.

145. Werne, S.: Studies in spontaneous atlas dislocation. Acta Orthop. Scand., *23* [Suppl.], 1957. (*This work is valuable for indepth understanding of the anatomy, kinematics, and clinical aspects of this region.*)

146. Westerborn, A., and Olsson, O.: Mechanics, treatment and prognosis of fractures of the dorso-lumbar spine. Acta Chir. Scand., *102:*59, 1951.

147. White, A. A.: Analysis of the mechanics of the thoracic spine in man. Acta Orthopaedica Scandinavica, *127* [Suppl.], 1969.

148. White, A. A., Panjabi, M. M., and Brand, R. A.: A system for defining position and motion of the human body parts. Med. Biol. Eng., *13:*261, 1975.

149. White, A. A., Southwick, W. O., DePonte, R. J., Gainor, J. W., and Hardy, R.: Relief of pain by anterior spine fusion for spondylosis. J. Bone Joint Surg., *55A:*525, 1973.

150. White, R. J., et al.: Spinal cord injury: sequential morphology and hypothermia stabilization. Surg. Forum, *20:*432, 1969.

151. Whitley, J. E., and Forsyth, H. F.: The classification of cervical spine injuries. Am. J. Roentgenol. Radium Ther. Nucl. Med., *83:*633, 1960. (*A good paper for correlating radiological findings with presumed mechanisms of injury.*)

152. Wickstrom, J., Martinez, J., and Rodrigues, J.: Cervical sprain syndrome: "Experimental acceleration injuries of head and neck" in the prevention of highway injury. Ann Arbor, Michigan: Highway Safety Research Institute, University of Michigan, p. 182, 1967.

153. Williams, T. G.: Hangman's fracture. J. Bone Joint Surg., *57B:*82, 1975.

154. Wiltse, L. L.: The etiology of spondylolisthesis. J. Bone Joint Surg., *44A:*539, 1962.

155. Wiltse, L. L., Widell, E. H., Jr., and Jackson, D. W.: Fatigue fracture: the basic lesion in isthmic spondylolisthesis. J. Bone Joint Surg., *57A:*17, 1975.

156. Wolf, B. S., Khilnani, M., and Malis, L.: The sagittal diameter of the bony cervical spinal canal and its significance in cervical spondylosis. J. Mt. Sinai Hosp., *23:*283, 1956.

157. Wood-Jones, F.: The ideal lesion produced by judicial hanging. Lancet, *1:*53, 1913.

158. Zatzkin, H. R., and Kveton, F. W.: Evaluation of the cervical spine in whiplash injuries. Radiology, *75:*577, 1960.

5 The Problem of Clinical Instability in the Human Spine: A Systematic Approach

"I don't know what you mean by 'glory'," Alice said.
Humpty Dumpty smiled contemptuously. "Of course you don't–till I tell you. I meant 'there's a nice knock-down argument for you'!"
"But 'glory' doesn't mean a nice knock-down argument," Alice objected.
"When I use a word," Humpty Dumpty said, "it means just what I choose it to mean, neither more nor less."
"The question is," said Alice, "whether you can make words mean so many different things."
"The question is," said Humpty Dumpty, "which is to be Master–that's all."
                                 Alice in Wonderland, Lewis Carroll

INTRODUCTION

During the time that one of the authors was preparing for his orthopaedic boards, he asked himself the following question: "How do you determine when the spine is unstable?" This question was most anxiety provoking, especially since the initial response was a recollection of a surgeon tugging up and down on the posterior elements of a lumbar vertebra and saying, " . . . yep, it's unstable, we'd better fuse it." The aspirant thus went frantically through the standard orthopaedic references in search of the answer. This study tended to reduce the anxiety level with regard to the ensuing examination, but it clearly raised some other, serious doubts. No one seemed to have a clear and valid answer to the question. In addition, it became apparent that making such a crucial determination in the clinical situation is extremely difficult. In many instances, such a decision can very significantly affect patient care. Misjudgment of one type may result in death or major neurologic deficits.

Misjudgment of another type may result in unnecessary surgery, again with death or other major complications. Evaluating a patient's condition erroneously can cause considerable needless inconvenience related to wearing complex encumbrances, such as Minerva casts or halo pelvic fixation devices. Correct judgment provides the patient with realization of the maximum recovery with an absolute minimum of risks and inconvenience. This chapter does not purport to provide physicians with ideal judgment and wisdom. It does, however, endeavor to present a systematic approach to the problem, based on current clinical and biomechanical knowledge.

Definitions

Many physicians, to some degree, have been like Humpty Dumpty in the "mastery" of the word stability, as it is used clinically. There are a number of stated and unstated definitions of the term, and if the definition of the condition is confusing, it can be expected that the diagnosis and treatment of the condition will reach progressively higher orders of ambiguity. One of the problems in the literature has been the absence of a clear definition. All physicians use the term stability, but they may have a variety of different concepts and definitions in mind as they use it. As a working definition for this chapter, we have chosen to employ the term "clinical instability."

Clinical instability is defined as the loss of the ability of the spine under *physiologic loads* to maintain relationships between vertebrae in such a way that there is neither damage nor *subsequent* irritation to the spinal cord or nerve roots, and, in addition, there is no development of *incapacitating deformity* or pain due to structural changes.

This is the working definition. The complexity of the subject matter demands a few qualifiers. *Physiologic loads* are those which are incurred during normal activity of the particular patient being evaluated. *Incapacitating deformity* is defined as gross deformity that the patient finds intolerable. *Incapacitating pain* is defined as pain unable to be controlled by non-narcotic drugs. Clinical instability can occur from trauma, disease, surgery, or some combination of the three.

Unless the term *clinical instability* or *clinical stability* is used, we are not referring to the preceding definition. Stability or instability alone is used when the term found in the literature is repeated and when other statements about it are reported. The term has rarely been defined in previous publications. Its connotations, however, occasionally overlap, to some extent, with the definition we have offered. When the term *clinical instability* is used, it refers to the preceding definition.

Background and Organization

In the diagnosis of clinical instability in any region of the spine, several crucial factors come into play. Anatomy is significant in terms of position and space relationships between neural structures and potentially damaging structures. It is also important because various structures provide different magnitudes and types of forces that are helpful in preserving stability. Biomechanical studies and information on kinematics

are presented whenever they are contributory. For each region of the spine, recommended methods of evaluation and management are discussed according to the outline below.

Basic Elements of a Systematic Analysis of the Problem of Clinical Stability in the Spine

Anatomic Considerations
Biomechanical Factors
Clinical Considerations
Treatment Considerations
Recommended Evaluation System
Recommended Management

Radiographic Magnification

The major practical consideration in the determination of clinical instability is the evaluation of the patient's radiographs. A good deal of emphasis has been placed on radiographic measurements to determine abnormal displacements and the likelihood of encroachment upon neurologic structures. By adopting standard distances, more meaningful measurements may be made from radiographs. Radiographic examination is currently the only objective means of determining the relative positions of the vertebrae in a potentially unstable spine. Therefore it is important to give some consideration to the accurate interpretation of linear radiographic measurements.

Linear Measurements. The parameters measured on radiographs are either linear, such as the distance between two points, or angular, such as the angle between two lines. The relative position of the radiographic source, the spine and, the film are the only factors that effect the magnification. A three-dimensional vertebra is transformed into a two-dimensional image on the radiographic film, as shown in Figure 5-1. A line AB on the object (vertebra) in a plane parallel to the film is imaged as A'B' on the film. The image is always bigger than the object. Let the magnification M be the percentage increase in length. The formula that shows the dependency of magnification on source, object, and film positions is

$$M = \frac{100 \times D_2}{D_1 - D_2}\%$$

where D_1 is the distance between the radio-

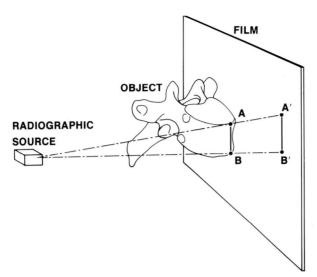

Fig. 5-1. Principle of radiographic magnification. The distance AB between two points on the vertebra becomes an image line A′B′.

graphic source and the film, and D_2 is the distance of the object (spine) from the film. These are shown in Figure 5-2.

The most commonly used value for the distance D_2 is 1.83 m (72 in). If the film is placed next to the shoulder, then the object-to-film distance D_1 in a lateral radiograph is half the shoulder width. Assuming this is 0.3 m (12 in) for the "average" person, the magnification, using the above formula, is 20 per cent. But the distance D_1 has not been standardized. Assuming a variation of 0.3 m (12 in) below and above the value of 1.83 m (72 in), the corresponding magnifications are 25 per cent and 17 per cent.

This range of magnification is for the "average" person. However, there is considerable variation of shoulder widths among individuals. For a nominal value for D_1 of 1.83 mm (72 in), the magnification factors for different shoulder widths (D_2) can be calculated. The results are shown in Table 5-1.

This table clearly shows that there is large variation in magnification introduced by the physical size of the person. The technique of holding the film next to the shoulder is responsible for this. If the two kinds of variation described above (source-to-object and object-to-film distances) are allowed to operate simultaneously,

*Table 5-1. Percentage Magnification of Image Associated With Different Spine-to-Film Distances***

Spine-to-film Distance, m(in)	0.15(6.0)	0.20(8.0)	0.25(10.0)	0.30(12.0)	0.36(14.0)
Magnification %	9	12.5	16	20	24

* Source-to-film distance = 1.83m(72 in)

then the range of magnification widens to 7.5 to 30 per cent.

The large variation in the magnification as shown above, of course, makes it nearly impossible to make any precise measurements from the radiographs when the distances D_1 and D_2 are unknown. An effort should be made to obtain radiographs in which the distances are known, so that, using the equation on page 192, one may easily calculate the magnification.

An even better procedure is to *standardize* the distances. This has several advantages. Templates can be prepared to utilize the standard distances; repeated computations to determine magnification for different patients are not necessary; and most important, it is then possible to compare different radiographs of the same

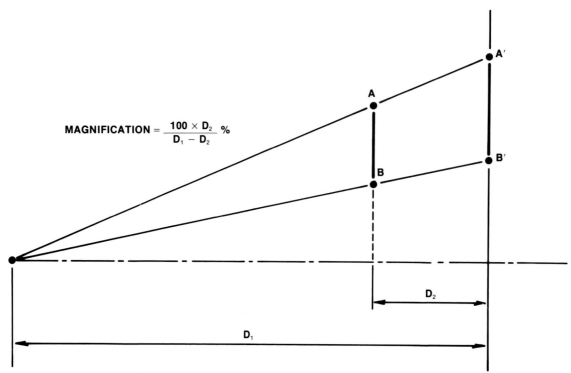

$$\text{MAGNIFICATION} = \frac{100 \times D_2}{D_1 - D_2} \%$$

Fig. 5-2.   In radiology, the image is always bigger than the object: A′B′ is greater than AB. The magnification M depends upon the source-to-film and object-to-film distances, D_1 and D_2, respectively.

patient, even if they were taken at different times. Based on these considerations, we suggest the following as standard distances:

Radiographic source-to-film distance,
$$D_1 = 1.83 \text{ m (72 in)}$$
Spine-to-film distance,
$$D_2 = 0.36 \text{ m (14 in)}$$

These two distances give a linear magnification, M = 24 per cent. The value of 1.83 m (72 in) was chosen because it is the one in most general use. The value of 0.36 m (14 in) for the distance D_2 was chosen to allow inclusion of practically all possible body widths.[A] The standard distances and the corresponding magnifications are depicted graphically in Figure 5-3.

Angular Radiographic Measurements. In contrast to linear measurements, angular radiographic measurements are true representations of the object. For example, the angle between two end-plates in the sagittal plane is precisely the same as the corresponding angle measured on a *true* lateral. One must bear in mind, however,

that if the radiograph is not truly lateral, the angular measurement will always be *larger* than the actual angle in the sagittal plane.

Muscle Forces

The role of the muscles in clinical stability remains obscure. Although an understanding would be useful, it is our view that the muscles offer a small amount of protection through splinting in the acute phases of injury. Furthermore, in the less acute situation, and against the normal range of physiologic loading, the muscles do not play a significant role. For example, in polio patients with total paralysis of cervical muscles, there is no loss of clinical stability as long as the bony and ligamentous structures remain intact.[72] Based on such examples, we feel justified in our endeavor to analyze clinical instability without full knowledge of the exact role of the muscle forces exerted. The physician cannot rule out the possibility that in the acute phase, voluntary and reflex muscle activity in response to pain may be operative.

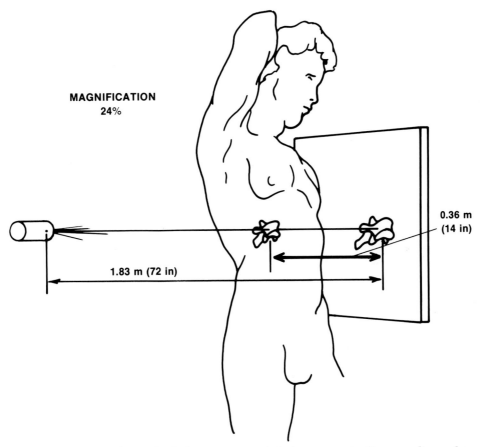

**MAGNIFICATION
24%**

0.36 m
(14 in)

1.83 m (72 in)

Fig. 5-3. Suggested standard distances to minimize errors in linear radiographic measurements.

Biomechanics of Spinal Cord and Nerve Roots

The biomechanics of the spinal cord and nerve roots are important in consideration of the potentially damaging effects of a clinically unstable spine.

An informative and excellently photographed study on the biomechanics of the spinal cord is that of Breig.[17] He showed that, contrary to popular belief, the cord *does not* slide up and down in the spinal canal during flexion and extension and other motions. The cord and its elements are elastic and deform like an accordion as the dimensions of its protective canal change with motion (Fig. 5-4). Dorsal extension tends to stretch the spine anteriorly and shortens it posteriorly, and, with lateral flexion, it stretches on the convex side and shortens on the concave side. This characteristic pattern of deformation seems

to be true of all the structures, including the axis cylinder, the blood vessels, the glial membrane, and all ligaments and meningeal components. Injuries to the cord and the nerve result from loss of elasticity of the cord, pathologic displacement between two or more vertebrae, or protrusions into the canal or posterior fossa. The spinal cord shows good elasticity and compliance in the axial direction. It is relatively much less able to accommodate deformation in the horizontal plane, which accounts for its high vulnerability to translatory displacements of the spine in that plane. The physiologic effects of cord trauma are discussed in Chapter 4. The main consideration is that one episode of force application can initiate a chain of events which beings with rupture of arterioles and venules, followed by hemorrhage, edema, and loss of spinal cord function.

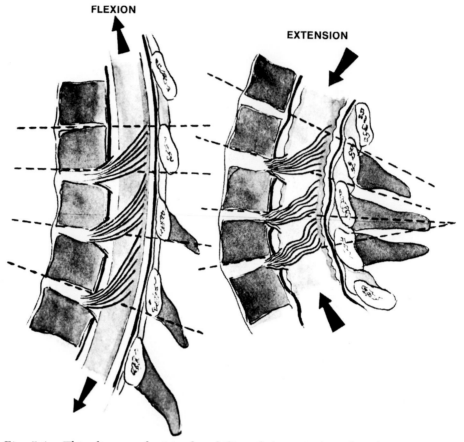

Fig. 5-4. This diagram depicts the ability of the spinal cord and nerve roots to accommodate to physiologic changes in measurement of the spinal column. The capacity of these structures to withstand the accordion-like deformation in the axial direction is an important biomechanical characteristic of the cord and its associated structures. (Breig, A.: Biomechanics of the Central Nervous System: Some Basic Normal and Pathological Phenomena. Stockholm, Almquist & Wiskell, 1960.)

Part 1: Occipital-Atlanto-Axial Complex (Ocp-C1-C2)

Occipital-Atlantal Joint (Ocp-C1)

With the possible exception of the terminal cocygeal joint, the occipital-atlantal joint has received less attention than any of the articulations in the axial skeleton. This generalization seems to hold for anatomic as well as biomechanical and clinical studies.

The anatomic structures that provide stability for this articulation include the cup-shaped configuration of the occipital-atlantal joints and their capsules (Fig. 5-5), along with the anterior and posterior atlanto-occipital membranes. The liga-mentum nuchae should be included here, although its significance as a stabilizing structure in the human spine is controversial.[33,51,52] Additional anatomic stability is gained through the ligamentous connections between the occiput and the axis. This is achieved through the tectorial membrane, the alar ligaments, and the apical ligaments, which are of dubious mechanical significance.[42] Based on structural characteristics, the authors believe that the occipital-atlantal joint is relatively unstable, at least in the child. There may be some increase in stability in adult

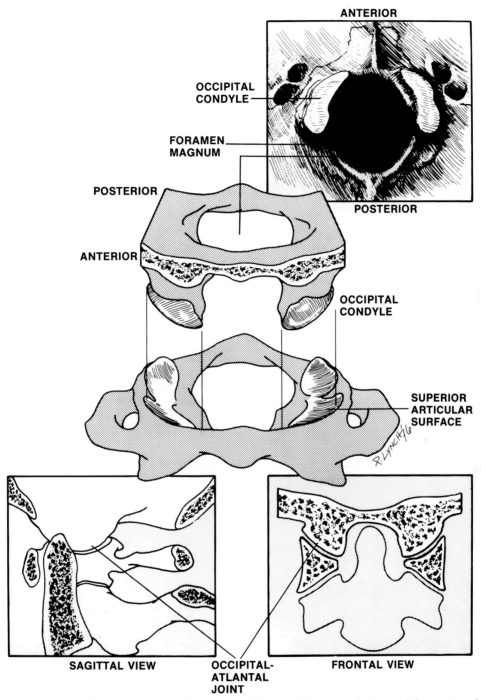

ANTERIOR

OCCIPITAL CONDYLE

FORAMEN MAGNUM

POSTERIOR

ANTERIOR

POSTERIOR

OCCIPITAL CONDYLE

SUPERIOR ARTICULAR SURFACE

SAGITTAL VIEW

OCCIPITAL-ATLANTAL JOINT

FRONTAL VIEW

Fig. 5-5. The three-dimensional anatomy of the cup-like articulations of the occipital-atlantal joints. The cup is relatively more shallow in the sagittal than in the frontal plane. Consequently, the joint is probably more unstable to anteroposterior displacement or dislocation than to lateral displacement.

life due to a decrease in elasticity of the ligaments. The limited studies of the mechanics of this articulation can be reviewed in Chapter 2. Dislocations of this joint are usually fatal. It seems likely that a number of these injuries are followed by instant death and are not discovered at autopsy. The level of the anatomic lesion is such that, unless resuscitation is instituted in a very short period of time, the victim dies. However, there is little in the literature to document the clinical characteristics of instability at this joint.

We are aware of one patient who has survived this injury for over one year (Fig. 5-6). He is a 14-year-old who was hit from behind by an automobile while riding his bicycle, and he is being sustained on a respirator. Cephalad progression of medullary damage destroyed the lower cranial nerves, rendering him unable to swallow, talk, or chew. Another case has been reported by Evarts.[31]

Based on our present knowledge of the structure of this joint, and the dangerous anatomic risks involved in its displacement, we suggest that any dislocation or subluxation be considered clinically unstable. The treatment that we recommend is posterior fusion, occiput to C2, followed by immobilization for 3 months in a halo device attached to a thoracic jacket.

Atlanto-Axial Joint (C1–C2)

The C1–C2 articulation is the most complex and difficult one to analyze. Both the basic and clinical literature concerning this area are highly controversial, and sometimes confusing. The most valid information relating to the problem of clinical instability in this area is discussed here.

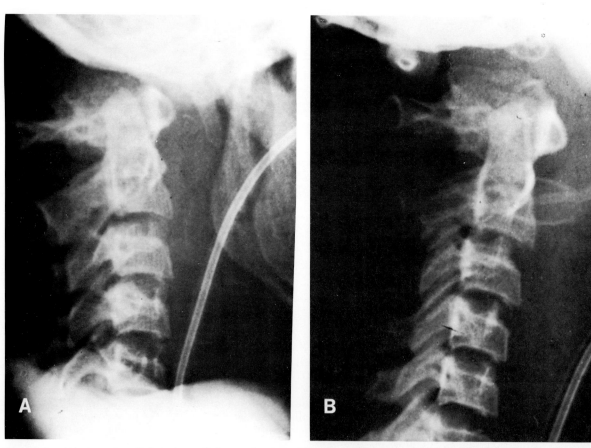

Fig. 5-6. (A) Anterior dislocation of the occiput on C1. (B) Axial traction resulted in +y-axis displacement suggestive of total disruption of the intervening ligaments. (Courtesy of Children's Hospital, Akron, Ohio.)

ANATOMIC CONSIDERATIONS

Various aspects of the anatomy of atlanto-axial region are presented in Chapters 2 and 4.

One of the key variables in the problem of clinical instability is that of allowable displacement without neurologic deficit. This is partially dependent upon the normal sagittal diameter of the spinal canal, which has been studied in 200 normal adult subjects by Wolf and colleagues.[103] These results are presented in Figure 5-7. Similar data for children is also available.[43]

The bony and cartilaginous articulations of the facet joints, with their biconvex configurations, are held together by a loose articular capsule designed to permit a large range of joint motion. Consequently, the capsule and osseous configuration contribute little to the clinical stability of the joint. Rather, the major mechanical stability of this articulation is provided through the dens and the ring formed by the anatomic structures surrounding it. This consists of the osseous portion of the atlas anteriorly and laterally and the transverse ligament posteriorly. Virtually all of the other anatomic structures play a secondary role in the stability of this joint. The strong yellow ligament is not present between C1–C2. Instead, there is the weaker atlanto-axial membrane.

Anterior Longitudinal Ligament

This structure is a continuation of the ligament that runs the entire length of the spine. It is well developed in the thoracic and lumbar regions and described as a thin translucent structure in the cervical region.[52] It runs from the anterior body of C2, attaches to the anterior ring of C1, and courses to the tubercle of the occiput. Little is known about the mechanical properties of this structure in this region of the spine.

The Anterior Atlanto-Epistrophical and the Atlanto-Occipital Ligaments

These structures are not shown in Figure 5-8. The atlanto-epistrophical ligament runs between the anterior portion of the body of C2 and the caudal portion of the anterior ring of C1. The atlanto-occipital ligament runs between the cephalad portion of the anterior ring of C1 and the tubercle of the occiput. Both constitute a continuation of the anterior longitudinal ligament.

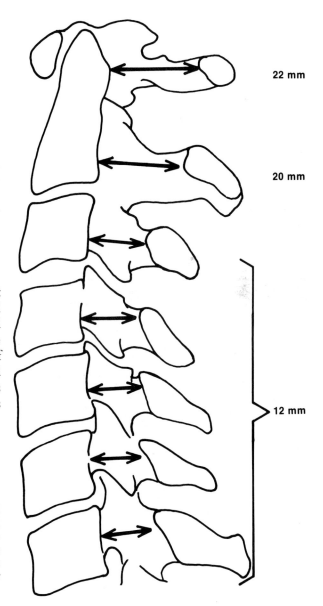

Fig. 5-7 The true sagittal plane diameter of the cervical spine canal. The upper portion has relatively more space for the spinal cord, even though the cord is larger there.

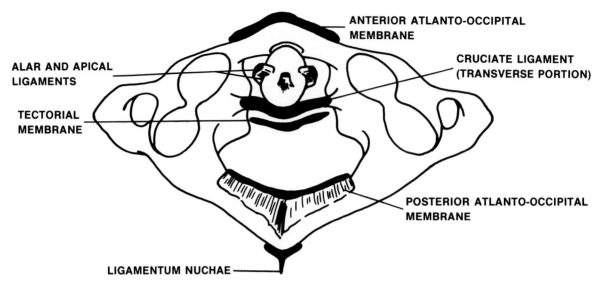

Fig. 5-8.   Schematic illustration of the major ligaments involved in the clinical stability of the upper cervical spine.

There have been no studies describing the mechanical properties of these structures. We can only observe that when they are both intact, they offer some modest mechanical advantage in preventing anterior displacement of C1 on C2.

Dentate (Odontoid) Ligaments

These ligaments consist of the alar ligaments and the apical ligaments. The alar ligaments are a pair of structures that are attached to the dorsolateral surfaces of the tip of the dens, and each runs obliquely to the medial surfaces of the occipital condyles (Fig. 5-8). The two structures form an angle of 140 to 180 degrees, the apex of which points caudally (Fig. 5-10C).[42] The left alar ligament limits rotation of C1 and the head to the right (−y-axis), and the right alar ligament limits rotation to the left. The apical dentate ligament connects the apex of the dens to the anterior edge of the foramen magnum. It has been described by Hecker as a fairly strong structure of fair development and of elastic consistency. Thus, it may be expected to contribute little to ocp-C1 stability, and nothing to C1–C2 stability.

The Cruciate Ligament

The major portion of this ligament is the transverse ligament, which is the most important ligament of the ocp-C1-C2 complex. This structure attaches to the two condyles of the atlas. There is an ascending and a descending band of this ligament. Both bands are triangular in shape. The ascending portion attaches to the anterior edge of the foramen magnum, and the descending portion attaches to the body of C2. The transverse band is the largest and the strongest. Its central portion has a thickness of 7 to 8 mm. The ascending and descending bands are 3 to 4 mm thick at the mid-portions (Fig. 5-10B).[42]

Tectorial Membrane

This structure is a continuation of the posterior longitudinal ligament. It runs from the body of C2 up over the posterior portion of the dens, and then makes a 45-degree angle in the anterior direction as it runs toward the attachment to the anterior edge of the foramen magnum (Fig. 5-10A). The anterior portion of the dura and the spinal cord completes the description of the anterior elements.

Posterior Atlanto-Occipital and Atlanto-Axial Membranes

These structures are anatomically analogous to the yellow ligament. However, they are considerably different in physical properties. The posterior atlanto-occipital membrane attaches to the posterior ring of C1 and the posterior portion of the foramen magnum (Fig. 5-8). The posterior atlanto-axial membrane attaches to the posterior ring of C1 and C2. The yellow ligament is first present between the lamina of C2 and C3. It then continues to the sacrum.

Nuchal Ligament

This is a triangular structure which is divided into a funicular and a triangular portion (Fig. 5-9). The funicular portion consists of a distinct band that runs from the posterior border of the occiput to the spine of C7. The lamellar portion divides the posterior neck into right and left halves. Its superior border attaches to the funicular por-

tion, and anteriorly it attaches to the posterior tubercle of the atlas, the spinous processes of the cervical vertebrae, and the interspinous ligaments.[33] Although this ligament is thought by some investigators to have biomechanical significance in the neck, the precise role has not yet been clearly delineated. It is doubtful that the structure is clinically significant.

Anatomic Interdependence and Clinical Stability

It is readily discernable from anatomic descriptions that there are a number of structures that provide some direct or indirect stability to both the occipital-atlantal joint and the atlanto-

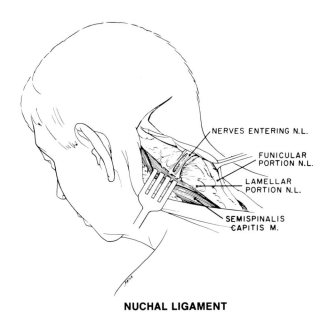

NUCHAL LIGAMENT

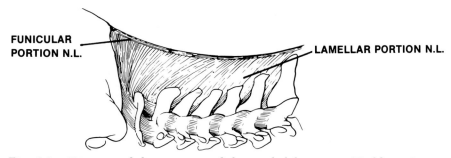

Fig. 5-9. Diagram of the anatomy of the nuchal ligament. (Fielding, J. W., Burnstein, A. A., and Frankel, V. H.: The nuchal ligament. Spine, *1*:3, 1976.)

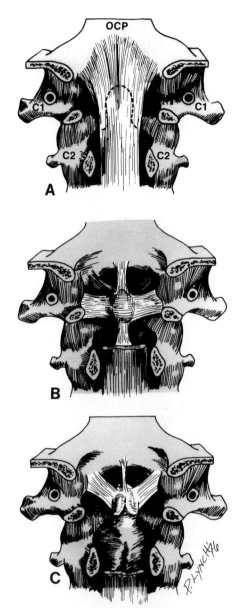

Fig. 5-10. Anatomic representation of the major stabilizing ligaments of the occipital-atlanto-axial complex. The structures may be separated into three layers. (*A*) *Layer one.* When the posterior osseous and ligamentous structures are removed, the tectorial membrane is visualized. (*B*) *Layer two.* The next structure, moving anteriorly, is the cruciate ligament. The transverse ligament is a component of the cruciate and is the most important stabilizing ligament of the atlanto-axial complex. (*C*) *Layer three.* Anterior to the cruciate lies the apical and alar ligaments, which serve as secondary stabilizers. These ligaments contribute to the interdependence in the occipital-atlanto-axial complex by way of anatomic attachments.

axial articulation. There are two groups of such structures. One group runs longitudinally, attaching to all three units, and includes the anterior longitudinal ligament, the tectorial membrane, the cruciate ligament, and the nuchal ligament. The other group offers some stability to both joints by skipping one segment and includes the alar and the apical ligaments (Fig. 5-10).

Present knowledge does not permit a complete analysis of the role of interdependence in clinical stability. However, it is known that with failure of the structures that run between the occiput and C1, at least some attachment of the occiput to the lower cervical spine remains through the apical and alar ligaments. Similarly, with the loss of only those structures between C1 and C2, some attachment of C2 to the occiput remains. Most clinically unstable injuries in this area probably destroy a number of structures in both articulations.

BIOMECHANICAL FACTORS

The basic kinematics of the occipital-atlanto-axial joints are presented in Chapter 2. This section reviews other biomechanical data that may have relevance in a systematic approach to the problem of clinical instability.

In flexion of the ocp-C1 joint, the limit is determined by impingement of the anterior margin of the foramen magnum on the dens. Additional flexion must then occur at the C1-C2 joint. This range is limited by the tautness of the tectorial membrane over the dens. Extension is also limited by the tectorial membrane.[94] Clearly, an additional amount of flexion would be expected to occur in this articulation upon failure of the tectorial membrane or failure of either the anterior portion of the foramen magnum or the dens. Werne confirmed these observations on a model that also showed little involvement of the tectorial membrane in inhibiting axial rotation.

Werne found that the cruciform ligament did not have any limiting effect on physiologic motion of the ocp-C1-C2 complex. The ascending band is too delicate. The descending band was shown to allow 6 to 7 mm of vertical (+y-axis) translation before reaching its limit. The alar ligaments function together to check movements in axial rotation and lateral flexion.[94]

The ocp-C1-C2 complex limits movement as follows. At ocp-C1 flexion $(+\theta x)$ is checked by osseous contact of the anterior ring of the foramen magnum on the dens. Extension $(-\theta x)$ is restricted by the tectorial membranes, and lateral flexion $(\pm\theta z)$ is checked by the alar ligaments. At the C1-C2 level, flexion is checked by the tectorial membrane, and extension is checked by the tectorial membrane and other posterior ligaments. Rotation is checked by the alar ligaments.[94] Although the cruciate ligament plays a small part in physiologic motion, Fielding showed that it is the most important structure in preventing abnormal anterior translation.[34]

Werne also carried out studies to evaluate the interdependence of the ocp-C1-C2 articulation. He studied rotation of the ocp-C1-C2 articulations in the sagittal plane before and after removal of the tectorial membrane. Although it was not true for all the specimens, the findings suggested that with loss of the tectorial membrane, there is an increase in flexion. Werne showed that if the alar ligaments were also transected, there was a *"luxation of the occiput."*[94]

Lateral flexion was studied in a similar manner, before and after transection of the tectorial membrane. There was an increased lateral flexion noted here also, but it was less convincing than in the flexion/extension studies. Axial rotation was also studied, and it was concluded that the alar ligaments are mainly responsible for the limitation of axial rotation.

When vertical translation was studied, the findings showed that this movement was greater after division of the tectorial membrane. The alar ligaments did not play a role in resisting vertical translation, except in a few specimens.

The studies of horizontal translation showed that an anterior dislocation of C1 on C2 can occur with an insufficiency of the transverse ligament only. The alar ligaments and the tectorial membrane were not found to prevent dislocation after the transverse ligament was transected. If the alar ligaments happen to be short, as may be expected in persons over 25, they may possibly offer some restraint against gross dislocation. The tectorial membrane depends upon an in-

tact transverse ligament to offer resistance to anterior translation. The biomechanical studies by Fielding on the transverse ligament showed that although the structure was very weak in some subjects, when present it prevented more than 3 mm of anterior displacement of C1 on C2. He also showed that the alar ligaments deform readily, and are not capable of preventing additional displacement under loads which would rupture the transverse ligament.[34]

CLINICAL CONSIDERATIONS

Communited Fracture of the Ring of C1 (Jefferson Fracture)

On the open mouth view of the odontoid, with the head in neutral rotation, the normal radiograph does not show any overhang of the lateral masses of C1 in relation to the lateral border of the body of the second cervical vertebra. However, with a Jefferson fracture there is overhang on both sides. If the total overhang from the two sides is as great as 7 mm, then there is presumably also a rupture of the transverse ligament (Fig. 5-11). When these conditions are present, there is clinical instability.[85]

Subluxations and Dislocations at the Atlanto-Axial Joint

With biomechanical experiments and a report on 11 cases, Fielding and colleagues showed that the clinical stability of the C1-C2 articulation depends upon an intact transverse ligament. This structure is, to some extent, supplemented by the alar ligaments, but in the absence of the transverse ligament the alar ligaments can not be expected to prevent abnormal anterior translation of C1 on C2. All of the patients studied sustained severe head injuries in addition to or associated with injury of C1–C2. They all complained of neck pain for a variable period of time following injury. Three of the patients had neurologic symptoms. The average anterior displacement upon radiograph in the patients was 7.2 mm. The investigators emphasized that fusion is probably the treatment of choice for this condition, since the potential risks of displacement in this area include quadraplegia and death.[34]

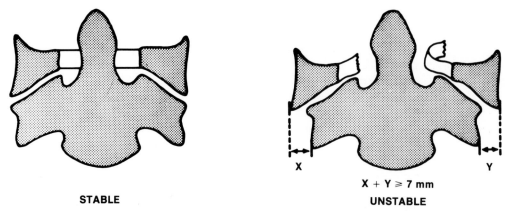

STABLE   **UNSTABLE**

X + Y ≥ 7 mm

Fig. 5-11. Jefferson fractures. When a communited fracture of C1 shows bilateral overhang of the lateral masses that totals 7 mm or more, a rupture of the transverse ligament has probably occurred, rendering the spine unstable.

The clinical problem of subluxation and dislocation at C1-C2 is extremely complicated, controversial, and difficult to diagnose. The possible types of displacement have not been completely described and documented.

Based on our review of the literature, and our own analysis and evaluation, we submit the following five patterns of abnormal displacement at the C1-C2 joint. Two of the patterns are primarily translatory, and the other three are mainly rotatory.

Patterns of Subluxations and Dislocations at the Atlanto-Axial Joint

Translatory
  Bilateral Anterior
  Bilateral Posterior
Rotatory
  Unilateral Anterior
  Unilateral Posterior
  Unilateral Combined Anterior and Posterior

Bilateral Anterior Displacement. This primarily translatory displacement may occur with a fractured or dysplastic odontoid, or an attenuated or ruptured transverse ligament (Fig. 5-12). There may be a history of a head or neck injury, or an impact to the trunk. In cases of transverse ligament inadequacy, there is usually a history of rheumatoid arthritis or an acute or chronic infection about the head or neck.[B]

The head may be in neutral, or due to muscle spasm in the "cock robin" position, with some degree of flexion along with lateral and axial rotation. Truly lateral radiographs of C1, axial tomography, or computerized axial tomography show an abnormal displacement of the ring of C1 anteriorly. These dislocations are clinically unstable when there is anterior displacement greater than 3 mm on radiographic examination with neurologic signs or symptoms. When they are due to transverse ligament disruption from pure trauma,

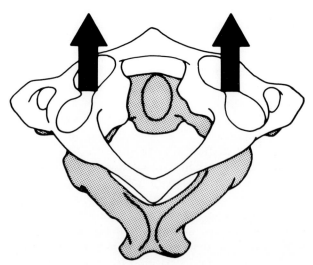

Fig. 5-12. Bilateral anterior translatory displacement of C1 in relation to C2. This may occur with transverse ligament rupture, and fractured, dyplastic, or aplastic odontoids.

they should be fused. If the laxity is secondary to infection, a trial of immobilization (halo apparatus) is recommended.[c] When the entity is associated with a fractured odontoid, either course is reasonable, depending on the probability of odontoid healing. The management of the various odontoid fractures is discussed in Chapter 4.

An unusual example of a type of bilateral anterior translatory displacement of C1 on C2 is shown in Figure 5-13. In this situation the displacement occurred in the presence of a normal, intact odontoid. With a clear history of trauma along with a loud snap, the displacement was obviously the result of a rupture of the transverse ligament. This type of displacement should be considered clinically unstable because of very high risks of spinal cord damage associated with additional anterior displacement in the presence of an intact odontoid. Moreover, the only remaining stabilizing structures are the accessory ligaments.[34]

Bilateral Posterior Displacement. This is an extremely rare, translatory dislocation (Fig. 5-14). It has been described in association with rheumatoid arthritis.[49] Such a dislocation is found only in the presence of a fractured dens, a dens destroyed by tumor or infection, a congenitally defective or absent dens, or a destroyed or congenitally absent anterior arch of the atlas. An example of this type of dislocation in the presence of a congenitally defective dens is shown in Figure 5-15. Sometimes patients with this condition provide their own clinical stability by holding the head with the hands. When this type of dislocation is seen with a fractured dens, it is treated according to the guidelines offered in Chapter 4. If the problem is due to an absent or destroyed dens, we suggest posterior fusion C1-C2.

Unilateral Anterior Displacement. This type of abnormal rotary displacement, between C1 and C2, is thought to be the most common. Either the left or the right articular mass moves anteriorly, and the axis of rotation is in the region of the articular facet that remains behind (Fig.

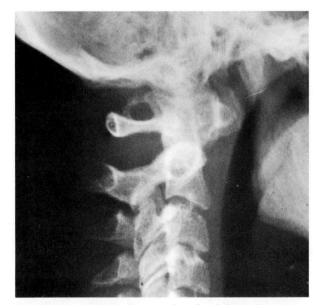

Fig. 5-13. A clinical example of a bilateral anterior translatory displacement of C1 on C2. This is a radiograph of a healthy 21-year-old female who fell 4 to 5 feet onto her head from a climbing bar. She heard a loud snap and immediately had pain in her neck. There were no neurologic signs or symptoms. The displacement between the anterior dens and the posterior portion of the anterior ring of C1 measured 7 mm. This bilateral anterior translatory displacement should be considered clinically unstable. The radiograph shows another interesting finding. The little arch on the posterior ring of C1 has no known clinical significance but is frequently observed. It has at least two names, *posterior ponticle* and *foramen arcuale.* It is never seen in children but is partially or completely present in 12 to 16 per cent of all adults.[91a] The vertebral artery passes under it before entering the cranium. (Courtesy of John Wolf, M.D.)

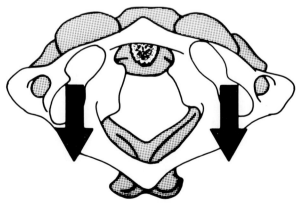

Fig. 5-14. Bilateral posterior translatory displacement of C1 in relation to C2. This may occur with fractured, dysplastic or aplastic, or otherwise diseased odontoids.

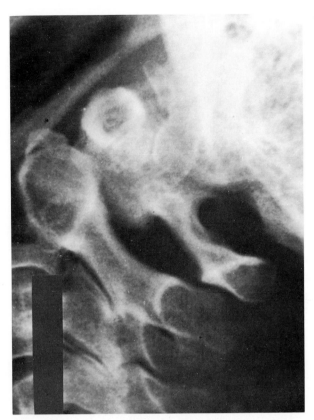

Fig. 5-15. This lateral radiograph shows a dysplastic odontoid. There is bilateral posterior translatory displacement of C1 on C2.

5-16). This usually occurs in association with various arthritic conditions or infections about the head and neck. Presumably, the pathology involves the transverse ligament as well as the articular capsule on the side of the subluxation.

The right unilateral anterior rotary subluxation shown in Figure 5-17 would be expected to have a torticollis with the head "cocked like a robin, listening for a worm." There is lateral bending of the head and neck to the right and rotation of the head to the left. Rotating the head away from the direction that it faces, toward the subluxed side (in this case rotation of the head to the right), is difficult, if not impossible. However, rotating it further in the direction that it faces, to the left, is not particularly difficult. The head is tilted toward the side of the subluxation or dislocation and rotated away from it. The muscles may or may not be in spasm. The syndrome is dis-

tinguishable from congenital torticollis by clinical history and by the absence of fibrosis of the sternocliedomastoid muscle. The anterior tubercle of the ring of C1 may be palpated on the posterior pharyngeal wall. In the case of a right unilateral anterior dislocation as described here, the tubercle is displaced to the patient's left pharyngeal wall.

In the unilateral right anterior rotatory subluxation, there are findings on the open mouth view that are compatible with normal rotation between C1 and C2. Specifically, there may be offsets or superimpositions of a lateral mass of C1 on C2. The key radiologic finding is seen on the true lateral view of the atlas (see Fig. 2-6). Here, there is a large displacement between the dens and the anterior ring of the atlas. This is shown diagrammatically in Figure 5-17. Unilateral offset is thought to be "normal."[29,44,70,83] Therefore, its presence alone is not diagnostic of abnormal displacement; there must also be an increased distance between the dens and the anterior ring of C1 in order to diagnose rotary subluxation. Axial tomography or computerized axial

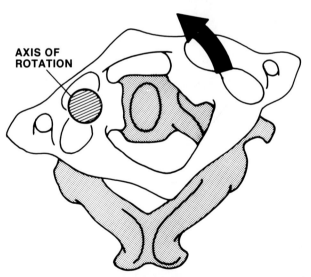

AXIS OF ROTATION

Fig. 5-16. Unilateral anterior rotatory displacement of C1 in relation to C2. The presumed axis of rotation is at or near the relatively stable lateral mass articulation. In addition to damaged or abnormal odontoids and transverse ligament damage, this type of displacement may have a unilateral articular capsule disruption on the anteriorly rotated side.

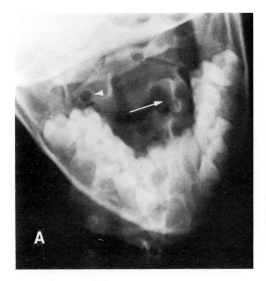

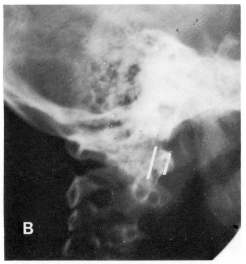

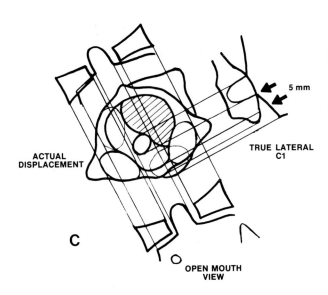

Fig. 5-17. Clinical example of unilateral anterior displacement of C1 in relation to C2. The patient has a typical torticollis with lateral flexion of the neck to the right, and the head is rotated to the left and held in slight flexion. (A) The open mouth radiograph shows deviation of the spinous process of C2 to the left (arrow), $-\theta$y-axis and apparent unilateral offset of the atlantal articular masses with respect to the foreshortened body of the C2. The foramen for the vertebral artery in C2 is readily visualized (arrowhead), signifying marked rotation ($-\theta$y-axis) to the right. Due to the flexion of the head and the angulation of the central ray, the atlanto-axial articular surfaces appear to overlap. The same radiographic manifestations are seen in torticollis. Therefore one cannot prove subluxation on the open mouth view alone. (B) The key diagnostic findings in true rotatory subluxation are seen on the true lateral view of the atlas; the distance between the anterior margin of the dens and the posterior margin of the anterior arch of the atlas measures 5 mm. (C) The line drawing depicts the radiographic findings. The patient's thorax faces the bottom of the page. The axis is rotated to the right secondary to the right lateral flexion of the neck. The head (and therefore also the atlas) is rotated to the left maximally with respect to the axis and moderately with respect to the thorax. The central ray is centered anteroposterior and lateral to the atlas. The key finding again is the increased distance from the dens to the anterior arch of the atlas. (Shapiro, R., Youngberg, A. S., and Rothman, S. L. G.: The differential diagnosis of traumatic lesions of the occipito-atlanto-axial segment. Radiol. Clin. North Am., 11:505, 1973.)

tomography shows anterior displacement of C1. Cineradiography may show absence of movement between C1–C2 on axial rotation.[32,35] Shapiro and colleagues have suggested that open mouth views of the dens in neutral, and with the head rotated 15 degrees in either direction, allow the diagnosis to be made if the spine of the axis remains on the same side of the midline after the voluntary rotation.[83]

These lesions, in the absence of odontoid fracture and neurologic deficits, are thought to be clinically stable. However, the persistence of severe symptoms of pain and/or deformity are indicators for surgical therapy. We suggest a 2 to 3 day trial of correction with adequate traction in extension, followed by C1–C2 fusion.

Unilateral Posterior Displacement. This is probably the most rare type of rotary injury.[35] It usually occurs with a deficient or a fractured odontoid. There may be neurologic symptoms, as with unilateral anterior displacement. One articular mass moves posteriorly, with the axis of rotation being in the region of the articulation on the opposite side (Fig. 5-18). There is torticollis and

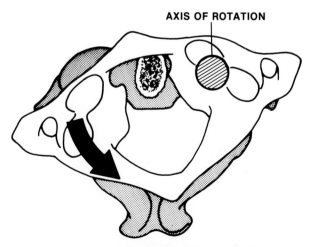

AXIS OF ROTATION

Fig. 5-18. Unilateral posterior rotatory displacement of C1 in relation to C2. The presumed axis of rotation is at or near the relatively stable lateral mass articulation. In order for this type of displacement to occur, there must be some abnormality of the odontoid (either congenital or acquired).

pain reported in the other types. In this entity, however, there is no abnormal separation between the dens and the anterior ring of C1. Lateral displacement of the dens may be seen on computerized axial tomography. Lack of C1–C2 motion may be apparent on cineradiography with axial rotation of the head.

The guidelines for treatment here are similar to those suggested for unilateral anterior displacement. We suggest that because this lesion is likely to be associated with a hypoplastic or fractured dens, it is more likely to be unstable.

Unilateral Combined Anterior and Posterior C1–C2 Subluxations and Dislocations. This situation occurs when there is abnormal rotary displacement, with one lateral mass dislocating forward and the other backward. The axis of rotation is in the region of the dens (Fig. 5-19). If either mass rotates completely off the normal articulation, then the deformity may become fixed. Pain and torticollis are manifested. The entity may also be associated with neurologic deficit. Radiographic findings are the same as those of unilateral posterior displacement. This lesion need not be presumed to be unstable. If the dens, the transverse ligament, and the tectorial membrane are intact, the loss of functional integrity of the capsular ligaments may not render the motion segment unstable. It can be difficult to recognize clinical instability in this type of subluxation. We suggest attempted reduction with traction. If this is not successful, and the symptoms are not tolerable, a C1–C2 fusion is recommended.

Computerized Axial Tomography of the Spine. This is a relatively new and exciting technique, which has considerable potential in the clinical evaluation of spine problems. It will be especially useful in helping to elucidate some of the complex displacements of C1 and C2. For a basic description and general information on the technique, volume *127* of the American Journal of Roentgenology, Radium Therapy and Nuclear Medicine, and the work of Hounsfield are recommended.[1,47]

In Figure 5-20, a unilateral anterior rotary subluxation of C1 is associated with a tumor involving the lateral masses and the facet articulation.

Although considerable work is needed to study normal relationships and recognize and corroborate abnormal findings, we are very optimistic about the usefulness of computerized axial tomography, which is reported to be 100 times more sensitive than standard radiography.

Discussion. The problems of the various subluxations and dislocations of the atlas need considerable work for documentation and clarification. These various entities have been presented as a complete theoretical listing of all possibilities. They have been summarized in Table 5-2. Werne and later Fielding have presented their own groupings of these entities.[35,94] In our opinion, the problem of definitive diagnosis and accurate analysis of the clinical stability has yet to be solved. We wish to reemphasize the limitations and speculative nature of information available on the subject.

Recommended Evaluation System. Little can be said about the clinical stability of C1–C2 subluxations and dislocations. We know that the transverse ligament, and one or more articular capsules, must be disrupted to allow abnormal rotary displacement. If there is abnormal sagittal plane (+ z axis) translation by radiographic measurement of greater than 3 mm in an adult or 4 mm in a child, or if there are neurologic signs or symptoms suggesting irritation to the spinal

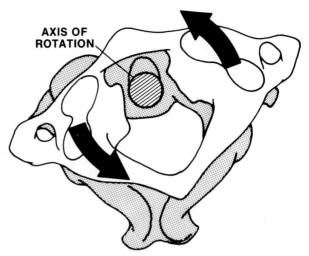

Fig. 5-19. Unilateral combined anterior and posterior rotatory displacement of C1 in relation to C2. The presumed axis of rotation is at or near the odontoid. Both lateral mass articulations are disrupted. This type of displacement is to be expected to least compromise the space available for the cord, because the axis of rotation is closest to the cord in this situation.

medulla, the situation should be considered unstable.

Recommended Treatment. We recommend treatment of these unstable injuries with traction in slight extension for 2 to 3 weeks, or until reduction is achieved. This is followed by fixation

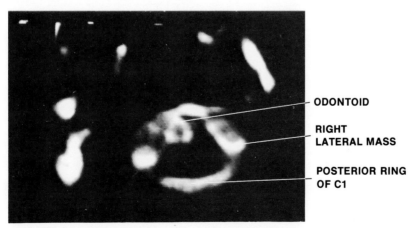

Fig. 5-20. Computerized axial tomogram of the C1, C2 articulation. There is a unilateral anterior rotatory displacement of C1 in relation to C2 of the type shown diagrammatically in Figure 5-16.

in a cervical orthosis of maximum control for an additional 10 weeks. If at that time there is no neurologic deficit, no torticollis, and no pain, the patient may progress to a cervical orthosis of intermediate control (four-poster brace with a thoracic support). If this is not the case, or should any of the above symptoms recur, a C1–C2 fusion is recommended.

A summary of the most cogent information on these conditions is provided in Table 5-2.

Table 5-2. Summary of C1–C2 Subluxations and Dislocations

Type	Causes and Displacements	Physical Findings	Radiologic Studies	Clinical Stability	Treatment
Bilateral Anterior	Dysplastic dens, trauma, infection, +z translation	Neutral or "cock robin" position of head	Lateral of C1, CT scan: anterior displacement of C1 on C2	Anterior displacement of 3 mm, neurologic deficit—clinically unstable	Fusion or trial of conservative therapy
Bilateral Posterior (very rare)	Fractured, absent, or destroyed dens; −z translation	Patient may hold head in hands	Lateral of C1, CT scan: posterior displacement of C1 on C2	Clinically unstable	Fuse C1–C2
Unilateral Anterior (most common)	Arthritic conditions and infections; ±y-axis rotation, IAR at opposite joint	"Cock robin" position of head. Difficulty in rotating head away from direction in which it faces. No difficulty in moving further in that direction. Anterior tubercle of C1 may be shown to be displaced laterally by palpation of posterior pharynx.	Lateral of C1, CT scan: anterior displacement of C1 on C2. A-P open mouth laminograms C1–C2: lateral masses in different planes. Cineradiography or several radiographs of axial rotation: no motion of C1 or C2	With no neurologic deficit, probably stable	Trial of reduction and conservative treatment. If symptoms require, fuse C1–C2.
Unilateral Posterior (rare)	Usually associated with a deficient or fractured dens; ±y-axis rotation, IAR at opposite sides	"Cock robin" position of head	Lateral of C1, CT scan: *no* anterior displacement of C1 on C2. A-P open mouth laminograms, C1–C2: lateral masses in different positions. Cineradiography or serial radiographs of axial rotation: no motion of C1 or C2	With no neurological deficit, probably stable	Attempt reduction and, if symptoms require, fuse C1–C2.
Unilateral Combined Anterior and Posterior	Trauma; ±y-axis rotation, IAR at dens	"Cock robin" position of head	Same as unilateral posterior	With no neurologic deficit, may be clinically stable	Trial of reduction and conservative treatment; if not satisfactory, fuse C1–C2.

CT = computerized axial tomography

Part 2: The Lower Cervical Spine (C2-C7)

This is the region of the spine that has received the most attention with regard to the problem of clinical instability. At the cervical spine, neurologic deficit is most frequently associated with trauma.[75] This section reviews the past and current biomechanical and clinical factors which relate to the problem of clinical stability in this region.

ANATOMIC CONSIDERATIONS

What anatomic structures are necessary to maintain clinical stability in the lower cervical spine? A schematic representation of the anatomy of the lower cervical spine is presented in Figure 5-21.

According to Bailey, "the most significant of the anatomic structures providing stability to

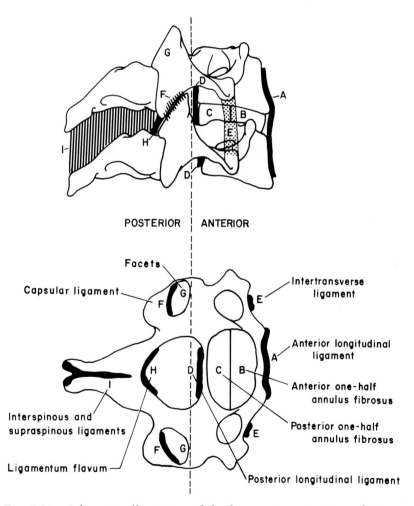

POSTERIOR | ANTERIOR

Facets
Capsular ligament
Intertransverse ligament
Anterior longitudinal ligament
Anterior one-half annulus fibrosus
Interspinous and supraspinous ligaments
Posterior one-half annulus fibrosus
Ligamentum flavum
Posterior longitudinal ligament

Fig. 5-21. Schematic illustration of the ligamentous structures that participate in the stabilization of the lower cervical spine. The components are divided into *anterior* and *posterior* elements. In the experiments on clinical stability, ligaments were cut in the alphabetical order indicated in the diagram from anterior to posterior and in reverse alphabetical order from posterior to anterior.

the cervical spine are the musculature and the firm bond between the bodies formed by the intervertebral disks."[4] He has emphasized the importance of the annulus fibrosus in other writings.[3] The role of the musculature is of considerable importance, but to our knowledge, its significance in clinical stability has not been studied. Munroe carried out experimental studies on cadaver spines and concluded that cervical spine stability comes mainly from the intervertebral discs and the anterior and posterior longitudinal ligaments.[63] Bedbrook suggested that the disc, with its two longitudinal ligaments, and the yellow ligament are the most important structures in maintaining stability.[8] This was based on his own study of 355 cases, the writings of Bailey,[3] and the experimental work of Roaf, who showed that in loading motion segments, bone injury occurs before disc or yellow ligament failure.[77]

Although Holdsworth emphasized the importance of the supraspinous and interspinous ligaments as well as the ligamentum nuchae, other investigators considered them to be much less significant.[45] Halliday and colleagues carried out anatomic dissections and observed that the interspinous ligaments are sometimes completely absent between one or more segments and that the ligamentum nuchae is quite delicate.[41] The latter observation was supported by the work of Johnson and colleagues, who carried out detailed anatomic studies of the ligaments of the lower cervical spine in 15 fresh specimens.[52] The more recent work of Fielding seems to offer considerable contradictory evidence, at least with regard to the anatomic structure of the ligamentum nuchae (see p. 201).[33]

BIOMECHANICAL FACTORS

Experiments have been carried out on cervical spine motion segments in high humidity chambers using physiologic loads to simulate flexion and extension.[68,98] The experimental arrangement is shown in Figure 5-22. The ligaments were cut in sequence from posterior to anterior in some motion segments and from anterior to posterior in others. The *failure point* was defined as the

point at which the upper vertebra suddenly rotated 90 degrees or was displaced across the experimental table. The *anterior elements* were defined as the posterior longitudinal ligament and all structures anterior to it. The *posterior elements* were defined as all structures behind the posterior longitudinal ligament (Fig. 5-21). Based on these studies, we suggested that if a motion segment has all its anterior elements plus one additional structure, or all its posterior elements plus one additional structure, it will probably remain stable under physiologic loads. In order to provide for some clinical margin of safety, we suggest that any motion segment in which all the anterior elements or all the posterior elements are either destroyed or are unable to function should be considered potentially unstable. Therefore, these studies show that the important anatomic structures for maintaining clinical stability are either all the anterior elements plus one posterior, or all the posterior elements plus one anterior.

CLINICAL CONSIDERATIONS

There are a number of important clinical studies that have considerable bearing on the analysis of clinical stability. Several of these are discussed below.

Incidence of Instability

The percentages reported by several authors are shown in Table 5-3. Overall, these reports show that previous investigators have chosen to

Table 5-3. Percentages of Nonfused Fractures and Dislocations of the Lower Cervical Spine Considered Unstable

AUTHOR(S)	NO. OF PATIENTS	% ESTIMATED AS UNSTABLE
Brookes (1933)	40	10
Durbin (1957)	63	12
Brav, et al. (1963)	156	10.9
Bedbrook (1969)	355	6
Cheshire (1969)	160	7.5
Burke, and Berryman (1971)	37	8

(White, A. A., Southwick, W. O., and Panjabi, M. M.: Clinical instability in the lower cervical spine. A review of past and current concepts. Spine, 1:15, 1976.)

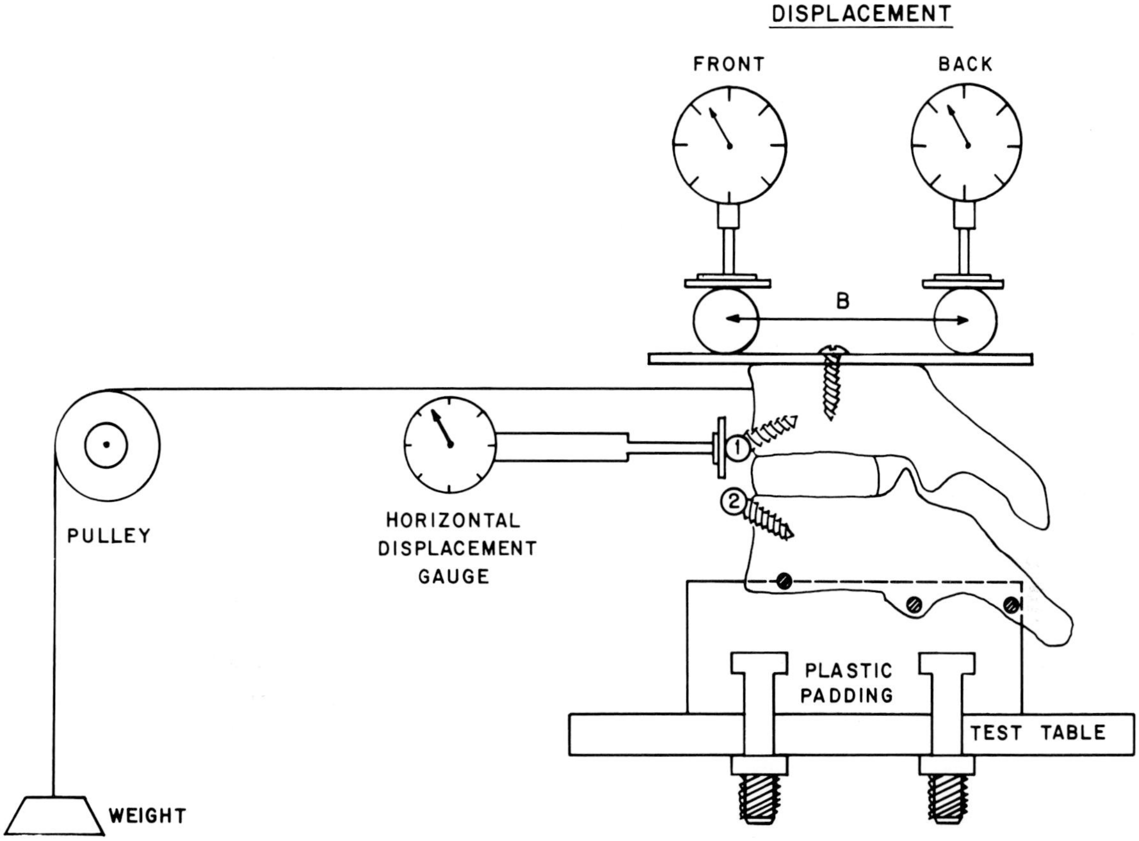

DISPLACEMENT

Fig. 5-22. The experimental setup. The vertical displacement of the balls at either end of line B measured angular displacement. Horizontal displacement was measured by the relative displacement of balls 1 and 2. This is the setup for testing flexion. When extension is tested, the motion segment is rotated 180 degrees on the vertical (y) axis. (White, A. A., Johnson, R. M., Panjabi, M. M., and Southwick, W. O.: Biomechanical analysis of clinical stability in the cervical spine. Clin. Orthop., *109:*85, 1975.)

call about 9 or 10 per cent of nonsurgically treated fracture dislocations unstable. The investigators have not defined instability in these series; however, these figures do provide an estimate of the percentage of injured spines that have been called unstable.

Structural Damage and Neurologic Deficit

Is there a correlation between recognizable structural damage to the spine and neurologic deficit?

Barnes notes that "one of the most puzzling features of injuries of the cervical spine is the lack of correlation between the degree of vertebral displacement and the severity of the spinal

cord lesion. There are cases with no radiographic evidence of bone injury in which the cord is irretrievably damaged; others, with gross dislocation, may have no paraplegia."[5]

Beatson was careful to compare the amounts of displacement in the sagittal plane that occur with unilateral and bilateral facet dislocation. Even though there is more displacement with bilateral facet dislocation, he did not document any consistent difference in the neurologic deficits.[7] On the other hand, Braakman and Vinken followed their observation of more displacement in bilateral facet dislocations with a convincing documentation of associated neurologic problems. They showed that the unilateral facet dislocations usually consist only of root symptoms, while the bilateral dislocations are associated with serious spinal medullary lesions.[15]

It is interesting to look at some additional aspects of this question. Brav and colleagues also studied the correlation between cord damage and degree of displacement. Patients were divided into four groups based on the amount of displacement in the sagittal plane (±z-axis translation). The observations were made on lateral radiographs. The investigators noted a correlation between displacement and medullary (cord) damage, and they observed that there was much more cord damage in injuries with posterior displacement of a dislocated vertebra as compared to anterior displacement.[16] Hørlyck and Rahbek reviewed 51 injuries in the lower cervical spine (C3–C7), and noted that except for the severely comminuted "bursting" fractures, the series did not show any correlation between the type of fracture and lesion of the spinal cord.[46] Iizuka reviewed 50 patients with fracture dislocations of the cervical vertebrae and remarked on the conspicuous absence of any correlation between the dislocation as seen on radiographs and the degree of spinal cord injury.[48] Castellano and Bocconi expressed the view that there is no relation between the severity of the morphologic lesion and the incidence of neurologic complication.[22]

An epidemiologic study of the incidence of cord injury with trauma to vertebrae in all regions of the spine resulted in some interesting data. When vertebral body fracture alone was present, the associated incidence of neurologic deficit was 3 per cent. However, if there was malalignment of 2 mm or more, or vertebral body damage plus posterior element damage, then the incidence of associated neurologic deficit went up to 61 per cent.[75] There are some other considerations that may relate to this question and account for some of the confusion. The experimental work of Gosch and colleagues on monkeys showed that it is possible for significant spinal cord damage to result from trauma without any fractures or ligamentous ruptures.[38] There is also the central cervical cord syndrome, described by Schneider and colleagues, in which there is paralysis of the upper limbs with function in the lower limbs and no radiologic evidence of fracture or fracture dislocation.[82] It was well documented by Marar that fracture dislocations in the lower

cervical region can go unrecognized (Fig. 4-33).[59] He reported on autopsy studies of four patients with extension injuries and transverse fractures of the vertebral body. The fractures reduced spontaneously after compressing the medulla between the upper portion of the fractured vertebra and the lamina of the subadjacent vertebra. The fracture was not visible on routine radiographic examination. The medullary damage in these four patients may have occurred in the presence of intact spinal elements. Similarly, there may sometimes be loss of continuity through failure of the annulus or its attachment to the vertebral end-plate.

When there is spontaneous reduction of such a dislocation and if there is no residual deformation at the time the radiograph is taken, the dislocation may go unrecognized.

There is usually a discrepancy between the damaging displacement, which occurs at the time of impact, and the *residual deformation*, which is what is actually observed on the radiograph. The presence of residual deformation shows that the motion segment as a whole was deformed into its *plastic range*. In addition, it is possible that the complex bony and ligamentous structure of the spine may conceivably deform enough to cause medullary damage, but remain entirely within its *elastic range*. In this case, the motion segment would recoil back to its normal position and condition.

Therefore, although there are exceptions, there is some correlation between neurologic deficit and the radiographic appearance of the spine following trauma. Bursting fractures of the vertebral body, especially with horizontal displacement and posterior element fractures, are highly correlated with spinal cord injury. The contrast between unilateral and bilateral facet dislocations has shown that, with the latter, more extensive injury, there is a greater neurologic deficit. Damage of the nerve roots, which may be independent of damage to the cord, has not been carefully distinguished and studied.

Neurologic Deficit and Clinical Instability

Is the presence of distinct medullary or root damage associated with spinal trauma evidence of clinical instability? This consideration can be confusing with regard to our definition of clinical instability. We have said that clinical instability concerns the prediction of *subsequent* neurologic damage. Therefore, what is the significance of the presence of *initial* neurologic damage to the probability of subsequent neurologic damage? We believe that if the trauma is severe enough to cause initial neurologic damage, the support structures probably have been altered sufficiently to allow subsequent neurologic damage, and thus the situation is clinically unstable. Some exceptions should be noted.

Since the work of Gosch and colleagues has shown that in animals it is possible to have medullary damage with intact supporting structures,[38] one must expect that this is also possible in humans. Such an occurrence is even more likely when there is a narrow canal, or encroachment by osteophytes or the yellow ligament, all of which are clearly feasible and may be operative in the central spinal cord lesion, as described by Schneider.[82] We believe, however, that in most instances where there is medullary or nerve root damage, instability should be suspected. This presumption, of course, must be weighed in relation to other clinical information about the particular patient under consideration. The following clinical problem exemplifies several crucial points related to clinical instability.

Case Report.   B.A. is a 19-year-old boy who was struck on the head from behind during a game of rugby. He developed an incomplete tetraparesis immediately following the injury. The radiographs on admission to the hospital showed an anterior subluxation of C4 on C5 (Fig. 5-23A). This was reduced with skull traction and the tetraparesis resolved quickly. Note that the extension film in Figure 5-23B shows almost complete reduction, except for slight separation of the laminae and spinous processes between C4 and C5. The patient was treated with a Minerva jacket for 3 months. Radiographs immediately after removal of the jacket, which included flexion/extension views, were reported to be normal. However, some 4 months later, an obvious resubluxation of an extreme degree was noted (Fig. 5-23C). Fortunately, this was reduced after a week of recumbency on a plaster bed. Subsequently, a successful posterior fusion was carried out (Fig. 5-23D).*

Discussion.   This case very nicely shows that

* Personal communication with T. McSweeney and W. Park.

even transient neurologic symptoms may suggest plastic deformation or complete failure of ligamentous structures. In this case, most likely there was extreme plastic deformation or rupture of all posterior ligaments, the posterior longitudinal ligament, and all or most of the annulus fibrosus, but with little residual displacement.

The stretch test (see p. 224) may have been helpful in demonstrating the loss of continuity of the damaged ligaments in this case. Also note radiographically the decrease in height or abnormal narrowing of disc space, a sign indicating probable disruption of the annulus fibrosus.[3] This is especially important when seen in a young patient whose other disc spaces are normal following trauma. Webb and colleagues have recognized a pattern for this type of situation. The findings are shown below. A review of Figure 5-23A shows the complete tetrad. This is a recognizable syndrome, which has a high probability of being clinically unstable. The findings correlate very well with Penning's description of kyphotic angulation.[71] The clinician should also look for disc narrowing at the interspace under analysis. The initial treatment in the previous case report was perfectly adequate and would have been successful had there been spontaneous fusion or satisfactory healing of the ligamentous structures.

A Recognizable Tetrad of Clinical Instability

Widening of interspinous space
Subluxation of facet joint
Compression fracture of subadjacent vertebra
Loss of normal cervical lordosis

(Webb, J. K., Broughton, R. B. K., McSweeney, T., and Park, W. M.: Hidden flexion injury of the cervical spine. J. Bone Joint Surg., 58B: 322, 1976.)

Clinical Stability of Unilateral Facet Dislocations

The clinical and experimental studies of Beatson are most instructive. He produced unilateral and bilateral facet dislocations and observed the sagittal plane displacement on lateral radiographs. These findings were correlated with anatomic studies of the associated ligamentous damage. On the lateral radiograph, a displacement of one-half of the anteroposterior diameter of the vertebral body or less indicates a uni-

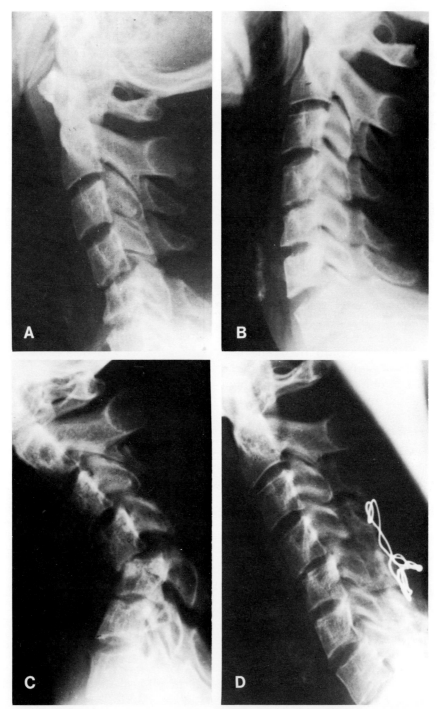

Fig. 5-23. Radiographs of a flexion injury in a 19-year-old with transient spinal cord symptoms. (See p. 215 for a case report.) Knowing the nature of the injury, could the resubluxation shown in *C* have been predicted from radiographs *A* (taken on admission) and *B* (taken after 3 months of treatment)? (*A*, *B*, and *D* courtesy of T. McSweeney and W. Park; *C* from Webb, J. K., Broughton, R. B. K., McSweeney, T., and Park, W. M.: Hidden flexion injury of the cervical spine. J. Bone Joint Surg., *58B*:322, 1976.)

lateral facet dislocation. If the displacement is greater than one-half of the diameter, it should be diagnosed as a bilateral facet dislocation.[7] Bedbrook suggested that with a displacement of one-half of the anteroposterior diameter of the vertebral body, the spinal canal is encroached upon by one-third of its anteroposterior diameter.[8]

Beatson also observed that with unilateral facet dislocation there is rupture of the interspinous ligament and capsule of the involved facet joint. There is only minimal damage to the annulus and the posterior longitudinal ligament on the dislocated side. He noted that it would be difficult to reduce this dislocation with straight longitudinal traction because of the resistance of the intact disc and capsule on the undislocated side.[7] Unfortunately, there is no mention of the status of the yellow ligament in this study; information about the fate of this important structure in the various facet dislocations would be valuable.

Cheshire reported on three patients with unilateral facet dislocations and spinal cord involvement. All were manually reduced and treated for 6 weeks in traction. Redislocation occurred while wearing cervical collars. These patients were then treated by surgical fusion to insure stability.[26] Braakman and Vinken reported on 37 patients with unilateral facet dislocations. Seven of these patients had nerve root involvement and 34 had medullary involvement. The investigators recommended conservative treatment and indicated a low incidence of late instability.[15]

Based on available clinical and experimental evidence, we make the assumption that only some unilateral facet dislocations are unstable. Generally, when there is neural involvement, especially with spinal medullary damage, enough displacement may have taken place to cause significant ligamentous damage. The observations of Beatson[7] showed that in at least some instances of unilateral facet dislocation, damage may occur to the anterior as well as the posterior elements.[7] Certainly, when there is an associated facet fracture, there is less stability. In general, unilateral facet dislocations associated with neurologic damage or facet fracture must be considered as clinically unstable. Other unilateral facet dislocations without neurologic deficit, especially when they are difficult to reduce (which

implies a largely intact annulus and yellow ligament), may be considered clinically stable.

Clinical Stability of Bilateral Facet Dislocations

In several reported clinical series, the bilateral facet dislocation is considered to be an unstable injury.[8,19,26] Beatson's experimental observations showed that in order to create a bilateral facet dislocation, it was necessary to rupture the interspinous ligaments, the capsules of both facet joints, the posterior longitudinal ligament, and the annulus fibrosus.[7] This would result in a clinically unstable situation. These injuries are prone to undergo abnormal translation along the z-axis. Experimental studies have shown that when flexion is simulated after removal (fracture) of the articular facets, there is a good deal more anterior translation (Fig. 5-24).[68] This factor, in connection with the relative vulnerability

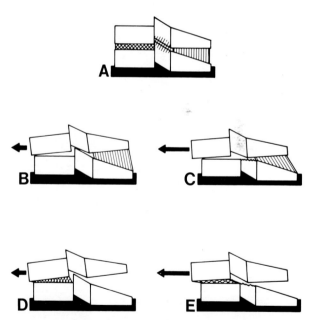

Fig. 5-24. This diagram is designed to show the role that the articular facets play in the anterior translation of a given motion segment. (*A*) The normal motion segment. (*B*) With all anterior elements removed, (*C*) there is more anterior translation after destruction of the facet articulation. (*D*) With all the posterior elements removed, (*E*) there is also more anterior translation after the facets are destroyed. The practical significance of this is that with bilateral facet fracture or dislocation, the tendency for anterior translatory displacement is much greater.

of the cord to damage by displacement in the horizontal plane, makes such an injury extremely unstable.

Laminectomy and Clinical Instability

This is an extremely controversial topic. We believe that the procedure is done too frequently, with improper indications, and with an astounding lack of appreciation of its effect on the mechanical function of the spine. In children there is a tendency for kyphosis, anterior subluxation, and "gooseneck deformity" to develop as a result of laminectomies in the cervical spine.[23] The growing spine is especially prone to deformity as the epiphysis responds to asym-

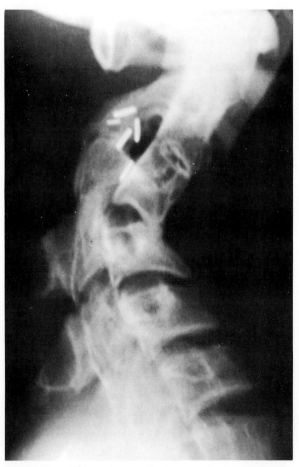

Fig. 5-25. This radiograph demonstrates clearly the role that laminectomy can play in contributing to the clinical instability of the spine. (Courtesy of Harry Gossling, M.D.)

metrical forces and causes wedging of the vertebral bodies.

Jenkins reported several cases of multiple laminectomies performed in the lower cervical spine without subsequent deformity or clinical instability.[50] Although there may not always be complications, we must emphasize that multiple laminectomies in the adult cervical spine may lead to clinical instability, with serious neurologic consequences. Clearly, the condition of the remaining structures following laminectomy is a significant factor in the outcome. The structure is less likely to be unstable if the facet articulations and their capsules are intact and the anterior elements are normal. If any of these remaining units are destroyed or nonfunctional, clinical instability is very likely to occur. The patient whose radiographs are shown in Figure 5-25 had laminectomies at C2 and C3, with the facet joints preserved and no anterior element surgery or injury. However, he developed a major neurologic defect and severe kyphosis.

In Figure 5-26, some important points about spine structure and clinical stability are demonstrated. The patient is a 38-year-old female who had an ependymoma removed from the lower cervical spine. Figure 5-26A shows the spine after total laminectomy of C4, total laminectomy and partial facetectomy of C5, and removal of all the posterior elements of C6. It appears as though the annulus fibrosus between C5 and C6 is degenerated. It is presumably fibrosed, partially ossified, and actually better able to resist translation than a normal disc. At C6 there are relatively larger loads applied, and the other interspaces are relatively more stable, since it was the only level at which *all* the posterior elements were removed. Predictably, the abnormal anterior translation and clinical instability occurred at the C6–C7 interspace, as shown in Figure 5-26A. Due to the spacial orientation and inclination of the interspace at this level, the abnormal translation was anterior. (This is in contrast to the posterior translation of L2 or L3 seen in the somewhat analogous situation on page 261). In Figure 5-26B a bone graft in the C6–C7 interspace is shown. This was not a good choice of surgical construct because it required removal of the anterior longitudinal ligament and the annulus fibrosus in order to

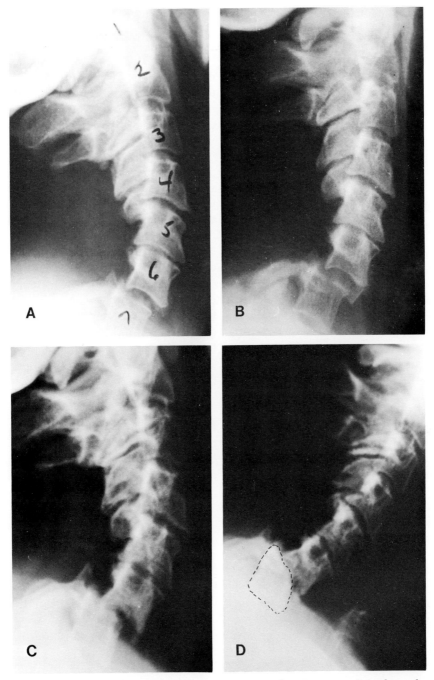

Fig. 5-26. These radiographs demonstrate several important points about the problem of clinical stability. Laminectomy and facetectomy that includes all the posterior elements renders the spine clinically unstable; the subsequent disruption of the anterior elements in order to insert a bone graft makes the situation even more grossly unstable; the two components of instability, translatory, shown in *B* and *C*, and in addition rotatory, shown in *D*, are graphically demonstrated by this case. (Courtesy of W. O. Southwick, M.D.)

219

insert the graft. The immediate postoperative stability was dependent on the posterior longitudinal ligament alone. This may be expected to result in a grossly unstable situation. The bone graft was partially reabsorbed and the predictable clinical instability is evidenced by the gross abnormal translation and rotation shown in Figure 5-26C, D. It was possible to reduce the severe subluxation and to achieve stability with the use of an anterior iliac trough graft and halo body cast fixation.

TREATMENT CONSIDERATIONS

Effects of Reduction on Prognosis

Does reduction of a fracture dislocation in the lower cervical spine favorably affect the prognosis? Rogers stated that progression of spinal cord symptoms was more likely to occur in unreduced injuries.[81] Burke and Berryman stated that a large number of patients showed improvement after manual manipulation.[19] However, these statements were not documented.

Dall, in a report of over 200 cases, emphasized that the major determinant of overall prognosis was the nature and magnitude of the *initial injury* to the spinal cord. He offered follow-up data on a large number of patients which supported his assertions that the type of bone injury, the lack of reduction, or even *redislocation* had no influence on spinal cord recovery.[27] Dall did not separate his findings into categories of cord and root symptoms. Thus, the evidence does not rule out the possibility that root recovery is related to achieving and maintaining reduction of the traumatized spine. Braakman and Vinken, reporting on 37 patients, were affirmative about the value of reduction in providing nerve root recovery in patients with unilateral facet dislocations.[15] These studies corroborated the generally expressed maxim of "rigorous therapy to preserve the root."

The Role of Manipulations

What is the value of manipulation in dislocations and fracture dislocations of the lower cervical spine? In the United States, there has apparently been a tendency to treat manipulation almost as though it were taboo, whereas in the United Kingdom it seems to be commonplace. Beatson has shown that axial traction is probably not of the most efficient method of reduction of bilateral or unilateral facet dislocations. He suggested techniques for the reduction of both injuries.[7] Other investigators have described techniques and management of manipulations for the treatment of spinal trauma.[*,14,19,26]

When reduction of unilateral facet dislocations without medullary damage is not achieved with 50 to 60 lb of axial traction, manual manipulation seems to be a desirable approach. Detailed reviews of the various techniques are available in the literature. The studies of Walton and Taylor constitute some of the earlier descriptions.[90,92] There are basically three types of loads applied to the head in manipulations for reduction. There is axial loading, as with ordinary traction; axial rotation, in which a torque is applied in the horizontal plane; and lateral bending, in which a torque is applied in the frontal plane. Axial rotation and lateral bending are applied in sequence and in either order, depending on individual preference.

We suggest that there is probably a place for the manipulative reduction of the unilateral facet dislocation in which there is no neurologic involvement. The pathoanatomic aspects of this entity have been well studied and the recommendations of previous investigators are available.[7,15,19,26]

The Role of Decompression

What about decompression? A detailed discussion of this controversy could fill as many pages as the topic of clinical instability. We are suggesting some guidelines and are aware of their limitations and controversial nature. The following are currently accepted indications for decompression: radiographic evidence of bone or a foreign material in the medullary canal, associated with medullary symptoms; evidence on air or contrast myelography of a discrete extradural block; and clinical judgment (e.g., in the presence of an incomplete progressive neurologic lesion, the surgeon believes that decompression would be beneficial). Generally, decisions about

---

* Personal communication, A. Brooks.

decompression should be made and carried out as soon as practical clinical conditions permit.

There are some cogent questions concerning decompression. Given the decision to decompress, should it be done from the front or from the back? Primarily this is determined by the location of the defect on myelographic study and secondarily, by the area in which there is the most structural damage, if there is no myelographic documentation. Decompression should be carried out whenever possible on the side of the defect. If that is impossible to determine, then most probably it is best to decompress where the major damage to the bony and ligamentous structure has occurred. Anterior decompressions for trauma are generally best achieved by total or partial excision of the vertebral body. The spine should be reconstructed with an appropriate bone graft (see Chapter 8). This is sufficient if the posterior elements are intact. If the posterior elements are not intact, they, too, should be fused and wired, preferably before anterior decompression. If the patient's condition and the surgeon's experience permit, the two procedures may be done in sequence under the same anesthesia.

With posterior decompression of one or two segments, leaving the facet joints intact, and with normal anterior structures, immediate fusion is not necessary. The patient should be followed carefully and observed for evidence of progressive instability with anterior displacement or for the development of posterior collapse (gooseneck) secondary to the loss of support structures. If decompression involves more than two levels, if there is any disruption of the facet joint integrity, or if the anterior elements are not intact, then bilateral posterolateral facet joint fusion and wiring should be carried out at the time of decompression.

Traditional Indications for Surgical Arthrodesis

It is necessary to determine, as precisely as possible, just what the indications for fusion are. There are few works that attempt to present the indications for fusion following fractures and fracture dislocations. Beatson suggested that bilateral facet dislocations were an indication for fusion.[7] Braakman and Vinken stated that a unilateral facet dislocation with a neurologic deficit should be fused.[15] We believe that only a unilateral facet dislocation requiring open reduction, with or without neurologic deficit, should be fused.

This rationale is based on three considerations. First, the previously described work of Beatson shows that there can be significant disruption of the anterior elements associated with the injury.[7] Secondly, there is the possible complication of delayed arthritis and pain associated with the disrupted joint. Thirdly, since the surgical exposure is performed in order to achieve reduction, it is possible to fuse and insure against future pain and instability with little additional surgical risk.

Dall described satisfactory results in his large series of patients with fracture dislocations treated nonsurgically (3 months of skeletal traction and 3 months of treatment with a cervical collar.) He considered progressive bone deformity with late pain or neurologic deficit to be an indication for fusion. In a series of 75 patients with fracture dislocations, only three were thought to need fusion. The work argues respectably for a nonsurgical approach.[28]

Rogers and Forsythe and colleagues wrote extensively on fusions for spinal trauma, but did not state their indications.[38,81] The indications given by Nieminen and Koskinen and Petrie are presented in Table 5-4.[66,73] These investigators addressed the problem and proposed some indications for fusion. Given the paucity of available knowledge, this is to be commended and appre-

Table 5-4. Indications for Surgical Arthrodesis after Cervical Spine Trauma

NIEMINEN AND KOSKINEN, 1973	PETRIE, 1964
Open reduction needed	Dislocation easy or *difficult* to reduce
Damage to the posterior longitudinal ligament	Bilateral facet dislocation with neurologic deficit
Multiple injuries of one vertebra	Progressive neurologic deficit
Injuries of *several* vertebra	Burst fracture with 3 mm decrease in spinal canal
Nerve root symptoms	Damage to two of the four following structures: vertebral body, pedicle, facets, lamina

ciated. However, there are limitations. Nieminen and Koskinen's third and fourth indications (see Table 5-4) lack specificity. How many injuries are "multiple" and how many vertebrae are "several"? Their second item entails determining the status of the posterior longitudinal ligament, but they do not suggest how this is to be done. Petrie is more specific, and his indications can be applied. The first listed, however, requires considerable judgment in defining "difficult."

White and colleagues propose that if, upon examination of flexion, extension, or resting lateral radiographs, there is a relative translation (anteroposterior displacement in the sagittal plane) greater than 3.5 mm, a relative rotation (more than either adjacent vertebra) greater than 11 degrees, or complete destruction and loss of function of all the anterior or posterior elements, then clinical instability after cervical spine trauma is present.[98] Although these criteria are precise and applicable, they, too, have limitations. They are based on *in vitro* experimental investigations rather than on *in vivo* clinical observations. For this reason and others, we have not recommended these three criteria alone serve as indications for fusion. However, a checklist has been developed that takes these criteria into consideration.

Incidence of Spontaneous Fusion

The high incidence of spontaneous fusion, which occurs without surgical intervention, leads to uncertainty about surgical fusion. Bailey and Bedbrook have both studied spontaneous fusions.[4,8] Table 5-5 shows some of the published figures of the incidence of spontaneous fusion reported by other investigators. Some are estimates, others are numerically documented. In any case, the incidence is high. To be able to predict which specific fracture dislocations will fuse spontaneously would solve the problem. Unfortunately, there is no published study that has attempted this.

Evaluation of Popular Arguments for Surgical Arthrodesis

The evidence in Table 5-5 argues well for the conservative approach of watching and waiting. Surgical enthusiasts deliberate about certain

Table 5-5. Incidence of Spontaneous Fusions Following Cervical Spinal Trauma

INVESTIGATOR	PER CENT SPONTANEOUSLY FUSED
Rogers '57	36
Brav, et al. '63	42
Robinson and Southwick '60	50
Hørlyck and Rahbek '74	66

(White, A. A., Southwick, W. O., and Panjabi, M. M.: Clinical instability in the lower cervical spine. A review of past and current concepts. Spine, 1:15, 1976.)

advantages of iatrogenic fusions. The most popular assertions are that surgical fusions reduce pain, improve stability, improve overall prognosis, facilitate nursing care, and reduce hospitalization time. Have fusions for fractures and fracture dislocations of the cervical spine been shown to reduce pain or improve stability? This question does not have a definitive answer, since pain is difficult to evaluate and stability has not been clearly defined. Munro reported that fusion reduced the incidence of pain in his patients by two-thirds, but there was no improvement in stability.[62] Rogers found no pain in a series of 39 patients who had undergone fusion.[81] Dall reported better reduction and stability in the few patients of his large series who were treated surgically.[28]

Effects on Nursing Care and Hospitalization Time. We found no studies in which this was investigated. The work of Brav and colleagues compared recumbency time of patients treated with and without fusion and observed no difference.[16] Norell and Wilson suggested that early anterior fusions reduce the time required for bed treatment, but they give no figures to support this.[67] Forsythe and colleagues, Durbin, Petrie, and Rogers asserted that fusion reduces the hospital stay.[30,36,73,81] Munro reported that patients treated with fusion did not have shorter periods of hospitalization.[62] Brav and colleagues actually compared figures in fused and nonfused groups and observed no difference in the period of hospitalization.[16]

Effects on Overall Prognosis. Forsythe and colleagues, Petrie, Rogers, Verbiest, and Durbin contend that patients treated with fusion have a better overall prognosis than those treated nonsurgically.[30,36,73,81,91] Munro vigorously argues to the contrary in a paper that reviews and reinterprets the data of other investigators.[62] The series of Brav and colleagues, the only study that actually compares a number of fused and nonfused patients, showed the overall prognosis to be virtually the same in the two groups.[16]

The arguments for cervical spine fusion following trauma may be summarized as follows: There is virtually no convincing evidence in the literature to support this procedure. However, there is also no significant evidence to the contrary.

RECOMMENDED EVALUATION SYSTEM

For experienced physicians, a checklist is not necessary. For the less experienced, however, it may be valuable. Certainly for the design of a prospective study, it can be useful. The care taken to construct the following checklist on the basis of a rational analysis of available evidence gives it validity. Of course, the reader has the option to accept or reject the system, based on personal judgment.

A point system has been included in order to standardize and objectify the checklist.

The Checklist

The system we propose is presented in Table 5-6. The patient is evaluated and each item that applies is checked. If the numbers assigned to the checked items total five or more, then the spine should be considered clinically unstable. It is not assumed that the information available on all patients will provide a definitive answer for each item on the list. It is recommended that when the evaluation of a given element leads the clinician to a borderline decision which can not be resolved, the value for that entity should be divided by two and added to the other points.

The evaluation of the first two entities, the status of the anterior and the posterior elements, is based on clinical history, evaluation of radiographs, and interpretation of flexion extension films, or the stretch test, if results are available. A history of disc removal does not necessarily indicate that all of the anterior elements are destroyed, but the situation may be suspect, since

Table 5-6. Checklist for the Diagnosis of Clinical Instability in the Lower Cervical Spine

ELEMENT	POINT VALUE
Anterior elements destroyed or unable to function	2
Posterior elements destroyed or unable to function	2
Relative sagittal plane translation >3.5 mm	2
Relative sagittal plane rotation >11°	2
Positive stretch test	2
Spinal cord damage	2
Nerve root damage	1
Abnormal disc narrowing	1
Dangerous loading anticipated	1
Total of 5 or more = unstable	

(White, A. A., Southwick, W. O., and Panjabi, M. M.: Clinical instability in the lower cervical spine. A review of past and current concepts. Spine, *1*:15, 1976.)

there is a possibility of disruption and weakening of the posterior longitudinal ligament from either surgery or degenerative disease. A separation of the vertebral end-plate following an extension injury, as described by Taylor,[89] or a transverse fracture of the vertebral body, as described by Marar,[59] may result in either the destruction of or the loss of the ability of the anterior elements to function. Although the study by Beatson did not mention the yellow ligament, it showed that with bilateral facet dislocations, virtually all of the anterior elements and all of the posterior elements may be destroyed.[7]

Radiographic Interpretations. With regard to posterior elements, it is wise to assume that bilateral pedicle fractures or bilateral facet and lamina fractures have negated all functional supports provided by the posterior elements. This is especially convincing considering the lack of strength and the not infrequent absence of the interspinous and supraspinous ligaments in such cases. Beatson found that unilateral facet dislocation results in a variable amount of anterior and posterior element damage, which is difficult to evaluate given present knowledge.[7] The stretch test is helpful in making this determination.

Radiographic Measurements. The measurement of translation is shown in Figure 5-27. This method takes into account variations in magnifications and should be useful when there is a tube to film distance of 1.83 m (72 in).[D]

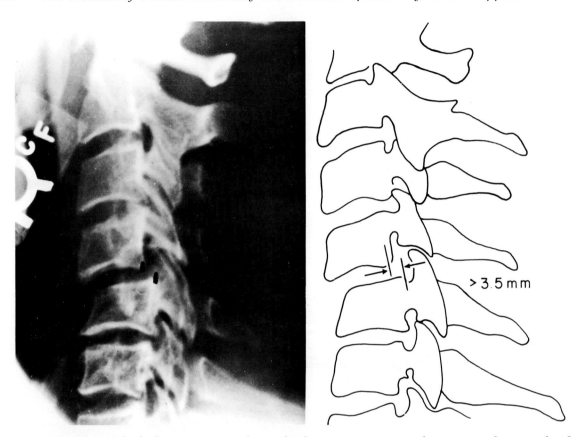

Fig. 5-27. The method of measuring translatory displacement. A point at the *posteroinferior* angle of the lateral projection of the vertebral body above the interspace in question is marked. A point at the *posterosuperior* angle of the projection of the vertebral body below is also marked. The distance between the two in the sagittal plane is measured. A distance of 3.5 mm or greater is suggestive of clinical instability.[D] (This distance is to be measured on lateral radiograph. It is computed from our experimentally obtained value of 2.7 mm and an assumed radiographic magnification of 30%.) (White, A. A., Johnson, R. M., Panjabi, M. M., and Southwick, W. O.: Biomechanical analysis of clinical stability in the cervical spine. *Clin. Orthop. 109:*85, 1975.)

The radiographic interpretation in general, especially for sagittal plane translation, is decidedly different in children up to at least 7 years of age.[24] It is risky to interpret radiographs of patients in this age-group without a knowledge of some of the normal findings that may appear to be pathological to the uninitiated.

There is no magnification problem in measuring rotation. Note that 11 degrees of rotation means 11 degrees greater than the amount of rotation at the motion segment above or below the segment in question. This standard of comparison takes into account the normal rotation between motion segments. The angles between these vertebral bodies are dictated largely by the existing lordosis and muscle spasm. Angular measurements are shown in Figure 5-28.[E] They are significant when measured on either flexion/extension or resting lateral radiographs. A discussion of radiographic standardization and analysis may be found on page 192.

The Stretch Test. The stretch test is still being developed. The validity of the concept has been well supported by laboratory studies and clinical observations, although a clinical series has not yet been provided.[69,98,99] The basic idea of the test is to measure the displacement patterns of the test spine under carefully controlled condi-

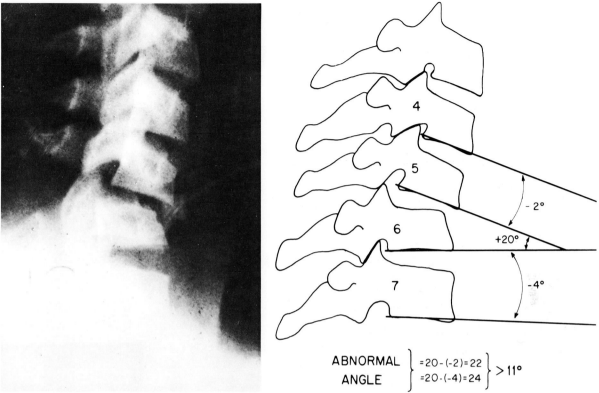

ABNORMAL ANGLE $\left.\begin{array}{l} =20-(-2)=22 \\ =20-(-4)=24 \end{array}\right\} > 11°$

Fig. 5-28. The angulation between C5 and C6 is 20 degrees, which is more than 11 degrees greater than that at either adjacent interspace. The angle at C4 and C5 measures −2 degrees, and the one at C6 and C7 measures −4 degrees. This finding of abnormal angulation is based on a comparison of the interspace in question with either adjacent interspace. This is to allow for the angulation that is present due to the normal lordosis of the cervical spine. We interpret a difference of 11 degrees or greater than either adjacent interspace as evidence of clinical instability. (White, A. A., Johnson, R. M., Panjabi, M. M., and Southwick, W. O.: Biomechanical analysis of clinical stability in the cervical spine. Clin. Orthop., *109*:85, 1975.)

tions and to identify any abnormalities in these patterns which may be indicative of ruptured ligaments.[E] Biomechanically, the spinal cord can tolerate considerable displacement in the axial (y-axis) direction. Thus, in the acute clinical situation, we believe that a test employing displacement in the axial direction is safer than less physiologic and potentially hazardous horizontal plane displacements.

Case Report. L. C. is a 23-year-old female who was involved in an automobile accident. She was unconscious for several minutes after the accident. When awake, she had neck and arm pain. However, the neurologic examination was within normal limits. Figure 5-29A shows a subluxation of C4 on C5. Figure 5-29B is a laminogram taken

with only 17 lb of axial traction. When that amount of axial displacement was noted, the traction was reduced. The patient's neurologic status remained normal.

Discussion. This case report illustrates several important points. The diagnostic value of axially directed traction to establish the presence of ligament disruption is demonstrated. Traction revealed that there was total disruption of all the anterior and posterior ligaments, which rendered the spine grossly unstable. The radiograph in Figure 5-29B exhibits dramatically the observations of Brieg, who found that the cord can withstand considerable axial displacement without structural damage and neurologic deficit.[17] The case report also shows the necessity of careful

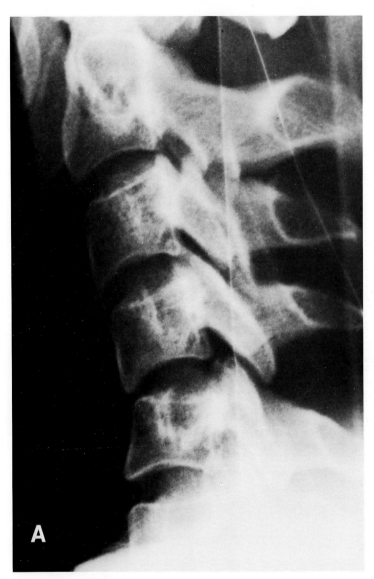

Fig. 5-29.   Radiographs of a patient with disruption of all ligaments between C4 and C5. (A) The spine in resting position.
(*Continued on facing page.*)

application of axial traction with close monitoring. While this patient had no additional damage
with this degree of displacement, certainly it is
not desirable to distract the cord and vertebral
column to such an extent. Therefore, we recommend, especially in weak-muscled individuals,
that the traction be applied in small increments
with frequent lateral radiographs to check the

position. The procedure in the case report was
not a formal stretch test. The protocol for the
stretch test is designed so that early minimal abnormal displacement can be recognized. Early
recognition permits demonstration of loss of
ligamentous continuity and avoids subsequent
damage, which may be imminent in Figure
5-29B.

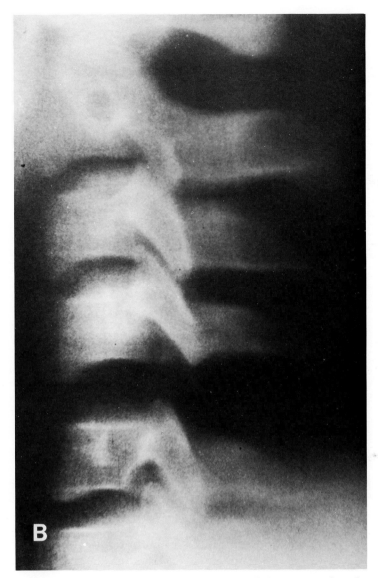

Fig. 5-29 (Continued). (B) Laminogram of the spine after the application of 17 lb of traction. There was no neurologic damage or irritation.

A detailed laboratory investigation of the patterns of displacement of the axially loaded cervical spine following ligament transections has been carried out. Figure 5-30 shows the experimental setup. The clinically relevant finding is as follows. Compared with the pattern of motion observed in the intact motion segment, an abnormal pattern of motion appears when all of the anterior structures or all of the posterior structures have been transected.[69]

The procedure for the stretch test is outlined briefly on page 229 and in Figure 5-31.

These guidelines based on studies of eight normals suggest than an abnormal stretch test is indicated by either differences of greater than 1.7 mm interspace separation or greater than 7.5

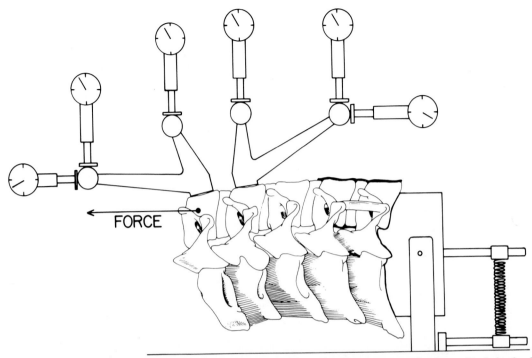

Fig. 5-30. The experimental arrangement in the stretch test. A force equal to one-third the body weight is applied; changes in rotation and separation of disc spaces as a function of ligament transection are measured by radiographs and the displacement gauges are attached to steel balls. The same schedules of ligament transections (anterior to posterior and vice versa) as those described in Figure 5-21 were used here. (White, A. A., Southwick, W. O., and Panjabi, M. M.: Clinical instability in the lower cervical spine. Spine, *1:*15, 1976.)

degrees of change in angle between vertebrae, comparing the prestretch condition with the situation after the application of axial traction equivalent to one-third body weight.[F] These are guidelines which will be improved with additional experience. It can be expected that with some cases abnormal separations may be seen and evaluated by clinical judgment without measuring.

Cord or Nerve Root Damage. Clinical evidence of cord damage indicates probable spinal instability, as discussed previously. Evidence of root involvement is, however, a less strong indicator of clinical instability. For example, a unilateral facet dislocation may cause enough foramenal encroachment to result in root symptoms but not enough ligamentous damage to render the motion segment unstable.

Disc Space Narrowing. Bailey remarked and we have observed that in the traumatized spine

there may frequently be narrowing of the disc space at the damaged motion segment.[3] We submit that this finding is modestly suggestive of disruption of the annulus fibrosus and of possible instability.

Dangerous Loading Anticipated. The final consideration involves the important individual variation in physiologic load requirements, especially with regard to differences in habitual activities. The clinician employs judgment in an attempt to anticipate the magnitude of loads that the particular patient's spine is expected to maintain after injury. Easy examples include an interior lineman on a professional football team and a sedentary retired seamstress.

Anticipating dangerous loads can be especially helpful when other available criteria are inconclusive. In situations where a particular life-style obviously exposes the patient to large physiologic loading, the desirability of surgical fusion is

Procedure for Stretch Test to Evaluate Clinical Stability in the Lower Cervical Spine

(1) It is recommended that the test be done under the supervision of a physician.

(2) Traction is applied through secure skeletal fixation or a head halter. If the latter is used, a small portion of gauze sponge between the molars improves comfort.

(3) A roller is placed under the patient's head to reduce frictional forces.

(4) The film is placed 0.36 m (14 in) from the patient's spine. The tube distance is 1.82 m (72 in) from the film.

(5) An initial lateral radiograph is taken.

(6) A 15-lb weight is added. (If the initial weight is 15 lb, this step is omitted.)

(7) Traction is increased by 10-lb increments. A lateral film is taken and measured.

(8) Step 7 is repeated until either one-third of body weight or 65 lb is reached.

(9) After each additional weight application, the patient is checked for any change in neurologic status. The test is stopped and *considered positive* should this occur. The radiographs are developed and read after each weight increment. Any abnormal separation of the anterior or posterior elements of the vertebrae is the most typical indication of a positive test. There should be at least 5 minutes between incremental weight applications; this will allow for the developing of the film, necessary neurologic checks, and creep of the viscoelastic structures involved.

(10) The test is contraindicated in a spine with obvious clinical instability.

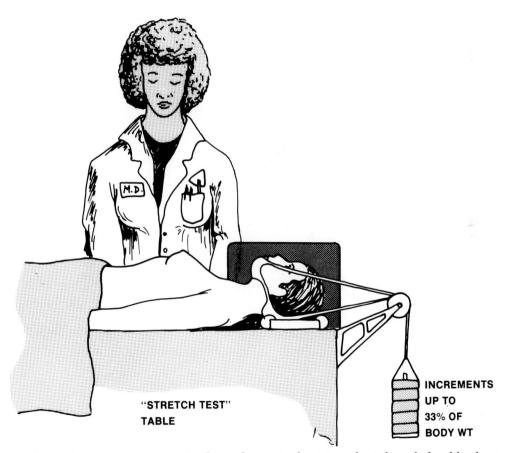

"STRETCH TEST" TABLE

INCREMENTS UP TO 33% OF BODY WT

Fig. 5-31. Diagrammatic synopsis of stretch test. A physician who is knowledgeable about the test is in attendance. The neurologic status is monitored by following signs and symptoms. Incremental loads up to 33 per cent of body weight or 65 lb are applied. Each lateral radiograph is checked prior to augmentation of the axial load. Note the neurologic hammer to symbolize neurological exam and the roller platform under the head to reduce friction. Despite the cartoon-like presentation, this is a serious test.

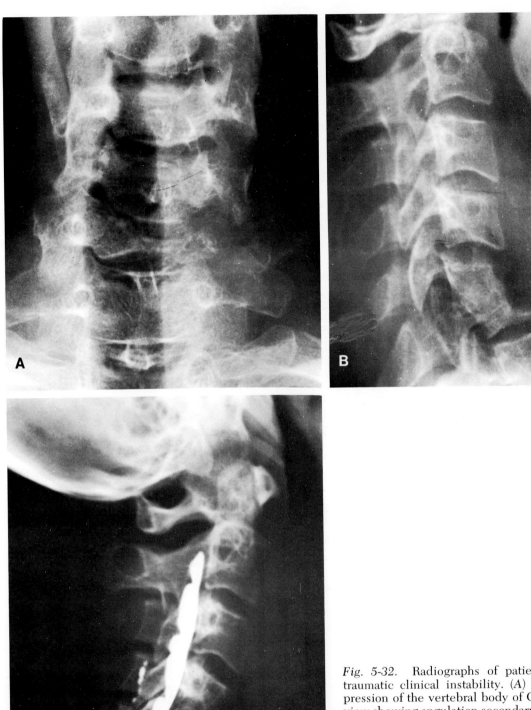

Fig. 5-32. Radiographs of patient with nontraumatic clinical instability. (*A*) Marked compression of the vertebral body of C6. (*B*) Lateral view showing angulation secondary to disruption of support function of anterior elements. (*C*) Myelogram showing myelographic block resulting from spinal canal encroachment due to vertebral collapse and angulation.

greatly increased. The strength of ligamentous healing in the human spine is not known. It is reasonable to assume that arthrodesis provides better stability than healed ligaments. The fusion may be thought of as protection against large anticipated loads. An active patient, such as the oarsman, would be better off with a fusion rather than depending upon ligamentous healing to withstand the anticipated loads.

Example of Clinical Stability Evaluation

Patient N. K., a 25-year-old male graduate student from India, complained of posterior neck pain with radiation into both arms. There was numbness in the left hand in the distribution of of the C5–C6 dermatome. Radiographs are shown in Figure 5-32. The anteroposterior view demonstrates collapse of the body of C6 and destruction of the lateral mass of C6. The lateral view shows the same, and in addition there is abnormal sagittal plane (z-axis) rotation of C5. The myelogram shows an incomplete block at the level of C5.

If the checklist is used to evaluate this patient for clinical stability, points would be given as follows: The anterior elements are distroyed and unable to function, 2 points; relative sagittal plane rotation is greater than 11 degrees, 2 points; there is root damage, 1 point. The total is 5 points, and the patient was thought to be clinically unstable.

The diagnosis was tuberculous osteomyelitis. The patient had laminectomies of C5 and C6 at another hospital. This procedure was associated with some relief of pain but rendered the situation even more clinically unstable. He was subsequently treated with posterior facet fusion and anterior resection with iliac graft to replace the vertebra. These resulted in a clinically stable, pain-free patient, with no neural defect.

Discussion

We have attempted to choose a number which would "set" the sensitivity of the system at just the proper level. In other words, if a score of 9 (4 above our "setting") were required in order to make a diagnosis of clinical instability, only those patients in such imminent danger as the person shown in Figure 5-33 would have insurance against the problems of instability. Physicians would almost never *overtreat* a patient for clinical instability. Such a high setting would leave a number of patients inadequately treated. Conversely, a low diagnostic score, such as 1 (4 below our "setting"), would result in a large number of clinically stable spines being *treated unnecessarily*. However, rarely would there be a neurologic catastrophe due to a clinically unstable spine being left untreated. A score of 5 avoids unnecessary surgery or too vigorous treatment, yet at the same time provides reasonable insurance against the unhappy development of additional root or cord damage (Fig. 5-33B). The system is presented to capsulize our views, to stimulate others, to develop better systems, and to help physicians to think about and use specific reproducible criteria for arriving at a diagnosis of clinical instability.

Relative Clinical Instability in Flexion or Extension

Experimental studies have shown that the anterior ligaments contribute more to stability of the spine in extension than the posterior ligaments.[98] The posterior ligaments limit flexion more effectively than the anterior ligaments. This information makes it possible to ascertain in some clinical situations whether a given spine is likely to be more unstable in flexion or in extension. For example, handling a patient with all the anterior elements destroyed, support of the patient to prevent extension is more important. This is also applicable to external support, as with transferring the patient and applying plaster immobilization or internal fixation. The converse is equally valid in the case of loss of the posterior elements. Figure 5-34 is a diagrammatic presentation of this basic concept.

RECOMMENDED MANAGEMENT

After defining and indetifying clinical instability in the lower cervical spine, how is it to be treated? Even when a particular spine has been determined to be clinically unstable, fusion is not

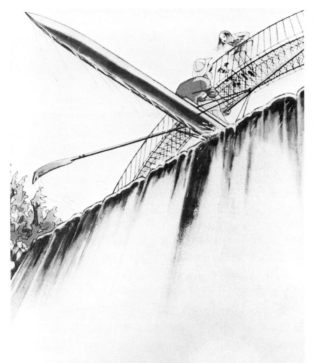

"My insurance company? New England Life, of course. Why?"

Fig. 5-33. (*Top*) Sometimes the need for insurance is obvious. With regard to clinical instability, one of the goals is to determine the less obvious needs for insurance and provide it through appropriate management of the patient who is in need of treatment. (*Bottom*) This is a theoretical graph depicting conceptually the choice of 5 as an "ideal" sensitivity setting. The ordinate shows percentages of *improperly treated* patients. The improper treatment could result in unnecessary surgery or unhappy catastrophe. The ideal setting should be the point at which the lowest percentage of patients are treated improperly. In our best judgment, that point is 5 on the *clinical stability scale*. We believe that this theoretical curve is correct; however, the real curve may be shifted to the right or to the left. For example, if it is shifted to the right as shown by the dotted curve, then a cut-off of 5 on the stability scale would result in a significantly large percentage of improperly treated patients. Assuming the curve is as indicated on the graph, a setting of 1 would involve a large percentage of unnecessary surgery and no unhappy catastrophe. A setting of 9 would avoid any unnecessary surgery, but permit a large percentage of unhappy catastrophes. (Cartoon courtesy of New England Life Insurance Company.)

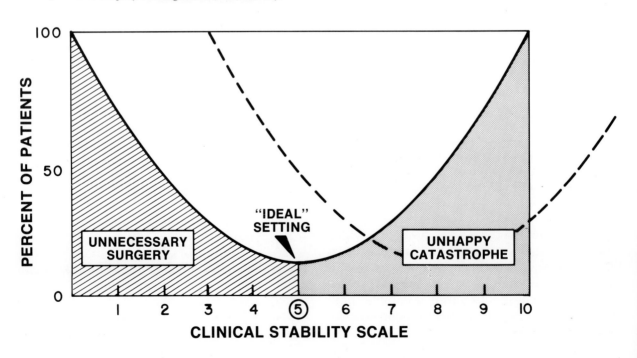

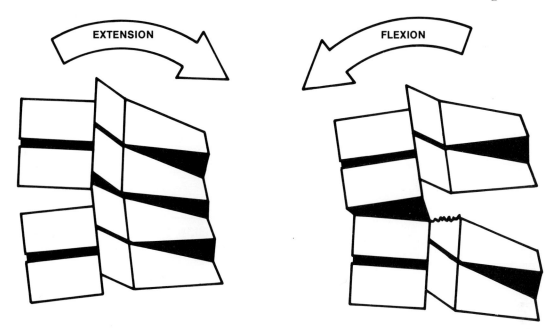

Fig. 5-34. If all other considerations are the same, (*A*) when the anterior elements are ruptured or cut the patient is more unstable in extension; (*B*) when the posterior elements are ruptured or cut the patient is more unstable in flexion.

necessarily the best method of treatment. The evidence in the literature is inconclusive on the relative merits of surgical and nonsurgical treatment. There is a paucity of information on the use of the various halo devices for the treatment of the unstable spine.

Flow Chart

A schematic organization of the management of clinical instability is presented in Figure 5-35.

Starting with patients with cervical spine trauma, initial treatment consists of bed rest for 1 to 7 days, in skeletal traction if there is evidence of severe injury. Patients with spinal cord involvement, with and without fractures or fracture dislocations, are considered to have major injuries. The patients without evidence of neurologic deficit who have either no fracture or only a minor compression fracture, without evidence of other damage, may be treated with head-halter traction. Minor injuries, such as strains, sprains, and muscle pulls, may be treated for symptoms and observed with subsequent radiographic examinations as indicated.

During the first week of traction patients are given a thorough clinical evaluation and whatever supportive care is required. After the patient is stabilized physiologically and evaluated for decompression, closed reduction with traction may be attempted, and if necessary, the various tests and maneuvers to rule out clinical instability may be performed.

It would be worthwhile to have a checklist to make a determination about decompression; however, at present, only the previously presented guidelines are available. Appropriate decompressions are carried out where indicated, and the patient is then evaluated for clinical stability using the checklist provided. If the decompression itself renders the spine clinically unstable, reconstruction and fusion may be carried out at the time of decompression.

All patients who are diagnosed as clinically stable can be treated with some modification of the following regimen. The assumption is that in 3 to 6 weeks, these patients will be comfortable and whatever damage they sustained will be healing. A four-poster cervical collar with a tho-

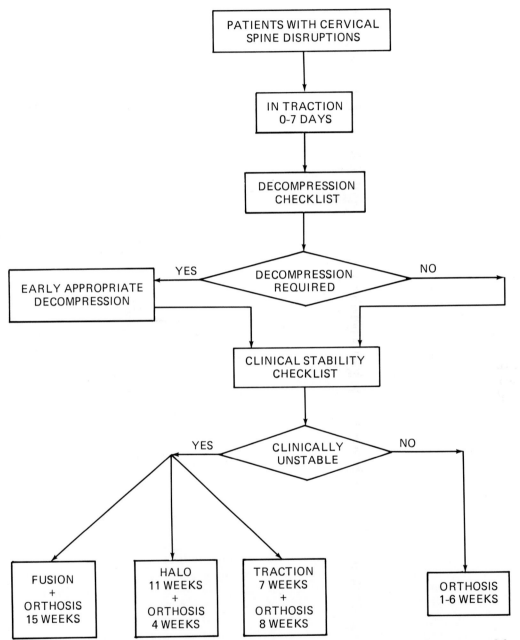

Fig. 5-35. Recommended flow diagram for the management of patients with disruptions of the lower cervical spine. Treatment regimens include occupational and physical therapy, as tolerated, and a follow-up schedule as outlined on page 235. (White, A. A., Southwick, W. O., and Panjabi, M. M.: Clinical instability in the lower cervical spine. A review of past and current concepts. Spine, *1:*15, 1976.)

racic attachment is desirable for adequate support and an effective intermediate range of control of movement. Such a device, along with the intrinsic stability of the spine, should be adequate to protect the patient from neurologic damage and allow injured structures to heal. It is possible that clinical instability may develop at a later time.

We have recommended below a basic schedule for follow-up of patients treated for problems of clinical instability in all regions of the spine. This schedule should allow cases of delayed instability to be recognized and treated before any complications occur. The visits are primarily for radiologic and neurologic evaluation. The frequency of the schedule is altered according to the individual patient's progress and prognosis.

Suggested Follow-up Schedule for Management of Clinically Stable and Unstable Spine Problems

(1) The schedule begins after the termination of initial treatment, surgical or nonsurgical (after removal of brace, cast, completion of bed rest, and initial physical therapy).

(2) The patient to be seen *3 weeks, 6 weeks, 3 months, 6 months,* and *1 year* after termination of initial treatment.

(3) If the appropriate clinical evaluation is carried out on this time schedule, all early and late complications should be recognized in time for treatment. Whenever possible, radiographic techniques should be standardized for purposes of comparison.

Treatment of Clinically Unstable Conditions

The three alternatives suggested provide clinical stability in the majority of patients. There is no convincing evidence in the literature that any of the three approaches is superior. The considerations are complex and have not been thoroughly studied. A successful fusion constitutes the strongest reconstruction for the unstable motion segment. However, it carries all the risks of spinal surgery in a seriously ill patient. Munro considered the risks to be significant.[59]

More recently, the halo apparatus has been used in the treatment of spinal trauma, with or without fusion.[55] This apparatus may have an important place in the treatment armamentarium of

this disease. The use of the halo apparatus (a halo attached to an outrigger stabilized on the body) may serve effectively as the primary treatment for some of these injuries. This method has promise and merits careful study in the management of clinical instability in the lower cervical spine.

The halo apparatus offers the best immobilization for the facilitation of ligamentous healing, and it may shorten hospitalization for the patient who has no major neurologic deficit. However, there has been no extensive experience with it as a primary treatment for clinical instability. The halo apparatus has its own complications. In addition, there is the unanswered question of whether ligamentous healing in any given case of spinal trauma is of satisfactory strength to withstand physiologic loads. The use of skeletal traction for a total of 7 weeks, followed by an orthosis of intermediate control for 8 weeks, is probably a more conservative approach and can be expected to be effective. We recommend 7 weeks of traction because Brav and colleagues showed that patients treated for 6 weeks or more had a redislocation rate of only 2.3 per cent.[16]

All of these regimens include careful clinical follow-up evaluations Lateral views of flexion/extension films are helpful for recognizing failed treatment or delayed or progressive subluxation or deformity. There are, of course, other combinations and regimens. Some surgeons prefer early or late Minerva casts. We believe that the halo apparatus gives better immobilization and that in most cases after 8 weeks of healing an orthosis of intermediate control is all that is required.

Each surgeon must choose from the various alternatives. The ideal would be to have some well controlled prospective clinical studies comparing the effectiveness of the different regimens. It would, of course, be essential to evaluate the various treatment levels in terms of effect on clinical stability. In addition, patient attitude, cost benefits, complications, rehabilitation, nursing care, and hospitalization time are all crucial variables to be evaluated before the best treatment regimen can be determined.

Because our experience has included a long tradition of success with surgical fusions of unstable spines, we recommend this procedure.

Part 3: The Thoracic Spine (T1–T10) and the Thoracolumbar Spine (T11–L1)

There are several unique considerations in the evaluation of clinical stability in the thoracic and thoracolumbar spine. This region of the spine is mechanically stiffer and less mobile than any of the other regions. There is less free space and a more precarious blood supply for the spinal cord in this region of the spine (Fig. 6-16). It is well stabilized by the articulation and the rib cage structure. Therefore, greater forces are required to disrupt it. The literature on the management of trauma to the thoracic spine contains abundant controversy. The selective presentation of one point of view does little service to the reader. We attempt to present all of the basic evidence, along with our interpretation of its significance.

ANATOMIC CONSIDERATIONS

There are several anatomic characteristics that relate to the biomechanics of this region and therefore affect its clinical stability. There is a normal thoracic kyphosis, which is due to the slight wedged configuration of both of the vertebral bodies and intervertebral discs. Because of this physiologic kyphosis, the thoracic spine is more prone to be unstable in flexion.

The Anterior Elements

The anterior longitudinal ligament is a distinct, well developed structure in the thoracic region (Fig. 5-36). Clinicians have noted that this structure is unusually thick in certain cases of abnormal thoracic kyphosis. This ligament is less developed in the cervical region.[52] The annulus, in this region as elsewhere, is one of the major factors in maintaining clinical stability. The posterior longitudinal ligament is also a distinct, well developed structure, which is of considerable importance in this region of the spine. The articulation of the ribs between vertebrae at the level of the intervertebral disc provides consid-erable additional stability to the thoracic spine motion segments. The radiate ligaments and the various costotransverse ligaments provide stability by binding adjacent vertebra to the interconnecting rib (Fig. 5-37).

The Posterior Elements

The yellow ligaments are thicker in the thoracic region. The capsular ligaments in the thoracic region, in contrast to those in the cervical region, are thin and loose, which is significant anatomically. It means that the support provided by these structures against flexion is minimal and is much less than might be expected in the cervical spine, where there are well developed capsules on the articular facets. Therefore, following multiple laminectomies in the thoracic spine, the usual support provided by the thick yellow ligament is lost, leaving the facet articulations, which can offer little support. This characteristic, along with the physiologic kyphosis, predisposes the thoracic spine to clinical instability after laminectomies at several levels. The rib articulation is able to provide some stability if it remains intact. The interspinous ligaments are not as thick in the thoracic as in the lumbar area. The supraspinous ligaments probably do not play a major role in the stability of this portion of the spine.

In addition to the effects of the capsular structure of the facet articulations, their spatial orientation has some significance. The kinematic factors are described in Chapter 2. In the middle and upper portion of the thoracic spine, the facets provide stability *primarily* against anterior translation. When the orientation changes, which may happen anywhere between T9 and T12, the facets provide less stability against anterior and posterior displacement. The joints are oriented more in the sagittal plane and therefore provide stability against axial rotation (Fig. 2-24). Therefore, in the presence of rotary displacement in the lower thoracic and thoracolumbar region, facet dislocations or fracture dislocations must be present.

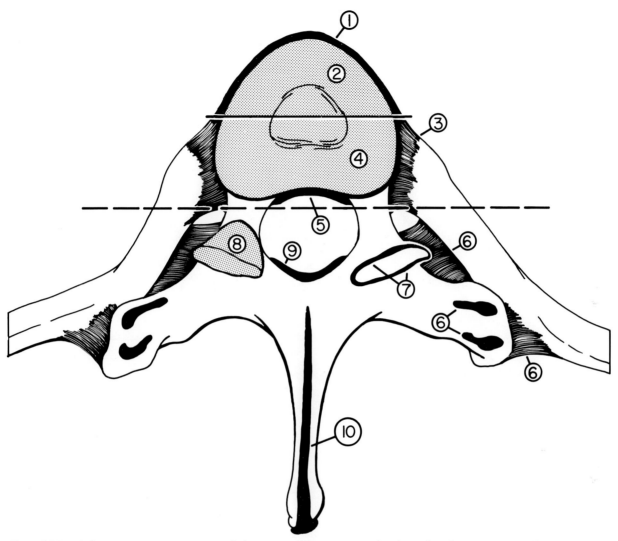

Fig. 5-36. Schematic representation of the major ligament involved in the thoracic spine. Ligaments are numbered according to the order in which they were cut in the biomechanics experiment referred to in the text. Anterior elements: *1*, anterior longitudinal ligament; *2*, anterior half of the annulus fibrosus; *3*, radiate and costovertebral ligaments; *4*, posterior half of the annulus fibrosus; *5*, posterior longitudinal ligament. Posterior elements: *6*, costotransverse and intertransverse ligaments; *7*, capsular ligaments; *8*, facet articulation; *9*, ligamentum flavum; *10*, supraspinous and interspinous ligaments.

BIOMECHANICAL FACTORS

Effects of Thoracic Spine Stiffness on Clinical Stability

There are two mechanisms through which the ribs tend to increase the stability of the thoracic spine. The first involves the articulation of the head of the rib to the articular facets of adjacent vertebral bodies (Fig. 5-37). The second is related to the presence of the entire thoracic cage. The thoracic cage effectively increases the transverse (x,z plane) dimensions of the spine structure. This increases the moment of inertia, resulting in added resistance to bending in the sagittal and frontal planes, as well as to axial rotation (Fig. 5-38). This has been well supported by

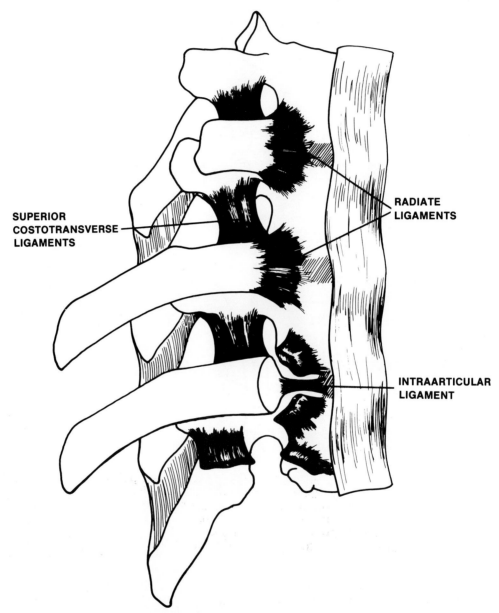

SUPERIOR COSTOTRANSVERSE LIGAMENTS

RADIATE LIGAMENTS

INTRAARTICULAR LIGAMENT

Fig. 5-37. This diagram highlights ligamentous structures in the costovertebral articulation that make some contribution to the clinical stability of the thoracic spine. Note the radiate ligaments attaching to the head of the rib and to *both adjacent* vertebral bodies. There are also the costotransverse ligaments, which may offer some secondary stability.

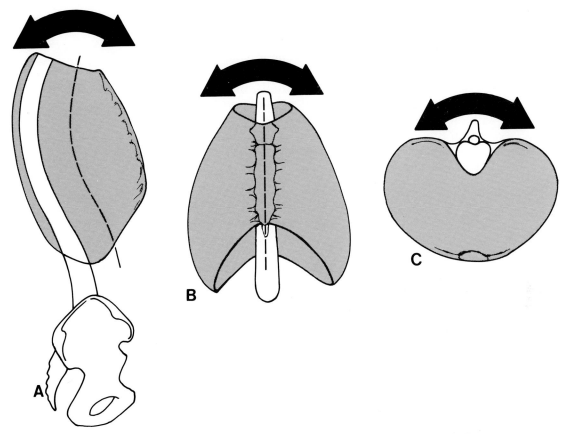

Fig. 5-38. The thoracic cage effectively increases the transverse dimensions of the spine structure. This in turn increases its moment of inertia and, therefore, its stiffness and strength in all modes of rotation: (*A*) bending in sagittal plane (flexion/extension); (*B*) bending in frontal plane (lateral bending); and (*C*) axial rotation.

studies of computer simulation of human spine models. The greatest increase in stiffness, as measured at T1 with respect to the pelvis, was 132 per cent during the motion of extension. The percentage increase in lateral bending was 45 per cent, and for flexion and axial rotation the increase was approximately 31 per cent.[2]

Biomechanical Analysis of Clinical Stability

Biomechanical studies have shown that the range of motion between thoracic vertebrae is altered by removal of the posterior elements.[97] Flexion, extension, and axial rotation were compared in individual thoracic spine motion segments before and after removal of the posterior elements. There was a statistically significant increase in the degree of flexion, extension, and

axial rotation following removal. These observations suggest that when the structures can no longer function as a result of surgery, trauma, or tumor, abnormal movement occurs. Such excessive displacement could be injurious to the cord.

We have completed some biomechanical investigations on the thoracic spine very similar to those described for the cervical region. In this study, thoracic spine motion segments with their rib articulations intact are examined. Flexion and extension are simulated with incremental loads up to 50 per cent of body weight. Anatomic components are then cut from front to back and vice versa, the sequence is shown in Figure 5-36. Flexion or extension was simulated in several motion segments for each loading modality. The initial results suggest the following: With all posterior elements cut, the segment remains stable in flexion until the costovertebral articulation is destroyed; all anterior ligaments plus at least one posterior component must be destroyed to cause failure; with the motion segment loaded to simulate extension, stability can be maintained with just the anterior longitudinal ligament intact; with the motion segment loaded to simulate flexion, stability can be maintained with just the posterior longitudinal ligament and the other anterior elements intact. The maximum physiological sagittal plane translation was 2.5 mm and the maximum sagittal plane rotation was 5 degrees.[41a,98a]

CLINICAL CONSIDERATIONS

Clinical Stability of Different Classifications and Fracture Types

Bedbrook and Edibaum suggested that if the initial observed displacement was one-half of the anteroposterior diameter of the vertebral body, the situation was unstable. They noted that in these situations, the reduced vertebra would redisplace and result in a final deformity. If the anteroposterior displacement was one-third or less, there was no development of gross deformity.[9] In Nicoll's report of 166 fractures, he suggested that wedge-shaped fractures were *unstable* when there is rupture of the posterior interspinous ligament. He defined stable fractures as those with no likelihood of increase in deformity or spinal cord damage and provided a listing of stable and unstable fractures. They are shown below.[65]

Nicoll's Classification of Stable and Unstable Fractures and Fracture Dislocations

STABLE	UNSTABLE
Anterior wedge fractures	Fracture subluxations with interspinous ligament rupture
Lateral wedge fractures	Fracture dislocations
Laminar fractures above L4	Laminar fractures of L4 and L5

(Nicoll, E. A.: Fractures of the dorso-lumbar spine. J. Bone Joint Surg., *31B*:376, 1949.)

Epidemiologic review of a large number of *fractures* suggests that the wedge fractures are generally stable because there is little risk of neurologic damage.[75]

The classification most frequently referred to in the literature is that of Holdsworth. It is shown below.

Holdsworth's Classification of Stable and Unstable Fractures and Fracture Dislocations

STABLE	UNSTABLE
Wedge compression fracture	Dislocations
	Extension fracture dislocations
Burst and compression fracture	Rotational fracture dislocations

(Holdsworth, F. W.: Fractures, dislocations and fracture dislocations of the spine. J. Bone Joint Surg., *45B*:6, 1963.)

Holdsworth expressed the view that the rotational fracture dislocation occurs only at the thoracolumbar junction and in the lumbar spine and is the most unstable of all vertebral injuries; the cord and roots are in grave danger (Fig. 5-39). He states that 95 per cent of all *paraplegias* at the thoracolumbar level have this rotational fracture dislocation.[45]

Roberts and Curtiss also offered a classification which is not related to stability. They considered a spine to be stable when there is little likelihood of progressive deformity with gibbus formation and neurologic damage. Their classification included three types based on the evaluation of the lateral radiograph.[78]

Roberts' and Curtiss' Classification of Fractures and Fracture Dislocations

Type I Wedge compression fracture with or without posterior element injury
Type II Compression burst fracture
Type III Rotational fracture dislocation

(Roberts, J. B., and Curtiss, P. H.: Stability of the thoracic and lumbar spine in traumatic paraplegia following fracture or fracture-dislocation. J. Bone Joint Surg., *52A*:1115, 1970.)

These classifications may be summarized in the following manner. Anterior wedge, lateral wedge, and bursting compression fractures are generally stable unless the posterior interspinous ligaments are destroyed. (The bursting fracture is

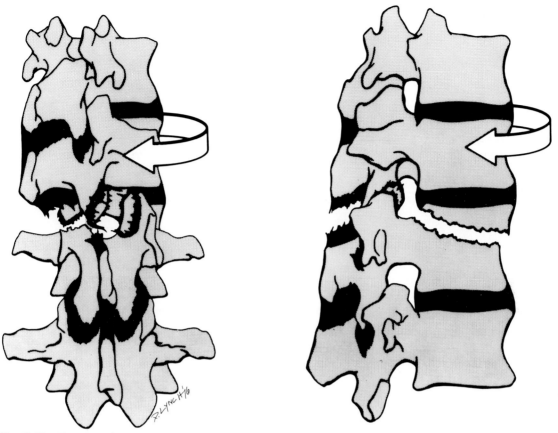

Fig. 5-39. Rotatory fracture dislocation of Holdsworth. The primarily horizontal failure line can occur either through the annulus fibrosus attachment to the end-plate or through the vertebral body as shown here. (*A*) Posterior view of two lower vertebrae. (*B*) Lateral view.

likely to undergo spontaneous fusion.) Dislocations and fracture dislocations were generally considered unstable, especially the classical fracture dislocation of Holdsworth (Fig. 5-39).

Although these classifications categorize various aspects of the problem, none of them deals comprehensively with all aspects. The definition of clinical stability with which we are concerned includes subsequent neurologic deficit and subsequent deformity and pain both short-term and long-term. The basic problems are to identify which injuries need to be treated to avoid instability and what that treatment should be.

Structural Damage and Neurologic Deficit

To what extent is structural damage to the vertebral elements correlated with neurological deficit?

Riggins and Kraus classified vertebral fractures in all regions of the spine into seven mutually exclusive categories, depending upon the grouping of three variables. The three variables are the conditions of the vertebral body, the posterior elements (structures posterior to the posterior longitudinal ligament), and the presence or absence of dislocation (any malalignment of the vertebral column greater than 2 mm). The seven groupings, along with the percentage of each type that was associated with neurologic deficit, are given in Table 5-7.

Some relevant conclusions can be drawn from this work. Fracture dislocations have a higher incidence of associated neurologic deficits. The remaining group, which includes fractures or dislocations alone, has a lower incidence of associated neurologic deficits. Riggins and Kraus ob-

Table 5-7. Association of Neurologic Deficit with Injury for All Regions of the Spine

	% WITH NEUROLOGIC DEFICIT
Dislocation only	17
Dislocation, posterior element fracture	27
Dislocation, body fracture	56
Dislocation, body and posterior element fracture	61
Posterior element fracture only	19
Body fracture only	3
Body fracture and posterior element fracture	11

(Riggins, R. S., and Kraus, J. F.: The risk of neurological damage with fractures of the vertebrae. J. Trauma, *17:*126, 1977.)

served that a simple wedge fracture is generally not associated with neurologic damage, while the rotatory fracture dislocation described by Holdsworth is generally involved with a neural deficit.[75] The high incidence of neural problems associated with this injury is due at least in part to the very high forces required to produce it.

It seems then that there is a tendency for structural damage to be associated with neurologic deficits. However, in any given patient there may be extensive destruction and displacement of the vertebral column without neurologic deficit.[9,37,75] The converse is also true. In a Northern California study it was reported that 13 per cent of patients showed neurologic damage without recognizable evidence of spinal column injury.[75]

What kind of structural damage is likely to result in neurologic deficit? This is a crucial problem. It has been shown that sagittal plane kyphotic deformities of 30 degrees or more are not associated with deterioration of neurologic function.[57] Roberts and Curtiss observed progressive deformity in their Type III fractures and some of Type I fractures. In determining the subsequent deformity of the wedge compression fracture, the status of the posterior ligamentous structures is important (see Chapter 4).

Neurologic Deficit and Clinical Instability

The incidence of spinal cord damage associated with injuries to the thoracic vertebrae is approximately 10 per cent. For the thoracolumbar region the figure is 4 per cent.[75]

In the thoracic and thoracolumbar spine, should one assume that all injuries that produce neurologic deficits are unstable? The rationale for such an assumption is as follows. If there is enough deformation at the time of injury to produce neural damage, there must also be sufficient structural damage to the vertebral column to render it clinically unstable. In the large majority of cases this is true. However, there can be neurologic deficit in situations in which there is either no structural damage or no recognizable damage.[38,59] The canal size in the thoracic region is relatively smaller in relation to the spinal cord size, than in other regions. Therefore deformation of ligaments within the Elastic range can allow enough displacement to deliver a detrimental impact to the neural structures. Although the large majority of cases with neural deficit in the thoracolumbar spine are clinically unstable, it is important to keep in mind the possibility of exceptions to the rule and the presence of unrecognized structural damage (Fig. 5-40).

TREATMENT CONSIDERATIONS

Effects of Reduction on Prognosis

Does surgical or nonsurgical reduction of dislocations and fracture dislocations in this region affect the prognosis? In North America there has been a trend to follow the dictates of Hippocrates, who believed that fractures should be anatomically reduced. Consequently, there has been advocacy of open reduction and instrumentation using various forms of internal fixation and surgical arthrodesis.[102] Nicoll and Leidholdt made observations on the prognosis of compression fractures. Nicoll studied patients with vertebral body compression fractures who were treated without plaster. A comparison of radiographs of the fractures on admission, discharge, and several years later revealed no significant increase in deformity. He concluded that there is no basis to assume that a good anatomic result is required for a good functional result, and he alluded to a patient who worked in the coal mine with an unreduced fracture for 30 years.[65] Leidholdt reviewed 204 patients and concluded that sagittal plane deformity of 30 degrees or even more did not affect prognosis. There was no suggestion that major deformities caused pain or decreased neurologic function.[57]

Nicoll and Leidholdt made another important observation. They noted that two paraplegic patients who had a deformity of 10 degrees or more in the frontal plane experienced difficulty with ulceration of the ischial spine from sitting. This obviously should be considered in decisions regarding surgical reduction and fixation in paraplegics.

Young conducted a thorough and careful study designed to ascertain any correlation between the severity of deformity of compression fractures of the thoracic and lumbar spine and the final clinical outcome in a group of workers. Severity of this fracture was measured by percentage of compression and loss of height of the vertebral body. Clinical outcome was gauged by categorizing the patients into three groups, those with no symptoms, those with symptoms that allowed them to return to their original work, and those with symptoms that resulted in retirement or taking a different job. Young observed no correlation of deformity with undesirable clinical outcome. There was no tendency for the original deformity to increase. Unlike the observations of Nicoll, who found that patients who were able to return to work in the coal mines showed spontaneous fusion,[65] Young found that spontaneous fusion occurred with the same frequency among patients with satisfactory and poor outcomes.[104]

Roberts and Curtiss, on the contrary, included in their report two patients who showed loss of recovery associated with progressive deformity of wedge compression fractures. In addition they pointed out the *undesirability* of the use of the circle electric bed in the management of patients with severe thoracic and thoracolumbar spine injuries. They observed that progression of deformity may be associated with loading to which the spine is subjected during turning if the patient is in a bed that goes beyond the upright position.[78]

Most of the evidence suggests that the presence of deformity itself is not associated with a poor prognosis. The evidence presented here raises questions about the desirability of employing vigorous methods purely for the purpose of correcting sagittal plane deformity.

Operative and Nonoperative Reduction

Lewis and McKibbin conducted a retrospective comparison of conservative versus operative treatment in a series of patients with paraplegic thoracolumbar spine injuries. Twenty-nine had surgery and 14 were treated nonsurgically. The following cogent quotation is from their work. "Support exists for both schools of thought and is sometimes expressed with great conviction; it is unlikely, however, that the relative merit of the two methods will ever be adequately appreciated unless they can be directly compared in a series of unselected cases."[58] According to their interpretation, their studies show that reduction and internal fixation is the preferred treatment. However, their data does not justify anything other than a tentative, meagerly supported conclusion. Lewis and McKibbin suggested that although surgery may offer little benefit with regard to the prognosis of neurologic deficit, it tended to help prevent pain and deformity.[58]

The significance of the status of the posterior ligaments in the probability of subsequent angulation is presented in Figure 5-41. The probability of posterior ligament disruption is greater in the wedged fracture. This is due to the fact that both the wedge and the posterior ligament disruption are likely to be the result of a significant flexion component in the injury mechanism.

Burke and Murry also compared two groups of patients, one treated conservatively and the other treated surgically. They found that 38 per cent of the surgically treated and 35 per cent of the conservatively treated patients showed neurologic improvement. These figures demonstrate no significant improvement in prognosis with surgery, despite the fact that the surgical group had more *incomplete* neurologic lesions, for which the prognosis is considered to be better. Significantly, the investigaters also observed that of the ten patients who had significant spine pain, eight had undergone surgery.[20] Frankel and colleagues reported that, out of 400 fractures of the thoracic and thoracolumbar spine, only two became unstable with nonsurgical treatment.[37]

The data from these studies do not demonstrate the superiority of either open or closed treatment of fractures and fracture dislocations in this region of the spine.

Several papers were presented in the 1978 meeting of the American Academy of Orthopaedic Surgeons on Harrington rod operative stabilization and arthrodesis of fracture dislocations of the dorsal lumbar spine. The general theme of these papers indicated that a better result was achieved with less expenditure of time and medical costs. These studies indicate that operative management of fracture dislocations may be preferable. However, additional experience, careful scrutiny, and some well designed controlled studies will be necessary to make a definitive conclusion.

The Role of Traction and Manipulation

We found little information on the use of either traction or manipulation for the treatment of vertebral column injuries in this region. Chahal reported on a group of seven patients that he had treated. He reported excellent results in those patients treated with the use of a pelvic girdle, through which he applied 40 to 45 lb of traction.[25] With regard to manipulations, Böhler reports a technique in which patients are suspended prone, with arms and legs on two separate chains, in order to achieve reduction through gravity, and a plaster cast is applied in the corrected position.[13]

The Role of Laminectomies and Anterior Decompressions

Laminectomies. This highly controversial procedure was first introduced by Paul of Aegina between 625 and 690 A.D. The use of this operation has, unfortunately, preceded and superceded the critical evaluation of its advantages and disadvantages. Laminectomies may contribute to clinical instability through the removal of supporting structures of the spinal column.[14,37,40,88] The basic biomechanics of the role of the posterior elements in the support of the spine is demonstrated in Figure 5-42. The procedure itself may be associated with additional neurologic deterioration.[21] In addition to its well documented attendant risks, the procedure itself is often not helpful. The posterior decompression does little or nothing to relieve anterior pressure (see Fig. 8-1).

Benassy reviewed 600 cases and showed that laminectomy was not helpful in most thoracic and lumbar spine injuries.[11] Morgan and Wharton compared a total of 198 injured spinal cords treated with and without laminectomy. They found that delayed laminectomy (more than 48 hours post-injury) produces an increased incidence of poor results compared to treatment by early laminectomy. Their basic conclusion was that the operation is only indicated when required for debridement of a compound wound or reduction of an otherwise irreducible fracture or dislocation. It is distressing and disappointing to observe how frequently this virtually useless and damaging procedure is inappropriately employed.

Anterior Decompression. With the development of anterior spinal surgery, there has been an increasing interest in anterior decompression through partial or total vertebral body resection. The basic biomechanics of the role of the anterior elements in the support of the spine is demonstrated in Figure 5-42. Proponents argue that when the block is anterior, posterior decompression is of little value. In addition, significant vascular compromise of the cord can readily occur as a result of anterior encroachment into the spinal canal. Anterior decompression of thoracic and thoracolumbar fractures has been recommended by Whitesides and Shah. They advocate posterior Harrington instrumentation for reduction, followed by anterior vertebral body resection, with iliac or rib bone graft replacement. They reported experience with five cases.[102] Although this treatment appears to have some advantages, it is hoped that a critical evaluation will precede and not be superseded by widespread use.

Evaluation of Popular Arguments for Surgical Treatment

Arthrodesis, Pain, and Deformity. Evidence of functional, painless spines after trauma without surgical arthrodesis has been presented. Some of these spines showed spontaneous fusions; others did not. The study of Burke and Murry reported a higher incidence of spine pain in patients who had undergone surgery than in those who had not.[20] Other studies have shown little or no progression of deformity without fusion, while Roberts and Curtiss noted that an increase did occur in the absence of surgical stabilization.[78]

Effects on Nursing Care and Hospitalization Time. There have been few studies designed to evaluate either of these considerations in the thoracic or the thoracolumbar spine. It appears a priori that surgical stabilization might be expected to reduce nursing care and hospitalization time. However, an accurate evaluation involves a number of complex considerations. For example, the intensive nursing care involved in the preoperative, operative, and postoperative periods is to be balanced against the less intense and possibly more prolonged nonoperative management. Moreover, nursing care of the complications associated with treatment methods should be studied. Comparative requirements of care by other members of the team, especially the physical therapist, also seem to merit consideration. There remains the important consideration of hospitalization. We believe that it is very worthwhile to have specific, active, nonoperative programs in conjunction with surgical management.

Effects on Overall Prognosis. This is an even more complicated issue. It brings into consideration cosmesis, psychological well being, attitudes toward rehabilitation, overall health, productivity, and activity levels achieved by the therapeutic programs under evaluation.

Obviously, all this information would be extremely expensive to obtain. Nevertheless, these considerations are presented to point out the need for more objective information and to show that it is not meaningful to assume certain advantages of operative intervention as if they were proven facts. We also wish to emphasize that a lack of proof does not necessarily invalidate indications for operative treatment in thoracic and thoracolumbar spine trauma.

A RECOMMENDED EVALUATION SYSTEM

The Checklist

We have presented here an objective system which will allow proper identification and treatment of the clinically stable and unstable conditions in the thoracic and thoracolumbar spine (see Table 5-8).

We suggest that injuries in this region be evaluated using laminograms in the anteroposterior and lateral planes, in addition to the regular anteroposterior and lateral radiographs. Here it is appropriate to emphasize the importance of and the difficulty in obtaining a good lateral radiograph of the C6–T1 area of the spine when evaluating a patient with spinal trauma. This issue has been well presented by Lauritzen, who recommends the use of lateral tomograms.[56] The swimmers view can also provide a satisfactory lateral radiograph of this region. Figure 5-40 stresses the importance of radiographs that satisfactorily show the vertebrae in this region.

Anterior Elements Destroyed or Unable to Function. The preliminary results of our laboratory studies suggest that with all the anterior elements cut, the loaded thoracic and thoracolumbar spine in extension is either unstable or on the brink of instability. In the rotary fracture dislocation, well known from clinical experience to be unstable, there is disruption of the anterior elements through the vertebral body, the annulus, or some combination of the two. With total or partial vertebral body resection for decompres-

Table 5-8. Checklist for the Diagnosis of Clinical Instability in the Thoracic and Thoracolumbar Spine

Element	Point Value
Anterior elements destroyed or unable to function	2
Posterior elements destroyed or unable to function	2
Relative sagittal plane translation > 2.5 mm	2
Relative sagittal plane rotation > 5°	2
Spinal cord or canda equina damage	2
Disruptions of costovertebral articulations	1
Dangerous loading anticipated	2
Total of 5 or more = unstable	

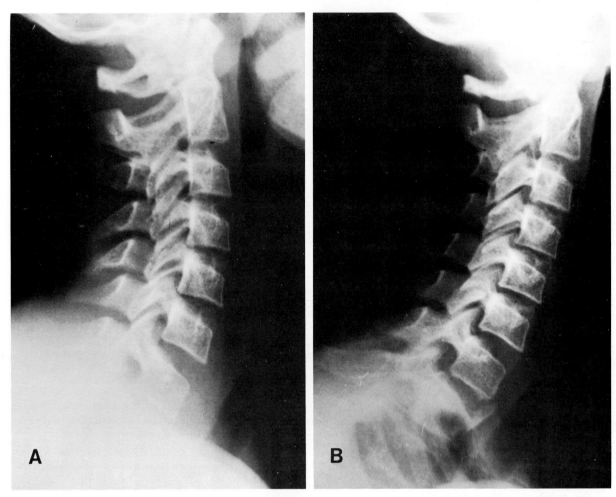

Fig. 5-40.   (A) A routine lateral cervical spine radiograph with a good view of C7 seems normal. However, the patient complained of back pain. (B) A radiograph taken with the shoulders pulled down. The fracture of the first thoracic vertebra is now obvious. These radiographs emphasize the necessity of careful and thorough examination of the cervical thoracic junction in any case of persistent undiagnosed neck or back problem following trauma to the spine. The fracture went undiagnosed for 3 months.

sion, these structures may also be lost or compromised.

There are some other important characteristics of the anterior elements that are worthy of consideration that relate to the status of the vertebral body. With regard to configuration, the sharply wedged compression fracture shown in Figure 5-41 is more likely to be associated with a clinically unstable situation than is the less severely wedged fracture with a more central, vertically directed, major injuring vector (see Chapter 4). There are several negative factors that are likely

to be associated with the wedged configuration of the vertebral body fracture. Aseptic necrosis, which has been observed following vertebral fracturing,[8] is more likely to occur in a highly *impacted*, severely wedged fracture, resulting in the loss of vertebral blood supply. When an injured vertebra undergoes aseptic necrosis, it can lose its ability to withstand compressive loads, especially during the stage of creeping substitution. The angulated compression fracture is more likely to be associated with progression of deformity. This is due not only to more efficient

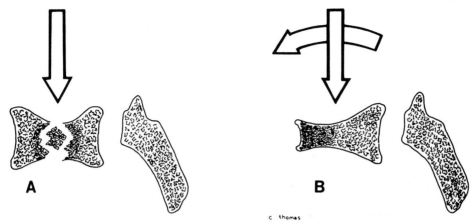

Fig. 5-41. Probable correlation between the mechanism of injury and configuration of vertebral body compression fracture. (*A*) Pure compression loading gives biconcave and communited type pattern. (*B*) When there is a significant bending moment, there is more of a wedge-like configuration. This type is more prone to subsequent angulation than that shown in *A*.

loading through a greater moment arm, but also to a possible collapse from asceptic necrosis. Although Leidholdt's clinical findings are reassuring,[57] from basic mechanics it is apparent that with increasing angulation, greater moments are applied per unit force (Fig. 5-42). Finally, the sharply angled compression fracture is more likely to be associated with significant posterior element disruption. The practical significance of this discussion involves biomechanical theory, which suggests that in the evaluation of the anterior elements, excessive wedging (approximately 50% or more of the estimated original anterior height) is suggestive of clinical instability.[G]

In the evaluation of the status of the anterior elements, special attention should be paid to the articulations of the ribs and vertebral bodies in laminographic studies. These articulations, through the linkages of vertebra, ligaments, and rib, provide considerable stability to the motion segments.

Posterior Elements Destroyed or Unable to Function. Key factors in making this determination are the physical examination and the evaluation of the position of the spinous processes on the anteroposterior radiograph. When there is extensive destruction of the posterior elements,

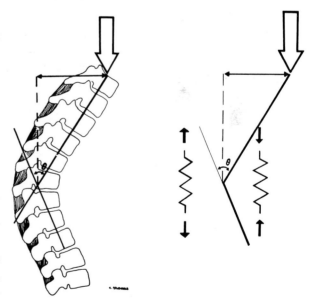

Fig. 5-42. This diagram is designed to illustrate several points about clinical instability and kyphotic deformity: The posterior elements contribute to stability primarily by resisting tensile loads; the anterior elements function primarily by resisting compressive loads; the greater is the load applied, the greater is Cobb's angle (θ); as Cobb's angle increases there is a greater moment arm, tending to cause kyphotic deformity.

there may be localized swelling, tenderness, edema, and a palpable defect under the skin. Wide separation of the spinous processes may be discernable. The anteroposterior radiograph shows wide separation of the spinous processes at the level involved. If there is a Holdsworth rotary dislocation, there will be an off-set of the spinous processes, showing axial rotation at the level of the injury. More subtle fractures, subluxations, and dislocations of the posterior elements are seen on the usual lateral films or laminograms.

The initial results of our experimental studies suggest that with all the posterior elements destroyed or unable to function, there is likely to be enough abnormal displacement to cause additional neural damage. Kinematic studies reported on page 77 showed that there can be abnormal movement in flexion, extension, lateral bending, and especially axial rotation when these structures are rendered functionless. All of these abnormal motions are potentially injurious to the cord. With the normal kyphosis of the thoracic spine, the posterior elements play a significant mechanical role by withstanding tensile loading in the erect position, as well as during forward flexion. The presence of a wedged compression fracture may be a clue suggesting that some posterior ligaments are torn. Thus the thoracic spine is probably more unstable in flexion when these structures are disrupted. The role of the posterior elements in the balance of the intact spine is shown in the theoretical model of Figure 5-42. The importance of the functional integrity of these elements in the thoracic spine is augmented by the normal kyphosis in this area.

Relative Sagittal Plane Translation.   A relative sagittal plane translation of greater than 2.5 mm is highly suggestive of thoracic spine clinical instability. This present criteria is based on experimental biomechanical studies completely analagous to those upon which the criteria suggested for the cervical spine were based.[42a]

Relative Sagittal Plane Rotation.   A relative sagittal plane rotation of >5 degrees is strongly indicative of clinical instability in the thoracic spine. This criteria is also based on the previously mentioned biomechanical study.[42a]

Spinal Cord or Cauda Equina Damage. One might consider giving this entity a full 5 points on the checklist. However, there are situations in which there is no recognizable structural damage and yet there is neurologic deficit. Some of these may be overlooked structural lesions, but it is also possible to have cord damage with a truly intact column. This, of course, would not be a clinically unstable situation. This entity is given a high value, but in such a manner that some other evidence of instability must also be present in order to make the diagnosis. Neural damage is also assigned a high value because in the thoracic region, the space occupied by the cord is such that there is minimal opportunity for any abnormal displacement to occur without damaging the neural structures. Therefore, once the structural integrity has been altered enough to cause damage, the risk of *subsequent* damage is very high, and the patient should be protected against this.

Dangerous Loading Anticipated.   This is the same as that recommended in the evaluation of the cervical spine. However, it is even more crucial in this region. The forces applied to this region are likely to be greater, because the superincumbent weight is greater, and the operative moment arms are greater, shown in Figure 5-42.

Discussion.   There is not as much clinical or experimental evidence upon which to base the checklist for the thoracic and thoracolumbar region as there is for that of the cervical spine. Given the currently available knowledge, this is a justifiable method for arriving at a diagnosis of clinical instability in this region of the spine.

RECOMMENDED MANAGEMENT

Flow Chart

The flow chart given in Figure 5-43 may be helpful as an outline of the major considerations in managing patients with disruption of the thoracic and thoracolumbar spine.

The patients may be placed in bed or on a turning frame. The latter should be used if there is significant neurologic deficit. The patient is

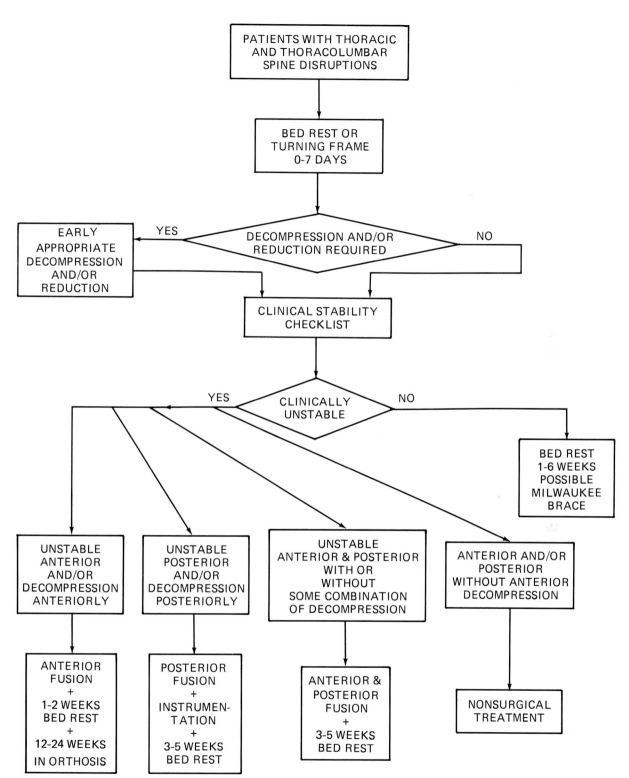

Fig. 5-43. A recommended flow diagram for the management of patients with disruptions of the lower cervical spine. All treatment regimens include occupational and physical therapy, as tolerated, and follow-up schedule (see p. 235).

given the necessary supportive therapy, and thoroughly evaluated through various neurologic and radiographic examinations and baseline laboratory studies. Within the first 48 hours, a decision about the indications for operative decompression is made and carried out as soon as the patient's condition permits. (The evidence suggests that the laminectomies should rarely be performed.) Decompression, which is preferably carried out anteriorly, is indicated when there is an incomplete neurologic deficit, with radiographic evidence of spinal cord compression. The patient, with or without decompression, is then evaluated according to the clinical stability checklist.

Treatment of the Clinically Stable Condition

Patients who have been evaluated and determined to be clinically stable are treated with 1 to 6 weeks of bed rest.[65] After termination of bed rest, they are then followed by radiographic and clinical evaluation, according to the schedule on page 235. The length of initial bed rest is determined by patient response and the severity of the injury. Once the patient can tolerate it, physical therapy may be instituted. The patients are given a series of treatments until they can stand erect. They are then taught to walk and are given exercises to strengthen the spinal and abdominal muscles. If there is prolonged or excessive pain or conditions suggestive of a possible increase in deformity, then we suggest a Milwaukee brace. The brace is prescribed using the three-point system, as in the treatment of adolescent kyphosis. This is the most effective orthosis for the treatment of these conditions. This brace offers support comparable to a cast and has the advantage of being readily adjustable.

Treatment of the Clinically Unstable Condition

There is no definitive study that convincingly shows the superiority of either operative or nonoperative therapy. Therefore, based on currently available information, we suggest that both approaches are justified. Clearly, we do not advocate any protocol that assumes that a diagnosis of instability is equal to an indication for surgery. There are, however, certain situations in which we strongly favor operative stabilization of an unstable spine. These are presented below. Surgical considerations are also presented in some detail in Chapter 8.

Indications for Operative Treatment of the Clinically Unstable Thoracic and Thoracolumbar Spine

Following anterior decompression with removal of complete vertebral body

Compelling conditions that demand immediate rehabilitation activity

---

Compelling conditions are situations in which the patient's mental or physiologic status is such that the required bed rest would obviously be detrimental or impossible.

In Figure 5-43, there are several types of clinically unstable situations included. As shown by the grouping clinically, instability may be present in several situations. It may be the result of anterior and/or posterior structural damage, as well as the result of anterior and/or posterior surgical decompression.

Clinically Unstable Anteriorly, With or Without an Anterior Decompression. We suggest anterior fusion, followed by 1 to 2 weeks bed rest and rehabilitation as tolerated. A plaster jacket with chin and occipital support or a Milwaukee brace is recommended. If there is instability at T6 or above, chin support is important. The individual is ambulatory in the orthosis for 12 to 24 weeks. The patient is then managed by the guidelines suggested in the follow-up schedule.

Clinically Unstable Posteriorly With or Without Posterior Decompression. When instability is primarily posterior due to disruption of the posterior elements from natural or iatrogenic disease, posterior fusion with instrumentation is indicated. Appropriate wiring or Harrington instrumentation is the best available method. There is room for additional improvement in instrumentation and techniques for open reduction and internal fixation of fractures in this region. We suggest that the patient be kept in bed for 3 to 5 weeks in a plaster jacket (including chin support if T6 or above), or a Milwaukee brace. The recumbency time will permit some degree of soft-tissue healing and allow reduction of cord edema. Following this, if possible, the patient is then treated with ambulation in the same device for 12 to 24 weeks. The rehabilitation and follow-up schedule is the same as that described on page 235.

Clinically Unstable Both Anteriorily and Posteriorly With or Without Anterior and/or Posterior Decompression. In some situations, posterior fusion alone is satisfactory, even when there is anterior and posterior instability. However, when there is a need for vertebral body removal, it is generally better to operate posteriorly first. Instrumentation or wiring can be used to provide some *immediate* postoperative stability, and posterior fusion can be applied with no additional loss of stability. Then the spine may be approached anteriorly, allowing decompression and fusion to be carried out with the insurance of some stability from posterior instrumentation. The regimen is carried out as follows. Posterior instrumentation and fusion is followed immediately or in 3 to 7 days by anterior decompression and/or fusion, as indicated. The postoperative regimen is the same as that of patients with posterior instability.

Clinically Unstable Anteriorily and/or Posteriorly Without Anterior Decompression. Except for clinical instability following anterior decompression by vertebral body removal, our interpretation of present knowledge suggests that other types of instability may also be treated by nonsurgical methods. These nonsurgical methods offer several justifiable alternatives. One may elect to proceed with postural reduction followed by additional bed rest and then some orthotic device.[40] Another approach is to simply have the patient rest in bed, or if there is significant sensory deficit, the patient may use a turning frame. After 6 weeks the patient may begin to walk using an orthosis for additional support.[9] With these and other nonsurgical regimens, physical and occupational therapy and appropriate exercises in bed are recommended. The patient is then given rehabilitation and activity as tolerated, and followed according to the suggested schedule.

Discussion. Several nonsurgical options have been offered here. There are a number of other regimens and combinations to be considered. Bedbrook and Edibaum, for example, suggested that possibly there should be trials of mobilization of some patients with neurologically involved spines after 3 weeks.[9] If such a series were shown to be successful, a number of the surgical "advantages" would be eliminated. The nonoperative regimens offered by us are all based on well documented experience and sound clinical biomechanics and rehabilitation. They all seem to be equally appropriate, and the non surgical regimens selected might well be determined by some equilibrium between the individual patient's and physician's needs and preferences, as well as the local practices and available facilties.

Part 4: The Lumbar Spine (L2–L5)

The problem of clinical stability in the lumbar spine has some unique considerations, related to both aspects of the definition of clinical instability. The associated neurologic deficits are relatively rare, less disabling, and more likely to recover. A large epidemiologic series of all spine injuries reported that only 3 per cent of patients with lumbar spine dislocations and fracture dislocations had neurologic deficits.[75] The second consideration is related to the phenomena of subsequent pain, deformity, disability, and the very high loads that must be borne by this region of the spine. The clinical biomechanical problem of pain and its management is discussed in Chapter 6.

ANATOMIC CONSIDERATIONS

Anterior Elements

The anterior longitudinal ligament is a well developed structure in this region. The annulus fibrosus, which has received an enormous amount of attention in the literature, constitutes 50 to 70 per cent of the total area of the intervertebral disc in the lumbar spine. As in other regions of the spine, it contributes in a major way to the clinical stability of the motion segment.

Posterior Elements

The posterior longitudinal ligament is less developed than is the anterior counterpart in the lumbar region. All the ligaments and the facet orientation are shown in Figure 5-44.

The facet joints play a crucial role in the stability of the lumbar spine. Usually a flexion rotation injury and displacement are required for dislocation to occur. The well developed capsules of these joints play a major part in stabilizing the motion segment against this type of displacement. When there is a fracture dislocation of the facet joints, there may be abnormal displacement, primarily axial rotation, and possibly lateral bending. When these displacements are observed, fracture or fracture dislocation of the facet articulations must be suspected. Figure 5-45 shows how the spatial orientation of the articular facets is designed to prevent excessive axial rotation. It is clear that these structures must fracture and/or dislocate in order to permit abnormal axial rotation. Moreover, Sullivan and Farfan showed in the laboratory that axial rotation of the lumbar spine of 30 degrees or more caused failure of the neural arch, progressing from facet joint dislocation to fracture of the articular process.[87] It seems obvious that with the forces involved in these kinds of disruptions and dislocations, there would also be injury involving the yellow ligament. With the relatively modest posterior longitudinal ligament and the degenerating and ruptured interspinous ligaments, it is readily apparent that the dislocations and fracture dislocations of the facet articulations tend to be associated with a loss of clinical stability.

Rissanen carried out an anatomic study of 306 cadavers, which resulted in some pertinent and interesting observations. The age distribution was from fetal life to 90 years, with significant representation throughout the range. He found that 21 per cent of those subjects over 20 years of

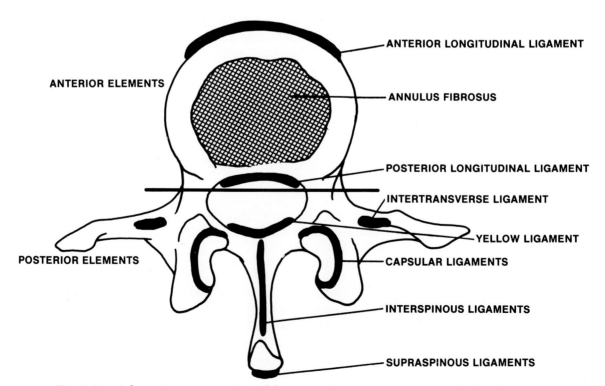

Fig. 5-44. Schematic representation of the major ligaments operative in the lumbar spine.

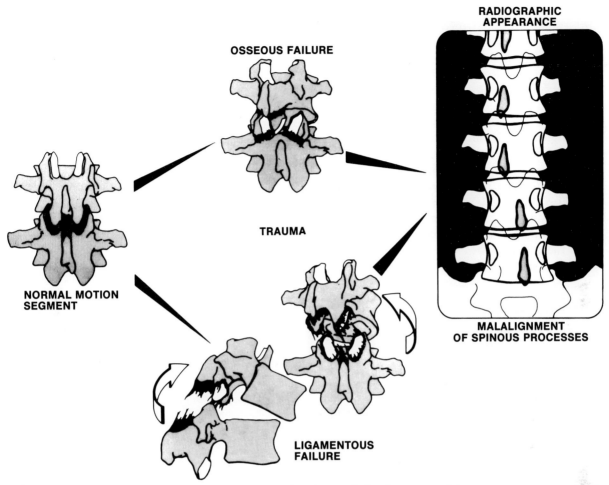

RADIOGRAPHIC APPEARANCE

OSSEOUS FAILURE

TRAUMA

NORMAL MOTION SEGMENT

LIGAMENTOUS FAILURE

MALALIGNMENT OF SPINOUS PROCESSES

Fig. 5-45. This diagram emphasizes that in order for abnormal displacement of the spinous processes in the lumbar spine to occur, it is necessary to have a dislocation of or a fracture in one or more facet articulations. The final radiographic view of the malaligned spinous processes may also show vertical separation of spinous processes and asymmetrical projection of the pedicles. These findings post-trauma are all suggestive of significant posterior element injury.

age had rupture of one or more of their interspinous ligaments, occurring mostly at L4–5 and L5–S1 motion segments. He also found that 75 per cent of the subjects between ages 31 to 40 showed cavitation where the ligaments are normally located.[76] These findings suggest strongly that the interspinous ligaments can be expected to make very little or no contribution to the clinical stability of the lower lumbar spine in the adult.

The status of the facet articulations is crucial in other ways. There is a consideration here that is similar to the observations of Beatson on the cervical spine.[7] Most probably, damage of the posterior longitudinal ligament and annulus fibrosus is associated with disruptions of the facet articulations. Such a correlation has not been demonstrated experimentally, but a study of the anatomic relationships with an evaluation of the amount of displacement involved in dislocation of the facets will support this hypothesis (Fig. 5-45).

The final consideration with regard to the posterior elements relates to the informative experimental setup that nature provides in the form of spondylolisthesis. The radiographs of a healthy,

17-year-old male are shown in Figure 5-46. This well known and well recognized entity demonstrates a situation in which the posterior elements are rendered unable to function due to a defect in the pars interarticularis. When this situation occurs, the remaining anterior structures may allow progressive displacement. This is due to plastic deformation of the anterior structures, the two longitudinal ligaments and the annulus fibrosus. The lateral radiograph shows graphically anterior displacement in the sagittal plane of approximately 50 per cent of the sagittal diameter. The oblique views clearly demonstrate the "Scotty dog sign," with the defect in the pars articularis that allows the forward displacement. The "broken neck" of the "Scotty dog" represents the actual defect. This spondylolisthesis shows that there can be clinical instability of the lumbar spine when the posterior elements are compromised.

BIOMECHANICAL FACTORS

The role of the muscles in clinical stability, as previously discussed, is difficult to evaluate. Certainly the lumbar region is well endowed with active muscles. The erector spine, the abdominal muscles, and the psoas are all actively involved in maintaining the functional upright and sitting stability of the lumbar spine.[6,61,64] They also contribute to the very high loads to which the lumbar spine is subjected. In this region, these well developed muscles and their characteristic load-

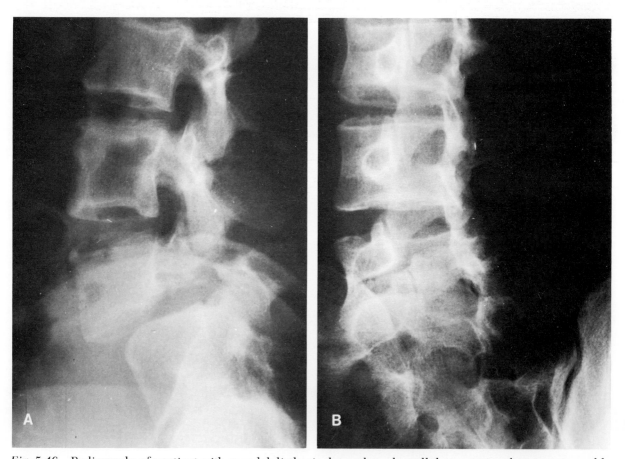

Fig. 5-46. Radiographs of a patient with spondylolisthesis shows that when all the posterior elements are unable to function, there may be abnormal displacement. (*A*) Lateral view and (*B*) oblique view, showing the "Scotty dog" sign.

ing patterns may render the lumbar spine less vulnerable to clinical instability. However, it must also be considered that the large and variable loads due to muscle and gravitational forces increase the likelihood that disruptions of the lumbar vertebral column will be associated with severe pain.

CLINICAL CONSIDERATIONS

In 1966, Kaufer and Hayes wrote the following: "Since lumbar dislocation is not uncommon and possesses special characteristics of therapeutic and prognostic significance, we were surprised that a search of medical literature failed to reveal a comprehensive report dealing exclusively with the special problem of lumbar dislocation or fracture dislocation."[54] More than ten years later, this statement remains essentially correct. The very thorough analysis of 21 cases by Kaufer and colleagues is still the major work that exclusively studies this region of the spine.

Incidence of Lumbar Injuries and Associated Neurologic Deficit

"Lumbar segments constitute 3 or 4% of all spine dislocations and fracture dislocations."[54] In the study by Riggins and Kraus, the incidence of neurological damage associated with lumbar spine injuries was just 3 per cent.[75] Kaufer and Hayes, however, reported an incidence of 53 per cent in their series of 21 cases.[54] Others have reported 60 to 70 per cent with neurologic deficit. These figures vary widely, depending on whether or not T12–L1 is included separately, or with the lumbar spine.

Structural Damage and Neurologic Deficit

In the study done in Northern California by Riggins and Kraus, there was a greater incidence of neurologic deficit in fracture dislocations, but here too there was no consistent correlation.[75] The radiographs in Figure 5-47 show quite dramatically the discrepancy between structural damage and neurologic deficit. This extreme fracture dislocation has no neurologic damage associated with it.

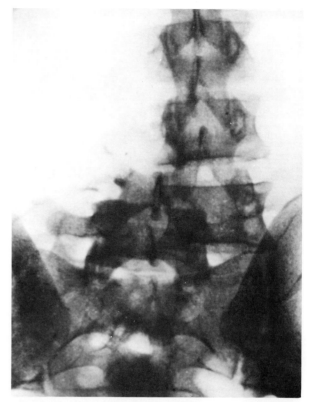

Fig. 5-47. Radiograph of a severely displaced L4–L5 fracture dislocation without neurologic damage. This is an astonishing example of the occasional gross lack of correlation between structural damage and neurologic deficit. This disassociation is more likely to occur in the lumbar region than in other regions of the spine. (Steinger, K. K.: Fracture-dislocation of the thoracolumbar spine with special reference to reduction by open and closed operations. J. Bone Joint Surg., 29:107, 1949.)

Neurologic Deficit and Clinical Instability

There is a relatively large margin of safety in the lumbar spine because the space available for the neural elements amply exceeds the space occupied by them. Therefore, the presence of neurologic deficit is very likely to be the harbinger of clinical instability. In other words, if there is enough displacement to cause neural damage then it must be assumed that enough displacement has occurred to cause significant ligamentous and/or bony failure. The pure vertically loaded compression fracture is an exception to this principle. The clinical observation of the study by Kaufer and Hayes, in which two patients progressed from mild to severe neurologic deficit between the time of injury and definitive treatment, supports this contention. These changes did not occur in transport but while the patients were hospitalized, during bed rest in Foster frames.

Classification System

Although Kaufer and Hayes did not expand upon the significance or use of their classification system, it was not related to prognosis or any treatment considerations. It is presented here because it is well thought out and contributes to the understanding and analysis of lumbar spine injuries. It also supports very nicely our assertion that the "key" to the evaluation of injuries in this region is the status of the articular facets.

Kaufer and Hayes' Classification of Fractures and Fracture Dislocations of the Lumbar Spine

Type I	Dislocation of both articular processes without associated fracture of the articular processes
Type II	Dislocation of articular processes and vertebral bodies with associated vertebral body compression fracture
Type III	Dislocation of both articular processes without dislocation of the vertebral body, but with disruption through the vertebral body
Type IV	Dislocation of only one pair of articular processes, disruption through the opposite pedicle or pars interarticularis, then through the intervertebral body or disc
Type V	No dislocation of either articular process, but dislocation of vertebral body with a posterior line of disruption through pedicles or pars interarticularis

(Kaufer, H., and Hayes, J. T.: Lumbar fracture-dislocation. A study of twenty-one cases. J. Bone Joint Surg., 48A:712, 1966.)

Considering these patterns of failure of lumbar vertebral motion segments in the clinical situation is most useful during the analysis of the clinical biomechanics of these injuries. In the course of radiographic examination it alerts the clinician to look for certain patterns of associated injury. The classification points out the importance of a careful radiographic evaluation of the status of the facet articulations. We suggest the addition of one more pattern to the classification of Kaufer and Hayes: the *unilateral* lumbar facet dislocation, which is frequently associated with a fracture of a lamina, a pedicle, or a pars interarticularis.

Pain and Disability Following Lumbar Spine Trauma

This region of the spine, because of socioeconomic reasons as well as biomechanical and pathophysiologic factors, is often a site of considerable pain and disability. Therefore, in evaluating clinical stability here, the prognosis with regard to pain becomes a more important consideration.

TREATMENT CONSIDERATIONS

Effects of Reduction on Prognosis

Reduction of these injuries is thought to help reestablish stability and may decompress the neural canal.[54] As yet, attempts at closed reduction have been associated with increases in neurologic deficits.[53,80] Kaufer and Hayes recommended open reduction, posterior fusion, and wire fixation of the involved motion segments. If one of the involved segments showed separation of the posterior elements, then fusion to the first intact segment on the other side of it was suggested. None of the patients treated by this method had severe back pain.[54]

The Role of Laminectomy

Laminectomy is rarely a useful procedure in fracture dislocations in the lumbar spine. Many of the injuries include decompression associated with the injury itself. Surgical exploration may reveal a subcutaneous hematoma which, when removed extends all the way to and exposes the dura or even the cauda equina (Fig. 5-48).[54] Clearly, there is no need for a laminectomy in this situation. Because of the anatomy and the available space for the cauda equina, mechanical pressure is rare, but when present it can usually be corrected by realignment of the vertebra. Certainly, if there is clear radiologic or other convincing evidence that some localized particulate matter is encroaching on the cord posteriorly, laminectomy is indicated.

Traditional Indications for Surgical Arthrodesis

The lonesome study by Kaufer and Hayes suggests that all lumbar spine dislocations and fracture dislocations with and without neural deficits are "unstable."[54] Therefore, they should be treated by open reduction, fusion, and internal fixation. The rationale is that without reduction, which achieves decompression and provides stability, all these injuries would progress to *subsequent* neurologic deficit. In the small series of patients so treated, they report no progression, but some recovery from neurologic deficit, no significant low back pain postoperatively, and better cosmetic appearance.

RECOMMENDED EVALUATION SYSTEM

The Checklist

There are comparatively very few biomechanical studies or clinical studies that can provide a solid basis for the systematic approach to the problem of clinical instability in the lumbar spine. The guidelines suggested here are therefore not as vigorously proposed as are those for other regions of the spine (see Table 5-9). Basically, we want to take full advantage of the recuperative power of the cauda equina and minimize the possibility of prolonged disability associated with low back pain.

Table 5-9. Checklist for the Diagnosis of Clinical Instability in the Lumbar Spine

ELEMENT	POINT VALUE
Cauda equina damage	3
Abnormal displacement (translation of 25% of sagittal or frontal plane diameter of subadjacent vertebral body)	2
Anterior elements destroyed or unable to function	2
Posterior elements destroyed or unable to function	3
Dangerous loading anticipated	1
Total of 5 or more = clinically unstable	

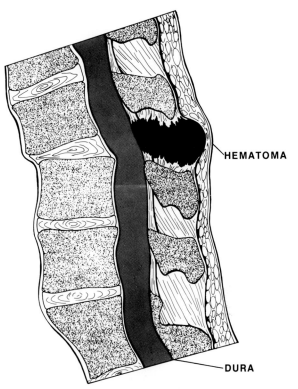

Fig. 5-48. Depiction of the lumbar spine flexion injury in which all the posterior elements are disrupted and the dura is separated from the outside by only hematoma and skin. This is hardly an indication for decompressive laminectomy. The hematoma is readily palpable between the spinous processes on physical examination.

The specific question has been raised concerning when the lumbar spine is clinically unstable following the various procedures for disc surgery. We recommend this checklist to make that determination. The use of this checklist will not indicate fusion of lumbar spine purely as a treatment for pain.

Cauda Equina Damage. Because there is ample space available for the cauda, when it is damaged by displacement it may be assumed that at the time of injury there was enough structural disruption to allow a large displacement.

Abnormal Displacement. When readily apparent residual displacement remains after the recoil and rebound of injury, the structural damage is obvious. However, when there is little or no residual displacement of the position of the vertebrae following injury to the cauda, clinical instability must be suspected. The physician should look for other evidence of clinical instability in order to make such a diagnosis when there is *no* residual displacement.

We do not have solid experimental or clinical evidence upon which to make this determination. It is simply our best opinion, based on our understanding of neuroanatomy, musculoskeletal anatomy, biomechanics, and clinical stability of this region. We suggest that if a vertebral body is displaced in the sagittal or frontal plane by one-fourth or more of the corresponding vertebral diameter in that plane, this is abnormal. The reference diameter is taken from the undisplaced subadjacent vertebra (Fig. 5-49). This criterion will also show significant displacement in axial rotation, which is an important variable in determining instability.

Anterior Elements Destroyed or Unable to Function. This situation occurs most frequently when there has been failure of the annulus fibrosus or a slice (shear) failure through the vertebral body, either of which may be part of the classic fracture of Holdsworth.[45] There are other specific instances in which the anterior elements may be unable to function. The vertically loaded vertebral body fracture may be a *bursting* fracture with multiple fragmentation, which excessively compromises the mechanical function of the structure in resisting compressive loads. If the pattern of loading results in major impacting of osseous structures, the blood supply may be irreversibly damaged, resulting in necrosis, creeping substitution, fragmentation, and loss of normal structural mechanics (the mechanical *advantages* of impacting are discussed on page 170).

Finally, there is the obvious loss of normal mechanical function due to infection, tumor, or surgery (see the list on p. 259).

Posterior Elements Destroyed or Unable to Function. A key factor in the evaluation of lumbar spine trauma is the relative position of the

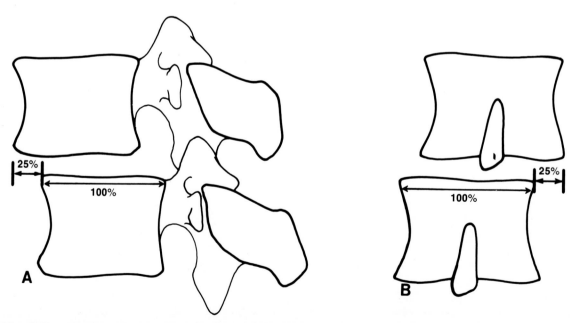

Fig. 5-49. Measurements to determine vertebral displacement in the lumbar spine. (*A*) A method for measuring *sagittal plane displacement.* If the displacement is as much as 25 per cent of the sagittal diameter of the subadjacent vertebra, it is considered to be abnormal. (*B*) In the frontal plane, if there is displacement of 25 per cent of the frontal diameter of the subadjacent vertebra from any combination of *frontal plane displacement* or *axial rotation,* it is considered to be abnormal. These criteria are included in Table 5-9.

Situations in Which the Anterior Elements Are Destroyed or Unable to Function

Failure of anterior ligamentous structures
   Increased forces
   Infection, tumor, disease
   Surgery

Failure of vertebral body
   Slice fracture
   Excessively comminuted fracture
   Aseptic necrosis
   Infection, tumor, disease
   Surgery

---

spinous processes. The position of these structures indicates the relationships of the posterior elements. Abnormal separation along the y-axis or the x-axis represents flexion and axial rotatory deformity, respectively.

The work of Kaufer and Hayes pointed out the importance of the status of the posterior elements by documenting in the classification the major patterns of structural failure that are associated with abnormal displacements of the facet joints.[54] Evaluation of the posterior elements fits very well with the observations of Holdsworth, who also pointed out the significance of malalignment of the spinous processes.[45] Although it is not known how much separation or axial rotation of the posterior elements is associated with failure of all posterior ligaments, it is a fact that any such residual displacement is indicative of at least some loss of mechanical support from these structures. When other considerations on the checklist are brought into the evaluation, they will either contribute to or detract from the significance of a given degree of spinous process displacement as an indication of clinical instability.

In the evaluation of the status of the posterior elements following trauma, there may be certain findings on physical examination that are helpful. There may be a painful, palpable defect in the midline, with a large hematoma between two widely separated spinous processes (Fig. 5-48). A subcutaneous hematoma that extended directly to the dura in 85 per cent of the cases was observed in the series of patients studied by Kaufer and Hayes at the University of Michigan.[54]

Nature has provided an interesting experimental model which allows us to make some assumptions about the role of the posterior elements in the clinical stability of the lumbar spine. Spondylolisthesis is an example of the loss of support function of the posterior elements due to a defect of the pars interarticularis. Obviously, other patterns in this area, such as different combinations of pedicle and laminar fractures, can result in similar structural failures. With this problem, there may be associated clinical instability.

Dangerous Loading Anticipated. This has been discussed previously. Because of the heavy loading in this region normally, and the socioeconomic considerations, this criterion is important in the evaluation of the clinical stability of the lumbar spine.

Examples of Clinical Stability Evaluations

Patient B.F. is a 23-year-old female who was involved in an automobile accident while under the influence of drugs. She sustained no neurologic damage and her only complaint was severe low back pain. The most demonstrative cuts of the anteroposterior and lateral laminograms are shown in Figure 5-50. At the level of L2–3 there is separation of the posterior elements, a fracture through the pedicle on the left, and a dislocation of the facet joint on the right. The lateral view suggests that there is a slice fracture or a separation of at least the posterior portion of the body. There is also some axial (y-axis) rotary displacement between L2 and L3. This injury in all probability was a result of incorrect use of a seat belt.

A checklist evaluation of the stability of this situation suggests that it is probably clinically stable. There is no cauda equina damage, no abnormal translation, and no dangerous loads anticipated. The posterior elements are destroyed, a value of 3 points, and since the anterior elements are only partially destroyed by an incomplete slice fracture, a value of only 1 or 0 points is assigned. The case was successfully managed as a clinically stable fracture.

Patient I.L. is a 35-year-old female who had severe, persistent lumbar spine pain. She subsequently had removal of the intervertebral disc

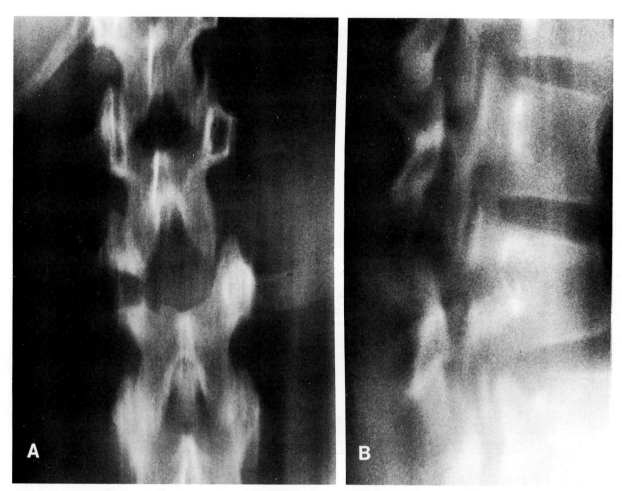

Fig. 5-50. Radiographs of flexion injury with slight axial rotation. (*A*) A laminogram clearly illustrates that significant abnormal separation of spinous processes occurs only with fracture and/or dislocation of the facet joint complex. On the left side there is a fracture and on the right side there is a dislocation. (*B*) A lateral laminogram shows that there is a fracture of the posterior portion of the vertebral body.

between L2 and L3 with good relief of pain. Recurrence of intolerable pain and neurogenic bladder symptoms developed, for which the final treatment was the construction of an ileal loop. The patient also had additional surgery on her back, which consisted of total laminectomy of L1–L3. Also, the facets at L2 and L3 were removed (Fig. 5-51A). During the year following her second spine operation, she developed progressive posterior dislocation of L2 on L3. This is shown in Figure 5-51B.

This patient's problems demonstrate two principles about clinical stability. The first and most important point relates to the fact that this patient's spine was compromised both anteriorly and posteriorly. The important function of the annulus fibrosus to resist translation was lost due to the disc excision. The laminectomies and facetectomies totally destroyed the posterior stabilizing elements. This resulted in a grossly unstable situation with subsequent subluxation. The other point demonstrated here involves the direction of the abnormal displacement. We suggest that the orientation of the intervertebral disc space is a determining factor in the direction of abnormal displacement. This orientation

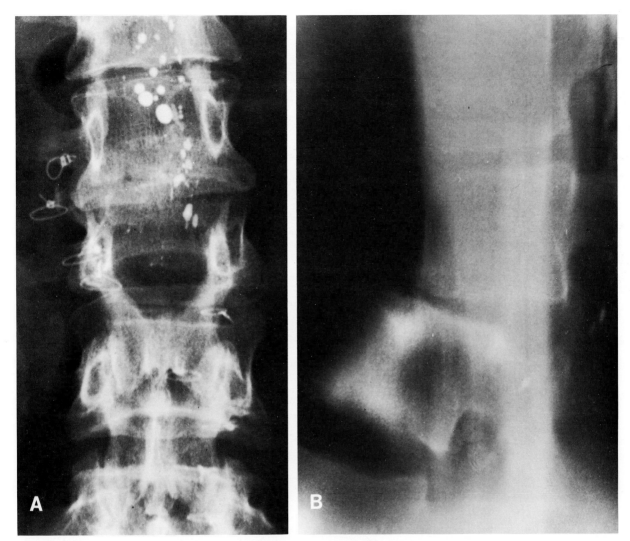

Fig. 5-51. Radiographs of a patient with clinical instability of the lumbar spine. (*A*) A wide laminectomy at L2, L3, and L4. (*B*) Abnormal posterior displacement of L2 on L3. In addition to surgery of the posterior elements, this patient also shows removal of the disc, which disrupted the stability anteriorly.

varies in different regions of the spine. In the upper lumbar region of the spine, the inclination of the L2–L3 disc space in the erect position is posterior in the sagittal plane (see Fig. 2-23). Thus, the gravitational loading tends to push the second lumbar vertebra posteriorly (-z-axis) as well as caudally (-y-axis).

When this patient is evaluated according to the checklist, we find the following. There are 2 points for abnormal displacement, 2 points for destruction of the anterior elements, and 3 points for ablation of the posterior elements. The total is seven and the spine is grossly unstable.

RECOMMENDED MANAGEMENT

Flow Chart

The flow diagram for management of these problems is shown in Figure 5-52. Patients are treated in bed if there is no neurologic deficit;

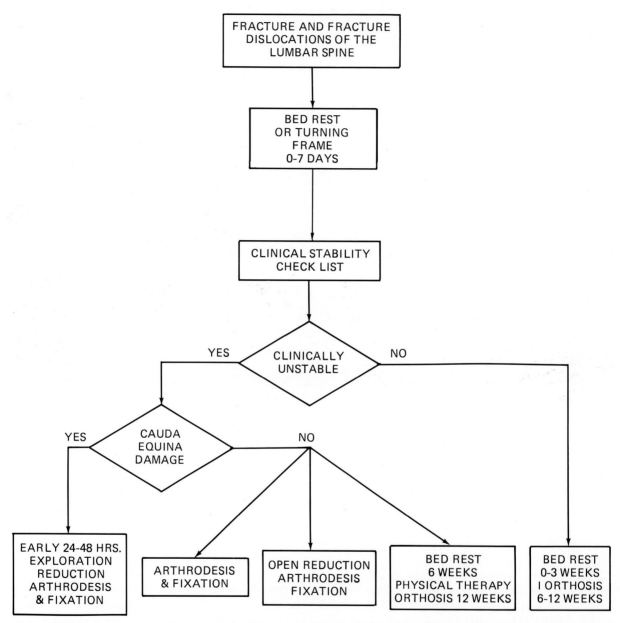

Fig. 5-52. A recommended flow diagram for the management of patients with disruptions of the lumbar spine. All treatment regimens include occupational and physical therapy, as tolerated, and follow-up schedule, page 235.

otherwise, they are treated on a turning frame. The patient is thoroughly evaluated clinically, and the necessary supportive and specific care is provided. Regular anteroposterior and lateral radiographs are taken. The clinical stability checklist is applied. In difficult judgements, anteroposterior and lateral laminograms are recommended for a detailed analysis of the status of the various anatomic elements.

Treatment of the Clinically Stable Condition

Patients that are found to be stable may be treated with bed rest until their symptoms allow initiation of gradual ambulation and exercises. Pain or fear of increasing deformity may lead the surgeon to prescribe an appropriate spinal orthosis. The schedule for follow-up of all the patients allows any progression of deformity to be recognized (see p. 235).

Treatment of the Clinically Unstable Condition

Conditions determined to be clinically unstable are separated into two groups, based on whether or not there is clinical evidence of cauda equina damage and evidence of a defect on a lumbar myelogram.

Cauda Equina Damage. If there is evidence of impingement upon the cauda equina or nerve roots, there should be early exploration, appropriate relief of the impingement, reduction, internal fixation, and arthrodesis. In view of the excellent recuperative potential of the cauda equina, we do not think that nonoperative treatment is justifiable in the presence of documented cauda equina impingement. Closed reduction of injuries in this group is not recommended, as there have been reports of additional neurologic damage with such attempts.[12,53,83,86] Laminectomy is generally a less effective means of decompression than open reduction. Kaufer and Hayes reported a situation in which laminectomy of four levels failed to relieve a block in a patient who subsequently recovered 1 week after open reduction and stabilization.[54]

No Cauda Equina Damage. If there is a diagnosis of clinical instability *without* neurologic deficit, the need for surgery is less urgent. The available objective evidence does not lead to the conclusion that all clinically unstable lumbar spines must be treated with surgery. We suggest that there are at least three currently justifiable alternatives. The first involves performing arthrodesis, with internal fixation as an elective procedure at a later time. This is done relatively early (7 to 21 days) or at a later time (several months to years) based on the patient's symptoms and the judgement of the surgeon. Both approaches seem justified by available objective information. Note that these two options do not include reduction of dislocations. The delayed approach to the fixation of these injuries is thought to be justified by the fact that the risk of initial neurologic damage is less in this region. This factor allows time for prolonged observation to determine whether or not pain will be a problem. In other words, the urgency for the establishment of early or immediate clinical stability is not as great in the lumbar spine as in other regions.

The second alternative is to include *open reduction* with internal fixation and fusion. This option should be exercised relatively early, at 7 to 14 days. In the opinion of some physicians, spondylolisthesis falls into this category. The necessity or desirability of reduction in spondylolisthesis is controversial. However, this can be surgically reduced months or years after its occurrence.

The nonsurgical alternative is justified in this group of clinically unstable lumbar spine injuries. Patients are treated with bed rest for 6 weeks, followed by gradual ambulation, physical therapy, and protected activity for another 6 to 12 weeks. A lumbar orthosis of intermediate control may be useful if symptoms of pain demand it. Even though this is contrary to the recommendation of Kaufer and Hayes, we believe it is a justifiable alternative for several reasons. First, their study is virtually the only one published, it includes a modest number of cases, and there is no controlled study that advocates surgery. Secondly, there is a generous portion of free space in the lumbar spine to accommodate the cauda equina without neural deficit. Thus, with adequate post-injury follow-up of the patient, surgical stabilization can always be done for pain, deformity, or neural irritation. The large powerful muscle mass lessens the risk of a sudden catastrophic displacement in the lumber spine. Moreover, the resistance to and the recuperative power from injury to the cauda equina is significantly greater than that of the thoracic or cervical spinal cord.

Part 5: The Sacrum

The clinical stability of the sacrum and pelvis poses a slightly different problem than in the previously described regions. The main concern here is the ability of these structures to perform their mechanical function after disruption from trauma, disease, or surgery.

ANATOMIC CONSIDERATIONS

The sacrum is stabilized in the pelvic ring by a somewhat unique, ear-shaped articulation, which is ingeniously reinforced by several structural characteristics. The joint is narrow and is provided with elevations and depressions. These characteristics limit motion and provide stability. It is fixed posteriorly and superiorly by a strong, stiff articular capsule. This capsule is further reinforced posteriorly and inferiorly by the sacroiliac ligaments, which are the strongest ligaments in the body.[84]

The major load bearing portion of the pelvic girdle has been described by the analogy of an arch with lateral pillars and a keystone (Fig. 5-53).[39] This construct is designed by nature for the support of very high loads. The vertical loads are resisted by the irregular surface of the joint and the wedge-shaped configuration of the sacrum. The separation of the pillars (the femora) is prevented mainly through the tension created by the tensile resistance of the large sacroiliac ligaments posteriorly and the interosseous ligament. The effectiveness of this coapting mechanism is due to the fact that it becomes increasingly stable with increasing loads.[H] There is a similar, secondary role played by the pubic symphysis anteriorly.

BIOMECHANICAL FACTORS

It is sometimes necessary that certain portions of the sacrum and ilium be removed to treat a tumor. Gunterberg carried out some tests on fresh autopsy specimens of the pelvis and sacrum to compare the load bearing capacity of the structures under different conditions. The available specimens were divided into three groups, with comparable age representation in each group. Group I was left intact. Group II and Group III were resected as described in Figure 5-54. Each specimen was loaded vertically at the top of the first sacral vertebra one to three times with a force up to twice the estimated normal physiologic load. The test specimen was then loaded to failure. As might be anticipated from the anatomic descriptions, these studies showed that the sacroiliac joint articulations remained intact. The failure occurred in the lateral parts of the sacrum, in both the resected and the unresected specimens. The data showed that with resection of the sacrum between S1 and S2, approximately 30 per cent of the ultimate load bearing capacity is lost, and with resection through S1, approximately 50 per cent is lost. The failure load was four to eight times the calculated upright standing load in the intact specimen, 1.5 to five times in the resection between S1 and S2, and about two times in the resection through S1. The investigators concluded that the residual strength of the

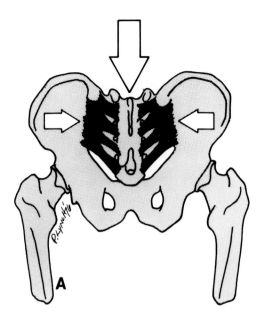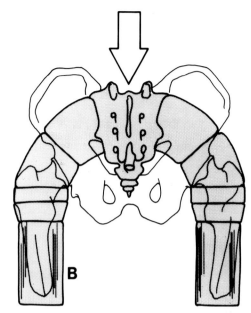

Fig. 5-53. (A) The posterior sacroiliac ligaments are oriented so as to provide additional stability to the sacroiliac articulations with increased loading. (B) The sacrum is analogous to the keystone of an arch by virtue of its shape and position.

pelvic ring is adequate following resection of the sacrum through S1, leaving some associated iliac bone to allow early ambulation with full weight bearing in the early postoperative period.[39]

CLINICAL CONSIDERATIONS AND MANAGEMENT

Instability in the sacral area may result from trauma, destruction by tumor, infection, and surgical resection or debridement. The question of management involves essentially bed rest versus ambulation. Evaluation of the ligamentous structures is difficult; moreover, there will almost never be instability within this region purely as a result of ligamentous failure. Fracture is really the only source of instability here. Thus, the main evaluation is with radiographic examination. The basic guideline is the previously described biomechanical study. This study suggests that as

long as the destruction leaves intact a fair portion of the first sacral body and its corresponding lateral structures and articulations, the patient may gradually ambulate. There is evidence that additional load bearing capacity may develop through biomechanical adaptation. Fractures or dislocations and other disruptions of the architecture of the pelvic ring anterior to the hip joint may be associated with severe pain, but they are rarely unstable with regard to ambulation.

SOME THEORETICAL CONSIDERATIONS ON THE BIOMECHANICS OF INSTABILITY

The basic mechanical phenomenon in instability is the abnormal displacement of portions of the spine under physiologic loads. The displacement may take the form of translation, rotation, or some combination of the two. Similarly, the

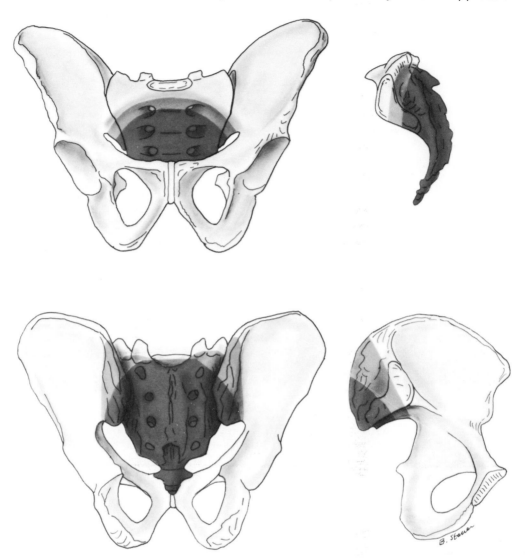

Fig. 5-54. Resections of two portions of the sacroiliac joints in an experimental study of the load bearing capacity of the partially resected sacrum. Resection A: resection between the bodies of S1 and S2. In addition, about one-third of the sacroiliac joint and corresponding ligaments were removed on both sides. This resection is indicated by the dark shading. Resection B: resection through the first body of S1. In addition, about one-half of the sacroiliac joint and corresponding ligaments on both sides were removed. This resection includes the dark-shaded structures plus the light-shaded structures. (Gunterberg, B., Romanus, B., and Hener, B.: Pelvic strength after major amputation of the sacrum: an experimental study. Acta Orthop. Scand., 47:635, 1977.)

physiologic load may be a force, a moment, or some combination of the two. In reality, the displacements and loads are combinations of these. However, for the purpose of analysis they may be thought of as separate entities.

Displacement

Translatory Displacement.   Study a motion segment. The lower vertebra is fixed. Physiologic loads are applied to the upper vertebra and displacement is measured. If the spine motion segment is biomechanically unstable, then the upper vertebra translates more than the corresponding vertebra of a stable motion segment subjected to the same physiologic force. This is depicted in Figure 5-55A. An example of translatory instability is anterior displacement of C5 on C6 after a bilateral facet fracture dislocation. An anteriorly directed physiologic force would be expected to produce greater anterior translation of C5 in the unstable spine than it would in a corresponding stable spine.

Rotatory Displacement. The situation is analogous for rotatory displacements. Here an unstable spine will show greater rotatory motion than a stable spine when the two are subjected to the same physiologic moments. This concept is depicted in Figure 5-55B. A suitable example of rotatory instability is a spine with unilateral facet fracture dislocation and partial rupture of the disc. When this spine is subjected to an axial torque, the upper vertebra may be expected to rotate about an axis near the intact facet joint.

Ligaments and Stability

For a basic understanding of the stability of the spine it is helpful to visualize the roles played by different ligaments. The intrinsic translatory and rotatory stability of the spine is provided by

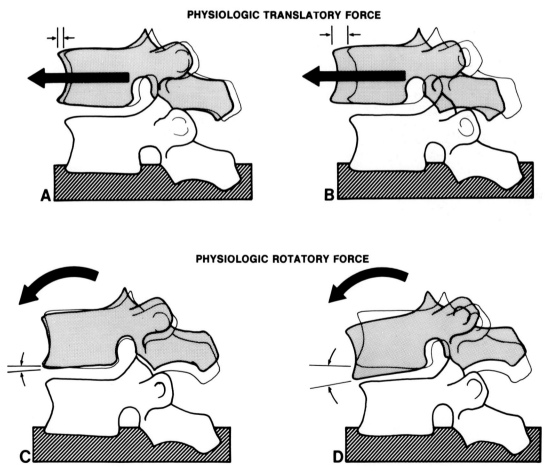

PHYSIOLOGIC TRANSLATORY FORCE

PHYSIOLOGIC ROTATORY FORCE

Fig. 5-55. (*A*) A stable spine motion segment which translates very little when subjected to an anteriorly directed force. (*B*) An unstable motion segment, which characteristically translates more under the same load. (*C, D*) Here the motion segments are being subjected to a physiologic bending moment. A greater angulation occurs in an unstable spine (*D*) as compared to a stable spine (*C*).

the ligaments. Contribution of a given ligament depends not only upon its particular strength, but also its location. Moreover, a given ligament may contribute relatively more to either translatory or rotatory stability, depending upon the loading circumstances. For example, the interspinous ligaments may contribute significantly toward the rotary stability in flexion ($+\theta x$) but little toward translatory stability in the anteroposterior direction.

Assuming that all ligaments are made of the same material, the strength of a ligament will be proportional to its corss-sectional area. A ligament with a larger cross-sectional area will provide greater stability and less displacement when the motion segment is subjected to physiologic loads. An example of this is the annulus fibrosus, which has much greater area as compared to the inter-

spinous ligament and therefore provides much greater stability.

Another factor that contributes to stability is the distance of a ligament from the center of rotation. An analysis of a single ligament may be done with the help of a simple mechanical model of a motion segment. The concept is depicted in Figure 5-56. The model, consisting of a block (upper vertebra) and a spring (the ligament under analysis), is shown in Figure 5-56A. The ligament in Figure 5-56B is closer to the center of rotation than is that of Figure 5-56C. As the moment M is applied to the two constructs, the resistance to motion is provided by the forces in the ligaments multiplied by their corresponding lever arms, L_1 and L_2, respectively. As L_2 is the larger of the two, the design of Figure 5-56C provides greater rotatory stability than does that shown in Figure

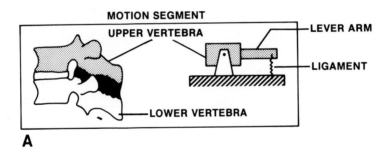

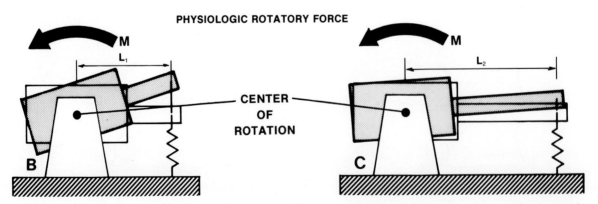

Fig. 5-56. The location of a ligament with respect to the center of rotation determines its contribution to the stability of the spine. (*A*) A model of a motion segment and a single ligament. The lower vertebra is represented by the white trapezoid. (*B*) The ligament that is located nearer to the center of rotation provides much less stability against bending than (*C*) a ligament that is further away from the rotation center.

5-56B. The example mentioned earlier may again be used to illustrate this point. The centers of rotation for flexion are in the posterior region of the vertebral body. This gives a greater lever arm for the interspinous ligaments as compared to the annulus fibrosus. Therefore, the contribution toward the rotatory stability due to the *location only* would be greater for the interspinous ligament. But, of course, the strength of the annulus outweighs this advantage many times over.

In discussing the stability of the spine and the various factors that contribute to it, the real situation has been considerably simplified for the sake of analysis. However, this helps one to make certain judgments about the stability of the injured spine in an objective manner. The analysis requires two types of information, the extent of structural damage to the spine and the physiologic loads. The former consists of identifying the ligaments that are nonfunctional, their cross-sectional areas, and their locations. The latter depends upon the anticipated physical activities of the patient. This type of analysis, together with the relevant clinical information, permits assessment of the clinical stability of a given spine.

Displacement and Cord Encroachment

What is the relationship between the displacement and the actual decrease in the vertebral canal space at the level of the displacement? It is important to determine the degree of this decrease because it is closely related to the potential for cord damage.

The unstable motion segment is represented by two identical rectangular blocks (vertebrae) with circular holes (spinal canal). The canal space is maximum with perfect vertebral alignment. Any relative displacement of the blocks results in a decrease in the space available for the spinal cord.

Figure 5-57A shows the situation in which, for a given angular displacement, there is the least possible decrease in canal space. This occurs when the center of rotation coincides with the center of the cord. In Figure 5-57B, a greater encroachment of the space is observed, although the same amount of rotatory displacement is present. This is due to the fact that the center of rotation is located away from the canal. An example is a fracture dislocation in which one of the facet joints is destroyed along with enough liga-

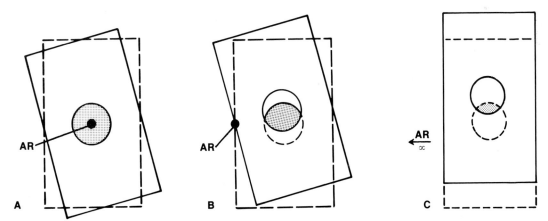

Fig. 5-57. Spinal cord encroachment is not only a function of how much angulation is produced when the spine is subjected to an axial moment. It is also dependent upon the location of the center of rotation in the horizontal (axial plane). This concept is exemplified here by a pair of blocks (vertebrae) with holes (canal space). (*A*) Minimum encroachment. One block is rotated with respect to the other around the center of the holes. For the circular hole (canal space), there is no decrease in the available canal space. (*B*) Intermediate encroachment. If the axis of rotation is shifted to the side, then for the same angulation, the available canal space is markedly decreased. (*C*) Maximum encroachment. Here the axis of rotation has been shifted far to the side (at infinity), producing near translatory displacement.

ments to allow rotation to take place about the relatively intact facet joint. Finally, there is the case in which the decrease in space around the cord is maximal (Fig. 5-57C). This occurs in association with a pure translation. An example is a fracture dislocation of both the facet joints, allowing a large translatory displacement in the anteroposterior direction. In such a situation, the displacement of the upper vertebral canal is equal to the displacement of the vertebral body translation. The three situations are well exemplified by the various types of dislocations and fracture dislocations at the level of C1–C2 (see Figs. 5-19, 5-16, and 5-12, respectively).

CONCLUSION

Our basic approach has been to take what is known of anatomy, biomechanics, and documented clinical experience and to analyze it in a manner that is clinically useful. A major anatomic consideration is the clinical significance of regional variations of several structural characteristics. Examples include the anterior longitudinal ligament, the yellow ligament, and the spatial orientation of the facet articulations and the disc in the standing posture. The relative size of the neural elements and the space in which they are enclosed is a cogent consideration. Regional variations also exist in mechanical properties such as kinematics, stiffness, and physiologic loads. We have emphasized the importance of a proper interpretation of the significance or neurologic deficit in the determination of clinical stability. Generally when a deficit is associated with significant structural damage, clinical instability should be suspected. The importance of standardization of radiographic techniques for more precise interpretation cannot be overemphasized.

The bony architecture and the ligamentous elements comprise the structural components of the spine. With all components intact the biomechanical function is normal. When sufficient anatomic disruption causes or threatens to produce an inability to function normally, we recommend that the spine be considered clinically unstable.

The goal of good patient management is to gain maximal recovery as rapidly as possible and avoid unneccessary treatment (surgical or nonsurgical) and at the same time prevent the unhappy tragedy of initial or subsequent neurologic damage. There is *no* convincing evidence that a diagnosis of clinical instability demands that the treatment should be surgical reduction, fusion, or fixation. However, the management of a patient with such a diagnosis should definitely differ from that of clinically stable patients.

The role of laminectomy in the management of spine trauma should be diminished and is indicated in only a few special situations. The indications for decompression need considerable elucidation.

Checklists, flow charts, and follow-up schedules have been presented to conveniently organize and summarize the information, to stimulate others to criticize and improve upon them, and to provide clinical protocols for systematic evaluation, management, and study. The concluding principle is that it is only through clear prospective clinical protocols that we can ever really improve our knowledge and base our decisions more on solid scientific evidence and less on well meaning speculation.

Without theory, practice is but a routine bore of habit. Theory alone can bring forth and develop the spirit of invention.

Pasteur

CLINICAL BIOMECHANICS

Standardization of radiographic techniques are important and specifications should be known when interpreting the significance of measurements.

The normal spinal cord has an ample range of elasticity when deformed in the axial direction. However, it is more prone to damage if displaced in the horizontal plane. Therefore, axial separation between vertebrae is safer than flexion/extension.

Occipital-Atlanto-Axial Complex

Dislocations at the ocp-C1 level are usually fatal and rarely present as a clinical problem of instability. Any patient who happens to survive is clinically unstable and should be fused, occiput to C2.

With transection of the tectorial membrane and the alar ligaments, there is an increased flexion of the units of the ocp-C1-C2 complex and a subluxation of the occipit.

The articular capsules between C1 and C2 are designed loosely, such that they allow a large amount of rotation and provide a small amount of stability.

The major stability is provided by the dens and the transverse ligament. The latter is the most important structure in preventing anterior translation.

The apical and alar ligaments may be expected to contribute little to ocp-C1 stability and almost nothing to C1-C2 stability.

Although the C1-C2 complex is clinically unstable after failure of the transverse ligament, the tectorial membrane, the alar and the apical ligaments probably provide some resistance against gross dislocation.

With 7 mm total lateral overhang following bursting fracture of the ring of C1 (Jefferson fracture), the transverse ligament is torn and the situation is clinically unstable.

The Lower Cervical Spine

The annulus fibrosus is the crucial stabilizing structure.

Clinical stability is lost or in danger when either all the anterior elements or all the posterior elements are destroyed or unable to function.

Although there are exceptions, there is a rough correlation between magnitude of structural damage of the spine and extent of neurologic deficit.

Although there are exceptions, the evidence suggests that when there are spinal cord or root symptoms or signs associated with spine trauma, a clinically unstable situation is to be suspected.

Unilateral facet dislocations when associated with fracture and/or neurologic deficits are probably unstable. Those that have no neurologic signs, symptoms, or fractures and are difficult to reduce are probably stable.

Bilateral facet dislocations and fracture dislocations are unstable. Abnormal anterior posterior displacements occur with relative ease following facet fractures.

The major factor in determining the overall prognosis for recovery from neurological deficit is the nature and magnitude of the initial trauma to the neurologic structures.

Based on the available knowledge and current biomechanical analysis, a checklist for diagnosis and a flow diagram for management of clinical instability has been provided.

Controlled, monitored axial traction, (the "stretch test") may be helpful in the evaluation of the integrity of the ligamentous structures of the lower cervical spine.

Patients with anterior elements destroyed are more clinically unstable in extension, while patients with posterior elements destroyed are more unstable in flexion.

Given the diagnosis of clinical instability, the patient may be adequately treated by surgical fusion, a halo apparatus with body attachment, or prolonged traction. There is no convincing evidence in the literature that any particular method is superior.

We usually employ surgical fusion because it has been successful in our experience.

The Thoracic and Thoracolumbar Spine

The thoracic spine is mechanically stiffer and less mobile than the other regions of the spine.

Thoracic spine stiffness, which is due to intrinsic qualities as well as the rib cage and its manner of articulations to the vertebrae, provides considerable stability.

As a result of normal kyphosis, the thoracic spine is more likely to be clinically unstable in flexion.

The anterior and posterior longitudinal ligaments, as well as the yellow ligaments, are well developed structures in the thoracic spine.

The ligaments of the facet joints are not well developed and offer little support following laminectomy.

Because of the anatomy and geometry of the

lower thoracic and thoracolumbar spine, radiographic evidence of local malalignment of the spinous processes in axial rotation is suggestive of dislocation or fracture dislocation of the facet articulations.

Removal or loss of function of the posterior elements of the thoracic spine allows for significantly more motion in flexion, extension, and axial rotation. Removal of posterior elements tends to make the spine unstable in flexion.

Removal or loss of function of the anterior elements tends to make the thoracic spine unstable in extension.

Extensive patient management experience and biomechanical evaluation both suggest that the rotational (axial rotation) fracture dislocation is one of the most clinically unstable injuries recognized.

Bursting fractures are likely to go onto spontaneous arthrodesis.

Although it is not always clear cut, it is more commonly the case that extensive structural damage tends to be correlated with neurologic damage.

The isolated vertebral body fracture is least likely to be associated with neurologic damage, and the fracture dislocation with body and posterior element damage is most likely to be associated with neurologic damage.

Most traumatic kyphotic deformities do not progress significantly. However, there are certain biomechanical considerations that indicate a likelihood of progression.

Paraplegics with 10 degrees or more of frontal plane angulation in the thoracic or thoracolumbar spine may be more prone to ischial ulcers from sitting.

There is no correlation between severity of stable compression fracture deformity and ultimate clinical outcome.

The theoretical probability of progression of deformity depends upon the continuity of the posterior elements, the sagittal plane angulation, the amount of wedging of the vertebral body, and the presence or absence of aseptic necrosis.

Laminectomy in the thoracic and thoracolumbar spine should be vigorously discouraged because it is of considerable detriment to the biomechanical functions of this region of the spine and offers little therapeutic value.

Anterior decompression is more rational biomechanically and shows promising results. However, the indications and benefits of this procedure need careful scrutiny to thoroughly determine its value.

The Milwaukee brace, designed to treat kyphosis, is thought to be the best orthosis for fixation of this region of the spine.

The Lumbar and Sacral Spine

Facet dislocations are suggestive of clinical instability and are associated with a variety of other bony and ligamentous injuries, including some of the anterior elements.

The supraspinous and interspinous ligaments in the adult lumbar spine are frequently absent, ruptured, or degenerated and can contribute nothing to stability.

The presence of neurologic deficit post-trauma is *strongly* suggestive of clinical instability.

Laminectomy to treat trauma in these regions is not usually helpful and should be discouraged.

Two key radiographic observations are abnormal rotatory alignment and abnormal separation of the spinous processes. Either or both of these alerts the observer to the possibility of clinical instability.

On physical exam, an obvious, palpable, subcutaneous hematoma between two abnormally separated spinous processes suggests a clinically unstable lumbar spine until proven otherwise.

Clinical and biomechanical evidence suggests that resection of a sizable portion of the first sacral body and its corresponding lateral structures and articulations, the patient may gradually begin to walk with clinical stability.

NOTES

[A] For exceptionally large patients, alternate values for the spine-to-film distance may be necessary. For these cases we suggest the alternate distance of 0.41 m (16 in), which will give a magnification of 29 per cent.

B The first verified case of C1–C2 dislocation due to rupture of the transverse ligament was described by Bell in 1830.[10] The patient had a syphilitic ulceration of the pharynx. The postmortem examination showed rupture of the transverse ligament and compression of the spinal cord as the cause of death.

C The management of bilateral anterior displacement in rheumatoid arthritis is controversial. We do not recommend surgery for the neurologically intact patients who have tolerable pain.

D A.L., a 39-year-old black male, fell down 9 steps striking the back of his head. On examination he complained of a stiffness of the neck but had no neurologic deficit. Plane, lateral radiographs of the neck revealed an anterior step-off of C4 on C5 of 2 mm which increased to over 4 mm with flexion (Fig. 5-27). Observation over the course of the next 3 weeks clearly indicated that this spine was unstable as progressive anterior subluxation and widening of the interspinous space at C4–5 occurred. Posterior interspinous fusion was required for stabilization. This patient demonstrates the fact that a spine can be unstable without immediately causing neurologic deficit. The presence of 4 mm horizontal displacement with flexion indicated the instability. Under these physiologic conditions, a spine that permits such displacement does not have an adequate margin of safety.

E J.S., a 20-year-old Caucasian man, sustained a traumatic paraplegia with loss of spinal cord function at C7 and below. Plane, lateral radiographs revealed angulation of C5 on C6, 20 degrees greater than the angulation of adjacent vertebrae (Fig. 5-28). Although this spine was clearly unstable, this patient was initially treated with only posterior decompressive laminectomy. Because of subsequent progression of the kyphosis at C5–6, he required a posterolateral facet fusion to correct the instability and prevent progression of the flexion deformity. Angulation is measured as shown in Figure 5-28 at the interspace(s) under evaluation for ligament disruption.

F Angulation is measured as shown in Figure 5-28 at the interspace(s) under evaluation for ligament disruption.

G The original anterior vertebral height is estimated by determining the average height of the anterior portion of vertebra above or below.

H The exceptional stability of the sacroiliac joints is due to two separate aspects of the anatomy, ligamentous and bony. The sacroiliac ligaments run, from ilium to sacrum, directed medially and caudally. The weight borne by the sacrum produces tension in these ligaments. The tension may be divided into its vertical and horizontal components. The vertical components support the downward weight. The horizontal components pull the sacrum equally in the left and right lateral directions, thus stabilizing it. A bending moment attempting to tilt the sacrum in the frontal plane will be effectively resisted by these stabilizing forces in the sacroiliac ligaments. The action of the ligaments is much like those of the oblique ropes tied to a flagpost for its stabilization. Seen from the bony aspects, the sacrum has two joint surfaces with the ilium. Although the surfaces are irregular, the main planes of the surfaces are slightly inclined to the sagittal plane, forming a wedge into the two iliac bones. Downward weight acting on the sacrum produces forces in the sacroiliac joint. These forces have two components, one along (frictional) and one perpendicular (normal) to the joint surfaces. Because of the small wedge angle, the frictional component is large. It is these large frictional forces that provide the bony stability to the sacrum. The wedging action of the sacrum is similar to the keystone in an archway.

CLASSIFICATION OF REFERENCES

Occipital-atlanto-axial complex
  Anatomy 33, 42, 43, 51, 94, 91a, 103
  Biomechanics 34, 94
  Clinical 10, 29, 31, 32, 34, 35, 44, 49, 70, 83, 85, 91a, 94
The Lower Cervical Spine
  Anatomy 33, 41, 43, 51, 52, 103
  Biomechanics 38, 63, 68, 69, 98, 99, 100, 101
  Clinical 3, 4, 5, 7, 8, 11, 14, 15, 16, 18, 19, 21, 22, 23, 24, 26, 27, 28, 30, 32, 36, 40, 46, 48, 50, 55, 56, 59, 62, 66, 67, 71, 72, 73, 75, 79, 81, 82, 89, 90, 91, 92, 93, 100
Thoracic and thoracolumbar spine
  Biomechanics 2, 17, 41a, 77, 97, 98a
  Clinical 9, 11, 12, 13, 20, 21, 23, 25, 37, 40, 41a, 45, 53, 57, 58, 60, 65, 75, 78, 80, 86, 88, 96, 98a, 102, 104
The Lumbar Spine
  Biomechanics 6, 17, 61, 64, 87
  Clinical 40, 45, 54, 57, 80, 104
Sacrum 39, 84

REFERENCES

1. American Journal of Roentgenology, Radium Therapy and Nuclear Medicine, Vol. *127*. (*This entire volume is devoted to computerized tomography and most of its uses. It is an excellent reference for introduction to various uses of the technique.*)

2. Andriacchi, T. P., Schultz, A. B., Belytscko, T. B., and Galante, J. O.: A model for studies of mechanical interactions between the human spine and rib cage. J. Biomech., *7*:497, 1974.

3. Bailey, R. W.: Observations of cervical intervertebral disc lesions in fractures and dislocations. J. Bone Joint Surg., *45A*:461, 1963. (*A very good presentation of some of the logical and practical aspects of this topic.*)

4. ———: Fractures and dislocations of the cervical spine: orthopedic and neurosurgical aspects. Postgrad. Med., *35*:588, 1964.

5. Barnes, R.: Paraplegia in cervical spine injuries. J. Bone Joint Surg., *30B*:234, 1948.

6. Bartelink, D. L.: The role of abdominal pressure in relieving the pressure of the lumbar intervertebral discs. J. Bone Joint Surg., *39B*:718, 1957.

7. Beatson, T. R.: Fractures and dislocations of the cervical spine. J. Bone Joint Surg., *45B*:21, 1963.

8. Bedbrook, G. M.: Are cervical spine fractures ever unstable? J. West Pac. Orthop. Assoc., *6*:7, 1969.

9. Bedbrook, G. M., and Edibaum, R. C.: The study of spinal deformity in traumatic spinal paralysis. Paraplegia, *10*:321, 1973.

10. Bell, C.: Physiologische und Pathologische Untersuchungen des Nervensystems, Berlin 1936. Translated by M. H. Romberg, M.D. Original title: The Nervous System of the Human Body. London, Longmans, Green & Co., 1830.

11. Benassy, J., Blanchard, J., and Lecog, P.: Neurological recovery rate in para- and tetraplegia. Paraplegia, *4*:259, 1967.

11a. Benner, J. H.: Thoracolumbar fractures and fracture dislocations treated by Harrington distraction rods and nonoperative methods. Paper No. 17. 45th Annual Meeting of the American Academy of Orthopaedic Surgeons, Dallas, February, 1978.

12. Böhler, L.: The Treatment of Fractures. ed. 5. New York, Grune and Stratton, 1956.

13. Böhler, L.: Operative treatment of the thoracic and thoraco-lumbar spine. J. Trauma, *10*:1119, 1970. (*A brief exposé of the author's beliefs concerning the indications for open reduction and anterior anthrodesis.*)

14. Braakman, R., and Penning, L.: Mechanisms of injury to the cervical cord. Int. J. Paraplegia, *10*:314, 1973.

15. Braakman, R., and Vinken, P. F.: Unilateral facet interlocking in the lower cervical spine. J. Bone Joint Surg., *40B*:249, 1967. (*The best paper on facet dislocations; a good, sound, insightful approach.*)

16. Brav, E. A., Miller, J. A., and Bouzard, W. C.: Traumatic dislocation of the cervical spine: army experience and results. J. Trauma, *3*:569, 1963. (*One of the few studies that evaluates and compares several management programs.*)

17. Breig, A.: Biomechanics of the Central Nervous system: Some Basic Normal and Pathological Phenomena. Stockholm, Almquist & Wiksell, 1960. (*An important, thorough, and very well illustrated presentation of the biomechanical anatomy of the spinal cord.*)

18. Brookes, T. P.: Dislocations of the cervical spine: their complications and treatment. Surg. Gynecol. Obstet., *57*:772, 1933.

19. Burke, D. C., and Berryman, D.: The place of closed manipulation in the management of flexion-rotation dislocations of the cervical spine. J. Bone Joint Surg., *53B*:165, 1971. (*Recommended for basic knowledge of cervical spine manipulation for reduction.*)

20. Burke, D. C., and Murry, D. D.: The management of thoracic and thoraco-lumbar injuries of the spine with neurological involvement. J. Bone Joint Surg., *58B*:72, 1976. (*A very good study which allows for some comparison of the two treatment methods.*)

21. Carey, P. C.: Neurosurgery and paraplegia. Rehabilitation, *52*:27, 1965.

22. Castellano, V., and Bocconi, F. L.: Injuries of the cervical spine with spinal cord involvement (myelic fractures): statistical considerations. Bull. Hosp. Joint Dis., *31*: 188, 1970.

23. Cattell, H. S., and Clark, G. L.: Cervical kyphosis and instability following multiple laminectomies in children. J. Bone Joint Surg., *49A*:713, 1967.

24. Cattell, H. S., and Filtzer, D. L.: Pseudo-subluxation and other normal variations of the cervical spine in children. J. Bone Joint Surg., *47A*:1295, 1965. (*This work augments the physician's ability to make crucial judgments about post-traumatic cervical spine radiographs in children. It is highly recommended reading.*)

25. Chahal, A. S.: Results of continuous lumbar traction in acute dorso-lumbar spinal injuries with paraplegia. Paraplegia, *13*:1, 1975.

26. Cheshire, D. J. E.: The stability of the cervical spine following the conservative treatment of fractures and fracture dislocations. Paraplegia, *7*:193, 1969.

26a. Convery, F. R., et al.: Fracture-dislocation of the dorsal-lumbar spine; Acute operative stabilization. Paper No. 16. 45th Annual Meeting of the American Academy of Orthopaedic Surgeons, Dallas, February, 1978.

27. Dall, D. M.: Injuries of the cervical spine: I. Does the type of bony injury affect spinal cord recovery? S. Afr. Med. J., *46*:1048, 1972. (*An important study of cord damage in trauma.*)

28. ———: Injuries of the cervical spine: II. Does anatomical reduction of the bony injuries improve the prognosis for spinal cord recovery? S. Afr. Med. J., *46*:1083, 1972. (*Recommended reading which thoroughly documents the outcome in a large number of patients treated nonsurgically.*)

29. Dankmeijer, J., and Rethmeier, B. J.: The lateral movement in the atlanto-axial joints and its clinical significance. Acta Radiol., *24*:55, 1943.

30. Durbin, F. C.: Fracture dislocations of the cervical spine. J. Bone Joint Surg., *39B*:23, 1957.

31. Evarts, M. C.: Traumatic occipito-atantol dislocation. Report of a case with survival. J. Bone Joint Surg., *52A*:1653, 1970.

32. Fielding, J. W.: Cineroentogenography of the normal cervical spine. J. Bone Joint Surg., *39A*:1280, 1957.

33. Fielding, J. W., Burstein, A. A., and Frankel, V. H.: The nuchal ligament. Spine, *1*:3, 1976. (*The best, the most useful, and well documented presentation of the anatomy of this ligament in the human spine.*)

34. Fielding, J. W., Cochran, G. V. B., Lansing, J. F., and Hohl, M.: Tears of the transverse ligament of the atlas, A clinical biomechanical study. J. Bone Joint Surg., *56A*:1683, 1974.

35. Fielding, J. W., and Hawkins, R. J.: Atlanto-axial rotary fixation. J. Bone Joint Surg., *59A*:37, 1977.

36. Forsythe, H. F., Alexander, E., David, C., and Underal, R.: The advantages of early spine fusion in the treatment of fracture dislocations of the cervical spine. J. Bone Joint Surg., *41A*:17, 1959.

37. Frankel, H. E., et al.: The value of postural reduction in the initial management of closed injuries of the spine with paraplegia and tetraplegia. Int. J. Paraplegia, *7*: 179, 1969. (*The eight authors of this work are all students and co-workers of Guttman. The article, which reports on 612 injuries, is written to commemorate Sir Ludwig's seventieth birthday and seeks to justify his method of treatment.*)

38. Gosch, H. H., Gooding, E., and Schneider, R. C.: An experimental study of cervical spine and cord injuries. J. Trauma, *12*:570, 1972.

39. Gunterberg, B.: Effects of major resection of the sacrum, clinical studies on urogenital and anorectal function and a biomechanical study on pelvic strength [thesis]. Uno Lundgren Tryckeri, A. B., Göteborg, 1975. (*This should be number one on the reading list of those who do surgery on the sacrum.*)

40. Guttman, L.: Management of spinal fractures. *In* Spinal Cord Injuries: Comprehensive Management and Research. Oxford, Blackwell Scientific Publications, 1973.

41. Halliday, D. R., Sullivan, C. R., Hollinshead, W. H., and Bahn, R. C.: Torn cervical ligaments: necropsy examination of normal cervical region. J. Trauma, *4*:219, 1964.

41a. Hausfeld, J. N.: A biomechanical analysis of clinical stability in the thoracic and thoracolumbar spine [thesis]. Yale University School of Medicine, New Haven, 1977.

42. Hecker, P.: Appareil ligamenteux occipito-atloido-axoidien: étude d'anatomie comparée. Arch. D'Anat., D'Hist, et D'Embryol., 1923.

43. Hinck, V. C., Hopkins, C. E., and Savara, B.: Sagittal diameter of the cervical spinal canal in children. Radiology, 79:97, 1962. (*A well done study and a very useful reference.*)

44. Hohl, M., and Baker, H. R.: The atlanto-axial joint. J. Bone Joint Surg., 46A:1739, 1964. (*An informative presentation of this topic.*)

45. Holdsworth, F. W.: Fractures, dislocations and fracture dislocations of the spine. J. Bone Joint Surg., 45B:6, 1963. (*A classical article so frequently referred to that it could be considered required reading for anyone interested in the question of clinical stability of the spine.*)

46. Hørlyck, E., and Rahbek, M.: Cervical spine injuries. Acta Orthrop. Scand., 45:845, 1974.

47. Hounsfield, G. N.: Computerized transverse and scanning (tomography): Part I Description of system. Br. J. Radiol., 46:1016, 1973. (*This article presents a description of the technique.*)

48. Iizuka, I. K.: Correlation of neurologic and roentgenologic findings in fracture dislocation of cervical vertebrae. Vopr. Neirokhir., 36:46, 1972.

49. Isdale, I. C., and Corrigan, A. B.: Backward luxation of the atlas. Two cases of an uncommon condition. Ann. Rheum. Dis., 29:6, 1970.

49a. Jacobs, R. R., Snider, R. K., and Asher, M. A.: Dorsolumbar spinal fractures: recurrent versus operative treatment. Paper No. 18. 45th Annual Meeting of the American Academy of Orthopaedic Surgeons, Dallas, February, 1978.

50. Jenkins, D. H. R.: Extensive cervical laminectomy, long-term results. Br. J. Surg., 60:852, 1973.

51. Jirout, J.: The dynamic dependence of the lower cervical vertebrae on the atlanto-occipital joints. Neuroradiology, 7:249, 1974.

52. Johnson, R. M., Crelin, E. S., White, A. A., and Panjabi, M. M.: Some new observations on the functional anatomy of the lower cervical spine. Clin. Orthop., 111:192, 1975. (*Review of some important aspects of the surgical and biomechanical anatomy.*)

53. Kallio, E.: Injuries of the thoraco-lumbar spine with paraplegia. Acta Orthop. Scand., 60 [Suppl.], 1963.

54. Kaufer, H., and Hayes, J. T.: Lumbar fracture-dislocation. A study of twenty-one cases. J. Bone Joint Surg., 48A:712, 1966. (*A lonesome article which thoroughly and informatively documents some important clinical characteristics of these injuries.*)

55. Keim, H. A.: Spinal stabilization following trauma. Clin. Orthop., 81:53, 1971.

56. Lauritzen, J.: Diagnostic difficulties in lower cervical spine dislocations. Acta Orthop. Scand., 39:439, 1968.

57. Leidholdt, J. D., et al.: Evaluation of late spinal deformities with fracture dislocations of the dorsal and lumbar spine in paraplegias. Paraplegia, 7:16, 1969.

58. Lewis, J., and McKibbin, B.: The treatment of unstable fracture-dislocations of the thoraco-lumbar spine accompanied by paraplegia. J. Bone Joint Surg., 56B:603, 1974.

59. Marar, B. C.: Hyperextension injuries of the cervical spine: The pathogenesis of damage to the spinal cord. J. Bone Joint Surg., 56A:1655, 1974.

60. Morgan, T. H., Wharton, G. W., and Austin, G. N.: The results of laminectomy in patients with incomplete spinal cord injuries. Paraplegia, 9:14, 1971.

61. Morris, J. M., Lucas, D. B., and Bresler, B.: The role of the trunk in stability of the spine. J. Bone Joint Surg., 42A:327, 1961.

62. Munro, D.: Treatment of fractures and dislocations of the cervical spine complicated by cervical cord and root injuries: a comparative study of fusion vs. nonfusion therapy. N. Engl. J. Med., 264:573, 1961.

63. ———: The factors that govern the stability of the spine. Paraplegia, 3:219, 1965.

64. Nachemson, A.: Electromyographic studies on the vertebral portion of the psoas muscle, with special reference to the stabilizing function of the lumbar spine. Acta Orthop. Scand., 37:177, 1966.

65. Nicoll, E. A.: Fractures of the dorso-lumbar spine. J. Bone Joint Surg., 31B:376, 1949.

66. Nieminen, R., and Koskinen, V. S.: Posterior fusion in cervical spine injuries: an analysis of fifty cases treated surgically. Ann. Chir. Gynaecol. Fenn., 62:36, 1973.

67. Norrell, H., and Wilson, C. B.: Early anterior fusion for injuries of the cervical portion of the spine. J.A.M.A., 214:525, 1970.

68. Panjabi, M. M., White, A. A., and Johnson, R. M.: Cervical spine mechanics as a function of transection of components. J. Biomech., 8:327, 1975.

69. Panjabi, M. M., White, A. A., Keller, D., Southwick, W. O., and Friedlaender, G.: Clinical biomechanics of the cervical spine. 75-WA/B10-7 Am. Soc. Mech. Eng., New York, 1975. (*Experimental basis for presumptions about the usefulness of the stretch test.*)

70. Paul, L. W., and Moir, W. W.: Nonpathologic variations in relationship of the upper cervical vertebrae. Am. J. Roentgenol., 62:519, 1949.

71. Penning, L.: Nonpathologic and pathologic relationships between the lower cervical vertebrae. American Journal of Roentgenology, Radium Therapy and Nuclear Medicine, 91:1036, 1964. (*An excellent article with which to gain accuracy and sophistication in reading cervical spine radiographs.*)

72. Perry, J., and Nickel, V. L.: Total cervical spine fusion for neck paralysis. J. Bone Joint Surg., 41A:37, 1957.

73. Petrie, G. J.: Flexion injuries of the cervical spine. J. Bone Joint Surg., 46A:1800, 1964.

74. Plaue, R.: Die mechanik des wirbel kompressionsbruchs [The Mechanics of Compression Fractures of the Spine]. Zentralbl. Chir., 98:761, 1973.

75. Riggins, R. S., and Kraus, J. F.: The risk of neurological damage with fractures of the vertebrae. J. Trauma, 17:126, 1977. (*A well done, well presented, and informative epidemiological study.*)

76. Rissanen, P.: The surgical anatomy and pathology of the supraspinous and interspinous ligaments of the lumbar spine with special reference to ligament ruptures. Acta Orthop. Scand., 46 [Suppl.], 1960. (*A revealing and exhaustive documentation of information not generally studied.*)

77. Roaf, R.: A study of the mechanics of spine injuries. J. Bone Joint Surg., 42B:810, 1960.

78. Roberts, J. B., and Curtiss, P. H.: Stability of the thoracic and lumbar spine in traumatic paraplegia following fracture or fracture-dislocation. J. Bone Joint Surg., 52A:1115, 1970.

79. Robinson, R. A., and Southwick, W. O.: Indications and technics for early stabilization of the neck in some fracture dislocations of the cervical spine. South. Med. J., 53:565, 1960.

80. Rogers, W. A.: Cord injury during reduction of thoracic

and lumbar vertebral-body fracture and dislocation. J. Bone Joint Surg., 20:689, 1938.

81. ———: Fractures and dislocations of the cervical spine: an end result study. J. Bone Joint Surg., 39A:341, 1957.

82. Schneider, R. C., Cherry, G., and Pantek, H.: The syndrome of acute central spinal cord injury. J. Neurosurg., 11:564, 1954. (*An important paper containing fundamental and essential knowledge.*)

83. Shapiro, R., Youngberg, A. S., and Rothman, S. L. G.: The differential diagnosis of traumatic lesions of the occipito-atlanto-axial segment. Radiol. Clin. North Am., 11:505, 1973. (*We highly recommend this excellent clinical radiological review of this complex region.*)

84. Solonen, K. A.: The sacroiliac joint in the light of anatomical, roentgenological and clinical studies. Acta Orthop. Scand., 27 [Suppl.], 1957. (*A very comprehensive reference and bibliography on many important aspects of this joint.*)

85. Spence, K. F., Decker, S., and Sell, K. W.: Bursting atlantal fracture associated with rupture of the transverse ligament. J. Bone Joint Surg., 52A:543, 1970. (*A useful paper which is helpful in the understanding of the clinical stability of Jefferson fracture.*)

86. Steinger, J. K.: Fracture-dislocation of the thoracolumbar spine with special reference to reduction by open and closed operations. J. Bone Joint Surg., 29:107, 1947.

87. Sullivan, J. D., and Farfan, H. F.: The crumpled neural arch. Orthop. Clin. North Am., 6:199, 1975.

88. Tachdjian, M. O., and Matson, D. D.: Orthopaedic aspects of intraspinal tumors in infants and children. J. Bone Joint Surg., 47A:223, 1965.

89. Taylor, A. R.: The mechanism of injury to the spinal cord in the neck without damage to the vertebral column. J. Bone Joint Surg., 33B:543, 1951.

90. Taylor, A. S.: Fracture-dislocation of the neck: A method of treatment. Arch. Neurol. Physchiat., 12:625, 1924.

91. Veribest, H.: Anterolateral operations for fractures and dislocations in the middle and lower parts of the cervical spine: report of a series of forty-seven cases. J. Bone Joint Surg., 51A:1489, 1969.

91a. Von Torklus, D., and Gehle, W.: The Upper Cervical Spine. Regional Anatomy, Pathology and Traumatology. A Systematic Radiological Atlas and Textbook. New York, Grune & Stratton, 1972. (*An excellent reference on this region of the spine.*)

92. Walton, G. L.: A new method of reducing dislocation of cervical vertebrae. J. Nerv. Ment. Dis., 20:609, 1893. (*Suggested for basic ideas of theory and technique of cervical manipulation for reduction of dislocations.*)

93. Webb, J. K., Broughton, R. B. K., McSweeney, T., and Park, W. M.: Hidden flexion injury of the cervical spine. J. Bone Joint Surg., 58B:322, 1976. (*These clinical observations constitute an important advancement in the recognition of clinical instability.*)

94. Werne, S.: Studies in spontaneous atlas dislocation. Acta Orthop. Scand., 23 [Suppl.], 1957. (*One of the most complete and thorough presentations of the biomechanical and clinical aspects of C1-C2.*)

95. Werner, B., Wehling, H., and Matthaes, P.: Vergleichende nachuntersuchungergebnisse aufgerichteter und konservativ behandedter wirbel frakturen der brust und lendenwirbelsaule. Bruns Beitr. Klin. Chir., 219:735, 1972.

96. Westerborn, A., and Olsson, O.: Mechanics, treatment and prognosis of fractures of the dorso-lumbar spine. Acta Chir. Scand., 102:59, 1951.

97. White, A. A., and Hirsch, C.: The significance of the vertebral posterior elements in the mechanics of the thoracic spine. Clin. Orthop., 81:2, 1971.

98. White, A. A., Johnson, R. M., Panjabi, M. M., and Southwick, W. O.: Biomechanical analysis of clinical stability in the cervical spine. Clin. Orthop., 109:85, 1975.

98a. White, A. A., Panjabi, M. M., Hausfeld, J., and Southwick, W. D.: Clinical instability in the thoracic and thoracolumbar spine. Review of past and current concepts. Presented at the American Orthopaedic Association Meeting. Boco Ratan, Florida, 1977.

99. White, A. A., Panjabi, M. M., Saha, S., and Southwick, W. O.: Biomechanics of the axially loaded cervical spine: development of a safe clinical test for ruptured cervical ligaments. J. Bone Joint Surg., 57A:582, 1975.

100. White, A. A., Southwick, W. O., and Panjabi, M. M.: Clinical instability in the lower cervical spine. A review of past and current concepts. Spine, 1:15, 1976.

101. White, A. A., Southwick, W. O., Panjabi, M. M., and Johnson, R. M.: Practical biomechanics of the spine for orthopaedic surgeons [Chapter 4]. Instructional Course Lectures, American Academy of Orthopaedic Surgeons. St. Louis, C. V. Mosby, 1974.

102. Whitesides, T. E., and Shah, S. G. A.: On the management of unstable fractures of the thoracolumbar spine; rationale for use of anterior decompression and fusion and posterior stabilization. Spine, 1:99, 1976.

103. Wolf, B. S., Khilnami, M., and Malis, L.: The sagittal diameter of the bony cervical spinal canal and its significance in cervical spondylosis. J. Mt. Sinai Hosp. N. Y., 23:283, 1956. (*A well done study and a very useful reference.*)

104. Young, M. H.: Longterm consequences of stable fractures of the thoracic and lumbar vertebral bodies. J. Bone Joint Surg., 55B:295, 1973. (*An excellent article highly recommended for the clinician interested in interpretation of significance of radiographic findings and their relationship to prognosis.*)

6 The Clinical Biomechanics of Spine Pain

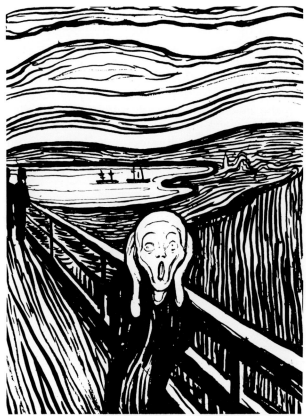

Fig. 6-1. "The Scream," 1895 Lithograph—OKK G/1 193. (Reproduced with permission from The Munch Museum.)

"I looked at the flaming clouds that hung like blood and a sword over the blue-black fjord and city . . . and I felt a loud unending scream piercing nature." So wrote Edvard Munch, creator of this expressionistic painting known as "The Scream" (Fig. 6-1).[123]

Few patients are so distraught or emotionally intense as this artist, but *all* of them to some extent have emotional and environmental factors affecting their particular response to spine disease. Not many patients have the talent to express their emotions so creatively, so physicians often must experience significantly less aesthetic aural manifestations of their inner turmoil.

The problem of pain has not only challenged the artist and physician, but it has always been an engaging topic for the psychologist, philosopher, and theologian. We may tend to become a bit philosophical in this chapter, although we are not philosophers and metaphysics is not the quest of our readers. In this chapter, the intent is to present what we consider to be some of the major reliable clinical and biomechanical information that may be helpful to the clinician in understanding the etiology, diagnosis, treatment, and prevention of spine pain.

In this chapter *spine pain* refers to cervical, thoracic, and lumbar pain that is not known to be related to infection, tumor, systemic disease, fractures, or fracture dislocation. The common neckaches and backaches that are so frequently encountered are discussed here.

It is well known that spine pain may be caused by tumor, trauma, infection, and a long list of systemic diseases. Psychologic, socioeconomic, biomechanical, biochemical, and immunologic factors also play a role. There may be any number of yet to be discovered causes.

Although there are unique considerations associated with spine pain in different regions of the spine, the information in this chapter, unless otherwise stated, is meant to apply to all regions of the spine. There has been considerable similarity between the problems of neck-shoulder-arm pain and low back-hip-leg pain. They both occur in the more mobile and lordotic portions of the spine. They have similar characteristics with regard to age of onset (30–50 years of age),[A] the frequency with which they affect the population, and their typical pattern of exacerbations and remissions.[72,73] Spine pain occurs most frequently in the lumbar region, followed by the cervical region, with the lowest incidence in the thoracic region.[71,72] Horal showed that there is a significantly increased incidence of cervical and thoracic spine pain found in individuals with low back disorders. Of patients who missed work with low back pain, 50 per cent of them had cervical spine pain, as compared with 38 per cent in controls. For thoracic spine pain, the respective percentages were 23 and 17.[71]

A discussion of pain should not continue without some information about the pain-sensitive structures in the spine. The posterior annular fibers and the posterior longitudinal ligament are innervated by the sinu-vertebral nerve (Fig. 6-2).[151] The capsular structures have a sensory innervation, as do the osseous structures through the autonomic nervous system. The paraspinous muscles have a sensory innervation also. Direct spine pain can come from physical, chemical, or inflammatory irritation of any of the previously described nerves. Nerve root pain is thought to come from any of the three types of irritation to the nerve roots. Finally, there is indirect or referred pain, which is not fully explained.

ETIOLOGIC CONSIDERATIONS

The exact cause of most spine pain remains unproven. Most of the theories impune the intervertebral disc through a variety of mechanisms, and consequently there are likely to be multiple causes. Information presented here may help to form some hypothesis about the causes of spine pain based on a synopsis of some of the most important current considerations.

"Gate" Control Theory of Pain

The "gate" control theory of pain is based on the work of Melzack and Wall.[101] Their historic article should be consulted for a full develop-ment, justification, and exposition. Although the theory is mostly unproven, it serves as a useful framework upon which to discuss pain. To follow is a freely interpreted and simplified synopsis of the theory as it may relate to spine pain. The essence of the theory is that within the substantia gelatinosa several factors are able to block or facilitate the transmission of pain producing impulses to the thalamus. The degree to which a theoretical gate is opened or closed to the transmission of these impulses depends upon blocking or facilitating influences from the cortex and/or midbrain, as well as upon influences within the spinal cord. There are fibers of small diameter that tend to open the "gate" and facilitate pain transmission. The fibers of large diameter are thought to close the "gate." The nerves in the latter situation are thought to be involved in the mechanism of pain relief with electrical stimulations. Acupuncture may have an effect of stimulating the midbrain to send efferent impulses to close the "gate."

More of our liberal interpretation of the theory is depicted in Figure 6-3A. The known anatomic pathways are shown in Figure 6-3B, and a number of clinically recognized phenomena are listed in relation to their possible mechanism with respect to the gate theory in Figure 6-3C. The various psychosocial and cultural influences are likely to be mediated either between the cortex and/or the thalamus or between the midbrain and the substantia gelatinosa. In a similar manner, the influences of transcendental meditation, hypnosis, placebo reaction, and psychomimetic and analgesic drugs may be mediated here.

Epidemiologic Factors

It is generally helpful in searching for the cause of a disease to study certain characteristics of a large group of individuals with the disease. In other words, how is spine pain related to age, sex, occupation, socioeconomic status, weight, or any other observable characteristic that can be studied?

Carefully designed and executed studies of the epidemiology of lumbar intervertebral disc diseases are rare. Such a study was done in the United States in the area of New Haven, Connecticut.[79,80,82–84] Some of the major observations are presented below.

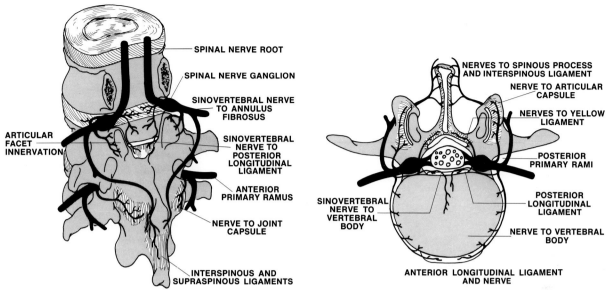

Fig. 6-2. This demonstrates clearly the sensory innervation of practically every anatomic structure in the spine. The annulus fibrosus, the major ligaments, the intervertebral joints and their capsules, the vertebral body, and all the posterior osseous structures are provided with sensory innervation. Thus, virtually any structure can be a potential source of spine pain.

Although the trends are not always consistent, it is interesting to discuss some of the mechanical considerations that may be operative in these findings. With regard to driving motor vehicles, the data suggests that men who spend 50 per cent

---

Relationship of Certain Epidemiologic Factors to Lumbar Disc Disease

Most important risk factors
   Driving of motor vehicles
   Sedentary occupations
   Previous full-term pregnancies
Suggestive but inconclusively related factors
   Male sex
   Chronic cough and chronic bronchitis
   Participation in baseball, golf, bowling
   Spring and fall seasons
   Lack of physical activity outside of work
Factors not related to an increase in risk
   Race (white vs. black)
   Smoking habits
   Sports other than baseball, golf, bowling
   Recent episodes of emotional stress
   Nonfull-term pregnancies
   Jobs involving lifting, pushing, pulling, or carrying
   Overweight

(Based on several studies by J. L. Kelsey and colleagues.)

or more of their work time driving a motor vehicle are three times more likely to develop a herniated disc than someone who does not have such an occupation.[83] Men or women who drive at work or elsewhere are more likely to develop a herniated disc than those who do not. It is known that sitting puts more pressure on the intervertebral disc.[76,107,108] This, in addition to the schedule of vibratory forces that are transmitted to the spine, may be a possible mechanism.[58] In addition, the position of the legs and the limited variety of optional sitting positions available to the driver may result in a predisposition to disc herniation. The study also showed that individuals with sedentary occupations were at significant risk of developing disc problems.[80] Driving a motor vehicle may qualify as a more sedentary occupation.

The suggestion of full-term pregnancy as a risk factor may be explained on the basis of the hormone relaxin and the increased load on the disc structures imposed by the increased weight of the uterus and its contents.[82] A study of 347 patients who had given birth to one or more children revealed that 39 per cent of the women developed symptoms of disc protrusion either

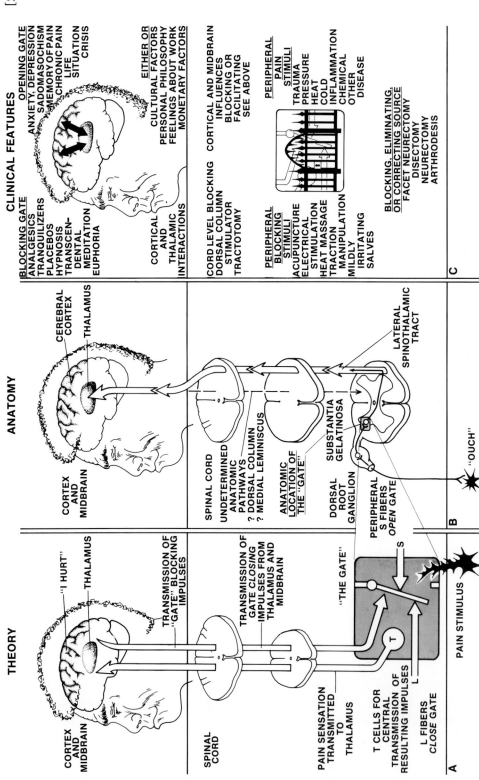

Fig. 6-3. (A) This is a diagrammatic sketch of the "gate" theory of pain. The intensity of the pain stimulus as ultimately experienced by the individual is dependent upon the extent to which the transmission of the stimulus is blocked. The S fibers tend to *open* the "gate" and facilitate the pain stimulus. The L fibers and also fibers that transmit impulses from the thalamus and the midbrain tend to *close* the "gate" and inhibit or reduce the pain. (B) This diagram shows *the anatomy* of the key structures involved in the "gate" theory of pain. The location of the gate shown in A is in the substantia gelatinosa. The lateral spinothalamic tract is the structure that transmits the T cell impulses to the thalamus. The specific location of the tracts through which the thalamus and midbrain exert their control on the gate is undetermined. (C) The clinical features may be viewed as an *interaction between painful stimuli and facilitating and inhibiting factors* that may operate through the "gate." Pharmacological, psychological, and socioeconomic factors probably have their origin in the cortex thalamus and midbrain but are to some extent mediated through the "gate" as shown in A and B. These factors also exert their influence to a considerable extent through interactions between the thalamus and cortex (*double arrows*). The therapeutic value of a number of treatments, such as heat and massage, may be interpreted in the context of the theory as peripheral stimuli that work through the spinal cord and midbrain and tend to close the "gate" and protect the T cells from painful stimuli.

during pregnancy or the puerperium.[115] The data in Kelsey's study suggested that the causative factor was related to the pregnancy rather than to the care of the children after pregnancy. Consequently, the lifting of children may not be an important consideration. This fits with other findings that showed little relationship between lifting on the job and the development of herniated lumbar discs.[80] However, it is important to keep in mind the fact that in altered, diseased, or irritated discs, the application of any incremental loads can not be expected to be desirable or helpful.

It is interesting to find that acute herniated lumbar disc disease was found to be a risk factor associated with sedentary occupations. This is consistent with the fact that sitting puts more pressure on the disc than either standing or lying down.[76,107,108] Also, there was no evidence that jobs involving heavy lifting, pushing, pulling, or carrying were significantly related to lumbar disc disease.[80] The effects of sedentary occupations did not appear before about 5 years of such work, and the influence is progressive after this time. The same study also showed a correlation with weekend sitting and disc herniation in males. Godsell studied 402 consecutive operations and from this review he expressed the opinion that heavy labor predisposes to disc rupture.[55] Other investigators have expressed a view that heavy labor is not a significant factor.[47,73] A controlled epidemiologic study of 429 subjects, divided into eight preselected occupational categories, provides some relevant data. Interestingly, the incidence of spine pain, not necessarily disc herniation, was positively correlated with the subjects' subjective evaluation of the type of work they were performing. There was more low back pain in subjects who thought their work was physically demanding.[96] It was found that a patient complaining of acute low back pain often gives a history of making a sudden unexpected exertion while carrying a heavy object.[97] The study also showed a significant association of low back pain with sitting and lifting weights when the spine is flexed as opposed to proper lifting when the spine is straight with hips and knees flexed. This observation fits with the experimental and simple biomechanical modeling data of Nachemson and Troup.[111,143]

A study by Magora showed that the subjects in the following occupations were most likely to experience low back pain at an early age: bank clerks, heavy industrial workers, farmers, and nurses.[98] In Kelsey's study, which involved only patients with herniated discs, weight lifting and bending were not among the factors frequently associated with radiculopathy.

Comments. With some studies, data is available on specifically herniated disc disease; in others, the data is simply related to back pain with or without sciatica. Nevertheless, there appear to be some general trends. The heavy laborer between the age of 30 and 40 is likely to get a herniated disc. Individuals who spend a good deal of time driving trucks or automobiles are likely to have back pain with or without sciatica. Women in the later stages of pregnancy or in early postpartum periods are prone to spine pain. The reader interested in a more detailed study of the epidemiology of spine pain is referred to a comprehensive review article by Kelsey.[81]

Many of these problems may be related to a mechanical etiology. The intervertebral disc, between the ages of 30 and 50 years, is changing from one of a rather healthy, resilient, high water content to a relatively dry, scarred disc characteristic of individuals over 50. The well hydrated, resilient disc under age 30 and the dry, scarred disc over age 50 may be mechanically less likely to fragment and displace. Obviously, other variables during these stages may also cause pain. Either the position of the spine or the patterns of the forces applied to it in driving a motor vehicle may well cause pain. A person whose job involves heavy labor, especially if he lifts improperly, can exert considerable forces on the structures of the spinal column, resulting in mechanical failure and/or pain. When the ligamentous structures of the pelvis and lower spinal segments alter their physical properties, mechanical disruption and pain may be the result.

There also may be a hereditary predisposition for a variety of different conditions that may lead to spine pain. This has been shown to be the case for spondylolisthesis and to a lesser extent for intervertebral disc disease.

The data on occupational and epidemiologic factors in back pain and disc disease is difficult to summarize. The more definitive relationships depend upon a clearer elucidation of the causes of low back pain and disc herniation. However, given present knowledge, it seems fair to suggest that sedentary occupations involving a good deal of sitting, especially driving a motor vehicle, are related to spine problems. Secondly, although it is not consistent, some types of heavy labor may be associated, but the relationship is not distinct.

Socioeconomic and Psychologic Factors

These factors obviously overlap considerably with epidemiologic factors; however, we have chosen to discuss them separately. Studies have shown that the tendency to report sick from work with spine pain is correlated with lower intellectual capacity, educational level, socioeconomic status, and the patient's own idea of "self-importance" on the job. Patients who missed work due to low back pain or sciatica tended to have

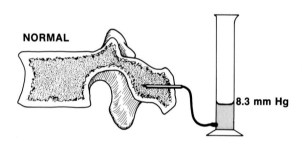

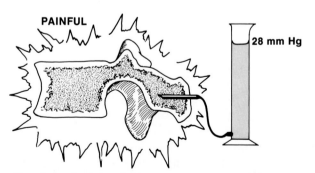

Fig. 6-4. Intraosseous pressure appears to be associated with spine pain. The differences between the two averages shown in the figure are statistically significant. (Based on data from Arnoldi, C. C.: Intervertebral pressures in patients with lumbar pain. A preliminary communication. Acta Orthop. Scand. *43:* 109, 1972.)

subordinate positions and to be less satisfied with their work. Moreover, parameters of social insufficiency, such as divorce rate, alcoholism, and various psychiatric disturbances, all tended to correlate with missed work and spine pain.[11,149]

It is well known that the complaint of pain or onset of illness may significantly be influenced by psychologic factors.[12,37,38,66,155] The secondary gain may be relief from guilt, responsibility, challenge, or the pain may be simply a manifestation of depression. Some of the recent psychiatric theories have generated evidence that a sado-masochistic patient may complain of spine pain in search of a surgical procedure.[10]

Spine Pain and Vertebral Pressure Dynamics

Many clinicians accept the hypothesis that hemodynamic abnormalities, mainly an increase in blood pressure in bone, can result in pain. It has been suggested that the success of just about any geometric configuration of osteotomy of the hip in diminishing pain may be the result of the relief of internal osseous pressure.[7] Arnoldi compared the intraosseous venous pressures in the spinous processes of 43 vertebra from ten subjects. The mean pressure was 8.3 torr. Twenty-two vertebrae from ten subjects with low back pain had an average venous pressure of 28.0 torr (Fig. 6-4). The difference was statistically significant (p<0.01).[5] The study and the results are preliminary, but they do suggest that increased intraosseous pressure may be a factor in low back pain.

Soft-Tissue Structures and Spine Pain

Spine pain has been attributed to trigger points in the skin, and relief has been reported from injections of the same. Back pain has been reported to be cured following resection of portions of deep facsia over the paravertebral muscles thought to be responsible for pain.[105]

Spasm of the muscles themselves is generally thought to be either a primary or a secondary source of back pain. This has resulted in the sale of a great quantity of muscle relaxing drugs and extensive use of massage administered by physical therapists and others.

Any of the numerous musculotendinous or ligamentous structures of the spine may suffer strain, sprain, or rupture. This may result in pain and inflammation, as well as a stimulus for paraspinous muscle spasm, a cause of considerable spine pain. The list below, based on the work of Wyke, names the various structures of the spinal column that are known to have pain receptors.[157] There are nerve fibers capable of transmitting pain present in the lumbodorsal fascia, the supraspinous and infraspinous ligaments, the vertebral periosteum, and the anterior and posterior longitudinal ligaments, as well as the outer layers of the yellow ligament and posterior annulus fibers.[64]

Sources of Pain Receptors in the Vertebral Column

Anterior and posterior longitudinal ligaments
Posterior annular fibers
Yellow ligaments
Interspinous ligaments
Intervertebral joint capsules
Periosteum of vertebrae
Fascia of vertebrae
Blood vessels of the vertebrae
Walls of epidural and paravertebral veins
Paravertebral musculature

(Wyke, B.: The neurological basis of thoracic spine pain. Rheumatol. Phys. Med., *10*:356, 1970.)

Posterior Elements

The intervertebral joints are cartilage-covered articulations, with a synovial and a fibrous capsule. Any disease of the cartilage or the synovial tissue can affect this joint as well as any other in the body. Ankylosing spondylitis and degenerative arthritis tend to involve the joint more often than some other diseases. These joints may be the source of a significant amount of spine pain. Hirsch and colleagues reported that injections of hypertonic saline in either the posterior annular fibers or the intervertebral joint areas produced similar clinical presentations.[63] However, when the annular fibers were injected, the clinical presentation was more characteristic of the lumbago seen spontaneously in patients.

The Etiologic Relationship of Some Radiologic Findings to Spine Pain

Which of the many radiologic irregularities seen in the spine can be presumed to cause spine pain? In order to convincingly demonstrate this,

it is necessary to show that patients with the particular radiographic irregularity have a significantly higher incidence of spine pain than individuals without the irregularity. This is no easy task, given all the subjectivity of complex variables involved in the complaint of pain and given the fact that about 80 per cent of the population at one time or another will have a complaint of back pain.[111] The radiographic conditions are listed below in three groups according to the probability of an association with spine pain (very likely, very unlikely, questionable). The information comes largely from the review article by Nachemson,[111] with some alterations substantiated from a variety of sources. This discussion is based on the assumption that there is no other clinically obvious explanation for spine pain.

Radiographic Irregularities of the Spine Likely To Be Associated With Spine Pain*

Very likely
    Spondylolisthesis (moderate or severe)
    Multiple, markedly narrowed intervertebral disc spaces
    Congenital kyphosis
    Scoliosis (severe)
    Osteoporosis
    Ankylosing spondylitis
    Lumbar osteochondrosis (Scheuermann's disease)
Very unlikely
    Spina bifida occulta
    Acute lumbosacral angle
    Single disc narrowing and spondylosis
    Facet arthrosis, subluxation, and trophism
    Disc calcification (except in thoracic spine)†
    Extra-cervical, extra-lumbar, or extra-thoracic vertebrae
    Sacralization of lumbar vertebrae
    Lumbarization of sacral vertebrae
    Hyperlordosis (moderate)
    Intravertebral body disc herniation (Schmorl's nodes)
    Accessory ossicles
Questionable
    Spondylolysis
    Spondylolisthesis (mild)
    Kyphosis (severe)
    Scoliosis (mild to moderate)
    Retrolisthesis of cervical, thoracic, or lumbar vertebrae
    Lumbar scoliosis (>80°)
    Hyperlordosis (severe)

---

* Based on data from Nachemson, A. L.: The lumbar spine, an orthopaedic challenge. Spine, *1*:59, 1976.
† Disc calcification in the thoracic spine should raise a high index of suspicion of a herniation.

A careful review of this list does not seem to reveal any patterns in the radiologic findings that might be related to some common factor, mechanical or otherwise. Perhaps the main value is to provide some helpful guidelines for the proper interpretation of the findings in the first two groups. It is also important to keep in mind that there can be marked disc degeneration in the absence of *any* radiographic changes.[64] When there is radiographic evidence of decreased disc space, sclerosis, and osteophytes, the corresponding disc is severely damaged but may not be painful. The plain radiographic findings are the same for disc degeneration as for disc herniation.[47]

The Intervertebral Disc

Ever since the milestone investigation by Mixter and Barr, most of the clinical and research work on spine pain has focused on the intervertebral disc.[103] Actually, the disc has been proven to be the cause of pain in only a very small percentage of patients. Many physicians agree that it has probably been overstudied and overrated as a cause of spine pain. Even though there are still a number of questions to be answered, there is a fund of anatomic, biomechanical, biochemical, immunologic, and clinical information on this structure. This data is valuable and useful. Other possible causes of spine pain have not been so vigorously studied. It is possible that the non-herniated intervertebral disc is the cause of much of the severe, clinically significant low back pain that is observed, but this may be difficult to prove. In support of this hypothesis, it is known that there is neural innervation to posterior annulus fibers and that the clinical pattern of low back pain tends to precede the herniated intervertebral disc. In opposition to this hypothesis, it is known that the spine pain that precedes herniation often has a course of gradual exacerbations and remissions that somehow belies a purely mechanical explanation. This phenomenon is not satisfactorily explained by movement of the disc in and out or into and away from the area of sensory innervation. This may be explained using a biochemical or immunologic basis, but current evidence is unconvincing and contradictory. The physician must accept that spine pain associated

with nerve root irritation can be caused by disc disease. Whether or not the disc can account for a significant portion of other spine pain remains in question.

In addition, there are a large number of other diseases and conditions that are known to be associated with radiculopathy, with or without spine pain. Most of these conditions are rare; however, they are important. Before focusing in detail on the disc, it is worthwhile to scan the list below.[1,81]

Conditions Other Than Intervertebral Disc Disease Known to be Associated With Radiculopathy

Osteoarthrosis of the spine	Poliomyelitis
Intraspinal tumors	Herpes zoster
Other tumors	Diphtheria
Epidural venous anomalies	Meningitis
Spondylolisthesis	Leprosy
Rheumatoid spondylitis	Tuberculosis
Generalized toxemia	Myelomeningocele
Alcoholism	Perineural cysts
Lead poisoning	Extradural or subdural cysts
Radiation radiculopathy	Root avulsion
Diabetes	Megacauda
Syphilis	Widening of nerve root socket
Sarcoidosis	Abnormal anatomic location of nerve root
Behcet's disease	

(Agnoli, A. L., et al.: Differential diagnosis of sciatica. Analysis of 3000 disc operations. *In* Wüllenweber, R., et al. [eds.]: Advances in Neurosurgery. vol. 4. New York, Springer-Verlag, 1977. Kelsey, J. L., and Ostfeld, A. M.: Demographic characteristics of persons with acute herniated lumbar intervertebral disc. J. Chronic Dis., 28:37, 1975.)

Normal Disc. This discussion refers to the normally functioning disc in a young individual, described in Chapter 1. The external loads create tensile forces in the peripheral annular fibers that are up to four to five times the superincumbent forces. There is a slight physiologic protrusion of the disc on the concave side of a physiologic curve, with a slight shift of the nucleus pulposus in that direction. Large tensile stresses are also applied to the peripheral annular fibers with torsional loading (y-axis rotation). This is thought to be especially true of the posterolateral annular fibers. As long as the nucleus is well hydrated, the annular fibers are well nourished, and there are no irritating or immunologically active chemical organic substances present, the intervertebral disc is healthy and causes no pain.

Pathologic Problems. As a normal process of use and aging, there are several phenomena that may take place. The water content of the disc diminishes, and the ability of its component structures to be nourished may be altered. There may be some element of fatigue failure of some of the annular fibers. These may undergo a variety of different degenerative and chemical decompositions.[50] The products of decomposition may be protein substances that stimulate immunologic responses and inflammatory activity.[11]

Other more purely mechanical possibilities relate to the peripheral annular fibers, which may rupture either from fatigue failure of some particular traumatic episode. It is known that sometimes episodes of a sudden unexpected load cause the onset of acute spine pain. This may be due to the sudden rupture of some of the fibers of the annulus fibrosus. As these various phenomena occur, they may be associated with a variety of clinical findings.

In 1952 Charnley wrote a stimulating and provocative paper in which he sought to describe the mechanisms of intervertebral disc pathology and to correlate the hypothesized pathoanatomic factors with the clinical presentation and treatment of acute low back pain and sciatica.[18] Here we attempt to update his hypotheses, 25 years later.

Acute Back Sprain (Type I). This is the acute back sprain that characteristically occurs when a laborer attempts to sustain a sudden additional load. There is immediate severe pain that may last for several weeks. The pain is primarily in the low back, without sciatica. This may be due to several factors. Charnley suggested the possibility of rupture of some of the deep layers of the annulus. We believe that while this is possible, the inner fibers are not innervated, and there is relatively less loading and deformation of the deeper fibers than of the periphery. There are several other possibilities. One is that peripheral annular fibers may be injured or ruptured along with any of the other posterior ligaments or musculotendinous structures. Also, there is the possibility that some of these injuries may involve rupture of muscle fibers or be associated with nondisplaced or minimally displaced vertebral

end-plate fractures (Fig. 6-5). The answer awaits further investigation. These conditions should respond to a period of rest, followed by a gradual resumption of normal activities.

Fluid Ingestion, Organic or Idiopathic? (Type II). It was hypothesized that an attack of low back pain and muscle spasm may be produced by the sudden passage of fluid into the nucleus pulposus for some unknown reason (Fig. 6-6).[18,112] Charnley suggested that this irritated the peripheral annular fibers, causing the characteristic pain. There is little to discredit the hypothesis 20 years later. Naylor suggests that increased fluid uptake in the nucleus is a precipitating factor in the biochemical chain of events that can lead to disc disease. Very indirect evidence suggests that increases in fluid in the disc structure may not cause spine pain. This is based on the observation that astronauts returning from outer space have heightened disc space but no back pain.* On the other hand, there is data, although inconsistent, which suggests that fluid injection into the normal disc causes low back pain.[60] This discrepancy may be partially explained by the differences in the *rate* of change in fluid pressure. The hypothesis of fluid ingestion fits with clinical data, because it is compatible with the characteristic clinical course of exacerbations and remissions, with or without progression to other clinical syndromes. In other words, movement of fluid in and out of the disc can explain the onset and resolution of the clinical symptoms. We suggest that this may be the explanation for spontaneous idiopathic organic spine pain (cervical, thoracic, or lumbar) unrelated to trauma, which accounts for a significant number of the many cases of spine pain.

Posterolateral Annulus Disruption (Type III). If there is failure or disruption of some of the annular fibers, posterolateral irritation in this region may cause back pain with referral into the sacroiliac region, the buttock, or the back of the thigh (Fig. 6-7). This is referred pain and is due to stimulation of the sensory innervation by mechanical, chemical, or inflammatory irritant. Thus, "referred sciatica," as Charnley called it, is distinguished from true sciatica by a negative

---

* Personal communication, L. Kazarian.

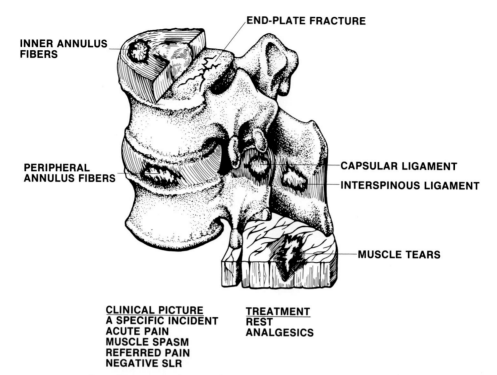

INNER ANNULUS
FIBERS

END-PLATE FRACTURE

PERIPHERAL
ANNULUS FIBERS

CAPSULAR LIGAMENT

INTERSPINOUS LIGAMENT

MUSCLE TEARS

CLINICAL PICTURE
A SPECIFIC INCIDENT
ACUTE PAIN
MUSCLE SPASM
REFERRED PAIN
NEGATIVE SLR

TREATMENT
REST
ANALGESICS

Fig. 6-5. A clinical picture of acute back sprain (Type I) may involve damage to any number of ligamentous structures, the muscle, or even vertebral end-plate fracture. SLR: straight leg raising test.

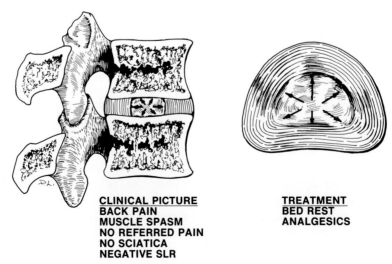

CLINICAL PICTURE
BACK PAIN
MUSCLE SPASM
NO REFERRED PAIN
NO SCIATICA
NEGATIVE SLR

TREATMENT
BED REST
ANALGESICS

Fig. 6-6. Organic or idiopathic fluid ingestion (Type II). This mechanism may account for a large portion of back pain for which no distinct diagnosis or etiology has been determined.

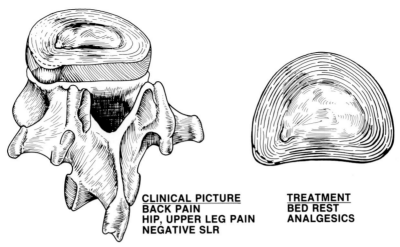

CLINICAL PICTURE
BACK PAIN
HIP, UPPER LEG PAIN
NEGATIVE SLR

TREATMENT
BED REST
ANALGESICS

Fig. 6-7. Posterolateral annulus disruption (Type III). The dotted line represents the original normal contour of the disc. Hip and thigh pain are referred pain rather than true sciatica.

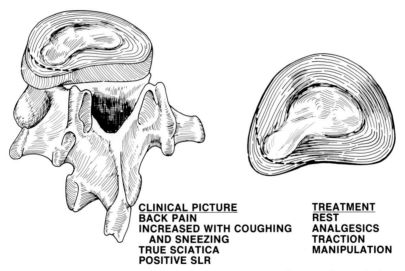

CLINICAL PICTURE
BACK PAIN
INCREASED WITH COUGHING
  AND SNEEZING
TRUE SCIATICA
POSITIVE SLR

TREATMENT
REST
ANALGESICS
TRACTION
MANIPULATION

Fig. 6-8. Bulging disc (Type IV). In this situation the annulus is bulging to such an extent that nerve root irritation has caused sciatica. The dotted line shows the normal position of the annulus rim.

straight leg raising test and a lack of any neuromuscular deficit. As suggested previously, this referred pain may be explained by the "gate" control theory. This situation may resolve itself through reabsorption or neutralization of the irritants and/or phagocytosis and painless healing of the disrupted annular fibers.

Bulging Disc (Type IV). Another proposed mechanism involves protrusion of the nucleus pulposus, which remains covered with some annular fibers and possibly the posterior longitudinal ligament (Fig. 6-8). There may be "true acute sciatica" with mechanical and still possibly chemical and/or inflammatory irritation of the nerve roots. The pain may include the back, buttock, thigh, lower leg, and even the foot. The pain may be increased with coughing and sneezing, and the straight leg raising test is positive. Radiographs in this situation usually do not indicate narrowing. It is feasible that traction or spinal manipulation may alter the mechanics in this situation and may possibly be therapeutic. With rest, the irritation may subside and remain stable or return spontaneously after mobilization.

Sequestered Fragment (the Wandering Disc Material; Type V). A theorized mechanical etiology is that of a sequestered nucleus pulposus and/or annulus fibrosus (Fig. 6-9). This may develop over a period of time associated with the normal degenerative processes of the disc and/or other presently unknown pathologic changes. This sequestrum may move about in a random fashion in response to the directions and magnitudes of forces produced at the motion segment by the activity of the individual. This movement may permit the sequestrum to irritate (by physical presence and/or chemical breakdown products) the annular fibers and to produce low back pain with or without referred sciatica. It may also produce a bulge in an area in which it can cause true sciatica. The sequestration may move about, such that in some positions it is either asymptomatic or causes some combination of spine pain, referred pain, or true radiculopathy. Because of

the movement of the sequestered fragment in response to forces at the motion segment, it may be possible that through axial traction or spinal manipulation of the motion segment, the sequestrum can be moved temporarily or permanently from a location in which it stimulates a nerve to one in which it causes no irritation. Subsequent motion of the disc fragment into areas of pain insensitivity or subsequent scarring may result in no recurrence. On the contrary, if there is no scarring, the random movement of the sequestered portion of the disc may include positions of subsequent nerve root irritation.

Displaced Sequestered Fragment (Anchored; Type VI). There is another clinical and mechanical situation that may develop. This is the displacement of a sequestrum of the annulus and/or nucleus into the spinal canal or intervertebral foramen (Fig. 6-10). The fragment is to some degree fixed in position. The nerve root irritation results from inflammation due to mechanical pressure, chemical irritation, or an autoimmune response or some combination of the three. There is true sciatica with positive straight leg raising tests. In association with a displaced portion of the intervertebral disc (sequestration), there may

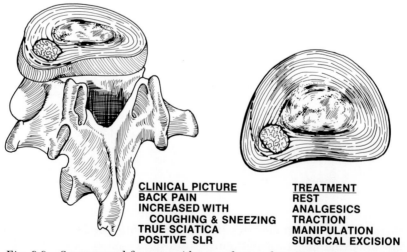

CLINICAL PICTURE
BACK PAIN
INCREASED WITH
    COUGHING & SNEEZING
TRUE SCIATICA
POSITIVE SLR

TREATMENT
REST
ANALGESICS
TRACTION
MANIPULATION
SURGICAL EXCISION

Fig. 6-9. Sequestered fragment (the wandering disc; Type V). The results of treatment with surgery are better than that of Types I to IV but probably not as good as that of Types VI and VII. The wandering disc is a possible explanation for the clinical picture of exacerbations and remissions that are so frequently encountered. It may also be a partial explanation of why some patients show a good response to traction or manipulation.

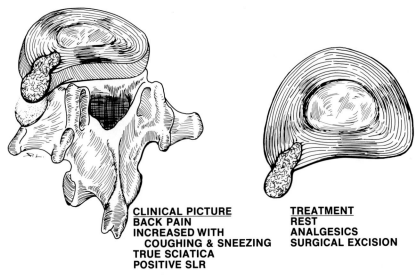

CLINICAL PICTURE
BACK PAIN
INCREASED WITH
**   COUGHING & SNEEZING**
TRUE SCIATICA
POSITIVE SLR

TREATMENT
REST
ANALGESICS
SURGICAL EXCISION

Fig. 6-10. With Type VI there is sequestration and displacement but some anchoring of the ligament, so that it cannot move about. This is less likely to be helped by traction or manipulation.

be narrowing of the interspace at the involved level. Axial traction, manipulation, or random movement is *unlikely* to help. Chymopapain injected into the disc space may never reach or affect the sequestrum, especially if there has been scarring or blockage of the hole in the disc structure. When this situation subsides spontaneously, we hypothesize that it is a result of phagocytosis and/or some physiologic adjustment of the neural structures to the irritation. These patients show the best results when treated with surgery, as suggested by Charnley and subsequently confirmed by Spangfort.[18,136]

Degenerating Disc (Type VII). Another stage may occur when the disc degenerates (Fig. 6-11). This involves a disruption of the normal annular fibers of the disc to such an extent that the disc is no longer able to serve an adequate mechanical function. This may be associated with degenerative arthritic processes of the vertebral bodies and/or the intervertebral joints. There may be chronic pain, intermittent pain, or such individuals may even be asymptomatic.

Organic Idiopathic Spine Pain. This is the type of pain present in patients who are diagnosed clinically as having organic spine pain without sciatica for which there is no known etiology. Pain may emanate from the disc, or it may come from increased fluid uptake by the disc (Type II), or any combination of the previously described etiologic factors, or some mechanism yet to be discovered.

Immunologic Factors in Spine Pain. The basic hypothesis is that during the degenerative processes of the intervertebral disc, one or more of the degradation products stimulate the autoimmune response. The associated inflammatory response is the cause of the spine pain, with and without nerve root irritation. Autoantibodies to autogenous nucleus pulposus have been experimentally demonstrated in both animals and humans.[11,119] Investigators have identified in humans through the leucocyte migration-inhibition test the presence of a cellular immune response in patients in whom a sequestered disc was found at surgery.[51]

Elucidating the possible mode of an immunologic inflammatory response is helpful in the explanation of several characteristics of disc disease. This hypothesized mechanism aids in accounting for the chronic course of exacerbations and remissions and the success of anti-inflammatory drugs, such as aspirin, phenylbutazone, and steroids (administered locally and systemically).

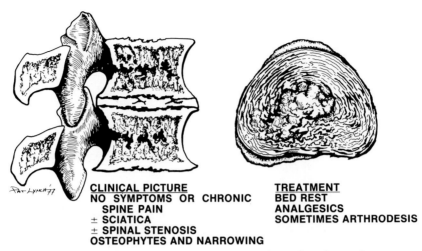

CLINICAL PICTURE
NO SYMPTOMS OR CHRONIC
SPINE PAIN
± SCIATICA
± SPINAL STENOSIS
OSTEOPHYTES AND NARROWING

TREATMENT
BED REST
ANALGESICS
SOMETIMES ARTHRODESIS

Fig. 6-11. A degenerated disc (Type VII) may be either the end process of the mechanical and biological effects of normal functioning or it may be associated with considerable pain and disability. There may also be arthritis in the intervertebral joints. It is important to emphasize that these various stages are a continuum. A given disc may move through several types or stages. The changes may accelerate or decelerate, stop, or in some instances they may even reverse.

The predominant neurologic symptom is *pain,* which implies irritation rather than *numbness,* a symptom compatible with simple chronic neural pressure. There have been gross and microscopic observations of inflammation, granulation, and fibrosis observed in excised discs.[13] Subsequent research will further explain and confirm or invalidate this hypothesis.

Biochemical Factors in Spine Pain. Naylor in a review article has presented an excellent summary of the biochemical and biomechanical factors that constitute a hypothetical explanation of the clinical phenomena of disc disease.[112] Although the disc is the largest avascular structure in the human body, there is considerable chemical interchange and activity there. The process is summarized in Figure 6-12. The initial change is thought to be a disruption of the balance between the synthesis of normal proteinpolysaccharide and its depolymerization. The disequilibrium is such that there is an increased depolymerization. There is an associated increased fluid content in the nucleus pulposus, resulting in greater intradiscal tension. The increase in discal tension alone as hypothesized by Charnley in 1955 can cause backaches. This may also be the cause of

organic idiopathic back pain. From this point, according to the Naylor hypothesis, the situation may develop in at least three different manners (Fig. 6-12). Processes 1 and 2 are set in motion when there is a cessation of the conditions that disturbed the equilibrum of synthesis, allowing it to be reestablished at a new but lower level. From this point the process can progress in one of two disparate directions. Process 1 involves *repeated cycles* of abnormal proteinpolysaccharide synthesis, accompanied by increased collagen fibrillation. The repeated cycles may explain the clinically observed course of intermittent attacks of spine pain that tend to follow their own schedule of exacerbations and remissions. This may continue on to extreme nuclear degeneration and a fairly rigid, scarred disc that cannot develop tension or prolapse. Presumably, this stage may be reached with or without either spine or radicular pain. In addition to or because of the abnormal nuclear synthesis, Process 2 involves disruption of the disc mechanics and damaging stress and results in disruption and failure of the annular fibers. The end point of Process 2 is prolapse of the nucleus pulposus and/or some portion of the annulus. In this situation, prior to frank pro-

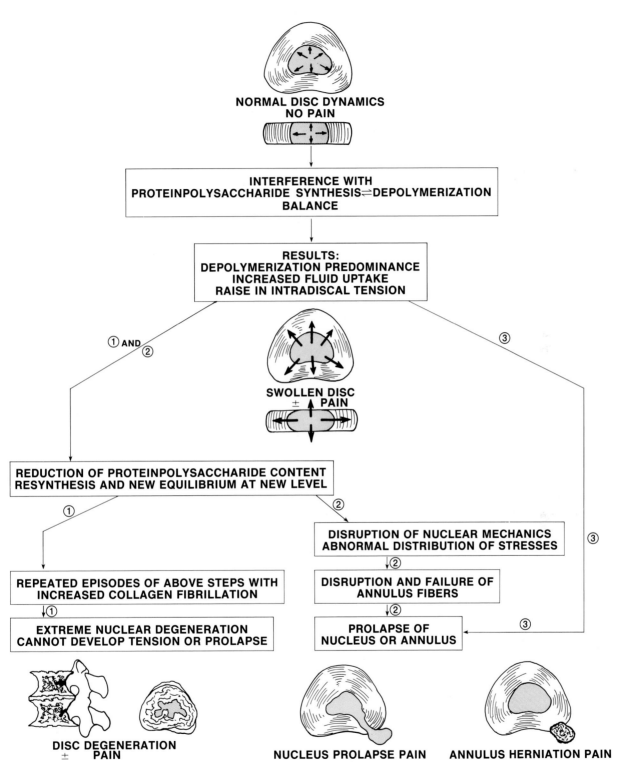

**NORMAL DISC DYNAMICS
NO PAIN**

INTERFERENCE WITH
PROTEINPOLYSACCHARIDE SYNTHESIS⇌DEPOLYMERIZATION
BALANCE

RESULTS:
DEPOLYMERIZATION PREDOMINANCE
INCREASED FLUID UPTAKE
RAISE IN INTRADISCAL TENSION

① AND ②

③

**SWOLLEN DISC
± ↑ PAIN**

REDUCTION OF PROTEINPOLYSACCHARIDE CONTENT
RESYNTHESIS AND NEW EQUILIBRIUM AT NEW LEVEL

①

②

③

DISRUPTION OF NUCLEAR MECHANICS
ABNORMAL DISTRIBUTION OF STRESSES

↓②

REPEATED EPISODES OF ABOVE STEPS WITH
INCREASED COLLAGEN FIBRILLATION

DISRUPTION AND FAILURE OF
ANNULUS FIBERS

↓①

↓②

③

EXTREME NUCLEAR DEGENERATION
CANNOT DEVELOP TENSION OR PROLAPSE

PROLAPSE OF
NUCLEUS OR ANNULUS

**DISC DEGENERATION
± PAIN**

NUCLEUS PROLAPSE PAIN

ANNULUS HERNIATION PAIN

Fig. 6-12. This flow diagram explains the biochemical hypothesis of the basic mechanisms of spine pain, disc prolapse, and degeneration. A number of mechanical factors mentioned in this chapter probably play a large role in the clinical presentation and outcome of these various biochemical phenomena. (Based on Naylor, A.: Intervertebral disc prolapse and degeneration; the biochemical and biophysical approach. Spine, *1:*108, 1976.)

lapse the patient would be expected to have a history of intermittent spine and radicular pain. Process 3 is a more direct progression to nuclear or annular prolapse following the initial biochemical and mechanical changes in the disc. This could be the pathophysiologic course followed by the patient with no spine pain who subsequently experiences rapid onset of radicular signs and symptoms, with or without spine pain.

As a simplified summary we suggest that Process 1 is normal disc degeneration, 2 is the subacute or chronic symptomatic degeneration, and 3 is the acute prolapse of a disc with varying degrees of degeneration. There may well be some overlap among the three hypothesized courses that a given disc may follow. This probably depends upon genetic factors, mechanical factors, treatment, or some combination of these or other presently unknown considerations. This theoretical analysis offers an explanation for a good deal of what is observed clinically.

Lumbar Spinal Stenosis

Spinal stenosis is defined as any type of narrowing of the central spinal canal or nerve canal excluding neoplastic and inflammatory disease. A classification of the various causes is provided below.

Spinal stenosis of the lumbar region is a condi-

Classification of Spinal Stenosis

Congenital developmental stenosis
  Idiopathic
  Achondroplastic
Acquired stenosis
  Degenerative stenosis
    Central canal
    Peripheral canal and neural canal
    Degenerative spondylolithesis
  Combined stenosis
    Herniated disc combined with combinations of the above
  Spondylolisthetic
  Postoperative stenosis
    Laminectomy, fusion, chemonucleolysis
  Post-traumatic stenosis
  Miscellaneous stenosis
    Paget's disease, fluorosis

(Arnoldi, C. C., et al.: Lumbar spinal stenosis and nerve root entrapment syndromes: definition and classification. Clin. Orthop., *115:4*, 1976.)

tion that is probably not recognized as frequently as it should be. Paine and Huang described 227 cases of the lumbar disc syndrome.[118] In this series disc herniation alone was present in 31 per cent of patients, developmental stenosis alone in 2 per cent, degenerative stenosis alone in 27 per cent, and combined lesions in 39 per cent of cases. This shows that spinal stenosis is frequently present and probably plays a significant role in low back pain and sciatica, in conjunction with disc disease as well as independently.

The clinical presentation may consist of constant or intermittent, vague, atypical complaints. The pain distribution and radiculopathy may be multilevel or unilevel, either bilaterally or unilaterally. One highly characteristic feature is that of intermittent claudication. Physicians should be highly suspicious of patients with a history of intermittent claudication who have no clinical evidence of occlusive vascular disease. "Drop attacks," sudden falling down without loss of consciousness due to leg weakness, is a rare finding but when present serves as a clue to the diagnosis.

The findings upon physical examination, like the clinical history, are likely to be mixed and vague. There may be a subtle suggestion of radiculopathy at several nerve root levels. The straight leg raising test may be weakly positive but not distinctive.

The diagnosis is made primarily on the basis of the bizarre nature of the history and physical findings and the radiographic evaluation. On the plain films, one may see osteoarthritic involvement of the posterior joints in which the anteroposterior and lateral diameters of the bony canal have been reduced. Myelography and computerized axial tomography are helpful in a more accurate evaluation of the size of the lumbar spinal canal.[148] There have been several attempts to measure and establish norms for the size of the osseous lumbar canal, but no highly accurate system has emerged. Current techniques are based largely on myelographic study, in which the lumbar region is filled with 30 ml of dye and films are taken with the patient erect. An anteroposterior diameter of less than 14 mm is suggestive of stenosis, as is streaking that looks like arachnoiditis or swollen nerve roots.[87] Some examples of spinal stenosis are diagrammed in Figure 6-13. The disease may present with the usual symptoms of disc disease or with low back pain and leg pain with no abnormal neurologic signs. Treatment includes nonoperative techniques, postural exercises, orthotic support, and spinal manipulation. Although these have been recommended in the literature, there is little reason to be optimistic about their efficacy. Surgical treatment is through decompression by laminectomy and root canal decompression if needed.[87,154]

Loads and Motion

In general, the cervical spine has the most intersegmental motion if one considers all the parameters of motion (see Fig. 2-24). However, the loads are relatively low in this region. In the thoracic spine there is relatively little intersegmental motion, and the stiffness is high due to intrinsic mechanical properties, the rib attachments, and the thoracic cage. The thoracic spine loads are intermediate between those found in the cervical and the lumbar spine. In the lumbar spine, there is an intermediate degree of intersegmental motion, but the loads applied are of the highest magnitude. It is in this region that patients most often experience pain.

A biomechanical analysis of the incidence of pain in the different regions of the spine suggests a relationship between *loads* and *motion*. The degree of motion is highest in the cervical spine, but the loads are small. It ranks second in incidence of pain. There is relatively little motion in the thoracic spine, and the loads in this region are moderate. It ranks third in incidence of pain. The lumbar spine undergoes a moderate degree of motion and very high loads. It ranks first in incidence of pain. These relationships are summarized in Table 6-1.

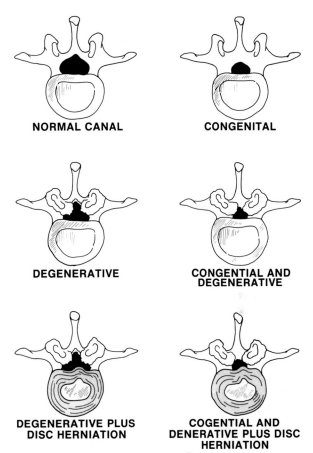

NORMAL CANAL   **CONGENITAL**

DEGENERATIVE   **CONGENTIAL AND DEGENERATIVE**

DEGENERATIVE PLUS DISC HERNIATION   **COGENTIAL AND DENERATIVE PLUS DISC HERNIATION**

Fig. 6-13. This diagram shows the normal canal and various combinations of conditions that may cause spinal stenosis. Congenital stenosis with disc herniation alone, not pictured here, is another possibility. (Arnoldi, C. C., et al.: Lumbar spinal stenosis and nerve root entrapment syndromes: definition and classification. Clin. Orthop., *115:*4, 1976.)

Table 6-1. Relationship Between Motion, Loads, and Pain in Regions of the Spine

	DEGREE OF MOTION (Rank)	MAGNITUDE OF LOADS (Rank)	INCIDENCE OF PAIN (Rank)
Cervical	1st	3rd	2nd
Thoracic	3rd	2nd	3rd
Lumbar	2nd	1st	1st

Because of the plane of orientation of the facet articulations in the lumbar area, there are relatively more shear forces on the intervertebral discs during axial rotation.[57] In addition, discs L4-5 and L5-S1 are subjected to high shear forces due to their high angles with the horizontal plane. It has been suggested that this may be a factor in the higher rate of development of disc herniation there. Farfan and colleagues have proposed that torsional loading causes failure of the annular fiber, which results in disc disease.[40] These factors may account at least in part for the high incidence of disc disease at L4–5 and L5–S1.

Comment

"Having engaged in research in the field for nearly twenty-five years and having been clinically engaged in back problems for nearly the same period of time, and as a member and scientific advisor to several international back associations, I can only state that for the majority of our patients, *the true cause of low back pain is unknown*" (Alf Nachemson, 1975).[110] Several possible mechanisms that may be involved in spine pain have been presented. The preceding quotation is included as a poignant reminder that the state of knowledge does not yet permit a full scientific understanding of spine pain. Although there are some good working hypotheses, a tremendous amount of research is needed to resolve this protean problem that frequently compromises the quality of life for so many people.

DIAGNOSTIC CONSIDERATIONS

This section focuses on factors that are of biomechanical significance or are crucial to the satisfactory evaluation of typical spine pain syndromes with associated neurologic problems. The discussion assumes that the physician has basic skills and knowledge in taking a general history, performing a physical examination, and maintaining the clinical management of an adult patient.

Clinical History

Cervical Spine Pain. A review of the salient clinical features of cervical spine pain follows.

Cervical spine pain is found in any combination of sites involving the neck, shoulder, and arm. The history of onset in the three regions may have any sequence. Usually, there is neck and interscapular pain, followed by pain in the other two areas. The location of arm pain and/or dysesthesia can be helpful in determining the level at which the pathology may exist. The neck or the brachial pain may be increased with coughing, sneezing, or Valsalva's maneuver (Fig. 6-14). There may be a history of whiplash injury, a strain of the neck with some active physical activity, or there may simply be a spontaneous onset, gradual or sudden. One of the common sites of

referred pain from the cervical spine is the interscapular region. There may be associated problems, such as frozen shoulder (28%), epicondylitis, or carpal tunnel. The reasons for the associations are not clearly understood. Epicondylitis and carpal tunnel may be related to the "double jeopardy" concept, in which it is suggested that when there are two sites of painful irritation of a nerve, they may reciprocally potentiate pain sensation associated with the two sites of irritation. In other words, the cervical nerve root disease lowers the threshold at which any irritation at the other sites may become symptomatic.

Thoracic Spine Pain. Thoracic spine pain syndromes, though relatively less frequent than in other regions, can be more serious if they are

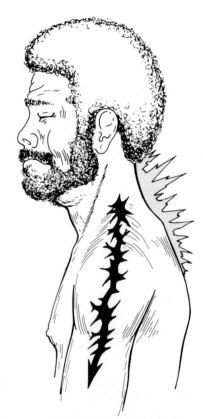

Fig. 6-14. Valsalva's maneuver, forced expiration against a closed glottis with tight perineal sphincters, increases venous and cerebral spinal fluid pressure. When there is cervical spondylosis or soft cervical disc disease, this maneuver may cause neck or neck-shoulder-arm pain.

associated with a herniated disc. There may be a dramatic onset of symptoms such that the patient drops to the floor with paralysis. The shoulder blade is a recognized location for pain associated with thoracic spine disease.[73] The data from this study also suggested that a history of heavy work before age 15 may contribute to the development of kyphosis, which is associated with thoracic spine pain.

The clinical patterns of presentation of a thoracic disc are quite variable. Many of the cases, however, show a rapid onset of thoracic or low back pain, followed by sensory disturbances and motor weakness; about 50 per cent of the patients have visceral dysfunction (bladder and bowel disturbances). The pain is increased by activities that constitute Valsalva's maneuver. Trauma is the precipitating factor in the onset of the symptoms in roughly one-third of patients.[142]

Lumbar Spine Pain. Spine pain of acute onset associated with a particular mechanical incident may be related to a strain or rupture of some of the annular fibers of the disc or other muscular or ligamentous structures. If there is associated sciatica, the presumption is strengthened. Spine pain with or without sciatica, occurring without specific incident even in sleep, does not rule out disc disease. It is known that disc degeneration occurs as a gradual process, and the ultimate displacement to the point of irritation may be a subtle insignificant event. As vascular, inflammatory, and biochemical factors may be operative in the production of pain, the onset may be gradual and progressive.

Lumbar disc pain is generally alleviated by rest, with the hips and knees flexed. The pain is accentuated by coughing, sneezing, and straining at stool. These phenomena are thought to be mechanically related. In the erect position, the disc pressure is greater and the disc tends to bulge about its periphery. It is also known that the venous system is connected with the ventricles and the subarachnoid space, and a Valsalva's maneuver (coughing, sneezing, or straining at the stool) can increase pressure in the subarachnoid space. This space extends out along the nerve roots just into the intervertebral foramen in the lumbar region. If there is inflammation and engorgement of this already crowded

space, the slightest change may constitute a pain stimulus. A slight increase in subarachnoid space pressure or a slight stretch of the nerve rootlet could easily trigger the pain-eliciting mechanism. It is for these biomechanical reasons that a Valsalva's maneuver tends to aggravate pain, and the position of flexed hip and knee, which gives the lowest intradiscal pressure and causes the least stretch of the sciatica nerve, tends to relieve pain.

Physical Examination: Cervical Spine

The physical examination of the spine has been well presented in other publications.[29,43,70,77] It is presumed that an adequate general physical and musculoskeletal evaluation will also be carried out. Aspects of the physical examination that have some biomechanical relevance are discussed here.

Comments. There should always be a thorough motor and sensory examination, with care to rule out any physical evidence of myelopathy. Pain to firm palpation or percussion over the spinous processes of the involved motion segment has been noted in the cervical spine, as in the thoracic and lumbar spine pain syndromes.[73]

Spurling's Test. This is a helpful test. The head is turned in maximal axial rotation facing, for example, first the patient's right. Then it is laterally bent maximally to the right. With the head in this position, a vertical blow is delivered to the uppermost portion of the cranium. With the head and neck in this position, the vertebrae are vertical, approximately, and the disc on that side bulges maximally into the intervertebral foramen, which is also at its smallest size in this position (Fig. 6-15). The blow to the head is transmitted to the disc, which spreads a bit further and causes maximum encroachment on the intervertebral foramen. The left side is then tested by axially rotating and laterally bending the patient's head to the left and delivering a new blow. This should stimulate any nerve root or other pain-sensitive structures related to disc disease and cervical spondylosis. A positive Spurling's test, then, would be a complaint of any combination of neck, shoulder, or arm pain when the blow is delivered with the head and neck in the described position.

Range of Motion. These tests offer some crude, indirect evidence of disease. During extremes of motion, pain similar to that which the patient generally suffers is some indication of disrupted mechanics, as with cervical spondylo-

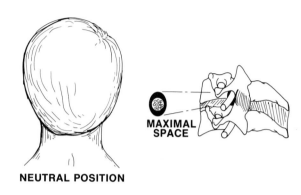

NEUTRAL POSITION

MAXIMAL SPACE

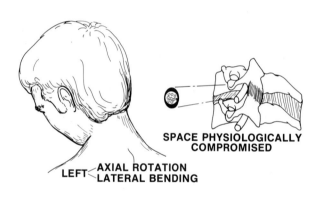

SPACE PHYSIOLOGICALLY COMPROMISED

LEFT〈**AXIAL ROTATION LATERAL BENDING**

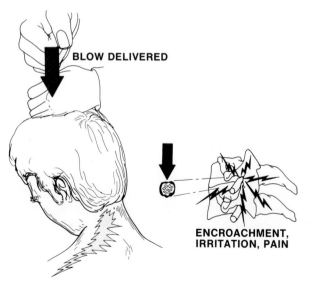

BLOW DELIVERED

ENCROACHMENT, IRRITATION, PAIN

sis. The other aspects of the physical exam are designed to localize dermatomic or myotomal dysfunction. The manual muscle tests, reflex changes, and sensory tests are carried out. When these findings correlate with the plain radiologic and myelographic evidence of the level of cervical spondylosis, the prognosis for a good or excellent result with surgery is very much improved.

Physical Examination: Thoracic Spine

There may be pain over the spinous processes of the involved motion segment. There is sometimes evidence of myelopathy. A sizable number of combinations of neurologic disturbances may be seen with thoracic disc disease.[142] No particular pattern appears to predominate. There may be abdominal level, sensory disturbances (numbness, parasthesis, and loss of vibratory strength), motion disturbances (paraparesis and paraplegia, muscle spasm, fasciculations, atrophy), and abnormal reflexes (hyperactive or hypoactive with or without symmetry). Some patients have had a positive Romberg's sign. All the varied combinations observed are presumably due to the distinct sensitivity of the spinal cord in the region. The vulnerability can be attributed to the minimal amount of free space available to the cord when it is impinged by displaced disc material. The spinal cord has less freedom of movement, and therefore there is a greater possibility for a contrecoup disruption and production of neurologic problems. Thus, the dorsal column signs and Brown-Séquard neurologic signs are sometimes present. Moreover, the blood supply of the cord in this region is precarious. Domissee showed

---

Fig. 6-15. Spurling's test is based on several biomechanical factors. If there is some pathological compromise or irritation of the nerve root, when the root passes through the intervertebral foramen the irritation is aggravated. In order to demonstrate this, the head is positioned as shown, and the coupled motions of axial rotation and lateral bending will further compromise the space available in the foramen. When the test is positive, a vertically directed blow of moderate impact produces an additional lateral bending moment that reduces this space, irritates the nerve root, and causes some combination of neck, shoulder, or arm pain. This does not occur in a normal person.

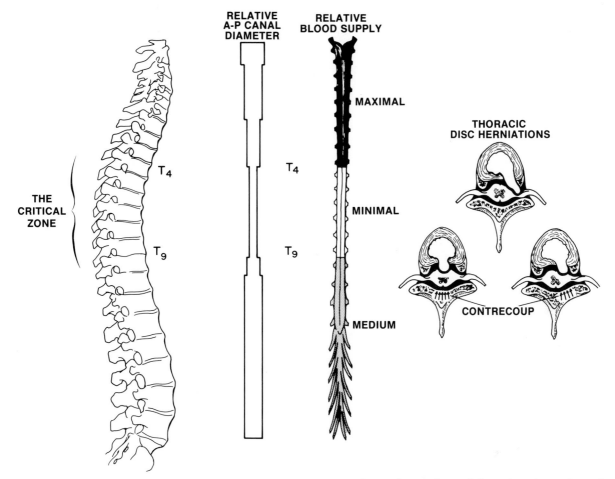

Fig. 6-16. This emphasizes several very important points in the understanding of thoracic spine pain and disc disease, as well as that of clinical stability in the thoracic spine. In the critical zone, the canal space and the free space between the spinal cord and the borders of the spinal canal are minimal. Although the thoracic cord is small, the relative free space is still minimal in the region of T4–T9. Moreover, the blood supply is less than elsewhere in the spinal cord. Therefore, this zone is doubly sensitive to any encroachment of the space available. A herniated disc not only readily causes spinal cord impingement, but there may be a contrecoup phenomenon in addition, so that both factors interfere with an already modest blood supply. It can be seen from the relative diameter of the anteroposterior canal that the situation is not quite as crucial in the highest and lowest regions of the thoracic spine. These considerations explain the catastrophic nature of thoracic disc disease and clinical instability in the thoracic spine.

lucidly that the thoracic spine between T4 and T9 exhibits the least degree of vascularity and space for the thoracic spinal cord.[31] Consequently, this is the region where there is the lowest threshold for spinal cord damage. This very important relationship of blood supply, available space, and the possible pathologic effects of mechanical disruption is shown in Figure 6-16.

Physical Examination: Lumbar Spine

There are characteristics revealed by physical examination that are helpful in the diagnosis of organic pain and in the recognition of disc disease. Findings that have a relevant mechanical basis are discussed here, along with some of the tactics that aid in diagnosing malingering and functional disease.

Body Stances.   The patient awaiting examination will consciously or subconsciously stand with the hip and knee both slightly flexed in the leg in which the pain resides (Fig. 6-17). This is a very reliable sign in our opinion, as the patient without realizing it has learned to stand in this position to relieve nerve root pressure. By slightly flexing the hip and knee there is less tension on the sciatic nerve. Often, if the patient is asked, "Why are you standing that way?" the response will be "Which way?"

There may be a list to either the ipsilateral or the contralateral side of the sciatica. Biomechanical considerations suggest the following: If the patient lists to the side of the sciatica, the disc herniation is in the axilla of the nerve root; if the patient lists away from the side of the sciatica, the herniation is lateral to the nerve root.[43] This hypothesis seems reasonable based on theoreti-

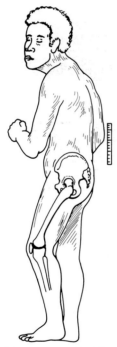

Fig. 6-17. The disc stance is highly suggestive of the presence of a herniated disc or some other form of mechanical nerve root irritation in the lower lumbar spine. The patient sometimes unconsciously stands in this position, usually with a straight back and hips and knees flexed. The former reduces the posterior buldge of the disc, and the latter minimizes the stretch on the sciatic nerve roots.

cal pathoanatomic evaluation. To our knowledge it has not been documented with clinical investigations. The rationale and interpretation are presented in Figure 6-18.

Camptocormia.   Occasionally, a modestly educated young male patient presents with a complaint of severe low back pain and an inability to straighten up. The patient is usually grotesquely bent forward and tilted to one side or the other. Attempts to have the patient actively or passively straighten up while standing are usually met with total failure. However, when he lies down on the examining table, the "deformity" is readily corrected. This is a unique and classic type of hysteria, the treatment of which is not in the realm of biomechanics but in the psychosocial.[93,126]

Muscle Spasms.   Unilateral or bilateral paraspinous muscle spasm is not diagnostic of a herniated disc, but if present and involuntary, it is suggestive of organic disease. Paraspinous muscle spasm associated with malingering or hysteria tends to relax on the side of the stance phase during ambulation. This can be tested by walking behind the patient with both hands on the paraspinous muscle masses.

Naphziger's Test.   When positive, this is a significant indicator of intervertebral disc disease with nerve root irritation (Fig. 6-19). The mechanism involves increased nerve root pain within a few seconds after bilateral jugular compression. This is due to increased pressure of the subarachnoid space at the intervertebral foramen. We have employed a slight modification of the test, which we find to be useful. While compressing the jugular, the patient is asked, "Does this make your leg pain go away?" If the patient responds "No, it makes it worse," the test is positive and suggestive of disc disease. If the patient says, "Oh yes Doctor, it feels better!" this is *suggestive* of malingering or functional disease.

Forward Bending.   The patient is then asked to bend forward. A cooperative attempt to do this along with simultaneous flexing of the hips and knees is suggestive of organic disease with or without nerve root irritation. With the attempt to bend forward, the lumbar region remains relatively fixed, while the rest of the spine moves above it. This is suggestive of organic disease.

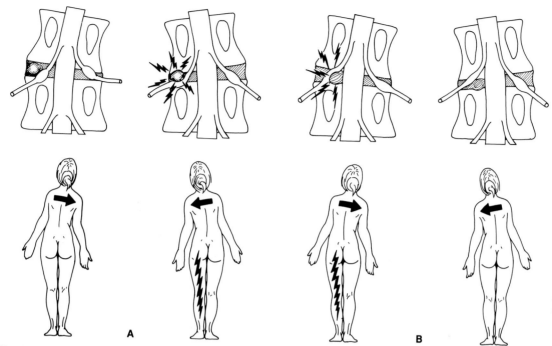

Fig. 6-18. Patients with herniated disc disease may sometimes list to one side. This is a voluntary or involuntary mechanism to alleviate nerve root irritation. The list in some patients is toward the side of the sciatica; in others it is toward the opposite side. A reasonable hypothesis suggests that when herniation is lateral to the nerve root (A) the list is to the side opposite the sciatica because a list to the same side would elicit pain. Conversely, when the herniation is medial to the nerve root (B), the list is toward the side of the sciatica because tilting away would irritate the root and cause pain. If this hypothesis could be documented in clinical practice, it would be helpful at the time of surgical exploration.

Dramatic refusal or half-hearted attempt is *suggestive of* nonorganic problems.

Percussion of Spinous Processes. Percussion over the spinous processes with a neurologic hammer sometimes elicits severe pain, localized maximally around two or three adjacent spinous processes. When this finding is consistent, it is suggestive of organic disease. There may be tumor, osteomyelitis, disc space infection, or a herniated disc. If increased vertebral fluid pressure does in fact cause spine pain, then this too would be stimulated by percussion.

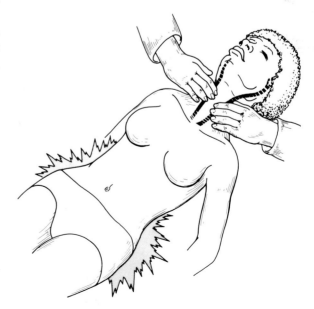

Fig. 6-19. Naphziger's test may be done while the patient is standing or lying down. The test is based on the hyphothesis that bilateral jugular compression increases cerebral spinal fluid pressure. The pressure increase in the subarachnoid space in the root canal may cause back or leg pain by irritating a local mechanical or inflammatory condition.

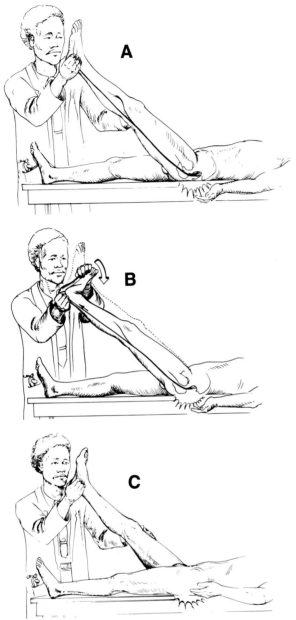

Fig. 6-20. The various straight leg raising tests are useful clinical signs. They are based on the mechanical principal of stimulating an irritable situation at the lower lumbar region of the nerve roots and the intervertebral discs. The sciatic nerve is readily stretched by flexion of the hip and ankle (when the knee is straight) due to its anatomic location away from the motion centers of the two joints. (*A*) Straight leg raising test. (*B*) Straight leg raising with ankle dorsiflexion. (*C*) Crossed straight leg raising test. (Hoppenfeld, S.: *Physical Examination of the Spine and Extremities*. New York, Appleton-Century-Crofts, 1976.)

Reflexes and Muscle Tests. Any gross muscle weakness from nerve root compression at L5 or S1 can be ruled out if the patient is able to first walk on the heels, fully extending the toes and then subsequently is able to walk on the toes. When the patient walks on the heels, the absence of toe extension on one side may indicate weakness of the extensor hallicus and an L5 myotomal paresis. Decreased reflex of the Achilles tendon is suggestive of nerve root irritation at S1. A diminished knee jerk may be indicative of nerve root irritation at L3 or L4.

In addition to the previously described muscle power tests, we suggest several additional manual muscle tests. With the patient supine and both ankles held at 90 degrees of extension, the examiner grasps a foot in each hand, holding them in the region of the metatarsal heads. The examiner then puts his feet together and with arms extended leans back so as to apply an equal force to the feet. This test will show weakness of the ankle dorsiflexors. The same test is done holding each of the patient's big toes. When these tests are positive, it is suggestive of nerve root irritation at L5. With both knees extended off the end of the table, the examiner can apply his weight equally to the dorsum, the anterior aspects of the distal tibias, and test the relative strength of the patient's quadriceps mechanism and the L3 and L4 root motor function.

Leg Raising Tests. There is some confusion about the consistent nomenclature of some of the leg raising tests for examination of the lumbar spine. Some physicians consider the Lasèque's test to be a simple straight leg raising test.[59] Others believe it to be flexion of the hip followed by extension of the knee.[29,43] Both interpretations are supported by reference to the original article by Lasèque.[88] This disagreement is of academic and historical interest, and no attempt will be made to resolve it.

The straight leg raising test is done with the patient in the supine position (Fig. 6-20A). Most normal subjects can have the hip joint flexed 80 to 90 degrees without back or leg pain. When there is back or ipsilateral leg pain, the test is considered positive. The sooner the pain occurs, the more definitive is the test. We do not think that the production of back pain without leg pain is as significant in this test as is the production of leg pain with or without back pain. If the test is consistent and associated with voluntary extension of the lumbar spine to reduce the sciatic nerve stretch, it may be thought of as significantly positive. The examiner should take care to distinguish the discomfort associated with the stretching of a normal but tight hamstring muscle from leg pain similar to that for which the patient is being evaluated.

Straight leg raising with ankle dorsiflexion is a very useful test that is helpful in documenting the presence of nerve root irritation. It may be regarded as a type of check or confirmation of the straight leg raising test and a maneuver which distinguishes posterior leg pain from pain that may be due to stretching of the hamstring muscles. With the patient in a supine position, the straight leg raising test is done. The angle of hip flexion at which posterior leg pain is elicited is found. The leg is then lowered to just below this level, so that the pain subsides. While the leg is held at that level, the ankle is slowly but firmly dorsiflexed to the maximum (Fig. 6-20B). If this maneuver causes the patient's characteristic leg pain, the test is considered positive and strongly indicative of nerve root irritation.

The crossed, straight leg raising test (Beckterew's test), although not often positive, is strongly indicative of a herniated disc or some other structure causing irritation of the nerve root.[136] This test is positive during flexion. The asymptomatic or relatively asymptomatic leg when flexed at the hip causes pain in the asymptomatic leg (Fig. 6-20C). The mechanism of this test is thought to be as follows: The inflammation or irritation of the nerve root of the symptomatic leg has sensitized it so much that the minute amount of motion produced by movement of the nerve root on the other side is enough to cause pain.

The Pedis Pulse Test. While the patient sits on the side of the examining table with hips and knees flexed, the examiner looks attentively at the dorsum of the foot, raises it by the heel with one hand, and carefully palpates for the dorsalis pedis pulse with the other hand (Fig. 6-21A). The heel is returned to its original position, and the same thing is done with the opposite side. This

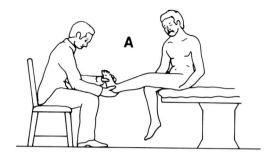

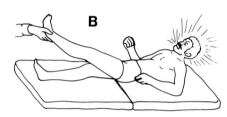

Fig. 6-21. (A) The patient is relaxed on the table while pulses are examined. The straight leg raising here is greater than 90 degrees. (B) Now that the patient is lying down, there is vigorous complaint with even less than 90 degrees of straight leg raising. This is inconsistent and suggestive of other than organic disease.

test provides considerable information. If both dorsalis pedis pulses are normal, it is highly unlikely that the patient's back or leg pain is due to occlusive vascular disease. (In order to be more certain of this, the examiner should determine that the femoral pulses are also present.) This maneuver also gives an excellent straight leg raising test, as the patient goes from a position of hips and knees flexed to one of a fully extended knee. This puts a large stretch on the L4–5 to S1 roots, which contribute to the sciatic nerve. A patient with real sciatic nerve root irritation on the side that is being so manipulated will *automatically* lean back on the examining table as the knee is extended, in addition to which, the patient may share various exclamations with the examiner (Fig. 6-21B). By leaning back, the individual is essentially *extending* the hip joint to compensate for and reduce the pain caused by excursion of the sciatic nerve. Another valuable aspect of this test is its potential to provide evidence supportive of malingering or functional disease. Consider the patient who sits quietly while the knees are extended to 180 degrees and with the hips flexed at 90 degrees as the pulses are being checked, but who complains vigorously of pain when the straight leg raising test is being done in the supine position. This may be thought of as a "positive pedis pulse test," *suggestive* of nonorganic disease.

Kernig's Test. When there is enough mobility of the neck and significant encroachment and/or irritation of the meningeal structures, this test may be positive. Even though there is considerable accordion-like folding of the cord, there can be sufficient motion transmitted to the cervical or lumbar region to cause neck, back, or leg pain with flexion of the neck (Fig. 6-22). Biomechanically and pathoanatomically, this test may be regarded as analogous to a leg raising test performed from the opposite end.

Of the tests discussed here, we consider the following to be most reliable: the crossed, straight leg raising test, the straight leg raising test with ankle dorsiflexion, protective flexion of the spine during the pedal pulse test and straight leg raising tests, the standing posture, deep tendon reflex changes, and distinct localized muscle weakness. Sensory examination is not discussed here. This, too, is important for a complete physical examination. However, it is often difficult to evaluate. Certainly, some of these other findings

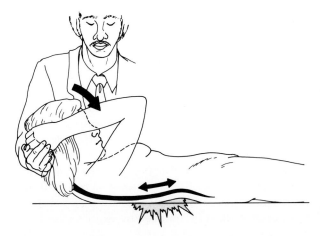

Fig. 6-22. Kernig's test is based upon the mechanism of increasing the tension in the meninges or the nerve roots by flexing the neck as shown. The test is positive when back, leg, or arm pain is elicited.

must be present in addition to sensory changes in order to convincingly indicate the presence of nerve root pathology.

Myelograms

This diagnostic test remains as the major laboratory test in the evaluation of spine pain. When the myelogram is positive, both the probability of finding a prolapsed disc and the probability of a good or an excellent result with surgery are increased. It has been suggested that there is approximately a 2 per cent incidence of false positives with this test.[64] The false negatives are thought to be significantly reduced with the use of the water soluble substance metrizamide for myelography. This substance is not yet on the market in the United States. It is available in Scandinavian countries where the fat soluble material Pantopaque has been taken off the market because of its association with arachnoiditis.[111]

Discograms

The term discogram is used with at least three different connotations. It sometimes refers to the amount of fluid that can be injected into a particular intervertebral disc. It also has to do with interpretations of the location and distribution of radiopaque fluids following their injection into an intervertebral disc. And finally, there is the use of injection as a clinical test of the extent to which this manner of irritation of the disc elicits the patient's characteristic pain.

The problem with discograms is that it is not possible to distinguish the distribution of the contrast media in the normal disc from that reported in the pathologic disc. Holt was able to do cervical and lumbar discograms on groups of volunteers from the Missouri State Prison. The study of cervical discograms was done with 50 subjects, ages 21 to 50, without histories of neck or arm pain or injuries to the cervical spine. In only ten disc spaces out of 148 injected did the contrast medium remain within the confines of the annulus. In addition, the volume of the injectable material was not a useful indication of an abnormal disc. Severe pain was produced by the injection of the contrast medium in every subject. This eliminated pain production as an indication of an abnormal disc.[67] Holt conducted a similar study in the lumbar spine. There he found 37 per cent false positives in 30 normal volunteer prisoners from Illinois.

Clearly, the ability of the intervertebral disc to retain a fluid within its confines is not related to its ability to cause spine pain. It does not appear that there is adequate evidence that discograms provide any useful diagnostic information with regard to localization of spine pain.

Electromyography

This test provides objective evidence of partial muscle dennervation. When this test is positive, it is thought to be of considerable significance in the accurate diagnosis of a herniated intervertebral disc. It may be helpful in the evaluation of a complex clinical picture in which evidence of radiculopathy is confusing or inconsistent. The presence of abnormal electromyographic findings can be crucial in the evaluation and management of a patient when compensation, litigation, and psychiatric problems are concerned. The test can not be positive within 4 days of the onset of root pathology.

TREATMENT OF SPINE PAIN

The problem of the evaluation of various treatment programs for spine pain is an extremely difficult one and should be approached with deference and humility. The numerous psychological and socioeconomic factors that are involved have been discussed. The issue is further complicated by two additional factors. The first is that in 30 to 35 per cent of patients there are placebo reactions to any form of treatment, including surgery.[30,138] The second is that the natural course of diseases that cause spine pain is such that 60 to 70 per cent of the patients will be cured with no treatment or any form of treatment.[59,73,136,147] It is therefore extremely difficult in many instances to know if a patient recovers because of a placebo response, the treatment rendered, or the natural course of the disease. In addition, for those patients who do not show good results, it is sometimes difficult to determine if it is because of incorrect diagnosis, the particular character of the

disease, insurmountable psychologic problems, malingering, or inappropriate, untimely, or ineffectively administered treatment. With this optimistic, inspiring background in mind, an attempt to review and evaluate some of the more widely used treatments for spine pain follows. Most of the information relates to low back pain and sciatica. However, the basic principles apply to both cervical and thoracic spine pain. The unique considerations related to cervical and thoracic pain are discussed when pertinent.

It is understandable that some physicians do not like to treat patients for low back pain. However, there are few diseases in which one is assured improvement in 70 per cent of patients in 3 weeks and 90 per cent in 2 months, regardless of the type of treatment employed.[111] Given the present state of knowledge and the objective information about the various forms of treatment for spine pain, it is possible to build an argument for withholding treatment. However, this is hardly feasible or practicable. Patients expect and demand to be "treated" and relieved of their misery. The physician is compelled to do something. Therefore, the main goal is to make the patient rest comfortably, to maintain confidence, and to insure against the occurrence of anything that is unnecessary and/or potentially harmful to the patient's physical and fiscal well being.

This evaluation applies to patients who have spine pain that has been adequately evaluated and diagnosed as a herniated disc or organic spine pain of undetermined etiology. The patients do not have tumors, infections, specific arthritis (e.g., rheumatoid arthritis, ankylosing spondylitis, lupus erythematosus), significant trauma, or some other systemic disease that is the cause of spine pain. This evaluation does include osteoarthrosis of the cervical, thoracic, and lumbar spine. There are certainly an ample number of treatment options that are available to the patient with spine pain (Fig. 6-23). Since it is sometimes difficult for the specialist to choose among them, one can be sure that the patient probably has even greater difficulty deciding.

Rest, Analgesics, and Anti-inflammatory Drugs

In most instances of spine pain, the patient improves in 2 to 3 weeks. Rest minimizes me

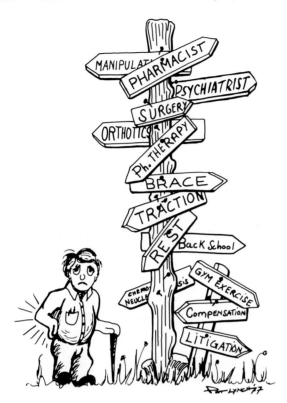

Fig. 6-23.   This cartoon includes most of the options currently employed by patients and therapists in the treatment of spine pain. There must be a *best* choice, and medical science should continue to search for it.

Results.   The results are usually successful in 1 to 3 weeks. Occasionally, the patient's condition will worsen or proceed to a protracted course. In either instance, additional, similar therapy may be continued, or some other treatment program may be substituted or added.

Complications.   There are the usual risks of bed rest in the middle-aged and aged. There are also the usual pharmacologic complications associated with the commonly used analgesics and anti-inflammatory drugs. The risk of addiction to narcotics is present, but this is not a high risk.

Comment.   Bed rest at home is inexpensive, low risk treatment that does no harm and generally is associated with relief of symptoms. It is a noninvasive treatment requiring no particular technical knowledge or experience. The use of medications in addition is a reasonable adjunct that makes the patient more comfortable and, in the case of the anti-inflammatory drugs, may accelerate the recovery rate. We recommend this regimen as the initial treatment of spine pain with or without sciatica.

The value of resting on a hard surface may simply be due to the more efficient, *immobilizing*

chanical irritation of what may well be a local inflammatory response. Anti-inflammatory drugs contribute to the alleviation of symptoms, as do analgesics.

Treatment.   In the acute situation, the patient may be treated with bed rest, preferably on a firm surface, and given analgesics. The position suggested is lying either on the back or the side, with hips and knees flexed (Figs. 6-24, 6-25). This effectively reduces the loads on the lumbar intervertebral discs.[111] The patient should assume the most comfortable position and level of activity. Some patients will be most comfortable on the side, lying in the fetal position with hips and knees flexed. This position obviously puts minimal stretch and irritation on the sciatic nerve. Some patients treated with bed rest will find that they are more comfortable if they can be up and about intermittently for minor activity.

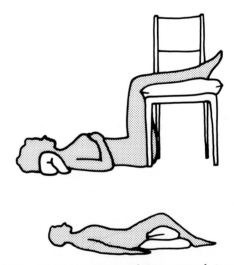

Fig. 6-24.   These positions have several important characteristics that should be beneficial to most patients with low back pain. The supine position reduces disc pressure. The straight back minimizes posterior disc bulging. With the hips and knees flexed, there is elimination of psoas muscle tension and thus disc pressure, and there is minimal stretch on the sciatic nerve.

capacity. By eliminating the bending of the spine that occurs because of a soft mattress, the patient is better able to attain and maintain a constant position of the spine without sagging and bending (Fig. 6-25).

In addition to the above regimen, there are a number of nonsurgical treatment programs of varying degrees of complexity, intensity, and risks that may be employed. They are used independently or in variety of combinations and sequences. Many of the conservative treatment modalities were evaluated in a study by Soderberg.[135] He found that 67 per cent of patients with sciatica treated with a combination of nonsurgical techniques, including bed rest, physiotherapy, plaster jacket, manipulation, local injections, and systemic medications, were symptom-free in an 8 year follow-up. A review of some information about the various treatment programs and some comments follow.

During the time interval when spontaneous remission of symptoms is being awaited, it is desirable to provide some medication to alleviate the pain. It is not within the scope of this presentation to discuss the pharmocology of pain medications. Most physicians tend to employ some combination of narcotic or non-narcotic analgesic, anti-inflammatory, muscle relaxant, and psychotropic drug. The choice of drugs is usually the result of some interaction between the knowledge and attitudes of the doctor and patient. We generally start with salycilates supplemented with codeine, if needed in the acute phase. Rest and reduction in pain with analgesics tends to relax the muscles. If the patient has psychiatric problems needing medication, the advise of a psychiatrist on the medications employed, as well as the general management of the patient, is recommended.

William's Exercises

The therapeutic goal of the classic William's exercises is to strengthen the lumbar spine flexors and stretch those muscular and ligamentous structures that tend to hold the spine in the extended position.[153] The premise is that the straight or slightly kyphotic lumbar spine is less painful and healthier. If the pain is from bulging of the posterior intervertebral disc, then it is

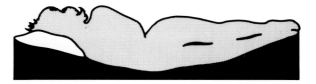

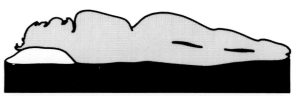

Fig. 6-25. (*Bottom*) The firm mattress allows one to splint the spine better and reduce the tension associated with excessive curves. If the patient lies on the side with hips and knees flexed on the firm mattress, he can maintain the position and accomplish essentially the same goals achieved when the hips and knees are flexed in the supine position. (*Top*) Bending in any plane maintained for a prolonged period of time can cause excessive stress of the disc.

reasonable to assume that the straight and flexed spine would be more comfortable than the extended spine. These exercises have been employed for years, and there are those who believe they are of value, as well as those who do not. Supporters argue that people who live in Asian and African cultures, where a good deal of time is spent in a squatting position with the lumbar spine flexed, do not have as high an incidence of spine pain.[39] We are not aware of an investigation in which cross-cultural and racial comparison has ever been satisfactorily studied.

On the contrary, there is the work of Gunnar, Nachemson, and colleagues which shows that the slightly extended spine is associated with electromyographic evidence of reduced paraspinous muscle activity and intradiscal pressure measurements that show reduced disc load in vivo in this position. If back pain is related to intervertebral disc mechanics and muscle spasm, then clearly the nonflexed, slightly extended position of the lumbar spine is likely to be therapeutic.

Another important point related to William's exercises should be discussed. Intradiscal pressure measurements during various activities showed that doing sit-ups (one of the William's exercises) resulted in intradiscal pressures of a high magnitude, as measured at the L3 disc. The observed pressures were the same as those recorded when the subject was lifting 20 kg (44 lb) by bending the back with the knees straight. This is hardly a task that the clinician should recommend as being therapeutic for a patient with low back pain. Of course, we are not sure that this organic, undiagnosed spine pain is due to disc disease, but assuming that it is, we consider sit-ups to be contraindicated in patients with acute or subacute lumbar spine pain and probably not advisable as part of an exercise program for people over 40 years of age.[c]

Treatment. The exercises are shown in Figure 6-26. They are usually prescribed in conjunction with other forms of physical therapy, such as heat and massage. The exercise program is more commonly used in the subacute and chronic low back pain syndromes.

Results. We are not aware of studies that specifically evaluate William's exercises. There is a considerable traditional enthusiasm for them, however. They have come to be the nucleus of most low back pain exercise programs in the U.S. It is suggested that the program be updated to eliminate back extension exercises and encourage isometric abdominal exercises.

Complications. There do not appear to be any documented examples of complications related to the use of William's exercises. However, based on the studies of Nachemson and subjective patient reports, it is suspected that certain exercises can be very painful and irritating in the acute and subacute phases of low back pain and sciatica.[111] We also hypothesize that the loads that are created on the discs by sit-ups can be expected to contribute to degeneration and failure of annular fibers.

Comment. These exercises are based upon the assumption that achieving and maintaining a flexed lumbar spine is preferred. This has not been proven and is contrary to evidence of studies in vivo of intradiscal pressure and electromyographic activity.[3] The sit-up exercise is contraindicated in individuals with degenerative lumbar disc disease. The loads exerted on the lumbar spine while doing a sit-up are comparable to those caused by improperly lifting 44 lb (Fig. 6-27). Should the therapist treat a patient with lumbar spine pain and sciatica by having him lift weights in this manner? Of course not! However, the forces on the lumbar spine during sit-ups are practically the same.

Miscellaneous Exercises

These exercises may or may not include William's exercises. However, they involve a number of exercises to strengthen the trunk muscles.

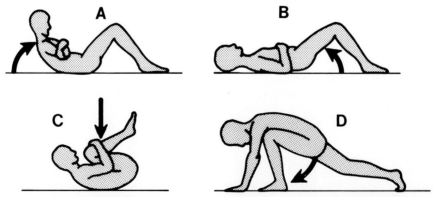

Fig. 6-26. The goal of these exercises is to attain a less extended and a more flexed position for the lumbar spine. Exercise A strengthens the abdominal muscles, which can increase flexion. Exercise B, the pelvic tilt, strengthens those muscles that rotate the pelvis (about the x-axis) so as to reduce lumbar extension. Exercise C is designed to stretch the posterior structures, which allows more flexion. Exercise D is designed to stretch the hip flexors, which, when tight, also contribute to an extended or lordotic position of the spine.

They are based on the general hypothesis that exercises are good and those that mobilize the spine and strengthen the back will allow a broader range of physiologic, pain-free function.

Treatment. Back extension exercises as well as range of motion exercises improve the range of flexion/extension, lateral bending, and axial rotation.

Results. The results of these programs are similar to those reported in general physical therapy programs. It is fair to say that approximately 60 to 70 per cent of patients improved with no demonstrated superiority over the numerous other forms of conservative treatment or no treatment at all.

Complications. Except for the discomfort and potential damage to the degenerating annular fibers associated with the large loads applied to the disc from back hyperextension exercises, there are no other complications associated with these exercises.[109]

Comment. We agree that exercises in general are good and that a gradual increase in the range of motion of a segment of the spine is desirable when the pain is not acute. Moreover, good muscle tone for the truncal and paraspinal muscles are desirable goals. We suggest that like sit-ups, hyperextension spine exercises should be avoided or prescribed only in a select group of patients, such as laborers or athletes who are not in the acute phase of spine pain and who must use their back muscles in an isotonic manner.

Isometric Truncal Exercises

The rationale for this form of treatment is based on several different observations. The load bearing capacity of the lumbar vertebrae in vitro is significantly less than the load bearing capacity in vivo;[8] a schematic analysis of the mechanics of the spine during lifting shows that the position and rigidity of an air- and fluid-filled column can efficiently and effectively reduce the weight on the lumbar spine.[143] It has been shown that the ability of a weight lifter to generate large thoracic and abdominal pressures is correlated with the amount of weight that can be lifted.[35,36] This is the evidence that demonstrates the role of the trunk in the stability of the spine. The use of exercises to develop truncal muscles is thought to aid in reducing the loads on the painful spine. Pain

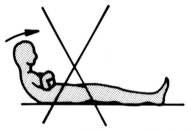

Fig. 6-27. Sit-ups with legs straight should not be prescribed for patients with low back pain. The loads to which the L3 disc is subjected during this activity are comparable to those associated with lifting 20 kg (44 lb) improperly, without bending the knees (see Table 6-6).

of any etiology or mechanism may be helped by reducing the stresses on the spine.

Truncal (abdominal and thoracic) muscle tone is of considerable importance in protecting the spine from the loads that are applied to it, especially when lifting. They also help to maintain the lumbar spine in the less lordotic, more therapeutic flat back position (Fig. 6-28). Intra-abdom-

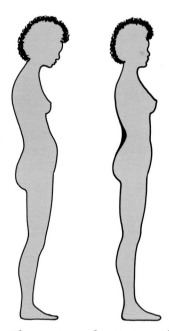

Fig. 6-28. The posture of patients with a lordotic spine (*left*) is associated with posterior bulging of the disc and also with greater intradiscal pressure. Both factors are reduced considerably by correct posture (*right*), which is maintained by good abdominal musculature, also of therapeutic value.

inal and thoracic cage pressure are important factors in providing strength and mechanical stability to the spine. We have suggested that this situation is somewhat analogous to a football in the abdomen (Fig. 6-29). The abdominal and thoracic air and fluid contents are compressed, creating turgor in the soft tissues and providing support. Thus it is suggested that these muscles be successfully toned and conditioned by isometric exercises.

Treatment. The isometric truncal exercises are done as follows. The patient is told to inhale normally, to close the windpipe and the rectal and urinary sphincters tightly, and to push hard with the trunk and abdominal muscles. In other words, the patient should push against the windpipe as though blowing up a hard balloon and push against the closed rectal sphincter as though constipated. The idea is to have the patient maximally compress the thoracic and abdominal contents against a closed glottis and perineal sphinc-ters with all available truncal musculature. This should be done at least 10 to 15 times, holding the contraction for 3 to 5 seconds, 3 to 4 times per day. Because of the ergonomic relevance of proper lifting, it has been suggested that quadriceps exercises be included in the exercise therapy for low back pain.[109]

Results. A double-blind study compared back extension exercises (strengthening paravertebral extensor muscles), mobilizing exercises (mainly involving flexion), and *isometric abdominal exercises*. There was a distinct and statistically significant superiority in the patients treated with the isometric abdominal exercise program.[85]

In another study, conventional physical therapy (i.e., heat, massage, extension and flexion exercises) was compared with a program that involved isometric abdominal exercises and axial pelvic traction. There was also a control group that received only heat treatment. Patients who were treated with isometric abdominal exercises

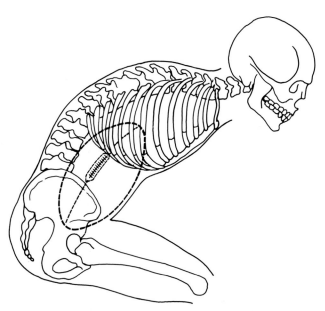

Fig. 6-29. The football shown here within the body cavities is analogous to the turgor created in the abdominal, pelvic, and thoracic cavities through the compression of fluid viscera and air by contraction of the truncal muscles, primarily the abdominals. (White, A. A., Southwick, W.O., Panjabi, M. M., and Johnson, R. M.: Practical biomechanics of the spine for orthopaedic surgeons (Chapter 4). *In* Instructional Course Lectures, American Academy of Orthopaedic Surgeons. St. Louis, C. V. Mosby, 1974.)

with traction did statistically significantly better than the other two groups.[91]

Based on the preceding studies as well as others examining the biomechanical functions of the spine, it is to be expected that the isometric abdominal exercises offer considerable support to the spine with minimal negative risks.[109,111]

Complications. The potential problems with this treatment are related to Valsalva's maneuver. If the patient is still in the acute phase of symptoms due to nerve root irritation, the exercise may cause considerable pain. The more important complication may occur in an individual with heart disease. In this situation, the alteration in pulmonary and myocardial circulatory dynamics associated with Valsalva's maneuver may cause myocardial ischemia. Thus, the exercise should be avoided in patients with heart disease. Such patients may have to use a well fitted thoraco-abdominal corset or some other spinal orthosis with an abdominal support.

Comment. For patients who can tolerate it, we believe that this is the best exercise for lumbar or thoracic spine pain, without true sciatica. There is considerable evidence of the role of the truncal musculature in protecting and assisting the spine in heavy lifting.[28,35] We hypothesize that that same role is crucial in protecting and improving the diseased symptomatic spine. As can be seen in Figure 6-28, the exercise also has the effect of placing the spine in a less lordotic position. Although there is controversy about the lordotic position as a cause of back pain and disc degeneration, it is true that the flat position is generally more comfortable and associated with about one half as much intradiscal pressure as is found in the lordotic position.[107]

Physical Therapy

This section includes an evaluation of massage and the various physical modalities of heat application.

There are several rationales that are used as the basis of these therapeutic modalities. Massage and heat application are soothing and relaxing, which makes the patient feel better and may have value in breaking up the cycle of muscle spasm, pain, and muscle spasm by alleviating the muscle spasm. Based on the "gate" control theory of pain

(see p. 278), it may also be suggested that sensory input from the heat and massage somehow plays a blocking or inhibitory role in the transmission of pain sensations. There is also the hypothesis that the heat is transmitted to the deep tissues and provides a curative function. Finally, physical therapy may be used for whatever placebo effect it can deliver.

Treatment. There is considerable work that has been done on the technology of massage and the various instrumentation that is employed to deliver heat. Such a discussion is not included here. The patients are generally given a few minutes of heat treatment and/or massage 1 to 5 times per week, for 1 or more weeks.

Results. The results of these treatments do not differ from the various other forms of nonsurgical therapy.

Complications. These are limited to the risks of skin burns from heat therapy of too high intensity and duration and any social complications that might result from massage.

Comment. Massage and heat application constitute a low risk form of therapy that satisfies the need on the part of physician and patient to treat and be treated. This is a fairly expensive emotional exercise that is worth avoiding if the patient can understand and tolerate a program of rest, isometric abdominal exercise, and education.

Basic Patient Education and Group Therapy Programs

Based on the hypothesis that in most instances the natural history of the disease is one of a satisfactory recovery for the patient, a treatment of "wait and see" is justified. Moreover, the results of virtually all forms of conservative therapy are the same. However, there is an implied or expressed demand by the patient that something be done. There are a number of practical, reliable "tips" that the knowledgeable patient can take advantage of to reduce the pain and improve the quality of life while getting well. Finally, there is the positive reinforcement, understanding, and sympathy that one can receive from a group of fellow sufferers. Put all of these facts together, and they constitute the rationale for a spine pain school. These have been in operation in Sweden for several years now.[111] Some similar ideas have been instituted in the U.S., with relatively more emphasis on the group dynamics. These have been used for patients in whom surgery is not thought to be of value.[104]

Treatment. The program in Sweden is called the Low Back School. The goals are to create self-confidence so that the patient may most effectively adjust to and manage the back condition; to avoid excess or potentially harmful treatment; and to decrease expenses.

The program consists of four 1-hour sessions, which are essentially teaching demonstrations. The patients are also given an exercise program as shown in Figure 6-30.[c] The course material is outlined below.

**Low Back School for Patients
(Course Outline)**

I   Anatomy and function of spine back pain
        Cause, incidence, treatment effects
II Biomechanics of spine
        Effects of various activities on intradiscal pressure
        Importance of decreasing loads on back
III Ergonomics and practical application
        Individual advise about working, resting, and other
            activities;
        Teaching isometric abdominal and back exercises
IV Repetition, synopsis and test
        Instilling self-confidence; encouraging sports and
            other activities

The program in the U.S. involved teaching and encouragement of exercises, activities, and weight loss when necessary, with social facilitation to achieve these goals. There are a number of useful booklets and "handouts" that are available to give to patients. Listed on p. 335 are some "tips" that, based on experience and current information, in our judgment are worthy of consideration.

Results. The Low Back School program has been shown, through a well designed and controlled investigation, to be superior to a placebo and moderately better than physical therapy. The patients treated in Low Back School reported less frequent absence from work than those treated with physical therapy. The physical therapy program, which consists mainly of manual therapy,

was also found to be more effective than a placebo.[9a]

Complications.   None were reported.

Comment.   Because of the large number of patients that are afflicted with spine pain, continuously increasing medical costs, the psychological overlay, and other considerations, this seems to be an approach worthy of consideration and trial.

Axial Traction

Continuous and intermittent traction has been used for treatment of spine pain. There are a number of hypothesized mechanisms through which axial (y-axis) traction is thought to offer some therapeutic benefit. Most of these mechanisms are listed below. It is probably true that none of these theories have been proven or have substantial evidence to support them.

**Some Theoretical Bases for Therapeutic
Mechanism of Pain Relief With Spinal Traction**

Enlargement of intervertebral foramen
Opening up of the intervertebral disc space
Separation of intervertebral joints
Stretching a tight or painful capsule
Release of entrapped synovial membrane
Freeing of adherent nerve roots
Production of central vaccum to reduce herniated disc
Production of posterior longitudinal ligament tension to
    reduce herniated disc
Relaxation of muscle spasm

Treatment.   Some of the various techniques and schedules for the application of cervical and lumbar traction are discussed, with information about their effectiveness.

There is considerable disagreement in the literature about the technique, degree and duration of traction that should be applied to the spinal column. The duration of traction recommended varies from 4 minutes to 1 hour. In the cervical spine the range of suggested forces is from 25 to 300 lb. Straight, axial traction is applied with the patient either supine or sitting. Varying degrees (0–30°) of neck flexion have also been employed.[23] In the lumbar spine the recommended forces range from 40 to 730 lb![22]

A traction weight of 30 lb for 7 seconds produces posterior separation of the cervical verte-brae. This appears to be the least weight and duration that effectively separate the vertebrae. Greater time causes additional discomfort with-out any significant increment of mechanical change. An increase in force to 50 lb increases the separation between vertebrae.[24] The greater the angle of neck flexion, the greater is the posterior elongation, and therefore the greater is the open-ing of the intervertebral foramen.[25] The greatest separation of the cervical vertebrae occurs at a flexion angle of 24 degrees. The amount of sepa-ration achieved with this degree of flexion is essentially as good with only 30 lb of traction as the separation obtained with 50 lb of traction without any flexion. The mechanical effects of traction are short-lived. It has been shown that with more than adequate cervical trac-tion techniques (25 minutes, 30 lb) there is no significant residual intervertebral foramen sepa-ration 20 minutes after completion of traction.[24]

Studies of the effects of traction on normal cervical spines showed that the axial stiffness of the spine in vivo was such that separation of the vertebrae was possible with an axial load of one-third of body weight. The range of separation observed was 1 to 2 mm.[128] This much displace-ment could separate the joint space, open the neural foramen, and conceivably result in several other theoretical conditions listed on page 310.

The problem of body-bed frictional resistance in the dissipation of traction forces is well eluci-dated in the work of Judovich.[74] His work is based on the study of one cadaver and three nor-mal subjects. By measurements before and after cutting through the cadaver at the L3–L4 inter-space, he was able to establish that the frictional resistance of the lower half of the body was about 26 per cent of body weight. Therefore, in order to apply traction to the lumbar spine, one must first overcome the *frictional resistance* of the lower body segment. Any traction force above this is then applied to the spine for whatever therapeu-tic benefit it can deliver. This problem of body friction may be overcome by adding the extra 26 per cent body weight or by a split bed-mattress technique, with wheels on the lower segment to reduce friction, or by vertical application of the traction. With vertical traction, the lower body

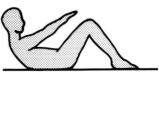

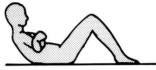

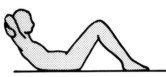

Fig. 6-30. The exercises shown here have been sug-gested as a method of strengthening the abdominal muscles. Note that the feet are always kept flat on the floor. The three exercises increase in difficulty from top to bottom. Greater abdominal muscle forces are required in the bottom exercises, as compared to the other two, because in this exercise the center of gravity of the upper body, due to the rearward posi-tion of the arms, is farthest away from the axis of motion. These exercises are done slowly and with the head raised initially, followed by a type of curling up of the upper trunk.

segment would, of course, add its own weight in traction force rather than dissipate the traction force through frictional resistance. Lehmann and Brunner described a hydraulically powered de-vice that delivered sufficient traction to the lum-bar spine to achieve separation of vertebrae along the y-axis. The force required, about 300 lb, was associated with "uncomfortable stretch." More-over, the mechanical effects were found to last only a short time after treatment.[90]

Lawson and Godfrey studied spinal traction and concluded that as much as 100 lb of cervical traction or 150 lb of lumbar traction resulted in no significant y-axis separation of the vertebrae. There was, according to these investigations, a slight temporary increase in height presumably due to a loss of cervical lordosis.[89]

However, other investigators showed that with the use of a split traction table and the hips flexed

70 degrees with the lower legs parallel to the floor, significant separation of the posterior elements of the lumbar vertebrae could be achieved with 50 lb. A weight of 100 lb significantly increased the vertebral separation more than that achieved by the 50-lb weight. The greatest separation occurred at the L4–5 and L5–S1 interspaces.

Results.   In a study of 212 patients with a variety of symptoms thought to be related to the cervical spine, it was found that patients with the symptoms most likely related to nerve root irritation benefited most from cervical traction.[144] In this group, 68 per cent of the patients were improved. The treatment consisted of heat and massage plus 3 to 13 kg of axial traction in slight flexion (sometimes intermittent motorized traction) 3 times per week for 4 weeks. Because the "nerve root" symptoms were relived better than were the other symptoms, it was thought that the study supported the hypothesis that the intervertebral foramina are enlarged by traction. It is extremely difficult to evaluate this series. We note that the cure rate is in the familiar range of 60 to 70 per cent, which makes it difficult to distinguish from placebo administration, the natural history of the disease, and most other forms of therapy.

Christie reported on the preliminary results of a study that compared the effects of traction with an oral placebo medication in acute and chronic low back pain with and without sciatica. There was no meaningful difference in the results of the two treatments.[20] Hood and Chrisman reported that 52.5 per cent showed good and excellent results with intermittent pelvic traction for lumbar disc disease.

Complications.   There have been complications associated with the use of axial traction. Eie and Kristiansen reported that about 33 per cent of a group of patients whom they were treating for lumbar spine pain had distinct aggravation of symptoms.[35] The major risk is neurologic damage secondary to overloading the spine beyond its tolerance limits.[48]

Comment.   It does not appear that axial traction is a superior modality for the treatment of spine pain. There is no convincing data to support a contention that the benefits are related to anything other than the improvement expected in time with the natural course of the disease or many other treatments.

Axial traction has been shown, at least temporarily, to separate either cervical or lumbar vertebrae. It can also reduce lumbar spine intradiscal pressure. There is no evidence that these changes are therapeutic or that this technique of treating spine pain with or without nerve root irritation is superior to any other. We note that it has certain associated risks. However, in patients who are not responding to other nonsurgical treatments, axial traction may be given a trial. The justification for this suggestion is based on the fact that axial traction is capable of at least temporarily altering the mechanics of the spine, such as with the Type IV or V disc pathology discussed on page 287. Should the pain happen to be emanating from a structure that can be altered by manipulation, there may be some benefit. As a therapeutic trial, we recommend two or three treatments per week for 2 to 3 weeks using the appropriate technical factors necessary to separate the vertebrae in the painful region of the spine.

Some investigators have expressed the opinion that traction should not be used if the patient is diagnosed as having a fully sequestered disc with sciatica.[18] However, the report of Hood and Chrisman showed that some patients with true sciatica improved with axial traction.[69] They have suggested that the position of neural encroachment upon the axilla of the nerve root may be a factor. If the impingement is in the axilla of the root, the patient tends to list to the side of the sciatica.[43] Such a patient may become worse with axial traction. The patient who leans away from the painful leg may show encroachment laterally and may achieve a beneficial result with axial traction (Fig. 6-31).

Spinal Manipulation

As part of the U.S. Senate Report on the Fiscal Year 1974, Appropriation for the National Institute of Neurological Diseases and Stroke (NINDS) of the National Institute of Health, there was a specification that ". . . this would be an opportune time for an 'independent, unbiased' study of the fundamentals of the chiropractic profession. Such studies should be high among the priorities of the NINDS . . ." In February, 1975, NINDS sponsored a workshop on "The Research Status of Spinal Manipulative Therapy."[54]

The following salient points are taken from the editor's summary of the workshop. There was no quantitative or qualitative reproducible description of "subluxation" either mechanically or anatomically. The concept of chiropractic subluxation remains a hypothesis yet to be evaluated experimentally. We believe that this has been one of the most frustrating aspects of certain views of the pathology that is purported to be altered with spinal manipulative therapy. When one is correcting a "subluxation" that cannot be perceived by independent scientific observers, it is difficult to convince those observers that the treatment is effective.

Spinal manipulation is one of the most controversial but frequently used methods of treating spine pain. The controversy is charged with no small degree of emotion or bias. We claim no unique monopoly on objectivity. Nevertheless, the attempt here is to present a synopsis of the current status of spinal manipulative therapy as related to spine pain and to offer some comments on the subject. Because of its controversial nature, popularity among lay people, and obvious biomechanical relevance, it is discussed in some detail.

There are a large number of maneuvers that may be employed in the manipulation of the spine.[99,114a] However, regardless of what the external manipulation may be, the movement of a vertebra is limited to the combinations possible with six degrees of freedom. Several of the best known and most used manipulations follow The simplest one is the manual application of forces directly to the spinous processes and posterior elements of a given vertebra. These structures may be loaded and displaced along the +z-axis, the ±x-axis, the ±y-axis, and along various combinations of these (Fig. 6-32). In addition to this, through indirect means (manipulation of the head) the cervical spine may undergo various motions, including flexion/extension, lateral bending, axial rotation, and a variety of combinations. It does not matter whether the displacement results from the direct forces applied to the spinous processes (Fig. 6-32), or through forces

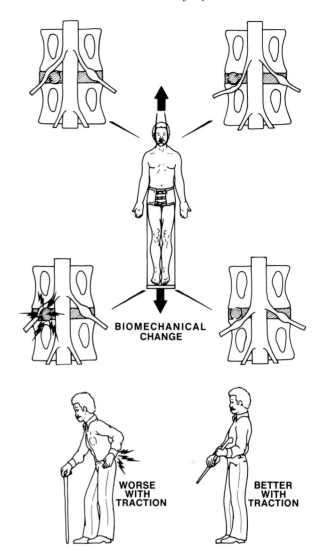

Fig. 6-31. This is a hypothetical explanation of why some patients may respond well to traction, while others may respond with more pain. When the disc is in the axilla of the nerve root, axial traction may irritate the problem. A correlation of this with Figure 6-18 shows that the patient that lists to the side of the sciatica is likely to be made worse by traction. Conversely, one who lists to the side away from the sciatica is likely to be made better by traction. A biomechanical explanation for this is offered. The traction produces bending, which converts the lumbar spine from its physiological lordotic posture to a more straight or flexed position. When this occurs, there is a relative displacement of the neural elements in the caudal direction. This results in either impingement by the herniated disc (*left*) or release of disc impingement (*right*).

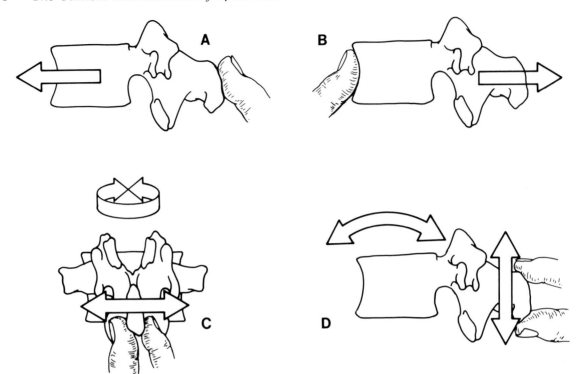

Fig. 6-32. These are all of the possible direct forces (except for skin interposition) that may be applied for the purpose of manipulating the spine. The various motions and some of the major associated coupled motions are shown. In the clinical situation the forces are not applied as shown here. However, it is possible to produce them with manipulation. (A) Direct +z-axis motion on the spinous process gives a forward translation (+z-axis). Since the spinous processes are just below the skin, this manipulation is possible in all regions of the spine. In the thoracic spine there may be x-axis rotation in addition to the z-axis translation. (B) Direct −z-axis motion can be achieved in the lower cervical spine by direct force application. When the neck is relaxed it is possible to palpate the anterior cervical spine, just anteromedial and deep to the carotid sheath. (C) The spinous processes may be directly manipulated in all regions of the spine, resulting in ±y-axis rotation and in the appropriate regions (cervical and upper thoracic) some amount of coupled ±z-axis rotation. (D) Here the spinous processes are manipulated in the sagittal plane in the ±y-axis direction. This results in ±x-axis rotation. These are the major motions that are possible with direct manipulation. It has not yet been determined whether or not these motions and forces are therapeutic.

applied by transmission through the ligaments and articulations of adjacent vertebrae (Fig. 6-33). The other variables available to the therapist are the rate of application of the forces and the magnitude of the forces. Of all the possible manipulations, those that appear to receive the most attention, at least in the medical profession, involve axial rotation.

What does manipulation do to the spine? From a study of the kinematics and physical properties of the spine, the basic constraints and patterns of motion of the spine are apparent. In Chapter 4

disruption of these patterns is shown to result in injuries when the normal tolerances of force or motion are surpassed. In order for spinal manipulation not to be harmful, it must not exceed certain tolerances, either in the normal or the diseased spine. In order for manipulations to be successful, they must somehow produce improvement using mechanical alteration, either directly or as a therapeutic stimulus to the diseased spine.

A more precise look at some structures that may be moved, stretched, stimulated, or relaxed by manipulation is necessary. Axial rotation is an

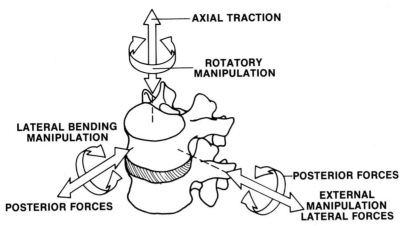

Fig. 6-33. It is possible to achieve motion along all six degrees of freedom in the clinical situation through transmission of forces to the vertebra by indirect methods of manipulation. All of the various motions may be achieved clinically by applying the appropriate forces. The rate and magnitude of the different forces may be varied. It should be kept in mind that no matter how complex or varied the external manipulation techniques, ultimately the vertebra is loaded and displaced according to some combination of these six degrees of freedom. The mechanism of their therapeutic benefit remains unknown. (Rotatory manipulation and posterior forces are illustrated in Figures 6-34 and 6-35.)

effective means of applying tensile forces to the fibers of the annulus fibrosus of the disc. Various bending modalities are capable of applying tension to the annulus fibrosus and other ligamentous structures, as well as altering a bulge in the disc. The anterior and posterior longitudinal ligaments, both of which are innervated with sensory fibers, can be effectively moved by rotation about all three traditional planes of movement. This is also true of the yellow ligaments and the various interspinous and the transverse ligaments. The importance of the fact that the intervertebral articulations are true synovial joints has been emphasized. Axial rotation effects considerable movement and displacement of these joints in the cervical and lumbar spine and a fair amount of impingement and force application in the lumbar spine (see Figs. 1-25, 2-24). The impingement forces are taken by deformation of the cartilage, the facets, and also displacement between the vertebral bodies anteriorly. There is a possibility that a synovial fold or some intra-articular material may be altered. Changes in the mechanical status may alleviate or eliminate any associated synovial inflammation.

The theories that relief of nerve pressure may result from such limited possibilities of displacement does not fit well with present knowledge. There is no reason to assume that manipulation and displacement of a motion segment through a normal range of motion can significantly move structures in or out of the intervertebral foramen.[B] This hypothesis has been studied in an experiment employing newborn cadaver material designed specifically to answer this question. The evidence from this study showed that this mechanism of nerve decompression is unlikely.[27] The work of Sunderland on adult anatomy tends to collaborate Crelin's findings in the newborn. Sunderland also warned against concentrating exclusively on the intervertebral foramen as the site of the pathological mechanism.[139] The importance of the posterior vertebral joints and ligaments as potential sources of neurovascular bundle entrapment must also be considered.

Treatment.   Treatments involve a number of manipulations, the details of which are available in the literature.[99,114a] The process may be repeated 1 to 5 times per week. Sometimes, manipulations are carried out under anesthesia. Prob-

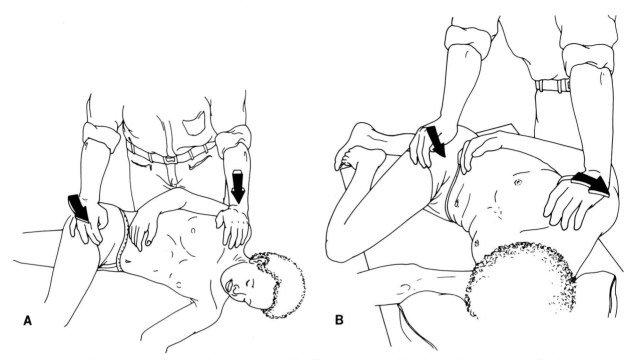

Fig. 6-34. This particular manipulation designed for the thoracic and lumbar spine appears to be the one most frequently employed by medical scientists. (*A*) This shows the technique from the frontal view. The major thrust comes from the therapist's right hand, rotating the pelvis forward and indirectly applying an axial torque (about the −y-axis) to the thoracic and lumbar spine. The left hand is used to sturdy the thorax by taking up the reaction forces. (*B*) This shows the same manipulation from a different vantage point to emphasize the axial torque that is applied. Nothing is known about the magnitude of the torques exerted on the spine, the motion imparted, or the changes (therapeutic or otherwise) that may be associated. The axial manipulation of the cervical spine is done through the application of y-axis rotations of the head.

ably, the most frequently employed manipulation is the axial torque of the cervical or the lumbar spine, shown in Figure 6-34. It is reasonable to assume that these manipulations can at least temporarily effect axial rotatory displacement of the cervical or thoracic spine. Direct manipulation is shown in Figure 6-35.

It has been pointed out in controlled experiments that sustained mechanical forces on axons or nerve trunks block rather than excite. This is the situation for transversely applied compressive forces as well as for longitudinally applied tensile forces. Transient, rapidly applied forces cause excitation.[120] If, indeed, the pathologic conditions exist at the nerve root level, then the relief of the compression or stretch by manipulation should not be expected to relieve the pain. This information does not rule out the possibility that some other mechanism may be possible for

the relief of back pain with spinal manipulation. It may be that there is associated inflammation, vascular engorgement, or chemical irritation of dural or ligamentous receptors that produces the pain. It is probably fair and accurate to indicate that at present there is no appealing substantial theory to explain the mechanism through which spinal manipulative therapy relieves pain, if in fact it does.

Results. Do manipulations help? As is the case with just about any form of treatment of spine pain, there is no well documented clinical evidence that manipulation alters the natural course of the disease. Also similar to other therapeutic modalities, there is enthusiastic anecdotal evidence from patients and highly optimistic reports from therapists. There is *absolutely* no data that substantiates a direct relationship between manipulative therapy and clinical improvement of *visceral disease* through the improvement of segmental neural interactions. There is considerable controversy over the question of the efficacy of spinal manipulative therapy in the treatment of pain, particularly low back pain and neck pain. The following is a review of some of the major studies related to the question of whether or not spinal manipulations help patients with spine pain.

Chrisman investigated 39 patients with herniated intervertebral discs who had myelograms before and after rotatory (axial) manipulation of the lumbar spine under general anesthesia. The patients had been previously treated with conservative therapy. About half of the patients (51%) had good or excellent results after the manipulation. The myelograms, whether initially positive or negative, were unchanged after manipulation. Although some of the patients with positive myelograms were good or excellent 3 years after manipulation, in general, the patients without positive myelograms did better with manipulations than those with positive studies.[19] These findings are the same as those of Mensor, who had a 51.2 per cent success with rotatory manipulation under anesthesia.[102] Chrisman recommended a pre-manipulation myelogram to avoid the dangers of manipulating a patient with a large herniated disc.

There are other studies in the literature that report that manipulative therapy is used for spine pain. One of these shows statistically significant evidence that this treatment is better than other nonoperative therapy. Coyen and Curwin compared 152 patients with acute low back pain randomly selected for treatment either with manipulation or with bed rest and analgesics. In the group that were manipulated, 50 per cent were symptom-free in one week and 87 per cent in 3 weeks. In the group that received analgesics, respective figures were 27 per cent and 60 per cent. However, the investigators stated that their figures were inadequate for statistical analysis.[26] In a randomized study, rotational manipulation was compared with de-tuned (simulated) short wave diathermy as a placebo. The patients were evaluated 15 minutes, 3 days, and 7 days after treatment. Both groups of patients were markedly improved; but for one factor, there was no de-

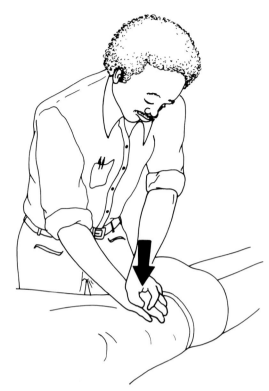

Fig. 6-35. This shows a frequently employed direct manipulation of the spine, which may be applied in either the thoracic or the lumbar region. As shown in Figure 6-32, it may result in ±z-axis translation and ±x-axis rotation.

monstrable difference between the two groups; the manipulated patients were better 15 minutes after treatment. It is also of interest that by subjective self-assessment, the patients in both the *placebo* and manipulated groups rated themselves as 70 to 93 per cent improved.[53]

Doran and Newell carried out a prospective, "blind" study to compare the efficacy of four different types of treatment. In this study 456 patients were randomly subdivided into four groups, according to the following treatments: manipulation, physiotherapy, a corset, or analgesic tablets. The patients were evaluated after 3 weeks, 3 months, and 1 year. There were never any important differences among the four treatment groups. However, as noted in other studies, *some* of the patients responded well and quickly to spinal manipulation.[32]

The work of Kane and colleagues is focal to the

question, does "manipulation" help? This study reviews 122 patients treated by chiropractors for back or spine problems and 110 patients treated by physicians for the same type of diseases.[75] With regard to patient perception of improvement and patient satisfaction, the chiropractors were at least as effective as the physicians. The two groups of patients were not significantly different with respect to demographic and socioeconomic factors, hypochondriosis, or their attitudes toward the medical profession. It was found that the patients treated by chiropractors responded more favorably to the personality of their practitioners. This was thought to be due to the fact that chiropractors seemed unhurried, sympathetic, communicated well with the patients, and treated them in an egalitarian relationship. These humanitarian considerations are important in all aspects of patient care, but they are especially crucial in the area of spine pain because the objective information is so meager and the subjective factors are so important.

Nachemson, pursuant to a thorough review of the literature, indicated that there is no clinically significant proof that manipulation for acute or subacute low back pain is superior to bed rest and salicylates.[108]

There is an important study by Edwards in which spinal manipulative therapy involved 184 patients who were divided in the following manner (Table 6-2).

The 46 patients in each of the groups were divided into those to be treated with heat massage and exercise and those to be treated with spinal manipulation. The salient results are reproduced in Table 6-3.

In Group I, the results were acceptable in 82.5 per cent for both treatments. However, they were achieved with spinal manipulation using about one-half the number of treatments that were needed for heat, massage, and exercise. In Group II, the results were slightly better with manipulation, and again they were achieved with about half as many treatments. In Groups III and IV, the manipulation therapy was statistically significantly better, and in Group IV, the results with manipulation were achieved with half as many treatments. If all groups are combined, the manipulative therapy is significantly better. This study certainly supports the efficacy of spinal

Table 6-2. Subject Groupings of Patients in Edwards' Study of Spinal Manipulative Therapy

GROUP	TYPE OF PAIN	TREATMENT
I (46 pts.)	Central low back pain only	23 HME* 23 Manipulation
II (46 pts.)	Radiation to one buttock	23 HME 23 Manipulation
III (46 pts.)	Radiation down back of thigh to knee	23 HME 23 Manipulation
IV (46 pts.)	Radiation down posterior leg to foot	23 HME 23 Manipulation

* HME = Heat, massage, and exercise.

manipulative therapy in comparison with heat, massage, and exercise. The results (80–95% satisfactory) are impressive in comparison with any form of therapy.

We suggest that the question is still unanswered. There is evidence that the use of spinal manipulation is beneficial for treating spine pain with or without sciatica. Its use in the treatment of other diseases, in our opinion, is *totally* fallacious.

Complications. Do manipulations harm the patient? The answer is yes, sometimes. There are some reported cases in the literature in which neurological damage was associated with spinal manipulation.[121,141] Poppen described four cases in which patients experienced paraplegia or cauda equina syndrome following manipulation. Two of the patients were manipulated by osteopaths and the other two by orthopaedic surgeons.[121]

Fisher reported a case of the precipitation of a large, midline L5 disc herniation, which occurred following manipulation of the low back by a chiropractor. The patient developed the clinical neurologic signs and symptoms of cauda equina tumor. The disc herniation was noted at the time of surgery and removed. The neurologic recovery was complete.[44]

Pratt-Thomas and Bergen reported two fatal cases of cerebellar hemorrhage and one fatal case of spinal cord injury following chiropractic manipulation.[120] Two additional patients suffered nonfatal vascular accidents following chiropractic manipulation of the cervical spine. One possible mechanism of vascular damage associated with

Table 6-3. Results of Edward's Study of Spinal Manipulative Therapy*

Group	Treatment	Total No. of Patients	Average No. of Treatments	Acceptable Results	
				No. of Patients	Percentage
I	H.M.E.†	23	9.7	19	82.5
	M.M.‡	23	4.8	19	82.5
II	H.M.E.	23	10.2	16	69.5
	M.M.	23	4.3	18	78.1
III	H.M.E.	23	8.5	15	65.2
	M.M.	23	6.2	22	95.7
IV	H.M.E.	23	13.3	12	51.7
	M.M.	23	6.4	18	78.5

* Edwards, B. C.: Low back pain and pain resulting from lumbar spine conditions: a comparison of treatment results. Aust. J. Physiother., *15:*104, 1969.
† H.M.E. = Heat, massage, and exercise.
‡ M.M. = Mobilization and manipulation.

axial torsion of the cervical spine is shown on page 68. It appears that these manipulations involve the application of high magnitudes of torsional loads to the cervical spine.[56]

Comment. As with other treatment modalities, there is the basic problem of demonstrating the effectiveness of spinal manipulative therapy over the improvement with a placebo that occurs in 33 per cent of patients and the improvement that occurs in the natural course of disease in 60 to 70 per cent. We suggest that additional patho-anatomical and biomechanical studies of the spine, including mathematical modeling, may provide a sound hypothetical basis for the mechanism of some types of spine pain. In addition, the development of theories explaining the therapeutic effects of manipulation is needed. The value of the therapy will have to be demonstrated by well designed prospective clinical studies. Spinal manipulation seems to be about as effective as most other treatments. There is a recurrent observation that on a short-term basis, a number of patients, usually by their own subjective reporting and sometimes based on a physician's evaluation, seem to do better with spinal manipulative therapy than with other forms of nonsurgical treatment. We must, however, keep in mind the risks of complications.

There remains the practical question of whether or not spinal manipulative therapy is to be recommended as a nonsurgical treatment for low back pain and sciatica. Present knowledge indicates that the risk-benefit factors are such that spinal manipulation that is not too vigorous is a justified, alternative, nonsurgical treatment. Prolonged, expensive, repeated manipulations that offer only brief, transient improvement do not make the best use of the patient's resources.

Orthotic Devices

The practical expectations and biomechanical aspects of orthotic devices are presented in Chapter 7. The rationale for their use in the treatment of spine pain is based on immobilization and abdominal support. Immobilization is for purposes of splinting, supporting, and resting the spine to reduce mechanical irritation and muscle spasm. The abdominal support assists in the development of adequate intratruncal pressures to support the spine. This may be done with certain braces, a corset, or a plaster cast. The mechanism of this support is described on page 353.

The results of orthotic treatment for spine pain have not been documented in the literature. With the use of a plaster cast, physicians should be on the lookout for the possible complication of superior mesenteric artery syndrome. Otherwise, there are no significant complications. There does not seem to be any major problem of muscle atrophy or weakness associated with the use of spinal braces.

In acute situations where there is poor abdominal muscle development, especially in the older age-groups, we recommend the use of an abdominal corset. Other physicians have employed a plaster body jacket with the patient in slight flexion. This is based on the desire to achieve abdominal compression and the undocumented assumption that flexion is good. For the more chronic conditions in which the possibility of development or redevelopment of good muscle tone is not feasible or cannot be expected, it is advisable to employ a spinal orthosis with an abdominal support (see Fig. 7-23).

Local and Regional Use of Drugs

The epidural injection of locally acting corticosteroids and Novocain has been employed in the treatment of spine pain with or without associated radiculopathy. Novocain is administered to control the immediate pain due to the procedure and also to break up any cycle in which a regional irritant is causing extensive muscle spasm. Cortisone is also at times injected into the intervertebral disc to reduce inflammation in and about the nerve root from any of several possible causes.[41]

The combination of Novocain with cortisone injections of the posterior elements (synovial joints) has been thought to be successful in tendons and joint compartments in other areas of the body; therefore it is also injected in the posterior intervertebral joints. These structures are well endowed with nerve supply and if inflamed may be expected to cause considerable pain.

Chemonucleolysis

This form of treatment, first proposed by Hirsch[61] is based on the assumption that lumbar spine pain and sciatica are caused by abnormalities of the nucleus pulposus. Chymopapain is a proteolytic enzyme that effects a rapid hydrolysis of the protein-mucopolysaccharide ground substance of disc material, mainly the nucleus pulposus.[52] The disc space is commonly narrowed

following injection of the material into the disc.[94,156] The intradiscal injection is given because the dissolution of the nucleus pulposus results in a relief of pain and nerve root irritation. The actual mechanism of pain relief is unknown.

Treatment. The technique has been well described by Brown and McCullough.[14,94] The patient rests on the side with hips and knees flexed. A needle is introduced into the diseased disc. A discogram is done to affirm the proper placement of the needle, and chymopapain is injected.

Results. Cervical spine chemonucleolysis has been done only rarely, and the reports are sparse. This discussion is limited to the treatment of lumbar discs. Macnab and colleagues reported on the use of chymopapain in 100 patients. The best results were in patients with positive myelograms whose major symptoms were pure sciatica of short duration. The overall success rate was 67 per cent.[95] A long-term follow-up series of 500 patients treated with chymopapain was reported by Wiltse and colleagues, and a similar study of 480 patients was reported by McCullough. In both groups 75 per cent had effective relief of symptoms.[94,156] In the review article by Watts, the range of satisfactory results using chymopapain in seven independent series was 49 to 75 per cent.[146] Higher incidences of satisfactory results were reported by Brown (82.5%), Orifine (83%), and Smith (90.7%).[14,116,133]

There have been studies in which chemonucleolysis was compared with surgical treatment of lumbar disc disease. In one study, 100 patients surgically managed prior to the availability of chymopapain were compared with an equal number of patients who had chemonucleolysis therapy. Chemonucleolysis resulted in a success rate of 74 per cent, while surgical treatment yielded a success rate of only 48 per cent.[114] Watts and colleagues compared the results in a group of 100 patients treated with chemonucleolysis with 174 patients who had undergone surgical disc removal. In the group of patients with a clinical picture compatible with a distinct posterolateral disc herniation including myelographic confirmation, chemonucleolysis gave better results than surgery. Satisfactory results were achieved 89 and 60 per cent, respectively. In the patients who had previous surgery and back pain with or without non-radicular leg pain, satisfactory results were achieved in 55 to 60 per cent with both types of treatment.[145]

The reports on the efficacy of the treatment of spine pain with chemonucleolysis may be summarized by saying that, with some exceptions, the results are not significantly better than with all of the other treatments of low back pain and sciatica. The patient who is most likely to show a good result with chemonucleolysis will probably also show a good result if treated surgically. In these carefully selected patients, there is suggestive evidence that chymopapain provides somewhat better results than surgery.

Complications. The major complications associated with chemonucleolysis are sensitivity reactions (some of which cause death), discitis, and arachnoiditis.[94,146] Experimental studies have shown that nerves exposed to chymopapain in clinically recommended concentrations for 2 hours may develop intraneural edema as an immediate result. With regard to long-term effects, investigators reported degeneration of nerve fibers, intraneural fibrosis, and impaired impulse transmission. Rydevik and Shealy also reported on neurotoxic characteristics of the drug.[121,131] Although there is other evidence attesting to the safety of the enzyme,[45,49,156] it is important to be aware of these observations.

Comment. There has been considerable controversy in the U.S. about the advisability of continuing clinical trials of chemonucleolysis and releasing the substance to a larger number of physicians. A prospective "double-blind" clinical study was carried out; the study compared chymopapain with a *placebo* that contained sodium iothalamate, cysteine hydrochloride, and ethylenediamine tetraacetic acid (EDTA). The results of the study showed that among the chymopapain-treated patients, the results were no better than among controls. Satisfactory results were noted in 60 and 50 per cent, respectively.[21] This study has been subjected to plausible criticism and deemed possibly invalid by Brown and Daroff.[15] They contend that the follow-up (code break) was too short, that there was an unreasonable dose limitation on chymopapain, and that since EDTA is an active ingredient, it could not have been an effective placebo control.

The usefulness of this drug is being further evaluated. The outcome is difficult to predict. Nevertheless, the evidence, experimental, radiographic, and clinical, shows that the enzyme is capable of significantly altering the disc. Clinical evidence suggests that it is at least as good and possibly better than a number of nonsurgical treatments. The risks and complications are not high as long as careful precautions are routinely taken for the treatment of anaphylaxis. The drug appears to have considerable potential. Its ultimate value will be determined by additional clinical investigations.

There is an interesting theoretical consideration about the use of the drug in the completely herniated disc. The problem is that intradiscally injected material may never reach a sequestered disc. Moreover, the material works primarily on the nucleus pulposus and not the highly collagenous annulus. McCulloch observed that a number of patients who clinically and myelographically were thought to have sequestered discs showed a successful result with chemonucleolysis.[94] It is possible that in some cases the disc is not truly sequestered and the material is able to reach the sequestration and to disintegrate the displaced annulus. This has been appreciated by Brown as well.[14] The therapeutic mechanism must be studied more extensively.

With the rather rapid narrowing of the intervertebral space that accompanies chemonucleolysis, there is an acute increase in the load bearing demands of the posterior articulations. This may result in some mechanical disruptions and back pain, especially in patients who have pre-existing facet joint disease. The same condition may occur following surgical removal of an intervertebral disc.

Disc Excision

Excision of all or part of the intervertebral disc is based on traditional surgical rationale. It is a diseased organ that is causing pain and disability to the patient, and it can be removed.

Treatment. There is some controversy about whether the disc or only the displaced fragment should be removed. In addition, there are questions about whether the disc removal should be done from the front or the back of the spine. And finally, there is the issue of whether or not the spine should be fused after removal of the disc. These considerations are discussed in Chapter 8. There are arguments to support all of these options and there is no definitive clinical or experimental evidence that supports one particular method.

Herniated fragment removal alone is thought to involve the least surgical trauma and to disrupt anatomy and function the least. The liability is that recurrent herniations at the same level are known to occur. We prefer removal of the offending disc, as it has already proven its ability to degenerate and herniate. The surgical approach is a matter of preference and practical considerations. In the cervical region the anterior approach is readily accessible and convenient. The thoracic disc should preferably be removed from an anterior approach, since the results with posterior removal are poor.[142] The posterior approach

in the lumbar spine is generally easier and associated with fewer complications than is the anterior approach. Spangfort found that for all age-groups the best result, success in approximately 90 per cent, was achieved in patients with complete herniation, followed by approximately 80 per cent in patients with incomplete herniation, and approximately 60 per cent in those with a bulging disc. This 60-per cent success rate is about the same as with most nonsurgical treatments. It is interesting to note that in those patients in whom there was no herniation found at surgery, the pain relief was about 35 per cent, the same as the placebo effect (Fig. 6-36). In the cervical spine we generally fuse at the time of disc excision (see Chapter 8). In the lumbar region arthrodesis is not required after single disc excision. Techniques and rationale for various decompressions and fusions are discussed in Chapter 8.

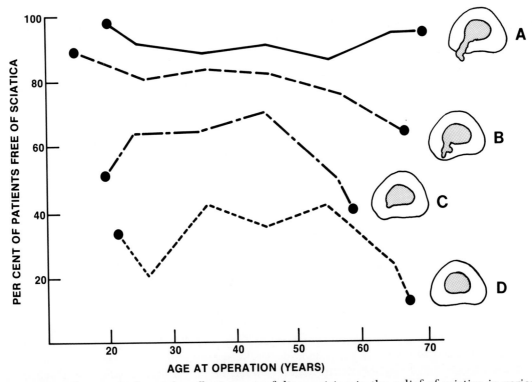

Fig. 6-36. This graph shows the effectiveness of disc excision in the relief of sciatica in various age-groups as a function of the actual pathology found at surgery. (*A*) Complete herniation; (*B*) incomplete herniation; (*C*) bulging disc; and (*D*) no herniation. (Modified from Spangfort, E. V.: The lumbar disc herniation. A computer-aided analysis of 2,504 operations. Acta Orthop. Scand., *142* [Suppl], 1972.)

Results. In the cervical spine, anterior disc removal with arthrodesis yields good or excellent results in 63 to 73 per cent of patients.[124,125,150,152] However, by selecting the patients in whom the myelographic defect corresponded to the level at which surgery was performed, the percentage of patients with good or excellent results is increased to 77 per cent in one series,[152] and to 91 per cent in another.[150] Here, as in the case of lumbar spine disease, the percentage of good results increased with more accurate selection of the distinctly herniated disc. Results comparable to the preceding groups (83% improved) have been reported with cervical disc disease treated with disc removal *without* fusion.[65]

The result of surgery for thoracic disc disease is generally not good.[136] This is due to the severity of the pathoanatomic disease process, the characteristic delay in diagnosis, and the relative lack of surgical experience in dealing with the problem. Patients without weakness, with a monoparesis or with absent or minimal sensory changes, generally show good to excellent results with surgery. Those with more severe neurologic deficit have a poor postoperative result.

The results with lumbar disc surgery have been carefully studied and have been shown to vary with the guidelines with which the patients are selected for the procedure. The trend noted in the cervical spine is distinctively demonstrated in the lumbar spine. If through a careful preoperative clinical evaluation the surgeon can select the patient with a complete herniation, the results with surgery are best.

Dunkerly operated on patients with a history and physical findings of disc disease, but without routine myelograms. The success rate among patients in that group was 75 per cent.[33]

Nachemson, in a comprehensive review of the literature, demonstrated convincingly the importance of a thorough preoperative evaluation in order to accurately diagnose a disc herniation.[111] Based on history and neurologic examination alone, a physician may expect to be correct 60 per cent of the time. If a positive straight leg raising test is observed preoperatively, a herniation is present 70 per cent of the time. Add a positive electromyogram to the evaluation, and the accuracy increases to 80 per cent. If, in addition to the preceding, there is also a positive *water soluble* contrast myelogram, the surgeon can expect to find a disc herniation in 90 per cent of patients (Fig. 6-37).

Complications. There are always the standard risks of medications, anesthesia, and blood transfusions that are a part of surgical therapy. Com-

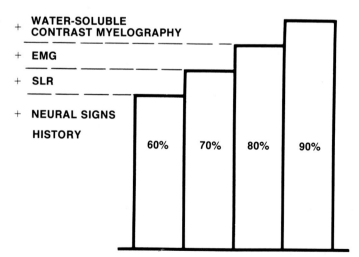

Fig. 6-37. This histogram shows how the percentage of accurate diagnoses of disc herniation can be increased as more aspects of the clinical evaluation are found to be positive. (Nachemson, A. L.: The lumbar spine, an orthopaedic challenge. Spine, *1*:59, 1976.)

plications associated with cervical spine disc surgery may be divided into major and minor. Minor complications subside without prolonged or vigorous treatment. They are hoarseness, dysphagia, and hematoma at the iliac donor site. Major complications include graft slippage, donor site problems, infections, pneumothorax, puncture of the esophagus or large vessels, and spinal cord damage.[150]

The lumbar complications include cauda equina damage, penetration of the aorta, vena cava, or iliac vessels, and wound infections.

Comment. Cervical and lumbar spine surgery is justified and indicated for carefully selected patients for whom the risk-benefit factor is appropriate. Surgery is mandatory for thoracic disc herniation once the diagnosis is made. Acute cervical myelopathy and cauda equina symptoms with bladder paralysis are situations in which immediate surgery is desirable. It is good to keep in mind that even though in elective, carefully selected lumbar disc surgery, 90 per cent of the patients will enjoy the relief of leg pain, as many as 60 to 70 per cent may continue to have some low back pain.[111] Subjective and objective information that should be of value to the clinician in discussions and deliberations about the surgical treatment of spine pain are provided below.

Who should do disc surgery? Selecki and colleagues studied a group of patients with low back pain and sciatica, some of whom were treated by neurosurgeons and others by orthopaedic surgeons. The percentage of patients in the two groups who were successfully treated were nearly identical, 59 per cent in the orthopaedic group and 63 per cent in the neurosurgical group. The neurosurgeons operated on a larger percentage of their patients than did the orthopaedic surgeons (75% vs. 56%). However, patients with radicular signs and symptoms tended to be in the neurosurgical group, whereas patients with only low back pain were more likely to be in the orthopaedic surgeons group.[130]

Table 6-4 includes a partial summary of the treatment discussed. We have attempted to rank the various treatment programs. There are some oversimplifications. The reported percentages successfully treated have been informally averaged. However, they reliably represent the trends found in the literature. The time span of treatment has not been standardized. It is known that with waiting and doing nothing, 70 per cent patients will be well in 3 weeks and 90 per cent in 2 months.[111] However, the table is based on reported results in the literature which evaluate and/or compare some of the different treatment regimens.

Table 6-4 also summarizes the relative risks of the different regimens, based on reported complications and the authors' opinions. Risk represents a combination of frequency as well as severity of complications associated with the various treatments.

Although expected results and relative risks are not the only factors involved in the selection of a given form of treatment, they are important considerations. Availability of facilities and techniques, and individual patient and physician

Table 6-4. Comparison of Treatment Regimens for Spine Pain

Relative Therapeutic Effectiveness	Risk Factors
Outstanding (> 80%)	*Serious*
Disc excision (conservatively selected)	Disc excision Chemonucleolysis
Good (70–80%)	*Moderate*
Isometric truncal exercises	Rest, analgesics, and anti-inflammatory drugs
Basic patient education and group therapy	William's exercises
Spinal manipulation	Spinal manipulation
Disc excision (not conservatively selected)	Local and regional use of drugs
Chemonucleolysis	
Average (60–70%)	*Minor or Insignificant*
Rest, analgesics, anti-inflammatory drugs	Isometric truncal exercises
William's exercises	Physical therapy (heat and massage)
Miscellaneous exercises	Basic patient education and group therapy programs
Physical therapy (heat and massage)	Axial traction
Axial traction	
Orthotic devices	
Local and regional use of drugs	
Disc excision (liberally selected)	

preferences are also major factors. For nonoperative treatment, isometric exercises and patient education rate highly with respect to effectiveness and low risk. If the situation demands that something be done, spinal manipulative therapy is effective, and there is only moderate risk. Other forms of conservative treatment may be employed. Obviously, drugs are frequently used effectively. Guidelines suggest that if the patient is not improved in 2 to 6 months with nonoperative treatment, surgery may be indicated, provided that the history, physical findings, and myelogram are indicative of a herniated, cervical, or lumbar disc or cervical spondylosis. As mentioned previously, the diagnosis of a herniated thoracic disc is an indication for anterior discectomy.

Well Doctor, what will happen if I don't have surgery? The study by Hakelius is of considerable help with respect to discussion with patients, decision making, and recommendations about the advisability of surgery in the presence of a herniated disc. The 583 patients in the study fit the subjective and objective clinical criteria for the diagnosis of disc herniation at the L4–5 or at the L5–S1 level. The patients had symptoms for no more than 6 months. Disc exploration and removal of the herniated fragment was accomplished through no more than a partial unilateral laminotomy in 166, or 28.5 per cent of the patients. The remaining patients were treated with varying degrees of relative immobilization. The conservatively managed and surgically treated patients were followed for an average of 7 years, 4 months.

The salient findings were as follows. When there is a distinct prolapse, the surgically treated patient experiences a speedier relief from sciatica and loses less time from work than the conservatively managed patient. The time away from work following surgery is likely to be less if the conservative treatment prior to surgery has taken less than 2 months. *However,* the study also showed that acute sciatica with neurologic symptoms is a transient condition and with few exceptions will subside with time. *Moreover,* in this study the results of the surgically and conservatively treated patients in this series were almost identical 6 months after the start of treatment. Table 6-5 shows the comparison of the two groups in more detail. The investigation reported that there were several points that indicated a slightly better prognosis for the surgically treated group of patients. These results are the patients' subjective evaluation of the improvement of their low back pain and sciatica. Also, follow-up treatment showed that the surgically treated patients took less sick leave for low back pain and sciatica than did the conservatively treated patients.[59]

But what about my leg, doctor? Will it be

Table 6-5. Comparison of Results of 166 Surgically Treated and 417 Conservatively Treated Patients With Herniated Discs

POST-TREATMENT RESULTS	SURGICAL REMOVAL OF DISC (%)	CONSERVATIVE TREATMENT WITH RELATIVE IMMOBILIZATION (%)
Reduced working capacity	12	15
Complete loss of working ability	0.75	1.5
Restrictions in leisure activity	15	15
Regular sleep disturbances	20	13
Sick leave for back pain-sciatica (90 days)	13	14
Pronounced residual sciatica	12	20
Pronounced residual paresis	20	16
Pronounced subjective motor symptoms	7	6
Pronounced subjective sensory symptoms	8	5
Objective sensory loss	34	33
Surgery for recurrences	5	6

(Hakelius, A.: Prognosis in sciatica. A clinical follow-up of surgical and non-surgical treatment. Acta Orthop. Scand., *129*[Supp.], 1970.)

weaker if I don't have surgery? A prospective study by Weber showed that 1 year following surgery, the surgically treated patients were no better than the conservatively treated patients with regard to objective measurements of motor function.[147]

All right, I need surgery, but when should we operate, doctor? How long can I wait without increasing the time lost from work? The amount of sick leave required after surgery is less if the preoperative conservative management lasts for *less* than 60 days.[59] This suggests that physicians should wait at least 2 months before recommending surgery. Moreover, 90 per cent of patients will be better by that time.[111] Patients who undergo surgery after 1 year of incapacity have roughly a 50 per cent less chance of gaining relief of symptoms than those patients treated by surgery sooner.[130] The poorer surgical results with long-standing preoperative disease may be contributed to by two factors, nerve root fibrosis secondary to long-standing compression and psychologic factors resulting from prolonged pain and disability.

Although this objective information is most helpful, there remains the problem of trying to weigh the disadvantages of exposing the patient to the risks of anesthesia and surgery against the pain, disability, and time away from work that may be involved in waiting. We have been especially attentive to the hypothesis posed by psychologists that, when a patient has had pain for as much as 1 year, the removal or correction of the organic source of that pain alone is not enough to free the patient of the pain. In addition to the surgical or other medical treatment, some psychologic treatment is also required.

Spine Fusions

The biomechanical rationale for arthrodesis to treat spine pain is based on the hypothesis that immobilization of the motion segment should reduce or eliminate any pain associated with that particular motion segment. The rationale, biomechanics, and indications for spine fusion are presented in detail in Chapter 8. The immobilization, or, more realistically, increased stiffness of the motion segment, is thought to eliminate or decrease irritation at the intervertebral disc, the intervertebral joints, or other pain-sensitive structures.

In the cervical spine, arthrodesis in addition to disc excision has not been proven to be superior to simple disc excision. However, with cervical spondylosis that involves osteophytes, joints of Luschka, and degenerative arthritis, arthrodesis is likely to give a better result. This observation has not been statistically documented, however.

In the lumbar spine the evidence seems to indicate that there is no particular advantage to routine arthrodesis at the time of disc excision.[113,130] The biomechanical studies of Rolander (see p. 418) demonstrated that even with solid union of the posterior elements there was sufficient motion between the vertebral bodies with physiologic loading to cause irritation of the disc. For lumbar spine pain in the absence of spondylolisthesis, arthrodesis is very unlikely to succeed in the eradication or even satisfactory alleviation of spine pain. This is based primarily on the overall lack of clinical success with this procedure.

There are some intriguing problems raised by observations of patients following spinal fusions. Pseudoarthroses are difficult to diagnose and when present are not always painful. In cervical spine fusions for spondylosis, patients with failure of fusion are sometimes relieved of pain.[150]

Newman observed that some treated surgically for lumbar spondylolisthesis had satisfactory relief of pain even though they developed pseudoarthrosis.[140] Shaw reported that 77 per cent of his patients with failed fusion were satisfied with their results.[140] Other surgeons have made similar observations.[130,140] The relationship of successful arthrodesis of the spine to the relief of pain remains obscure. Spinal fusion for the treatment of spondylolisthesis and *some* of the other radiographic entities that are very likely to be associated with spine pain appears to produce the most consistently good results with regard to pain relief. As shown in Chapter 8, the results of fusion alone for the treatment of other spine pain is variable and unpredictable.

Salvage Procedures

This is a discussion of the advisability of performing surgery for a painful spine on a patient who has had two or more such operations. It is generally accepted that the probability of a satisfactory result is 1 in 10 or less. Yet, in a neurosurgical, orthopaedic, or pain referral center, one may encounter a patient who has had as many as 13 operations for low back pain.* When should a physician give up, when should a so-called salvage procedure be done, what should the procedure be, and what is the prognosis? These questions are unanswered at present. Given the complexities of treatment and corresponding results, it is obviously imprecise and unobjective to generalize about multiple operations on the back.

The third operation is generally one of extensive decompression of cord or cauda equina and nerve roots including their course through the neural foramen. This is usually done in conjunction with fusion of all involved motion segments. A group of 54 patients who had had two unsuccessful disc operations were studied at the Mayo Clinic. One-half of the patients were treated conservatively and the other half had a third operation. The patients were not assigned to the two groups on either a matched or a random basis. Thus, there was no statistical evaluation. The conservative therapy consisted of various spine orthoses, rest on hard mattress, limitation of activity, heat massage, and special exercises. The surgery involved disc removal and/or spinal fusion. The patients treated by salvage surgery tended to show a better result. However, this group had a higher incidence of complaints of sciatica prior to the salvage procedure than the conservatively treated group. This may account for the better results observed in the surgically treated group.[78]

Another report on salvage surgery for low back pain emphasized certain factors in the selection of patients. Patients with psychiatric problems, and patients involved with compensation and litigation were not as likely to achieve an acceptable result with yet another operation. However, the history of a 1-year, pain-free interval following the last surgery was highly correlated with a successful salvage procedure.[42]

The fact that *recurrent* disc protrusion was found to be a problem in this series may be considered an argument for removal of the entire

disc as well as the displaced fragment at the initial operation. Some investigators have recommended excision of the displaced fragment only.[59,111]

Each patient is, of course, evaluated and managed as an individual. A thorough psychologic evaluation should precede any salvage procedure. If the history indicates the patient returned to work after previous procedures, there may be a more optimistic prognosis. When a specific pseudoarthrosis is to be treated, there may be a greater chance for success. The basic surgical procedure adequately frees the nerve roots from scarring, impingement, or compression and reduces motion with arthrodesis. Thus, once all of the involved discs have been removed, the nerve roots freed through their course in the neural foramina, and the involved segments fused, there should as a general rule be no more spine surgery in the region. It is certainly desirable to avoid contributing one or more episodes to the saga of the painful, unhappy, totally disabled patient who has undergone multiple spine operations. Determining how to manage the patient who has undergone two or more back operations requires considerable additional basic research and some well designed prospective clinical studies.

Transcutaneous and Dorsal Column Stimulators

These therapeutic modalities are mentioned for completeness and are discussed briefly. The "gate" theory of pain transmission suggests that if it is in some way possible to create a sensory overload at the dorsal root areas that are transmitting pain impulses, this will block or diminish the pain signals and prevent characteristic discomfort. The block may be developed by placing an electronic device on the dorsal column of the spinal cord of the region involved and stimulating it with an electrical current. The alternative technique is to employ a transcutaneous electrical stimulation in order to achieve the same results. We are not aware at the present time of any studies that convincingly demonstrate the usefulness of these techniques.

A Regimen to Consider

Following a thorough diagnostic evaluation, any specific diagnosis that is made is treated appropriately either directly or by referral to the

---

* Personal communication, F. D. Wagner.

appropriate specialist. The remaining patients have a diagnosis of nonspecific organic low back pain and/or a herniated intervertebral disc. Both groups are treated essentially the same way, by waiting 3 to 6 months and employing one or more forms of conservative therapy. During that time, rest, activity, and anti-inflammatory narcotic and non-narcotic drugs are prescribed as indicated. We believe that *time* is the most important factor. However, any combination of physical traction and/or manipulation may be employed, depending on the physician's clinical judgment and evaluation of the particular patient. If 2 to 3 weeks of one form of conservative therapy is not effective, it is advisable to switch to some other program. This is true even with bed rest. Sometimes a patient who does not improve with bed rest will do better with moderate activity and/or some other form of treatment. For the reasons previously discussed, it is very difficult to determine why a particular patient improves.

When both the patient and the doctor decide that it is time to give up (the suggestion may come from either individual), the patient is then hospitalized for a myelogram. If the study is positive, the entire intervertebral disc and any ectopic fragments are removed. If the study is not positive and the surgeon is convinced that there is disc pathology, one or two interspaces are explored. If there is uncertainty, then the prehospitalization program is reinstituted. This continues until the patient gets well with or without surgery, adjusts to the pain, or goes to another doctor or practitioner.

For cervical spine pain, the management is essentially the same. The nonsurgical treatment may include a cervical orthosis of *intermediate control*. Elective surgery in the absence of an abnormal myelogram involves disc excision and Smith-Robinson fusion at either one level or the two adjacent levels that best fit the clinical data.[150] This depends upon pain distribution, evidence of sensory and neuromuscular deficit, and location of cervical osteophytes in the intervertebral foramen.

Before surgery, especially in the case of normal myelograms, we suggest some type of psychologic screening test. The MMPI or an interview with a psychologist or psychiatrist is suggested.

The patients with a long and complex history of spine pain who are involved in compensation or litigation are more difficult to cure. It is only the *very* exceptional or unusual patient in this group that should be considered for surgery in the absence of a positive myelogram, spondylolisthesis, or clearly recognizable structural deformity secondary to trauma.

PROPHYLAXIS AND ERGONOMICS

How can spine pain be avoided once a patient has been so afflicted, and how can the severity and probability of recurrence be minimized?

Certainly, it is reasonable to assume that spine pain resulting from most causes can be aggravated by mechanical factors. Prophylaxis and ergonomics are obviously intimately related to treatment, and there is some overlap with physical therapy, exercise, and low back pain school.

Prophylactic measures for avoiding spine pain are numerous. Those related to trauma involve all of the well documented practices of street, road, and highway safety, which are generally well known. The value of seat belts and head rests is discussed in Chapter 4. Some of the epidemiologic data suggests that truck driving and automobile commuting may predispose certain people to the development of disc disease. A patient with spine pain that is related to disc disease should be advised to limit automobile riding and especially driving. Sports injuries are another significant source of spine trauma. The basics of good conditioning, coaching, and proper supervision are of obvious benefit. Proper equipment and changes in rules may be helpful in preventing some of the sports injuries. Education of the public concerning recreational dangers, proper conditioning, and the use of "common sense" is valuable in the reduction of spine pain from trauma. It has also been suggested that some of the present compensation laws are such that the quality of life, all things considered, is better for the person who *has* pain and even *surgery* than for the person who does not *have* pain or *surgery*. Therefore, perhaps changes in some of the compensation laws and practices may be a form of prophylaxis against spine pain.

Postural Biomechanics

The issue of ergonomics and prophylaxis calls attention to the question concerning the comfortable and desirable position of the lumbar spine. Some physicians suggest that the reason bars have bar rails is so that while the customers enjoy conviviality and ethanol, they may be more comfortable with the back in the slightly flexed, relatively straight or non-lordotic position (Fig. 6-38). We have reviewed the cultural hypothesis that states that this position is used more frequently in populations that complain less frequently about low back pain. However, this statement is not documented. Experimental studies show that there is more of a posterior bulge of the disc with extension than with flexion. In contrast, there is evidence that shows that the reclined, slightly extended, and relatively unloaded spine has less pressure in the intervertebral disc and less activity in the paraspinous muscles. These studies are reviewed in the next section. Although this biomechanical data sup-

ports the use of a reclined, slightly extended position at least for sitting, the definitive resolution of the question requires additional information. Meanwhile, we suggest that the most comfortable posture for each patient be determined and that the patient be advised and taught to maintain it.

Biomechanics and Sitting

There has been some interesting biomechanical information related to the question of sitting. This data is important both to prophylaxis and ergonomics as workers often perform their job in the sitting position. The investigations have analyzed the effects of back rest inclination and lumbar support on L3 intradiscal pressure and quantitated electromyographic recordings.[4] The goal was to determine the seat type and reclining angle that was associated with the lowest disc pressure and the least paraspinal muscle activity. The hypothesis is that these characteristic seat types and angles might be the least stressful and

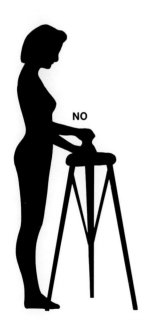
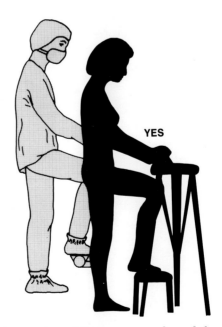

Fig. 6-38. Flexion of the hip reduces the tension of the psoas muscle and the lordosis of the lumbar spine, both of which tend to reduce loads on the lumbar spine. This bit of ergonomic advice is particularly important to the surgeon who may stand for several hours on occasion at the operating table. The housewife is advised to assume the work position shown as much as possible. This is a valid ergonomic principle.

most therapeutic for the spine. The subjects also reported their subjective feelings about the comfort of the seats following several alterations of the two variables. A number of important points come from this study. It is assumed that the lowest disc pressure and the least electromyographic activity of the paraspinal muscles are the most desirable situations. The lowest electromyographic and intradiscal pressure recordings were found with a back rest inclination of 120 degrees and a 5-cm lumbar support. The highest intradiscal pressure was found in the situation in which there was no lumbar support and a 90-degree inclination (i.e., a straight back; Fig. 6-39).

In view of the studies by Kelsey and colleagues in which the vehicle driver was found to be at a risk to develop sciatica,[83] we recommend that a lumbar support be used by the frequent or the symptomatic driver. The study showed that the use of arm rests as well as lumbar supports reduced intradiscal pressure. The use of arm supports in addition to lumbar supports is recommended for the symptomatic and frequent driver.

Thigh support and adequate space for alteration of position are also positive factors in the ideal seat design. An example of good seat design is shown in Figure 6-40. Obviously, for the worker there are practical considerations about where the person must look and what he or she does with the arms and legs. These and other factors may require design adjustments that might interfere somewhat with the use of the ideal seat.

Biomechanics of Work Activity

Ergonomics is important in many ways to prophylaxis in different work situations.[132] Crucial to ergonomics is the question concerning the proper way to lift an object. The loading mechanics of the lumbar spine, for example, are such that any increased load that is anterior to the vertebral

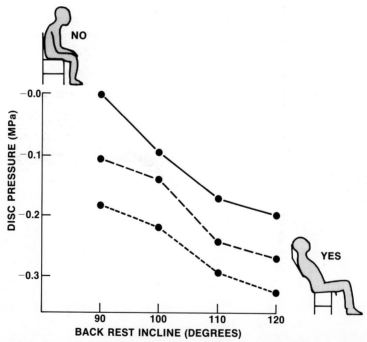

Fig. 6-39. This graph depicts the effects of the variables of back rest inclination and size of lumbar support on intradiscal pressure. The solid line represents no lumbar support; the large dashed line represents a 3-cm support; and the small dotted line represents a 5-cm lumbar support. (Nachemson, A. L.: The lumbar spine, an orthopaedic challenge. Spine, *1*:59, 1976.)

bodies greatly increases the forces that are exerted on the lumbar spine. This is due to the forces that must be extended by the paraspinous muscles in order to maintain equilibrium. The resultant forces at the fulcrum, which is the lower lumbar motion segment, are very high. This is shown in Figure 6-41.

Although there has been suitable emphasis of the importance of leg lifting as opposed to back lifting,[108,111] the distance of the object from the body at the time of lifting has also been shown to be a very important ergonomic consideration.[2-4,106,117] Simultaneous electromyogram, and truncal and intradiscal pressure measurements were made while normal subjects went through different types of lifting procedures. These studies showed that with all three procedures, the distance of the weight away from the body was directly related to high measurements. This is due to the high forces necessary to maintain equilibrium because of an increased lever arm

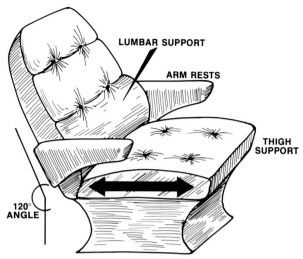

Fig. 6-40. The current available knowledge suggests that this is the biomechanically ideal chair for comfort and relaxation (not desk work). This takes into consideration the proper inclination, lumbar support, arm rests, thigh support, and space to move around and change position.

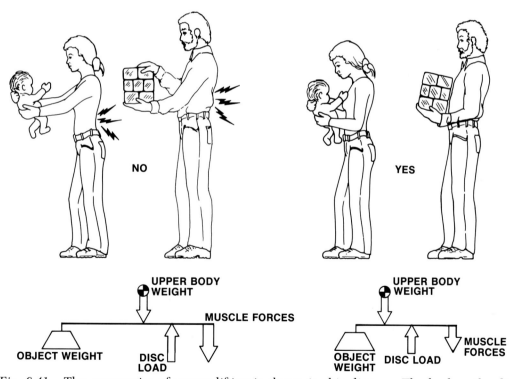

Fig. 6-41. The ergonomics of proper lifting is shown in this diagram. The load on the discs is a combined result of the object weight, the upper body weight, the back muscle forces, and their respective *lever arms* to the disc center. On the left, the object is farther away from the disc center compared to the situation on the right. The lever-balances at the bottom show that smaller muscle forces and disc loads are obtained when the object is carried nearer to the disc.

(Fig. 6-41). There is a larger joint reaction force (high intradiscal pressure), a greater force required by the erector spinae muscles (high electromyographic activity), and a need for greater truncal support to protect the spine (high truncal pressure).[2–4] This shows the significance of lifting with the object close to the body. It is of considerable importance in both industrial and domestic ergonomics.

There have been several experiments carried out in order to correlate abdominal and/or thoracic cage pressure with quantity of weight lifted by different subjects.[28,36,86] These studies showed a correlation between the ability to increase the fluid pressure in the two cavities and the amount of weight lifted (Fig. 6-42). This attests to the value of abdominal and thoracic cage muscles in supporting the spine when it is carrying heavy loads. Based on this work we suggest good muscle tone, especially for the abdominal muscles. However, the strength is *not* to be developed by sit-ups. Isometric abdominal exercises achieve the same goals without excessive intervertebral disc loading. In addition, this work is partial justification for the use of a spinal corset or a brace with an abdominal corset in situations where development of the abdominal and thoracic muscles (truncal pressure) are not feasible. The use of a corset is associated with the risk of further weakening the abdominal muscles. Therefore, its prolonged use is not recommended for patients who are capable of strengthening their muscles.

It has been shown that intratruncal pressures increase when heavy weights are lifted. The pressure increase is greater when heavier weights are lifted and it is also increased when the speed of weight lifting is faster.[28,86] Studies of simultaneous intrathoracic and intra-abdominal pressures comparing pulling, pushing, and lifting were carried out. The results show the largest pressures were recorded when subjects were pushing and the smallest ones occurred during pulling.[28] It was also observed that during pulling the back muscles were tense (Fig. 6-43A), while during pushing the rectus abdominis muscle was tense (Fig. 6-43C). Thus, the intratruncal pressures probably reflect the tension in the abdominal muscles. The biomechanical explanation for the reduced disc load in pushing versus that in

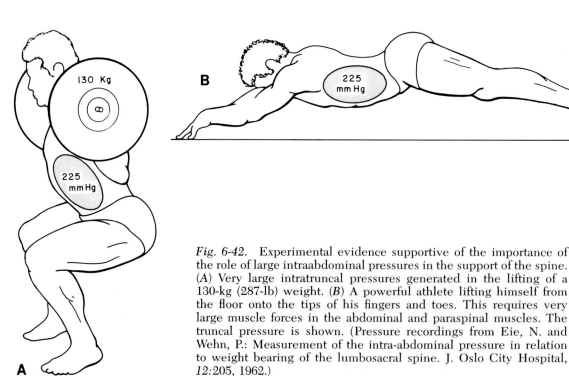

Fig. 6-42. Experimental evidence supportive of the importance of the role of large intraabdominal pressures in the support of the spine. (*A*) Very large intratruncal pressures generated in the lifting of a 130-kg (287-lb) weight. (*B*) A powerful athlete lifting himself from the floor onto the tips of his fingers and toes. This requires very large muscle forces in the abdominal and paraspinal muscles. The truncal pressure is shown. (Pressure recordings from Eie, N. and Wehn, P.: Measurement of the intra-abdominal pressure in relation to weight bearing of the lumbosacral spine. J. Oslo City Hospital, 12:205, 1962.)

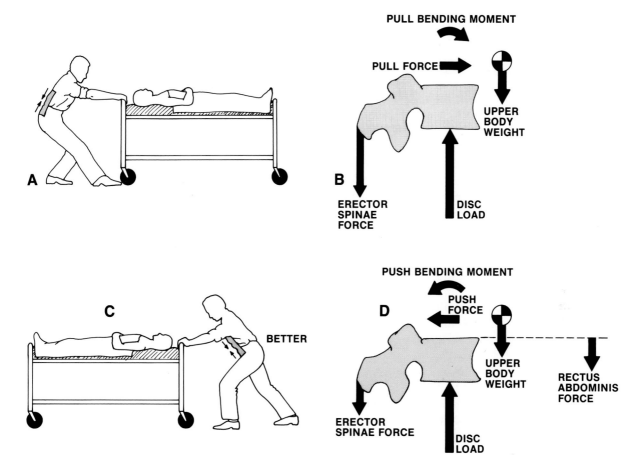

Fig. 6-43. The ergonomics of pulling and pushing and the probable forces and bending moments involved. (*A, B*) During pulling the erector spinae muscles resist the bending moment created by the horizontal pull force. (*C, D*) On the other hand, during pushing rectus abdominis resists the bending moment produced by the pushing force. Because this muscle has a much larger lever arm than the erector spinae muscles, its force requirement is relatively smaller. Therefore, the load on the disc is smaller during pushing than during pulling.

pulling is depicted in Figure 6-43. The probable loads acting on a lumbar vertebra during pulling are seen in Figure 6-43B. The pull force, directed anteriorly, increases the bending moment and the erector spinae force considerably because of the short lever arm this muscle group has with respect to the axis of rotation. Thus, the disc load is also increased. The situation is different in pushing (Fig. 6-43D). The horizontal push force is now directed posteriorly. Its bending moment is counterbalanced by the rectus abdominis force. Because this muscle has a larger lever arm as compared to the erector spinae muscle, its force

is relatively smaller. Thus, there is a smaller increase in disc load with pushing than with pulling.

A study has been carried out to determine whether or not an isometric strength test of a person's ability to lift weights is correlated with the incidence of low back pain.[17] The results showed that workers who were doing jobs in which their isometric test strength did not equal the strength required by their jobs had a much higher incidence of job-related low back signs and symptoms. The proper use of this type of testing and information can be most useful in the ergonomics and the prevention of spine pain. For the present, it is suggested that a patient returning to work involving lifting should have a thorough and well executed program of isometric exercises beforehand.

Activities to Avoid

We believe that the following recommendations are well supported by the data depicted in Figures 6-44, 6-45 and Table 6-6. Patients with spine pain may be expected to aggravate their condition by coughing, straining, and laughing. Also, activities such as bending forward and lifting are associated with large increases in intradiscal pressure. A variety of exercises are prescribed in physical therapy for patients with back pain. Sit-ups with or without the hips flexed cause large loads to be exerted on the lumbar spine. The intradiscal pressure generated by sit-ups with or without the hips flexed is comparable to pressure generated by bending forward 20 degrees holding 20 kg, hardly an exercise that a physician would suggest for a patient with low back pain.[c] An examination of Figure 6-45 shows that the patient with spine pain should also avoid straight leg raising exercises and lumbar hyperextension exercises. The least loads are exerted on the lumbar spine in the supine position with 30 kg of traction,

or in the semi-Fowler's position (Fig. 6-24). The spine is also flexed, an excellent resting position for the patient with low back pain.

In one study, pressure-sensitive needles were injected into the third lumbar intervertebral disc of subjects who subsequently performed a number of tasks. Some of the most important activities are depicted in Figure 6-44. The chart is presented so that the various activities may be compared on the basis of percentage of standard. The standard selected was that of the force on the third lumbar disc recorded with the subject involved in normal standing. A large amount of valuable information has come from this data. The actual measurements are given in Table 6-6. A good deal of our prophylactic and ergonomic recommendations are based on and supported by this data.

Obesity greatly increases both the direct vertical compressive load on the spine and also significantly increases the anteriorly acting loads, which through the action of the muscles create very large joint reaction forces. The panniculis in Figure 6-46 is presented to emphasize this point. Consequently, obesity should be avoided.

A list of tips is shown on page 335 for patients who have or have had spine pain. Of course, *none* of them apply to all patients.

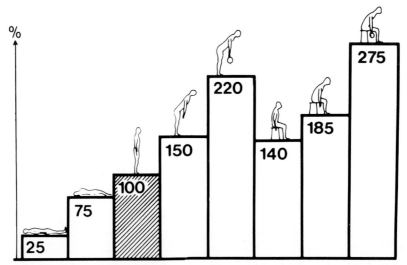

Fig. 6-44. A diagrammatic comparison of in vivo loads (disc pressures) in the third lumbar disc during various activities. Note that sitting pressures are greater than standing pressures. (Nachemson, A. L.: The lumbar spine, an orthopaedic challenge. Spine, *1:*59, 1976.)

Table 6-6. Nachemson's Data on Loads in the Third Lumbar Discs During Various Positions and Activities[107,108,110]

ACTIVITY	LOAD (kgf)
Supine in traction	10
Supine	30
Standing	70
Walking	85
Twisting	90
Bending sideways	95
Upright sitting, no support	100
Coughing	110
Isometric abdominal muscle exercise	110
Jumping	110
Straining	120
Laughing	120
Bending forward 20°	120
Bilateral straight leg raising, supine	120
Active back hyperextension, prone	150
Sit-up exercise with knees extended	175
Sit-up exercise with knees bent	180
Bending forward 20° with 10 kg in each hand	185
Lifting of 20 kg, back straight, knees bent	210
Lifting of 20 kg, back bent, knees straight	340

Prophylactic and Ergonomic Tips For Patients With Spine Pain

Exercise to maintain painless range of motion and muscle tone.

Avoid improper sit-ups and back extension exercises.

When sitting, use a lumbar support.

Use arm rests when possible.

Move around within the seat; also, get out of the seat occasionally.

Determine whether the flexed or extended lumbar position is better.

Use this position in walking, standing, sitting, and lying.

Avoid excessively high-heeled shoes.

When lying in bed, during severe pain flex hips 90°.

Try sleeping on the floor on three blankets during severe pain.

Use a flat firm bed otherwise.

Lift with legs and with object close to you while doing a Valsalva's maneuver.

Develop truncal muscles with isometric abdominal exercises.

Be careful about opening and closing windows.

Avoid sudden jerks or incremental loads when lifting or carrying.

Avoid heavy lifting and strenuous activity when the back is symptomatic.

Swimming is generally a good exercise.

Avoid obesity.

Sit on the bed or use a high table for changing diapers.

Avoid pain-related activities.

When standing for a long period of time, elevate one foot on a footrest.

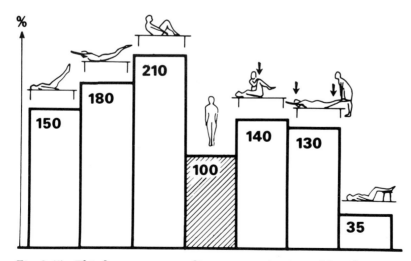

Fig. 6-45. This figure compares disc pressures in vivo at L3 with various exercises and positions. Note pressures during sit-ups with legs bent, hyperextension exercises, and back lying with hips and knees flexed. (Nachemson, A. L.: The lumbar spine, an orthopaedic challenge, Spine, *1*:59, 1976.)

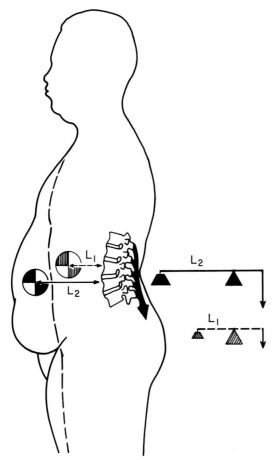

Fig. 6-46. The mechanics here are the same as those in Figure 6-41, except that the weight here is adipose tissue rather than an external object. In the latter case, it is much easier to correct the lever arm. However, this diagram does emphasize yet another prophylactic and therapeutic value in avoiding or eliminating obesity.

CLINICAL BIOMECHANICS

Etiologic Considerations

From the biomechanical vantage point, most information is about the intervertebral disc, which is focal to spine pain. However, other anatomic factors are important, and there are numerous psychologic and socioeconomic factors that are crucial to the clinical evaluation and management of spine pain.

Epidemiologic studies suggest somewhat para-doxically that individuals involved in sedentary occupations as well as those who are heavy laborers are equally prone to spine pain and/or radiculopathy. Those who spend a good deal of time driving motor vehicles and those who experience full-term pregnancies are also at risk. Vibration may be a factor in the former group and increased loads associated with alterations in the mechanical properties of the ligaments may be accountable for the problem in the latter group.

It has been shown that patients with back pain had intraosseous vertebral fluid pressures that were significantly higher than pressures found in subjects with no spine pain.

The following radiographically demonstrable conditions are thought to be causes of spine pain: spondylolisthesis, multiple, narrowed intervertebral discs, congenital kyphosis, scoliosis, osteoporosis, ankylosing spondylitis, and lumbar osteochondrosis. There does not appear to be any biomechanical thread that is common to these conditions.

Fibers of the annulus fibrosus during the process of maturation and aging may undergo fatigue failure or rupture during degeneration.

The acute back sprain is probably due to sudden loading that causes rupture of peripheral annulus fibrosus fibers or some of the other ligamentous or musculotendinous structures associated with the spine. A nondisplaced or minimally displaced vertebral end-plate fracture may also be responsible.

Low back pain or cervical spine pain may be caused by irritation of the peripheral annular fibers associated with the passage of fluid into the nucleus pulposus.

Referred hip and thigh pain associated with back pain may result from irritation of the posterolateral annular fibers. This may occur in the absence of true radiculopathy, which results from irritation of the nerve root.

When there is significant bulge of the disc posterolaterally, there can be true sciatica or radiculopathy in addition to the low back pain.

The actual sequestered portion of the disc that can move randomly about, depending on the direction and magnitude of forces involved, may either be asymptomatic or cause any combination of spine pain, referred pain, or true radiculopathy. This pathologic condition may respond to axial traction or manipulation.

When there is a displaced sequestration, partially or completely fixed, the clinical picture is less changeable. If there is radiculopathy, it is distinct and more persistent. Axial traction or manipulation seem unlikely to be helpful in this situation, although both have been used with reported success.

A degenerating disc is associated with mechanical disruption, and there may be evidence of degenerative changes of the intervertebral joints.

There is evidence that the increased disc pressures associated with and combined with the biochemical changes in the nucleus pulposus may lead to pathologic disruption and failure of the annular fibers and ultimately disc herniation.

Of considerable importance in the problem of spine pain are all the various factors and combinations of factors that can compromise the space available for the neural elements and result in spine and radicular pain.

There is some biomechanical correlation between loads, motion, and pain. The lumbar spine carries the heaviest loads, exhibits the second largest range of motion, and has the highest incidence of pain.

Diagnostic Considerations

Thoracic kyphosis, which is associated with heavy work before age 15, is also associated with thoracic spine pain.

Irritation of any painful structure adjacent to the subarachnoid space (nerve root, peripheral annular fibers) may be caused by any alteration of venous pressure. Thus, coughing, sneezing, or straining at stool may cause severe spinal or radicular pain.

In Spurling's test, one takes advantage of the knowledge of cervical spine kinematics to position the vertebra so as to lower the threshold of sensitivity in order to irritate the nerve root in the intervertebral foramen. For the nerve root at the right intervertebral foramen, the patient should look and bend to the right. The opposite should be done for the left side. In each case, additional impact further compromises the foramen by approximating the vertebra and causing the disc

to bulge. This causes radicular pain from the nerve that is compromised in a crowded foramen.

The sensitivity and complexity of neurologic problems in the thoracic spine due to disc disease are largely explained by the paucity of spinal cord blood supply and free space in the canal.

The patient with lumbar disc disease and sciatic nerve root irritation may stand with hip and knee slightly flexed, because this puts the least stretch on the nerve root at the site of irritation.

There may be a correlation between the direction of a patient's list with respect to the side of the sciatica and the position of the disc herniation with regard to the axilla of the involved nerve root.

The patient with camptocormia is able to straighten his spine in the reclining but not in the standing position because psychological, not biomechanical factors are involved.

Naphzier's test is based on the secondary pressure changes in the subarachnoid space around the irritated nerve root due to manual compression of the patient's jugular veins.

The leg raising tests, in which pain is elicited by sciatic nerve movement, are important and reliable indicators of nerve root irritation.

The patient with a "positive pedal pulse test" is able to flex the hip to 90 degrees without pain when sitting but not when supine because of psychological and/or socioeconomic, not biomechanical factors.

Based on sound clinical studies and pathoanatomic and biomechanical analysis there seems to be little data to support the clinical usefulness of discograms.

Treatment of Spine Pain

Rest reduces mechanical irritation and is especially useful during the acute phase of the symptoms.

The goal of William's exercises is to maintain the spine in the straight or flexed position. This seems to be reasonable, but tradition appears to have inflated the value of these exercises far beyond that which is justified by solid supportive evidence.

Sit-ups and active hyperextension exercises

exert forces on the lumbar spine that are comparable to *improperly* lifting 20 kg (44 lb), hardly a therapeutic exercise for a patient with low back pain.

Hyperextension exercises may be required by the athlete or laborer who is over the acute phase of spine pain and must prepare for isotonic activity of the posterior spinous muscles.

There is ample theoretical, clinical, and experimental biomechanical evidence to convincingly support the advisability of isometric truncal exercises for patients with lumbar spine pain. The development of strong muscles to compress the contents of the truncal cavities provides enormous mechanical support to the spine.

Physical therapy (heat and massage) has not been shown to have any particular biomechanical effect on the spine. The therapeutic response is satisfactory for about 60 to 70 per cent of patients.

Spine pain school relies on patient education directed toward an understanding of the problem and practical advice about how to best care for oneself. Erognomic advice based on sound biomechanical knowledge is provided.

It has been shown that it is possible with appropriately applied axial traction to increase the separation between vertebrae and consequently enlarge the neural foramen in the cervical and lumbar region of the spine. However, the separation does not persist when the traction is released. This form of therapy gives satisfactory results in 60 to 70 per cent of patients. Certain specific pathologic conditions may be expected to respond better than others to axial traction.

Regardless of how the forces are applied and transmitted to a vertebra, it can only move within some combination of six degrees of freedom.

Only the magnitude of the forces and their rate of application may be altered by the therapist.

It has been shown that axial rotatory manipulation does not alter the size of the intervertebral foramen.

Based on current traditional anatomic, pathologic, and physiologic scientific knowledge, there is no basis for any assumption that spinal manipulation is therapeutic for visceral disease.

Spinal manipulation is as effective as a number of other forms of therapy that offer satisfactory results in 60 to 70 per cent. There is a suggestion that there is an immediate but transient post-treatment benefit, and one study showed manipulation to be superior to heat massage and exercise, with satisfactory results in 80 to 95 per cent of patients.

The evidence indicates that a herniated disc is not a contraindication to this form of therapy, although there are risks involved.

Cervical spine manipulation can be fatal.

Orthotic devices reduce spine motion to some extent. This has the value of reducing irritation. If the orthosis has an abdominal component, it can further reduce irritation by providing support to the spine.

The enzyme chymopapain is capable of hydrolyzing and at least partially dissolving the intervertebral disc. Several studies report results that are significantly better than the good to excellent results commonly observed in 60 to 70 per cent with other treatment. Some series suggest that chemonucleolysis produces better results than surgery.

The risks of using chymopapain, in addition to possible death from anaphylaxis, include the possibility of neural damage, discitis, and arachnoiditis.

Chymopapain injected into the nucleus pulposus may be ineffective in the treatment of a sequestered portion of disc material. The enzyme may not pass from the nucleus to the displaced, sequestered material.

When patients are carefully selected by extensive preoperative evaluation to ascertain the presence of a herniated disc, the results are satisfactory in 90 per cent. The results are best in patients with lumbar spine disc herniations. In the cervical spine the results of treatment are not quite as good, and they are generally not good in the thoracic spine.

In the surgical excision of a herniated disc, the radiculopathy tends to improve more than the spine pain.

Once the diagnosis of herniated disc disease (cervical or lumbar) is made, the patient is generally better served by surgery at least 3 months after onset of the disease and not more than 1 year after onset of the problem. The advantages and disadvantages of surgery at any given point in the course of the disease obviously vary with the individual patient.

Fusions may be employed on the assumption that decreasing mobility of the motion segment reduces irritation of all related structures and alleviates or eliminates pain.

It has been shown that posterior fusion reduces but does not eliminate motion.

A *third* spine operation in the same region should thoroughly free all neural elements, fuse the involved segments, and should be the last operation.

Prophylaxis, Ergonomics

There is indirect pathoanatomic evidence that the slightly flexed or straight back position of the spine is less painful and more comfortable. This is controversial, and the desirable position may be best determined for each individual patient.

There is solid biomechanical evidence that shows that a back rest inclination of 120 degrees and a 5-cm lumbar support constitute the ideal seat. Arm rests, adequate thigh support, and space within which to comfortably alter position are some additional biomechanically important factors in design.

When an object is being lifted, the distance that it is held away from the body has been shown to be the factor of major importance in the ergonomics of lifting. To greatly reduce forces on the lumbar vertebrae, objects should be held close to the body when lifting.

The ability to generate large intratruncal pressures through the use of powerful abdominal muscles significantly protects the spine as well as increases the capacity to lift heavy loads. It is recommended that patients with spine pain have a program of isometric abdominal exercises before returning to work that involves significant lifting.

Flexing the knees and hips and lifting with the legs while maintaining a straight back are also important in the ergonomics of lifting. However, these factors may not be as important as are the two preceding considerations.

It is suggested that patients with acute, subacute, or chronic lumbar spine pain avoid sit-ups and hyperextension exercises because these activities exert such large forces on the lumbar spine. The exception is the worker or the athlete who must perform isotonic flexion or extension muscle activity.

NOTES

[A] The onset of cervical disc disease is later than that of lumbar disease.[71] Patients in the age range of 30 to 39 years are most likely to have lumbar disc surgery, as opposed to age 40 to 49 for cervical disc surgery.[79,84]

[B] It is possible that Type V disc pathology may respond to spinal manipulation. This constitutes an exception to the statement that manipulation and displacement of a motion segment through a normal range of motion cannot significantly move structures in or out of the intervertebral foramen.

[C] This statement apparently conflicts with the recommendations of the Low Back School (see Fig. 6-30). In an attempt to resolve this, M. Zachrisson-Forssell was consulted. The discrepancy was acknowledged, but it was suggested that the exercises are not performed in the acute phase of spine pain and that they are very carefully taught and supervised. The technique is one of a slow curving upward, starting with the head, followed by the shoulders, upper thoracic spine, and the lumbar spine. Although there are no measurements, this is thought to be associated with much lower loads than the ones recorded in the studies conducted by Nachemson. Despite the findings of Nachemson, some physical therapists state that partial sit-ups, with hips and knees flexed, do not cause any detrimental loads or irritations. It is more generally agreed, however, that sit-ups with legs straight (Fig. 6-27) are to be avoided in patients with back pain. With this type of sit-up, the lumbar spine is loaded by the erector spinae, psoas, and abdominal muscles.

CLASSIFICATION OF REFERENCES

Etiology 1, 5, 6, 7, 11, 18, 50, 58, 63, 81, 99, 105, 110, 119, 157

Epidemiology 55, 71, 72, 73, 79, 80, 81, 82, 83, 84, 96, 97, 98, 115

Socioeconomic, psychological topics 9a, 10, 12, 37, 38, 66, 93, 96, 97, 98, 111, 126, 149, 155

Radiographic variations and anomalies 47, 64, 111

The intervertebral disc 11, 13, 18, 40, 47, 50, 56, 57, 58, 76, 103, 107, 108, 111, 112, 118

Diagnostic considerations (history, physical exam, laboratory) 29, 43, 59, 64, 67, 68, 70, 72, 73, 77, 87, 88, 111, 126, 136, 142, 148

Treatment 9a, 30, 59, 73, 111, 136, 138, 147

Rest, exercise, physical therapy 3, 8, 9a, 28, 35, 36, 39, 85, 91, 107, 109, 111, 135, 143, 153

Patient education 9a, 104, 111

Traction 18, 20, 22, 23, 24, 25, 35, 44, 48, 69, 74, 89, 90, 128, 144

REFERENCES

1. Agnoli, A. L., et al.: Differential diagnosis of sciatica. Analysis of 3000 disc operations. *In* Wöllenweber, R., et al. (eds.): Advances in Neurosurgery. vol. 4. New York, Springer-Verlag, 1977.
2. Andersson, G. B. J., Nachemson, A., and Örtengren, R.: Measurements of Back Loads in Lifting. Spine, *1:*178, 1976.
3. Andersson, G. B. J., Örtengren, R., and Nachemson, A.: Quantitative studies of back loads in lifting. Spine, *1:*178, 1976.
4. ———: Intradiscal pressure, intra abdominal pressure and myoelectric back muscle activity related to posture and loading. Clin. Orthop., *129:*156, 1977.
5. Arnoldi, C. C.: Intervertebral pressures in patients with lumbar pain. A preliminary communication. Acta Orthop. Scand., *43:*109, 1972.
6. Arnoldi, C. C., et al.: Lumbar spinal stenosis and nerve root entrapment syndromes: definition and classification. Clin. Orthop., *115:*4, 1976.
7. Arnoldi, C. C., Lemperg, R. K., and Linderholm, H.: Immediate effect of osteotomy on the intraosseous pressure of the femoral head and neck in patients with coxarthrosis. Acta Orthopaed. Scand., *42:*357, 1971.
8. Bartelink, D. L.: The role of abdominal pressure in relieving the pressure on the lumbar intervertebral disc. J. Bone Joint Surg., *37B:*718, 1957.
9. Belytschko, T., Kulak, R. F., Schultz, A., and Galante, J.: Finite element stress analysis of an intervertebral disc. J. Biomech., *7:*277, 1974.
9a. Bergquist-Ullman, M., and Larsson, U.: Acute back pain in industry. A controlled prospective study with special reference to therapy and confounding factors. Acta Orthop. Scand., *170*[Suppl.], 1977.
10. Blummer, D.: Psychiatric considerations in pain. *In* Rothmann, R. H., and Simeone, F. A. (eds.): The Spine. vol. 2, chap. 18. Philadelphia, W. B. Saunders, 1975. (*One of the most comprehensive and clinically useful works on the psychopathologic aspects of spine pain.*)
11. Bobechko, W. P., and Hirsch, C.: Auto-immune response to nucleus pulposus in the rabbit. J. Bone Joint Surg., *47B:*574, 1965.
12. Breuer, J., and Freud, S.: Studies on hysteria. The Standard Edition of the Complete Psychological Works of Sigmund Freud, vol. 2. London, The Hogard Press, 1895.
13. Brown, M. D.: The pathophysiology of disc disease. Orthop. Clin. North Am., *2:*359, 1971.
14. ———: Chemonucleolysis with disease, technique, results, case reports. Spine, *1:*115; 161 [erratum], 1976. (*A very good reference for the "how to" aspects of this form of treatment.*)
15. Brown, M. D., and Daroff, R. B.: Double blind study comparing disease to placebo. Spine, *2:*233, 1977.
16. Brown, M. D., and Tsaltas, T. T.: Studies on the permeability of the intervertebral disc during skeletal maturation. Spine, *1:*240, 1976.
17. Chaffin, D. B.: Human strength capability and low back pain. J. Occup. Med., *16:*248, 1974.
18. Charnley, J.: Acute lumbago and sciatica. B. Med. J., *1:*344, 1955. (*This work is a classical exposition on the topic. There is a clear theoretical presentation of the mechanism, diagnosis and treatment of the various combinations of back pain and sciatica. Highly recommended for both the primary care physician and the specialist.*)
19. Chrisman, O. D., Mittnacht, A., and Snook, G. A.: A study of the results following rotatory manipulation in the lumbar intervertebral disc syndrome. J. Bone Joint Surg., *46A:*517, 1964. (*An informative clinical study of spinal manipulative therapy.*)
20. Christe, B. G. B.: Discussion of the treatment of backache by traction. Proc. R. Soc. Med., *48:*811, 1955.
21. Cloud, G. A., Doyle, J. E., Sanford, R. L., and Schmitz, T. H.: Final Statistical Analysis of the Disease Double Blind Clinical Trial. Biostatistical Services Department, Travenol Labs., Inc., Feb., 1976.
22. Colachis, S. C., and Strohm, B. R.: Effects of intermittent traction on separation of lumbar vertebrae. Arch. Phys. Med. Rehabil., *50:*251, 1969.
23. ———: Cervical traction: relationship of traction time to varied tractive force with constant angle of pull. Arch. Phys. Med. Rehabil., *46:*815, 1965.
24. ———: Effect of duration of intermittent cervical traction on vertebral separation. Arch. Phys. Med. Rehabil., *47:*353, 1966.
25. ———: A study of tractive forces and angle of pull on the vertebral interspaces in the cervical spine. Arch. Phys. Med. Rehabil., *46:*820, 1965. (*A good bibliography and synopsis of the literature.*)
26. Coyer, A. B., and Curwen, I. H. M.: Low back pain treated by manipulation. A controlled series. Br. Med. J., *1:*705, 1955.
27. Crelin, E. S.: A scientific test of chiropractic theory. Am. Sci., *61:*574, 1973.
28. Davis, P. R., and Troup, J. D. G.: Pressures in the trunk cavities when pulling, pushing and lifting. Ergonomics, *7:*465, 1964.
29. DePalma, A. F., and Rothmann, R. H.: The Intervertebral Disc. Philadelphia, W. B. Saunders, 1970. (*An excellent review of the clinical problem of disc disease.*)
30. Dimond, E. G., Kittle, C. F., and Crockett, J. E.: Comparison of internal mammary artery ligation and sham operation for angina pectoris. Am. J. Cardiol., *5:*483, 1960. (*A convincing example of the placebo effects of surgery.*)
31. Domissee, G. F.: The blood supply of the spinal cord. A critical vascular zone in spinal surgery. J. Bone Joint Surg., *56B:*255, 1974. (*A lucidly and beautifully illustrative work of major importance.*)
32. Doran, D. M. L., and Newell, D. J.: Manipulation in treatment of low back pain: A multicenter study. Br.

Med. J., 2:161, 1975. (*A well designed and well executed study, the results of which are of considerable importance.*)

33. Dunkerley, G. E.: The results of surgery of low back pain due to presumptive prolapsed intervertebral disc. Postgrad. Med. J., 47:120, 1971.

34. Edwards, B. C.: Low back pain and pain resulting from lumbar spine conditions: a comparison of treatment results. Aust. J. Physiother., 15:104, 1969. (*A well designed, executed, and analyzed study.*)

35. Eie, N., and Kristiansen, K.: Komplikasjoner og farer ved traksjonsbehandling av lumbale skiveprolaps. T. Norske Laegeforen, 81:1517, 1961.

36. Eie, N., and Wehn, P.: Measurement of the intra-abdominal pressure in relation to weight bearing of the lumbosacral spine. J. Oslo City Hosp., 12:205, 1962. (*An interesting, well executed, informative, and well presented study.*)

37. Engel, G. L.: Psychogenic pain and the pain prone patient. Am. J. Med., 26:899, 1959.

38. ———: Applied physiology and clinical interpretation. *In* MacBryde, C. M. (ed.): Signs and Symptoms. ed. 5, chap. 3. Philadelphia, J. B. Lippincott, 1970.

39. Fahrni, W. H.: Conservative treatment of lumbar disc degeneration: Our primary responsibility. Orthop. Clin. North Am., 6:93, 1975.

40. Farfan, H., et al.: The effects of torsion on the lumbar intervertebral joint: The role of torsion in the production of disc degeneration. J. Bone Joint Surg., 52A:468, 1970.

41. Feffer, H. L.: Treatment of low back pain and sciatic pain by injection of hydrocortisone into degenerated intervertebral disc. J. Bone Joint Surg., 38A:585, 1956.

42. Finnegan, W., et al.: Salvage spine surgery. Proc. Am. Acad. Orthop. Surg. J. Bone Joint Surg., 57A:1034, 1975.

43. Finneson, B. E.: Low Back Pain. Philadelphia, J. B. Lippincott, 1973.

44. Fisher, E. D.: 1943 Report of a case of ruptured intervertebral disc following chiropractic manipulation. Kentucky Med. J., 41:14, 1943.

45. Ford, L. T.: Experimental study of chymopapain in cats. Clin. Orthop., 67:68, 1969.

46. Frazier, E. H.: Use of traction in backache. Med. J. Aust., 2:694, 1954.

47. Friberg, S., and Hirsch, C.: Anatomical and clinical studies of lumbar disc degeneration. Acta Orthop. Scand., 19:222, 1949.

48. Fried, L. C.: Cervical spinal cord injury during skeletal traction. J.A.M.A., 229:181, 1974.

49. Garvin, P. J., Jennings, R. B., Smith, L., and Gesler, R. M.: Chymopapain: a pharmacological and toxicological evaluation in experimental animals. Clin. Orthop., 41:204, 1965.

50. George, R. C., and Chrisman, O. D.: The role of cartilage polysaccharides in osteoarthritis. Clin. Orthop., 57:259, 1968.

51. Gertzbein, S. D., Tile, M., Gross, A., and Falk, R.: Autoimmunity in degenerative disc disease of the lumbar spine. Symposium on the Lumbar Spine. Orthop. Clin. North Am., 6:67, 1975.

52. Gasler, R. M.: Pharmacologic properties of chymopapain. Clin. Orthop., 67:47, 1969.

53. Glover, J. R., Morris, J. G., and Khosla, T.: Back pain: A randomized clinical trial or rotational manipulation of the trunk. Br. J. Industr. Med., 31:59, 1974. (*An important, informative, well-designed and well-executed study.*)

54. Goldstine, M. (ed.): The research status of spinal manipulative therapy. HEW Publication No. 76, p. 998. Bethesda, 1975. (*This publication does an excellent job of presenting a large amount of current information on this topic, including several points of view. The document does not answer the question of effectiveness of spinal manipulative therapy nor does it resolve controversy.*)

55. Goodsell, J. O.: Correlation of ruptured lumbar disc with occupation. Clin. Orthop., 50:225, 1967.

56. Green, D., and Joynt, R. J.: Vascular accidents to the brain stem associated with neck manipulation. J.A.M.A., 170:522, 1959.

57. Gregersen, G. G., and Lucas, D. B.: An in vivo study of the axial rotation of the human thoraco lumbar spine. J. Bone Joint Surg., 49A:259, 1967.

58. Gruber, G. J., and Ziperman, H. H.: Relationship between whole-body vibration and morbidity patterns among motor coach operators. HEW Publication No. 75-104, p. 51. Office of Technical Publication, Cincinnati, 1974.

59. Hakelius, A.: Prognosis in sciatica. A clinical follow-up of surgical and non-surgical treatment. Acta Orthop. Scand., 129[Suppl.], 1970. (*Highly recommended for those therapists involved in the treatment of patients with low back pain and sciatica.*)

60. Hirsch, C.: An attempt to diagnose the level of disc lesion clinically by disc puncture. Acta Orthop. Scand., 18:132, 1948.

61. ———: Studies on the pathology of low back pain. J. Bone Joint Surg., 41B:237, 1959.

62. ———: Low back pain. Etiology and pathogenesis. Appl. Ther., 8:857, 1966.

63. Hirsch, C., Ingelmark, B. E., and Muller, M.: The anatomical basis for low back pain. Acta Orthop. Scand., 33:1, 1963.

64. Hirsch, C., and Nachemson, A.: The reliability of lumbar disc surgery. Clin. Orthop., 29:189, 1963.

65. Hirsch, C., Wickbom, I., Lidström, A., and Rosengren, K.: Cervical disc resection. A follow-up of myelographic and surgical procedure. J. Bone Joint Surg., 46A:1811, 1964.

66. Holmes, T. H., and Masuda, M.: Life Change and Illness Susceptibility. Separation and Depression. AAAS Publication, No. 94, p. 161, 1973. (*A fascinating and thoroughly documented demonstration of the relationship between the onset of life crises and disease.*)

67. Holt, E. P.: Fallacy of cervical discography. Report of 50 cases in normal subjects. J.A.M.A., 188:799, 1964.

68. ———: The question of lumbar discography. J. Bone Joint Surg., 50A:720, 1968. (*This work seems to conclusively lay the question of the usefulness of lumbar discography to rest as a diagnostic tool.*)

69. Hood, L. B., and Chrisman, D.: Intermittent pelvic traction in the treatment of the ruptured intervertebral disk. J. Am. Phys. Ther. Assoc., 48:21, 1967.

70. Hoppenfeld, S.: Physical Examination of the Spine and Extremities. New York, Appleton-Century-Crofts, 1976. (*A very instructive, pleasant and well illustrated book.*)

71. Horal, J.: The clinical appearance of low back disorders in the city of Göthenburg, Sweden. Comparison of

incapacitated probands with matched control [Thesis]. Acta Orthop. Scand. *118*[Suppl.], 1969.

72. Hult, L.: Cervical, dorsal and lumbar spinal syndromes. Acta Orthop. Scand. *17*[Suppl.], 1954. (*An important and frequently referred to work, highly recommended.*)

73. ———: The Munkfors investigation. Acta Orthop. Scan., *16*[Suppl.], 1954.

74. Judovich, B. D.: Lumbar traction therapy. Elimination of physical factors that prevent lumbar stretch. J.A.M.A., *159*:549, 1955.

75. Kane, R. L., et al.: Manipulating the patient. A comparison of the effectiveness of physician and chiropractor care. Lancet, *1*:1333, 1974. (*This is suggested as required annual reading for every physician involved in the care of patients with spine pain.*)

76. Keegan, J. J.: Alterations of the lumbar curve related to posture and seating. J. Bone Joint Surg., *35A*:589, 1953.

77. Keim, H. A.: Low Back Pain. Ciba Clinical Symposia. vol. 25, no. 3, 1973. (*Another Ciba classic*).

78. Kelley, J. H., Voris, D. C., Svien, J. H., and Churmley, R. K.: Multiple operations for protruded lumbar intervertebral disc. Proc. Staff Meet., Mayo Clin., *29*:546, 1954.

79. Kelsey, J. L.: An epidemiological study of acute herniated lumbar intervertebral discs. Rheumatol. Rehabil., *14*:144, 1975. (*A thorough well controlled and statistically analyzed study.*)

80. ———: An epidemiological study of the relationship between occupations and acute herniated lumbar intervertebral disc. Int. J. Epidemiol., *4*:197, 1975.

81. ———: Epidemiology of radiculopathies. Adv. Neurol. [In Press]. (*A highly recommended review article on the epidemiology of spine pain.*)

82. Kelsey, J. L., Greenberg, R. A., Hardy, R. J., and Johnson, M. F.: Pregnancy and the syndrome of herniated lumbar intervertebral disc; an epidemiological study. Yale J. Biol. Med., *48*:361, 1975.

83. Kelsey, J. L., and Hardy, R. J.: Driving of motor vehicles as a risk factor for acute herniated lumbar intervertebral disc. Am. J. Epidemiol., *102*:63, 1975.

84. Kelsey, J. L., and Ostfeld, A. M.: Demographic characteristics of persons with acute herniated lumbar intervertebral disc. J. Chronic Dis., *28*:37, 1975.

85. Kendall, P. H., and Jenkins, J. M.: Exercises for backache. A double blind controlled trial. Physiotherapy, *54*:154, 1968.

86. Keith, A.: Man's posture, its evolution and disorders. Br. Med. J., *1*:587, 1923.

87. Kirkaldy-Willis, W. H., Paine, K. W. E., Cauchoix, J., and McIvor, G.: Lumbar spinal stenosis. Clin. Orthop., *99*:30, 1974. (*This very important article is highly recommended. A thorough review of the literature that brings forth some cogent considerations in the etiology, diagnosis and treatment of spinal stenosis.*)

88. Lasèque, C: Considérations sur la sciaticque. Arch. Gén. Med. 2:558, 1864.

89. Lawson, G. A., and Godfrey, C. M.: A report on studies of spinal traction. Med. Serv. J. Can., *14*:762, 1958.

90. Lehmann, J. F., and Bruner, G. D.: A device for the application of heavy lumbar traction: Its mechanical effects. Arch. Phys. Med., *39*:696, 1958.

91. Lidström, A., and Zachrisson, M.: Physical therapy on low back pain and sciatica. An attempt at evaluation. Scand. J. Rehabil. Med., 2:37, 1970.

92. Lora, J., and Long, D.: So called facet denervation in the management of intractable back pain. Spine, *1*:121, 1976.

93. Luck, V.: Psychosomatic problems in military orthopaedic surgery. J. Bone Joint Surg., 28:213, 1946.

94. McCulloch, J. A.: Chemonucleolysis. J. Bone Joint Surg., *59B*:45, 1977. (*One of the most important and well presented investigations on this topic.*)

95. Macnab, I., et al.: Chemonucleolysis. Can. J. Surg., *14*:280, 1971. (*A useful concise review of the most cogent literature and some suggestions about the indications for the use of chymopapain.*)

96. Magora, A.: Investigation of the relation between low back pain and occupation. Ind. Med. Surg., 39:504, 1970.

97. ———: Investigation of the relation between low back pain and occupation. 4. Physical requirements: Bending, rotation, reaching and sudden maximal effort. Scand. J. Rehabil. Med., *5*:186, 1973.

98. Magora, A., and Taustein, I.: An investigation of the problem of sick-leave in the patient suffering from low back pain. Ind. Med. Surg., 38:398, 1969.

99. Maitland, G. D.: Vertebral Manipulation. ed. 3. London, Butterworth, 1973.

100. Massie, W. K., and Stevens, D. B.: A critical evaluation of discography. Proc. Am. Acad. Orthop. Surg. Scientific Exhibits, J. Bone Joint Surg., *49A*:1243, 1967.

101. Melzack, R., and Wall, P. D.: Pain mechanisms: A new theory. Science, *150*:971, 1965. (*A classic. Also an excellent review of the literature on the psychophysiologic aspects of pain.*)

102. Mensor, M. C.: Non operative treatment including manipulation for lumbar intervertebral disc syndrome. J. Bone Joint Surg., *37A*:925, 1955.

103. Mixter, W. J., and Barr, J. S.: Ruptures of the intervertebral disc with involvement of the spinal canal. N. Eng. J. Med., *211*:210, 1934.

104. Mooney, V.: Alternative approaches for the patient beyond the help of surgery. Orthop. Clin. North Am., *6*:331, 1975.

105. Morotomi, T.: Affections of spine. *In* Amako, T. (ed.): Orthopaedics. Tokyo, Kanehara, 1960.

106. Morris, J. M., Lucas, D. B., and Bresler, B.: Role of the trunk in stability of the spine. J. Bone Joint Surg., *43A*:327, 1961.

107. Nachemson, A. L.: The influence of spinal movement on the lumbar intra discal pressure and on the tensile stresses in the annulus fibrosus. Acta Orthop. Scand., *33*:183, 1963.

108. ———: In vivo discometry in lumbar discs with irregular radiograms. Acta Orthop. Scand., *36*:418, 1965.

109. ———: Physiotherapy for low back pain. A critical look. Scand. J. Rehabil. Med., *1*:85, 1969. (*An excellent review article highly recommended for anyone interested in physical therapy treatment.*)

110. ———: A critical Look at the Treatment for Low Back Pain. The Research Status of Spinal Manipulative Therapy. DHEW Publication No. (NIH) 76-998:21B, Bethesda, 1975. (*An excellent review article.*)

111. ———: The lumbar spine, an orthopaedic challenge.

Spine, *1*:59, 1976. (*An outstanding, well written review of all aspects of current state of knowledge. There is an excellent bibliography.*)

112. Naylor, A.: Intervertebral disc prolapse and degeneration; the biochemical and biophysical approach. Spine, *1*:108, 1976. (*A superb, comprehensive review article, which elucidates the hypothesis clearly.*)

113. Nichlas, I. W.: End-result study of the treatment of herniated nucleus pulposus by excision with fusion and without fusion. Res. Com. Acad. Orthop. Surg. J. Bone Joint Surg., *34A*:981, 1952.

114. Nordby, E. J., and Lucas, G. L.: A comparative analysis of lumbar disc disease treated by laminectomy or chemonucleolysis. Clin. Orthop., *90*:119, 1973.

114a. Nwuga, V. C.: Manipulation of the Spine. Baltimore, Williams & Wilkins, 1976.

115. O'Connell, J. E.: Lumbar disc protrusion in pregnancy. J. Neurol. Neurosurg. Psychiatry, *23*:138, 1960.

116. Onofrio, B. M.: Injection of chymopapain into intervertebral disc. J. Neurosurg., *42*:384, 1975.

117. Örtengren, R., and Andersson, G. B. J.: Electromyographic studies of trunk muscles, with special references to the functional anatomy of the lumbar spine. Spine, *2*:44, 1977. (*An excellent, concise and comprehensive review of the literature on the functional significance of muscle activity in the biomechanics of the spine.*)

118. Paine, K. W. E., and Huang, P. W. H.: Lumbar disc syndrome. J. Neurosurg., *37*:75, 1972.

119. Pankovich, A. M., and Korngold, L.: A comparison of the antigenic properties of nucleus pulposus and cartilage protein polysaccharide complexes. J. Immunol., *99*:431, 1967.

120. Patton, H. D.: Summary of general discussion: What do the basic sciences tell us about manipulative therapy? The research status of spinal manipulative therapy. HEW Publication No. 76-998, p. 213, Bethesda, 1975.

121. Poppen, J. L.: The herniated intervertebral disc. An analysis of 400 verified cases. N. Eng. J. Med., *232*:211, 1945.

122. Pratt-Thomas, H. R., and Berger, K. E.: Cerebellar and spinal injuries after chiropractic manipulations. J.A.M.A., *133*:1947.

123. Reinhold, H.: Munch the scream. New York, Viking Press, 1972.

124. Riley, L. H., Robinson, R. A., Johnson, K. A., and Walker, A. E.: The results of anterior interbody fusion of the cervical spine. Review of ninety-three consecutive cases. J. Neurosurg., *30*:127, 1969.

125. Robinson, R. A., Walker, A. E., Ferlic, D. C., and Wiecking, D. V.: The results of anterior interbody fusion of the cervical spine. J. Bone Joint Surg., *44A*:1569, 1962.

126. Rockwood, C. A., and Eilert, R. E.: Camptocormia. J. Bone Joint Surg., *51A*:553, 1969. (*A neat synopsis of the entity, with a good bibliography.*)

127. Rydevik, B., et al.: Effects of chymopapain on nerve tissue. An experimental study on the structure and function of peripheral nerve tissue in rabbits after local application of chymopapain. Spine, *1*:137, 1976.

128. Schlicke, L., et al.: A quantitative study of vertebral displacement in the normal cervical spine under axial load. [In Press].

129. Schwetschenau, P. A., et al.: Double blind evaluation of intradiscal chymopapain for herniated lumbar disc. J. Neurosurg., *45*:622, 1976.

130. Selecki, B. R., et al.: Low back pain: A joint neurosurgical and orthopaedic project. Med. J. Aust., *2*:889, 1973. (*A fascinating and informative study highly contributing to better understanding between the two specialties.*)

131. Shealy, C. N.: Tissue reactions to chymopapain in cats. J. Neurosurg., *26*:327, 1967.

132. Singleton, W. T.: Introduction to Ergonomics. Geneva, World Health Organization, 1972. (*A good synopsis of the field.*)

133. Smith, L.: Chemonucleolysis. Clin. Orthop., *67*:72, 1969.

134. Smyth, M. J., and Wright, V.: Sciatica and the intervertebral disc. J. Bone Joint Surg., *40A*:1401, 1958.

135. Soderberg, L.: Prognosis in conservatively treated sciatica. Acta Orthop. Scand. Suppl., *21*:1, 1956.

136. Spangfort, E. V.: The lumbar disc herniation. A computer-aided analysis of 2,504 operations. Acta Orthop. Scand., *142*[Suppl.], 1972. (*An excellent paper for the evaluation and interpretation of the significance of various physical findings.*)

137. Stern, I. J.: Biochemistry of chymopapain. Clin. Orthop., *67*:42, 1969.

138. Stolley, P. D., and Kuller, L. H.: The need for epidemiologists and surgeons to cooperate in the evaluation of surgical therapies. Surgery, *78*:123, 1975. (*Recommended reading for individuals making decisions about the "value" of a given surgical procedure.*)

139. Sunderland, S.: Anatomical perivertebral influences on the intervertebral foramen. The research status of spinal manipulative therapy. HEW Publication No. 76-998, p. 129, Bethesda, 1975. (*A well illustrated review.*)

140. Symposium on lumbo-sacral fusion and low back pain. J. Bone Joint Surg., *37B*:164, 1955.

141. Thibodeau, A. A., and McCombs, R. P: Backache. Ther. Conf. Bull. N. Eng. Med., *11*:34, 1949.

142. Tovi, D., and Strang, R. R.: Thoracic intervertebral disc protrusions. Acta Chir. Scand. Suppl., *267*:1, 1960. (*A highly recommended and useful reference on this relatively sparsely written about topic.*)

143. Troup, J. D. G.: Relation of lumbar spine disorders to heavy manual work and lifting. Lancet, *1*:857, 1965. (*A good synopsis and excellent review of the literature on the biomechanics of lifting.*)

144. Valtonen, E. J., and Kiuru, E.: Cervical traction as a therapeutic tool. A clinical analysis based on 212 patients. Scand. J. Rehabil. Med., *2*:29, 1970.

145. Watts, C., Hutchinson, G., Stern, J., and Clark, K.: Comparison of intervertebral disc disease treatment by chymopapain. J. Neurosurg., *42*:397, 1975.

146. Watts, C., Knighton, R., and Roulhac, G.: Chymopapain treatment of intervertebral disc disease. J. Neurosurg., *42*:374, 1975. (*An informative and thorough review of the historical, pharmacologic, experimental and clinical aspects of chemonucleolysis.*)

147. Weber, H.: The effect of delayed disc surgery on muscular paresis. Acta Orthop. Scand., *46*:631, 1975.

148. Wedge, J. H., Kinnard, P., Fley, R. K., and Kirkaldy-Willis, W. H.: The management of spinal stenosis. Orthop. Rev., *6*:89, 1977.

149. Westrin, C. G.: Low back pain sick listing. Ansological

and medical insurance investigation. Scand. J. Soc. Med. Suppl., 7:1, 1973. (*An enlightening and important study.*)

150. White, A. A., et al.: Relief of pain by anterior cervical spine fusion for spondylosis. J. Bone Joint Surg., *55A:* 525, 1973.

151. Wiberg, G.: Back pain in relation to the nerve supply of the intervertebral disc. Acta Orthop. Scand., *19:*211, 1950.

152. Williams, J. L., Allen, M. B., Jr., and Harkness, J. W.: Late results of cervical discectomy and interbody fusion: Some factors influencing the results. J. Bone Joint Surg., *50A:*277, 1968.

153. Williams, P. C.: Lesions of the lumbosacral spine. Part II. Chronic traumatic (postural) destruction of the lumbosacral intervertebral disc. J. Bone Joint Surg., *19:*

690, 1937. (*The rationale for the use of Williams exercises are well explained. However, we respectfully disagree with the sit-ups.*)

154. Wiltse, L. L., Kirkaldy-Willis, W. H., and McIvor, G. W. D.: The treatment of spinal stenosis. Clin. Orthop., *115:*83, 1976.

155. Wiltse, L. L., and Rucchio, P. D.: Preoperative psychological tests as predictors of success of chemonucleolysis in treatment of the low back syndrome. J. Bone Joint Surg., *57A:*478, 1975.

156. Wiltse, L. L., Widell, E. H., and Yuan, H. A.: Chymopapain. Chemonucleolysis in lumbar disc disease. J.A.M.A., *231:*474, 1975.

157. Wyke, B.: The neurological basis of thoracic spine pain. Rheumatology and Physical Medicine, *10:*356, 1970.

7 Spinal Braces: Functional Analysis and Clinical Applications

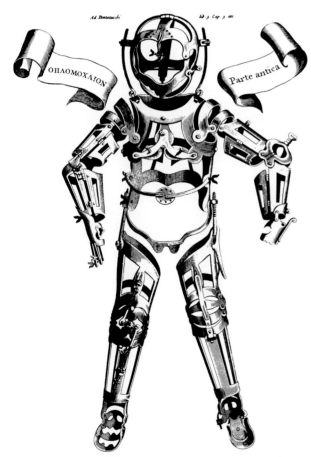

Fig. 7-1. This shows how easily the skill of the armorer can be transfered to the fabrication of orthoses. With modest imagination, one can extrapolate the components of almost any brace directly from this picture. (Reproduced from Orthopaedic Appliances Atlas, vol. 1. American Academy of Orthopaedic Surgeons, Ann Arbor, J. W. Edwards, 1952. Original from Heironmus Fabricus ab Aquapendente. Opera Chirurgica. Patavii, Bolzetti, 1641. Courtesy of the Armed Forces Institute of Pathology.)

Unfortunately, there has been very little actual research done in the area of spinal orthotics. Thus, a significant portion of this chapter is based on "arm chair science" and inferences from objective information about physical properties of the tissues involved. The end result is not hard science, but a rational approach based on the available biomechanical knowledge and concepts.

The names of the various spinal orthoses are complex, confusing, and frustrating. Hopefully, this chapter will not add to the appellative turmoil, but will alleviate it through an analytical approach that emphasizes components and functions rather than cities, states, and eponyms.

HISTORICAL BACKGROUND

This section is based largely on information from the *Orthopaedic Appliances Atlas*.[16] *Corpus Hippocraticum*, a sifting of all contemporary medical knowledge as well as a humanistic approach to medical ethics, was written by Hippocrates in the first century A.D. Two of his books, *On Fractures* and *On Articulation*, dealt with methods of treating orthopaedic problems.

Galen (131–201 A.D.) was the first to employ the terms scoliosis, kyphosis, and lordosis. Because of his experiments with animal dissections, he is given credit for the first attempt at active correction of spinal deformities based on his broad concept of physiology and morbid anatomy. He advocated breathing exercises, singing, and chest strapping for the correction of scoliosis. In the Middle Ages during peace time, when the armorers were not involved in military endeavors, their talents were displayed in brace making. Figure 7-1 readily shows the similarity of orthotic appliances and armor. It is difficult to resist the suggestion that the spirit of these armorers may have been the precursor of the contemporary spirit of bioengineers, motivated to employ their knowledge and expertise for humane rather than martial purposes. There are certain observable patterns, even in these crude, old armor-like braces, which have molded pelvic supports and spinal uprights.

Ambrose Paré (1509–1590) is considered a pioneer in the modern art of brace making. Among his inventions were metal corsets, leather walking splints, and different types of shoes for sufferers of club feet. In the 17th century, though orthopaedics was far from a recognized specialty, supportive appliances, slings, and extension devices were being improved far beyond the advancements of previous centuries. Nicholas Andry (1704–1756), professor of medicine at the University of Paris, led many of these advances and combined the words which gave this field of medicine its name: *orthos*, meaning straight, and *paidios*, meaning child. Two of his colleagues, Lorenz Heister and Levache, made substantial contributions in the development of brace making. Heister is credited with the development of the first crude spinal brace. This apparatus was quite aptly known as the "iron cross" (Fig. 7-2). Note the "halo-like" head piece and the support for the sling, both principles of which are still currently employed. Levache devised a suspension brace by elongating the posterior bar of a spinal brace over the head ("jury mast"), attached firmly to a snug fitting cap. This same principle, although often revised, is now used in a different manner with the halo traction apparatus.

Dr. Lovett wrote the following:[16]

. . . although the period at the middle of the 18th century . . . was one of considerable activity and progress, in the development of scoliosis, at about this time, there began and there lasted for over 100 years, the dreariest and most confusing period in the history of the affectation. The theorist and the apparatus inventor went mad, and every form of device appeared. Braces and corsets, infinitely complicated, worse than useless, appeared by the dozen. Beds, especially constructed chairs, slings, swathes, belts, levers and the like all found their advocates and theories as to causation also ran riot, but on the whole, the invention and the elaboration of apparatus held the center of the stage.

Notwithstanding Lovett's views, this period of epidemic creativity yielded several valuable principles or devices in the nonsurgical treatment of scoliosis, such as the plaster jacket, the thigh attachment, pressure pads, pelvic pads, pelvic bands, axillary supports, and the important concept of dynamic bracing.

An analysis of contemporary orthotics reveals that there have not been very many significant changes in the basic concepts and mechanisms of bracing. There have been some worthwhile refinements, however. The 19th century witnessed the emergence of modern medical science. Surgery became more established on a scientific basis rather than as a craft. Along with this change there were the corresponding refinements in the design of mechanical appliances. As the orthopaedist of the 19th century was not primarily a surgeon, his reputation grew in proportion to his ability to effectively utilize *mechanical principles*. Probably the most famous orthopaedist of this period was Hugh Owen Thomas, a prolific inventor of appliances and one whose influence and simplicity of design are still present in modern orthotics. This dedicated, energetic chain-smoker is credited with the development of the frequently used and generously modified Thomas cervical collar. He established his own workshop where braces and splints were fashioned, and his work represents the beginning of the fusion between the mechanical and surgical phases of orthopaedic treatment.

Another advance is credited to Anthonius Mathijsen who used a plaster of paris bandage in 1852 as a substitute for the cumbersome splints which had been used to immobilize limbs. Lewis Sayer (1820–1901), considered the father of orthopaedic surgery in the U.S., was the first to apply a plaster of paris jacket. It was not long before the principle of uninterrupted rest was appreciated, and plaster supplemented many techniques.

The science and technique of brace making have been largely influenced by other American surgeons who devoted much of their time and study to the improvement of existing designs. The last 50 years have seen tremendous strides in the facilities made available to orthopaedic patients, and ongoing research programs continue to discover new materials and techniques which will contribute to more effective spinal bracing. During this period the highlight has been the development of the Milwaukee brace by Schmidt and Blount.

FUNCTIONS OF SPINAL ORTHOSES

The clinical science of spinal orthotics is essentially that of the application of forces to the spine in order to control it. The goals may be any combination of the following: support, rest, immobilization, protection, or correction. The application of forces alters the existing patterns of deformation and kinematics of the spine. To rest the spine, the orthosis must substitute for or assist the actions of muscles. The rationale may be to limit the range of motion when certain positions or movements are painful to the patient. It may be desirable to protect the vital cord and nerve roots immediately following surgery or after injury. In this instance, the brace carries out a function that either the intrinsic structure of the spine or the muscles normally achieve. If inappropriate judgment is employed and erroneous assumptions are made, there is potential danger to the patient. The brace can sometimes function purely as a psychologic reminder; when the patient moves, his brace touches or irritates him in some way, serving as a stimulus to limit that particular activity. Finally, there are the correctional uses of spinal orthoses, as in the treatment of scoliosis and kyphosis.

BIOMECHANICAL FACTORS

Physical Characteristics of the Spine

The spine may be viewed mechanically as a series of semirigid bodies (vertebrae) separated by viscoelastic linkages (discs and ligaments). Elasticity is exemplified by a spring. If a load is

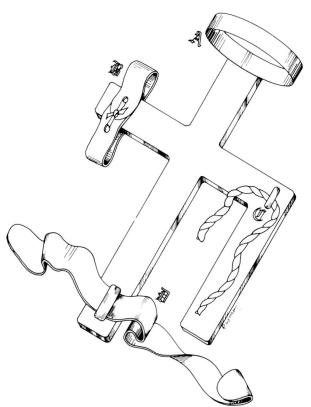

Fig. 7-2. An interpretation of the "iron cross." Lorenz Heister, a student of Professor Andry is credited with having developed this *first spinal brace* in the 18th century. In the art of bracing, variations are prolific and originality is precious. In this construction one can see some basic components. (*A*) A halo-like structure. (*B*) An axillary sling. (*C*) Shoulder straps with splint for the upper arm. (*D*) A waist or pelvic band.

applied, there is an immediate deformation. When the load is released, the spring goes back to its original position. A syringe may be used to describe viscosity. When a load is applied to the plunger, it does not return to its original position upon removal of the load. The rate of application of the load on the plunger is related directly to resistance. Viscoelasticity is a combination of viscosity and elasticity, a syringe-like spring-like phenomenon. An engineering analysis of biologic materials has suggested a model of the linkage for the tissue between vertebrae. This is shown in Figure 7-3.

The clinician is working with a series of linkages suspended in the body, with viscoelastic

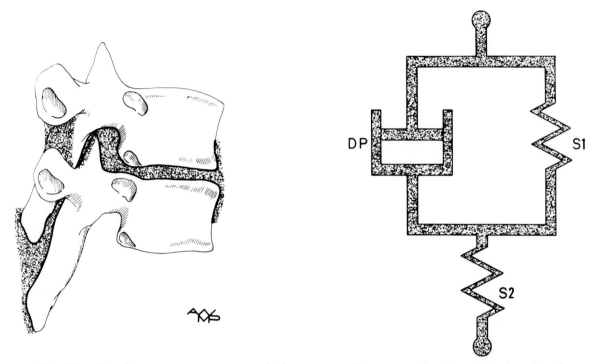

Fig. 7-3. The ligamentous structures which connect adjacent vertebrae may be thought of biomechanically as viscoelastic linkages. The linkage is symbolized by a three-element model consisting of a dashpot (DP) and a spring (S1) in parallel connected to a second spring (S2) in series.

structures of various stiffness attached to it. In the cervical spine, the vertebrae and the linkages are surrounded mostly by muscle. In the thoracic spine, they are encased by muscles, ribs, air, and the lungs. In the lumbar spine, there are the muscles, air, water, and the viscera. Skin and subcutaneous fat are involved, to some degree, in all three regions. The materials encasing the structures have different moduli of elasticity and viscous properties. Materials adjacent to the spinal column are all of fairly low stiffness, except for the ribs, which are significantly stiffer. The ribs stiffen the thoracic spine by forming a box-like construction. It has been calculated by Andriacchi and colleagues that ribs increase the stiffness of the thoracic spine in bending by 200 per cent.[1]

All of these elements may be viewed as sitting in a cylinder, the body. The goal of the orthotist is to transmit force through the cylinder to the spinal column. A force is a quantity necessary to accelerate a mass, to push or to pull, and may be represented by a vector. A vector has three characteristics: magnitude, direction, and point of application.

The Transmitter Problem

In the science of orthotics, the force is not applied directly to the spine but must be transmitted. Whether the goal is support, immobilization, or correction, the mechanism will depend on the transmission of forces. The major mechanical factor that limits the transmission of forces to the spine is the *stiffness* of the structures through which the forces must be transmitted. If a feather is used to push a deformity, very little force is transmitted. This is true regardless of the amount of force that is available. The feather has a low stiffness and will deform. Thus, essentially no force is transmitted. If, on the other hand, a steel rod is employed to push the deformity, it will transmit the force almost completely (Fig. 7-4). The same principle holds when there is an attempt to apply forces to the spine with an orthotic appliance.

The basic biomechanical problem of spinal orthoses is one of transmitting sufficient forces to a series of vertebrae through low stiffness, viscoelastic transmitters. The stiffness of these transmitters varies considerably; the ribs (though not especially stiff) probably represent the stiffest available transmitter. Fat, which has a much lower stiffness, is at the other end of the continuum. The overall biomechanical problem of spinal bracing is summarized schematically in Figure 7-5. These factors are of considerable importance to the clinician in his evaluation of the forces that can be expected to be transmitted to any particular region of the spine in order to achieve a desired therapeutic goal. It is possible to more effectively apply forces to a thoracic scoliosis than to one in the lumbar region because the ribs are better (stiffer) transmitters than the muscles and viscera of the lumbar region. It is known that the Milwaukee brace is less effective for holding or correcting lumbar curves than for that of thoracic curves.

Other Limiting Factors

The pain sensitivity of the skin and the deeper tissues must be considered. Also, there are biologic functions of the skin that have a limiting influence. The skin must be freed of dirt, debris, and its own excretions. It must also be ventilated. These factors limit the magnitude and the duration of pressures that may be applied to the skin. As a result, the clinician is able to apply forces to the spine with most orthoses but is not actually able to control it with complete reliability.

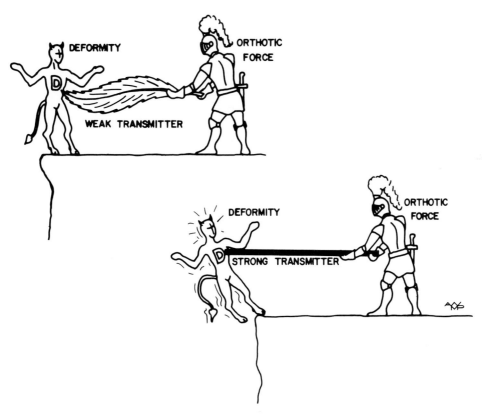

Fig. 7-4. The feather is a weak or a very *low stiffness transmitter.* Thus, no matter how much force the Knight applies, the deformity moves little. With strong or very *high stiffness transmitter,* practically all force is transmitted to the deformity, which readily moves. The Knight's sword may be thought to symbolize the option of surgery should the externally applied forces fail to take care of the deformity.

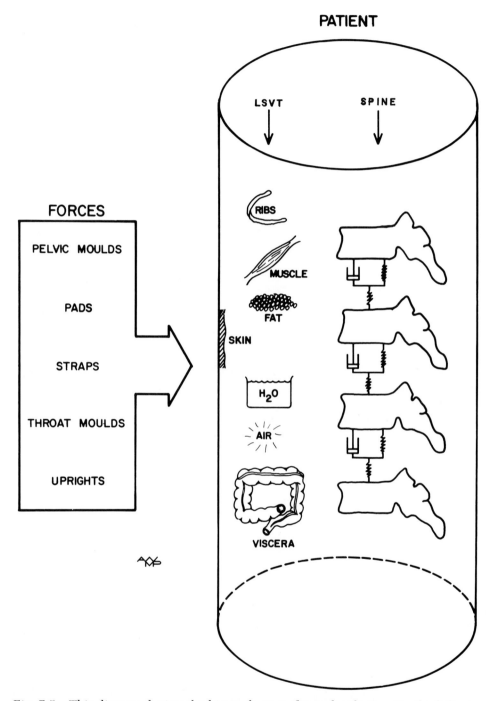

Fig. 7-5. This diagram depicts the biomechanics of spinal orthotics. On the left are the various orthotic components through which forces are applied to the patient on the right. The anatomic components are divided into various low stiffness viscoelastic transmitters (LSVT), and the spine, a series of rigid bodies separated by viscoelastic linkages (see Fig. 7-3). The mechanics of bracing involve the process of transmitting forces to the spine through low stiffness viscoelastic transmitters in order to exert various controls on the vertebrae.

The characteristic elasticity of bone is a limiting factor. Rolander carried out experimental cement fusions of the laminae and spinous and transverse processes of motion segments and observed motion between the vertebral bodies under loads that did not exceed the physiologic range.[18] This was due to the elasticity of the unfixed portion of the vertebra, the pedicles, and the body. Although this experiment has limited application to the spine in vivo, it points out the improbability of completely immobilizing a motion segment with an orthosis when a direct fusion may not do so (see Chapter 8).

In a similar sense, it is important to be aware of the limitations of a brace in protecting an osteoporotic vertebra. (The weakened vertebral body in osteoporosis is discussed in Chapter 1 on page 32). It should be recognized that a brace will be significantly limited in its ability to compensate for the very large loss of supporting elements in the osteoporotic vertebra.

The Normal Kinematics

An analytical approach to the biomechanics of orthotics involves some additional considerations. It is worthwhile for the clinician to keep in mind the *normal* kinematics of the spine as bracing problems are approached. The cervical spine is the most mobile. There is generally more flexion than extension. Most of the motion is in the sagittal plane, and that occurs in the mid-portion (C5–6). The C1-C2 joint, however, has the greatest axial rotation in this region. There is strong coupling of axial rotation and lateral bending in the lower cervical spine, and there is a generous amount of axial rotation in this region. In the thoracic spine, there is significant motion, but it is certainly less mobile than either adjacent region. Here, too, flexion is greater than extension. The amount of rotation in the sagittal plane progressively increases cephlocaudally. The coupling has the same characteristics as that in the cervical spine, but it is not as strong or as consistent. There can be a transition to the kinematic pattern of the lumbar spine anywhere between T9 and T12. There is also an axial rotation in the thoracic region which decreases cephlocaudally. In the lumbar spine, there is little axial rotation. Most of the motion is in flexion/exten-

sion (x-axis rotation). At the lumbosacral joint, there is relatively more rotation. Also, any pelvic motion will move the lumbosacral spine.

For the most complete evaluation of the controls that a clinician can apply to the spine with a brace, two factors should be considered. First, there should be a consideration of the characteristic regional kinematics involved. Then an analysis with respect to the six degrees of freedom should be carried out (see Chapter 2). This includes evaluation of probable translation along each of the three coordinates and rotation about each of the three axes. The clinician then decides which movements he wants to restrict and then selects the appropriate orthosis to achieve that control.

The clinician is usually most concerned with only two or three of these six degrees of freedom. However, an awareness and analysis of all six is desirable. Consider a patient with low back pain. If an orthosis that effectively discourages flexion and extension (rotation about the x-axis) but allows considerable axial rotation (rotation about the y-axis) is prescribed, this may cause difficulty. If the patient has a significant synovitis of the facet joints, the axial rotation may irritate the joints and elicit significant pain, despite the fact that they remain reasonably well protected in flexion and extension.

When orthotics are employed to compensate for instability, a basic understanding of clinical instability is of value. It is necessary to consider which structures have been rendered nonfunctional so that appropriate support may be instituted. Spines that are unstable as a result of the loss of the functional integrity of the anterior elements are more unstable in extension. Spines unstable due to disruption of the posterior elements are more unstable in flexion (see Chapter 5). Certain orthoses protect better against anterior displacement and others protect better against posterior displacement. Here again, all six degrees of freedom should be considered, and decisions concerning the type of motion to be controlled are necessary. Attention is then given to the question of how rigid the fixation should be. The clinician must be certain that it is possible to compensate for the instability with an orthotic device, and that the device selected is most appropriate for the particular instability under treatment.

Creep and Biomechanical Adaptation

The creep phenomena is based on the characteristic of viscoelasticity. It manifests itself in the form of additional deformation over a period of time that may vary from several seconds to several days. Somewhere during this period, probably between 1 and 72 hours, it is predominantly the creep phenomenon that is operative. After this period, biomechanical adaptation comes into play. *Biomechanical adaptation* may be defined as biologically mediated changes in mechanical properties of tissues (material properties and/or structural changes) in association with the application of mechanical variables to these tissues. For example, if the hardness of skin under the pelvic band of a Milwaukee brace was measured

after the first and the 99th day, the values would no doubt be different. The change would be due to biomechanical adaptation.

In long-range responses to forces, there are differences in the configuration of ligaments and bone. The so-called giraffe-necked women of the Padang tribe of Indonesia demonstrate biomechanical adaptation (Fig. 7-6). A radiograph of such a person shows shoulders are pushed caudad; however, there is an intrinsic loss of physiologic cervical lordosis and some exaggerated elongation and separation of vertebral bodies. Another example of adaptation to long-range forces is the change seen in Scheuermann's disease with Milwaukee brace treatment (Fig. 7-22). Here the actual configuration of the spine changes. The alterations are more readily mediated in the growing skeleton, where Heuter Volkmann's laws can operate through the epi-

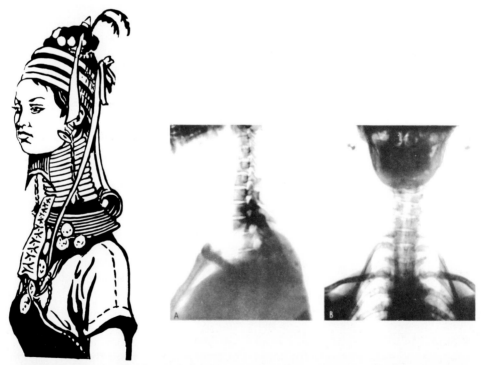

Fig. 7-6. This is a demonstration of *biomechanical adaptation*. In the Padang tribes of Indonesia, rings are placed about the neck, added in gradual increments, and left over a long period of time. The shoulders are pushed down, which adds to the appearance of length. Biomechanical adaptation also is shown by the loss of normal cervical lordosis and more than the usual separation between vertebrae. (Roaf, R.: Scoliosis. Edinburgh, Churchill Livingstone, Ltd., 1966.)

physis. In early gradual correction and also in long-range biologic adaptation, time is an important consideration in the use of spinal orthotics.

Five Principles of Spinal Orthoses

Balanced Horizontal Forces. Horizontal forces are eminently suitable to provide efficient bending moments for the correction of lateral curvature, derotation of vertebrae, and immobilization of the spine. Most of the loading situations in braces can be shown to be mediated through a three-point loading system; this is analyzed in some detail below.

Three horizontal forces are applied at points along the length of the spine. Two are in one direction, and one is in the opposite direction (Fig. 7-7A). There are some fundamental characteristics of this force system. Since the system is in equilibrium, the sum of the forces and the sum of the bending movements they create must be equal to zero. Therefore, the site of application of the forces and their magnitudes are interrelated.

In a general case shown in Figure 7-7, the forces at points B and C have to be in inverse proportion to their perpendicular distances, D_B and D_C, from point A. Further, the sum of the forces at points B and C must always be equal to the force at point A. Thus, with the perpendicular distance D_C being twice that of D_B, the magnitudes of forces at points A, B, and C must be in the ratio of 3 : 2 : 1.[A]

This information has clinical relevance. In order to adjust the skin pressure at the three force points, the pad sizes must be proportioned according to the force magnitudes. In the case of the Jewett brace, shown in Figure 7-8, with two anterior pads placed at an equal distance from the posterior pad, the force at the posterior pad is twice that of the anterior pads and therefore should have twice the pad area in order to have the same skin pressure.

Another important characteristic of this three-point force system is the bending moment applied to the spine. Actually it is the bending moment and not the forces that produces the angular correction. The bending moment at the various intervertebral spaces varies. It is maximum at the level of the middle force F_A, and linearly decreases to zero at the level of the two

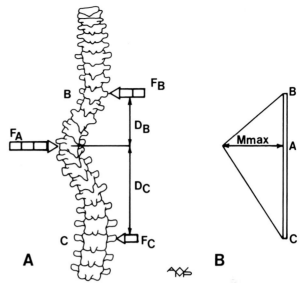

Fig. 7-7. (A) A three-point force system is formed by forces F_A, F_B, and F_C. Relative verticle (y-axis) distances dictate the relative magnitudes of the three forces. (The lengths of the arrows correlate with the relative forces.) (B) The bending moment diagram for the three-point force system is a triangle with its apex at the level of the middle force. The maximum corrective potential or control is thus applied at that point.

end forces, F_B and F_C (Fig. 7-7B). By placing the middle force at the apex of the curve, the clinician maximizes the correctional efficiency of this force. It can be further shown that forces F_B and F_C should be located as far away from F_A as possible.[A]

Fluid Compression. It is possible to use soft tissues (muscles, fascia, and tendons) to support a compressive load. Nature has used the diaphragm and abdominal muscles to compress its contents and employ the turgor of fluid under pressure to support or splint the spine. The orthotist makes valuable use of this concept by applying compression externally, through the use of a corset or an abdominal support, either attached to an appliance or worn alone. A Williams brace is one that uses this corset effect anteriorly on the abdomen to achieve additional support for the spine. This technique is especially effective in resting and unloading the lumbar spine. This mechanism was no doubt operative when fashions were different and the woman would note

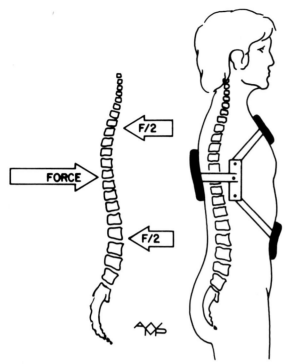

Fig. 7-8. The Jewett brace functions on a three-point force system. As is shown, the posterior pad has been placed midway between the two anterior pads. Therefore each of the anterior forces is one half of the posterior force.

that her back felt better when she "had on her foundation."

Distraction. By the application of tension through distraction, it is possible to achieve a certain amount of immobilization and stability of the spine. The value of distraction as a form of fixation can be readily appreciated with an ordinary sheet of paper held vertically stretched between the two hands. The paper becomes rigid due to this tension and can resist a lateral force. Without tension applied to the two ends, the paper has negligible lateral stability.

Sleeve Principle. Essentially this involves the construction of a cage around the patient. There are basically two semicircular fixation points, one above the other. Then, between the two, there are various uprights. The uprights may be at the sides of the patient, or they may be posterior and paraspinous. These uprights serve as a sleeve, a splint, a distractor, and as a point for attachments

of various accessory devices such as localizer pads, axillary slings, or abdominal pads.

Skeletal Fixation. This is another useful orthotic technique. The prime and perhaps only examples are the halo fixation and the halo pelvic fixation devices. These appliances provide the most effective methods of applying reliable controls to the spine.

CLINICAL REVIEW OF SPINE REGIONS AND THEIR SPECIFIC ORTHOSES

After the clinician makes a diagnosis, he determines the specific mechanical goals that are to be achieved, whether to support (rest, assist), immobilize (protect), or correct the spine. An analysis of the six degrees of freedom in which the involved vertebra or vertebrae can move is carried out. The clinician then determines which degrees of freedom are to be controlled as well as the manner and extent to which they are to be altered.

When these determinations are made, the orthosis which is best able to achieve these goals can be selected. The authors have not chosen to present this section of material as a catalogue of diseases and braces recommended for treatment. The major types of orthoses are reviewed. In an attempt to systematize, these arbitrary groupings have been chosen, based on the effectiveness of control applied by the orthosis: *minimum control* (least effective); *intermediate control* (a broad range with some effectiveness); *most effective control* (the best in the group). A more precise classification is desirable; however, present knowledge dictates this somewhat arbitrary classification. The list on page 355 outlines a systematic clinical analysis of the biomechanics involved in the selection of a spinal orthosis.

Cervical Region

Experimental Studies. An in vivo study by Hartmann and colleagues has provided some relevant guidelines about the effectiveness of immobilization by cervical spine orthoses.[5] These investigations evaluate normal motion and motion in five different orthoses using moving pictures and cineradiography. Their findings are shown in Table 7-1. The most difficult motion to

Systematic Analysis for the Selection of Orthoses

(1) Determine the goal of orthosis:
  Support (rest, assist)
  Immobilization (protection)
  Correction
(2) Determine how many degrees of freedom are to be altered:
  Flexion
  Extension
  Lateral bending
  Axial rotation
  Axial distraction
(3) Determine the magnitude of control:
  Minimum
  Intermediate
  Most effective

restrain was rotation that occurred between the occiput and C2. Therefore, an effective cervical orthosis must fix the head directly or hold the occiput and mandible through effective molding.

An evaluation of cervical braces by Johnson gives some additional information about their immobilizing efficiency. He placed normal subjects in four different orthoses and made photographs and radiographs of their cervical spines in full flexion and extension. The total motion between C1 and C7 was studied. Angles were drawn as shown in Figure 7-9. The findings are shown in Table 7-2.

In a quantitative study of cervical orthoses by Johnson and colleagues, there were several cogent findings.[6a] Increasing the length and rigidity of a cervical orthosis generally improved the effectiveness of its control of motion. There was not very effective control of lateral bending or axial rotation of the cervical spine by the conventional orthosis. The most effective conventional braces were able to restrict C1-C2 flexion/extension by only 45 per cent of normal. The halo apparatus restricted the same motion by 75 per cent. The major quantitative findings from this study are shown in Table 7-3.

Several generalizations may be made from these studies. The soft collar does little in the way of immobilization. The efficiency of fixation at the chin and occiput are major elements in the design of a cervical orthosis. For the most satisfactory immobilization in this group, the use of some type of shoulder and thoracic fixation and support should be added to the cervical and chin occipital components of the brace. When the chest support not only rests upon but is fixed to the thorax, the immobilizing efficiency is even greater.

Minimum Control. Since the time of Sir Thomas, collars have been popular for the treatment of a variety of problems in the cervical spine. They vary in height and in rigidity. They may be altered or worn so as to limit either flexion or extension relatively more than the other. If the high portion of the collar is worn anteriorly, there is relatively less flexion. If the high portion is worn posteriorly, there is relatively less extension. The cervical collars have the advantages of being inexpensive, convenient to use, and easily fabricated. Although they do little to immobilize or unload the spine, they provide warmth as well

Table 7-1. Effectiveness of Cervical Spine Orthoses in Immobilization*

| | APPROXIMATE % RESTRICTION OF RANGE OF MOTION C1–C7 | | | | | |
| | *Motion Picture* | | | *Cineradiograph* | | |
ORTHOSES	FE†	LB†	AR†	FE	LB	AR
Soft cervical collar	5–10	5–10	0	0	0	0
Hard plastic collar (Thomas)	75	75	50	75	75	50
Four-poster cervical	80–85	80–85	60	85	85	60
Long two-poster	95	90	90	90	90	90
Guilford two-poster	90–95	90–95	90–95	90	90–95	90
Halo devise	Essentially no motion					

* Based on data from Hartman, J. T., Palumbo, F., and Hill, B. J.: Cineradiography of the braced normal cervical spine. Clin. Orthop., *109*:97, 1975.
† FE: Flexion/extension (x-axis rotation)
  LB: Lateral bending (z-axis rotation)
  AR: Axial rotation (y-axis rotation)

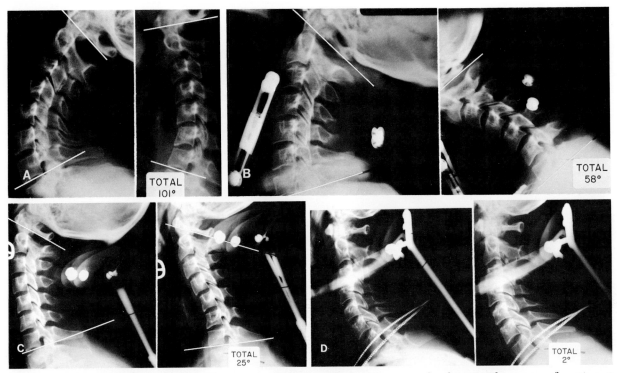

Fig. 7-9. The actual radiographs of the range of motion achieved by normal subjects. The range of motion at C1–C7 achieved by these subjects is shown for the different cervical orthoses. (*A*) Soft cervical collar. (*B*) Hard plastic collar. (*C*) Four-poster cervical orthosis. (*D*) Duke orthosis with occipital chin and chest piece. (Courtesy of R. M. Johnson, M.D.)

*Table 7-2. Efficiency of Cervical Braces in Immobilization**

ORTHOSES	TOTAL MOVEMENT FROM FULL FLEXION TO FULL EXTENSION† (degrees)
Soft cervical collar	101
Hard plastic collar (Thomas)	58
Four-poster cervical	25
Duke (occipital, chin, and chest piece)	2

* Based on personal communication with R. M. Johnson.
† The median normal is approximately 90 degrees.[9]

as psychologic comfort and support. These devices are useful in a broad variety of conditions, such as minor sprains and strains, some whiplash cases, cervical spondylosis, and postoperative management when the spine is clinically stable.

It has been observed that the long-term use of a cervical collar can prevent or reduce a "double chin." This little cosmetic aside is an example of biomechanical adaptation.

Intermediate Control. There are a variety of modifications of the cervical collar. Within this range of intermediate control there are different degrees of effectiveness. For slightly more restriction, a beefed-up cervical collar, such as the Philadelphia collar, may be employed (Fig. 7-10). Through its rigidity and the anterior and posterior reinforcement under the chin and the occiput, it is able to offer better restriction, especially in flexion and extension (x-axis rotation).

In order to achieve greater degrees of control of the cervical spine, it is necessary to have some purchase on the shoulders and the thoracic cage, as well as fixation of the mandible and the occiput. This in effect is an addition to the simple cervical collar in the caudad direction. This lengthens the sleeve and provides more effective anchoring and purchase. For example, suppose a

Table 7-3. Rigid Conventional Braces that Provide the Best Control of Flexion and Extension at Different Levels of the Cervical Spine

SEGMENTAL LEVELS	FLEXION-EXTENSION		FLEXION		EXTENSION	
	BRACE	MEAN MOTION ALLOWED (degrees)	BRACE	MEAN MOTION ALLOWED (degrees)	BRACE	MEAN MOTION ALLOWED (degrees)
C1–C2	(Halo)	3.4	Somi	2.7	Cervicothoracic	2.5
C2–C3	(Halo)	2.4	Somi	0.9	Four-poster	2.0
	Four-poster	3.7	Four-poster	1.6	Cervicothoracic	2.1
	Cervicothoracic	3.8	Cervicothoracic	1.8		
Middle (C3–C5)	Cervicothoracic	4.6	Somi	1.7	Cervicothoracic	1.8
			Four-poster	2.0		
			Cervicothoracic	2.8		
Lower (C5–T1)	Cervicothoracic	4.0	Cervicothoracic	1.5	Cervicothoracic	2.5
			Somi	2.9	Four-poster	2.5

(Johnson, R. M., et al.: Cervical orthoses. A study comparing their effectiveness in restricting cervical motion in normal subjects. J. Bone Joint Surg., 59A: 332, 1977.)

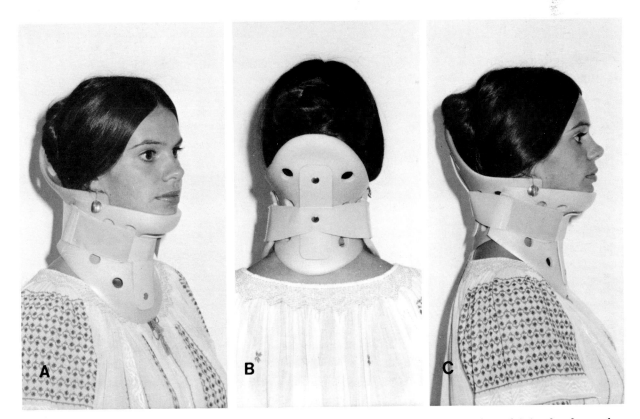

Fig. 7-10. The Philadelphia collar in three views: anterolateral (A); posterior (B); lateral (C). The device has some purchase on the upper chest and back but no fixation there. It is stiff enough to allow some distraction. Note the anterior and posterior splints. There is some degree of support and fixation of the mandible and occiput, which should reduce axial rotation. This orthosis has been classified as exerting controls in the *intermediate range.*

patient has had an elective anterior cervical spine fusion at two levels. There is essentially adequate stability, but there is a need in the early postoperative period to prevent excessive cervical spine motion. In this situation a well fitted cervical brace with shoulder or chest and shoulder fixation would be satisfactory. There are several braces that fit into this category: the four-poster brace (Fig. 7-11A), the Duke brace, the Guilford brace, and others (Fig. 7-11B). It should be kept in mind that shoulder supported fixation and unloading are most valuable and necessary in the erect position. However, in the supine position or any situation where there is considerable rotation of the shoulders and spine, the directions of the forces are altered and the appliance may not be as effective.

Most Effective Control. If the clinician determines that there has been a significant loss of stability through destruction or removal of supporting structures in the cervical spine, then the maximum amount of immobilization and unloading is desirable. Major control is needed in all six degrees of freedom.

For more effective fixation the Thomas collar may be extended in both directions and made more rigid. Thus, one employs the Minerva cast, which includes the forehead and goes high upon the occiput and extends all the way to the pelvis.

This device is appealing, if for no reason other than its glorious and powerful appellation from the highest echelons of Greek mythology. Minerva was born by popping from the head of Jupiter fully armored. (Knowing how she was born, it is challenging to speculate about how she may have been conceived.) This cast, which constitutes a sizable portion of armor, encases the head, shoulders, thorax, abdomen, and pelvis. This device does indeed offer considerable control and is especially useful for protection of an irresponsible patient. It should be kept in mind, however, that a few degrees of cervical spine motion is present even in the carefully applied Minerva jacket.[19] The limitations of force that may be applied depend somewhat on the ease with which talking and eating is to be permitted. Opening the mouth requires either space for the mandible to move caudad or for the head to ex-

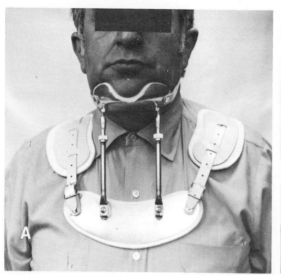 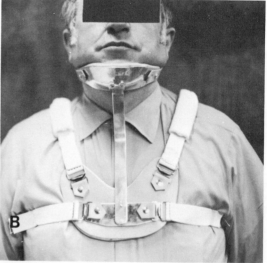

Fig. 7-11. (*A*) The four-poster cervical brace. This is adequate mandibular and occiput fixation. There is purchase on the thorax anteriorly and posteriorly. The four posts may be adjusted to alter distraction. The anterior and posterior pairs may be adjusted to determine the amount of flexion and extension. (*B*) The Guilford, Duke, or long cervical brace prototype. There is fixation of mandible and occiput as well as straps to anchor the purchase on the chest. These devices have both been classed as exerting *intermediate control*. The long cervical braces with thoracic anchoring have been shown to be the most effective in the intermediate range. (Courtesy of J. T. Hartmann, M.D.)

tend. Either of these motions allows a displacement of the occiput and thus some motion at C1-C2.

In precarious clinical situations where extensive disease or surgery renders the cervical spine dangerously unstable, the use of the halo apparatus should be considered. This devise allows skeletal fixation at the skull (Fig. 7-12). It may be used in several ways. It may be attached to a molded removable waist-length jacket, a plaster waist-length jacket, a plaster jacket molded about the pelvis, or to a pelvic hoop. All of these offer good fixation and are listed in order of increasing effectiveness. The combination to be employed depends on the problem, the involved region of the spine, and the clinician's preference and judgment. There are complications associated with the use of the halo. These include penetration of the skull, brain abscess,[22] and abducens, glossopharangeal, and facial nerve palsies. When a patient is in large magnitudes of skeletal traction, applying axial loads to the spine on daily rounds should include requests for the patient to smile, to roll the eyes, and to stick out the tongue at the doctor. If the patient is not able to do any of the three activities, then careful neurologic evaluation is indicated (see Chapter 8).

Thoracic Region

Minimum Control. In this grouping there are the long thoracic corsets. Some of these orthoses when well fitted can offer significant immobilization. However, they do not serve as effectively as some of the other appliances. Probably their main indication would be for chronic, benign, thoracic pain, in which the orthosis gives good "symptomatic" relief.

Intermediate Control. The hyperextension brace is sometimes referred to as the Jewett or Griswold brace (Fig. 7-8). It is designed for resistance of motion primarily in flexion. This brace has fixation points at the manubrio-sternal area and at the pubis, and it employs counterpressure between these two pads from the posterior to the anterior direction, thus achieving a three-point fixation. The advantage of this brace is that there is the possibility of adjusting the levels at which maximum fixation can occur, thus it is possible to better immobilize a particular region of the thora-

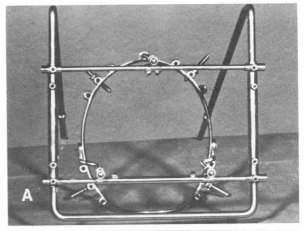

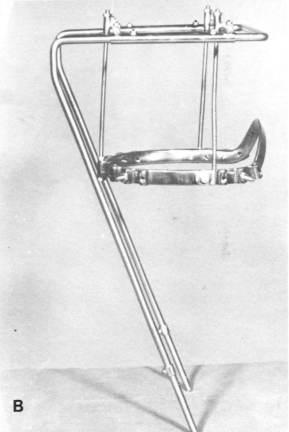

Fig. 7-12. The halo apparatus. The device achieves skeletal fixation of the skull and thus indirectly fixes the spine through pins attached to the stainless steel rim. The outrigger which holds the rim is attached to a fitted jacket or a molded plaster body jacket, with or without including the hips. There are other outrigger designs that have more degrees of freedom or options for adjustment.

columbar spine. This brace is less effective in restricting rotation in the coronal plane (about the z-axis) and there is virtually no resistance to axial rotation (y-axis rotation). When this brace can be adjusted to obtain some degree of hyperextension, it is reasonable to assume that it is capable of shifting the weight bearing axis more toward the posterior elements of the vertebra. Thus, it may be helpful in diminishing stresses on the vertebral body and the anterior elements. Most probably this orthosis cannot be relied upon to prevent additional collapse of a severely comminuted thoracic spine fracture. If this is a major concern, a full body cast should be applied in hyperextension. It is also important to bear in mind that the decrease in the strength of the vertebral bodies in osteoporosis is such that the orthosis is not likely to be completely effective in protecting them from collapse. Vertebral strength is studied in Chapter 1.

The Taylor brace is one of the standards for the thoracic and the thoracolumbar spine (Fig. 7-13). This brace consists of a pelvic band with two long posteriorly applied bars extending to the shoulders and joined with a transverse bar. There are straps that pass from these uprights

around the shoulders and under the axilla. There is also a full-length abdominal pad which is attached to the uprights. Thus, it consists of a pelvic band and an axillary band attached by two rigid posterior uprights. The sleeve principal is employed for a splinting effect. The points of attachment at the axilla and the pelvis, with the abdominal pad anteriorally, constitute a three-point fixation. The immobilizing efficiency of this brace is good in the lower thoracic area, especially with regard to motion in the sagittal plane (x-axis rotation). The resistance against lateral bending is less effective because there are no lateral bars to prevent that motion. Although there are axillary shoulder attachments, resistance to axial rotation is not very satisfactory. This type of orthotic design functions largely as a reminder to resist excessive motion in flexion and extension. There are other models of this brace which enhance its usefulness in limiting other types of movement. To limit lateral bending, lateral uprights are added. They anchor the pelvic and thoracic bands and restrain lateral trunk bending (Fig. 7-14).

Sometimes there is a therapeutic indication to minimize axial rotation (y-axis rotation). This

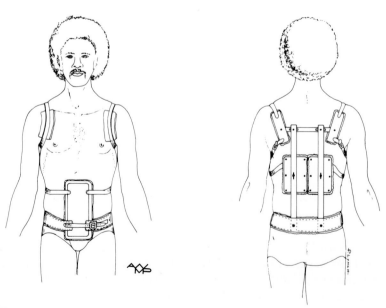

Fig. 7-13. The Taylor thoracolumbar brace is one of the standards. Its components are described in the text. This orthosis offers *intermediate control* to the thoracic and the thoracolumbar spine.

could be of primary importance in a patient in whom there was extensive pain explicitly elicited by that particular movement. For this, the clinician adds to the lumbosacral, anteroposterior, and lateral control brace bilateral subclavicular pads anchored to the lateral uprights (Fig. 7-14). This device provides some resistance and serves as an irritant and therapeutic reminder to the patient. There is no definite evidence that this devise is superior to the axillary supports in resisting axial rotation.

Most Effective Control. A tightly worn Milwaukee brace and a well molded Risser plaster jacket should be included in this category. Both of these appliances exert control against axial rotation as well as effective control of flexion/extension and lateral bending. The Risser cast controls axial rotation through its molding about the pelvis, the thoracic cage, the chin, and the occiput. The Milwaukee brace exerts its control through the pelvic mold, the localizer pads, and the axillary sling.

The most effective immobilization of the thoracic spine, as with all regions of the spine, is with the halo pelvic apparatus (Fig. 7-15). With the skeletal fixation this apparatus offers maximum control in all six degrees of freedom. Due to the viscoelastic properties of the spine and the strength of the bone to which the device must be fixed, it is not possible to apply enough tension to the spine to *completely* immobilize it even with this orthosis (see Chapter 8).

The Milwaukee Brace in the Treatment of Scoliosis

The usual halo-hoop device has a turn buckle mechanism in each of the uprights for displacing the halo on the y-axis with respect to the hoop. Distraction is produced by adjusting the turn buckles. However, there is no way to determine the magnitude of the forces shared by the four uprights and the total force that is applied to the spine. A halo-hoop apparatus developed in Hong Kong and reported by Clark and Kesterton solves this problem in a neat and simple manner. They have incorporated a spring at the base of each of the four uprights so that the force in a given upright is transmitted to the hoop by way of the spring. By measuring the length of the previously

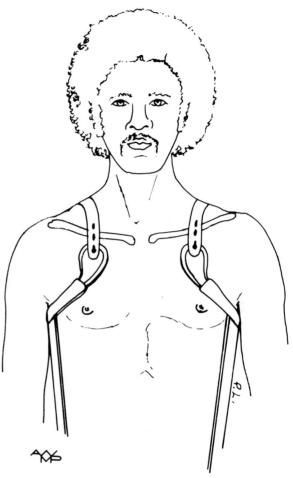

Fig. 7-14. In any thoracic or lumbar brace where it is desired to exert an *intermediate control* of lateral bending, (z-axis rotation) laterally placed uprights may be added to the basic Taylor orthosis shown in Figure 7-13. If the requirement is to control axial rotation (y-axis) the clavicular pads and straps shown here are recommended.

calibrated spring, an accurate measure of the force is obtained. The total force applied to the spine is the sum of the four upright forces.[3] In the halo-hoop without measuring springs, an unknown amount of force is applied to the spine. In order to avoid the possibility of injuring the spine, the clinician may apply suboptimum levels of force. With the halo-hoop designed by Clark and Kesterton, a near optimum level of force can be applied and maintained. Use of this device results in a highly efficient controlled form of distraction.

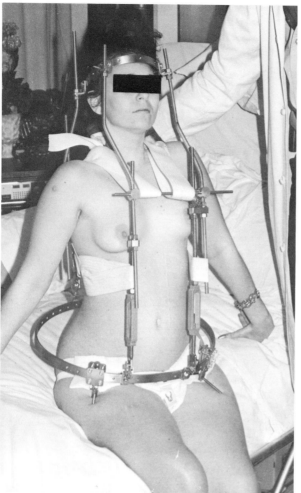

Fig. 7-15. At present the halo pelvic apparatus offers the best external fixation and control of any portion of the spine for all the six degrees of freedom. The white straps are part of an improvised sling to resist any tendency for additional posterior angulation of the kyphosis, since this patient was supine most of the time. There has recently been developed a spring device which is incorporated in the vertical uprights. This provides for the patient the great advantage of allowing the clinician to monitor the forces applied with this apparatus. (Courtesy of C. West, M.D.)

The Milwaukee brace represents a high degree of sophistication and elegance in the art of bracing. This complex apparatus embodies a number of mechanisms and principles involved in the clinical science of orthotics. When the mechanism of this device is fully understood, the discipline has been mastered.

The principles involved in the brace and the technical considerations involved in fulfilling these principles are discussed here. The Milwaukee brace and the spine form a complex three-dimensional structure which is subjected to both passive and active loads. The correctional effect is on a long-term basis and involves not only immediate mechanical effects but also biologic adaptation. Any mechanical analysis and optimization of such a system is extremely complex. The complexities include elements as divergent as the variability of the stiffness of the spine and the equilibrium of the enthusiasm between the therapist and the patient.

To gain some understanding of the mechanics involved the Milwaukee brace and spine system may be studied in the grossly simplified manner shown in Figure 7-16. The real situation is modeled as a plane curved bar subjected to a set of forces. Forces F_1 and F_2 are the mandibular-occipital pads and the pelvic support forces which seem to correct the spine deformity by stretching. (Actually the angular correction is obtained by producing bending moments in the scoliotic spine.) Forces F_3 (thoracic pad), F_4 (axillary sling), and F_5 (pelvic support) form a neat three-point force system. The purpose of these three forces is to bend the spine into a curvature opposite to that of the scoliotic curve, and thus correct it. The two force systems may be applied separately or together. In the combined situation they are interdependent. The results of this interplay are studied in Chapter 3.

The brace is built to fit what would be expected to be the normal body of the patient. The normal mold is made with the body in the position of maximum attainable correction. This is achieved by the following procedures. In order to compensate for any functional or real leg length discrepancy, the pelvis is balanced by employing lifts on the short side. Any lordosis is then minimized by having the patient stand with the knees slightly bent in order to rotate the pelvis in the saggital plane and minimize the amount of lumbar lordosis. Also, in order to gain maximum correction of the supple growing scoliotic curve, the patient is suspended in a head halter traction apparatus. These important techniques are shown in Figure 7-17.

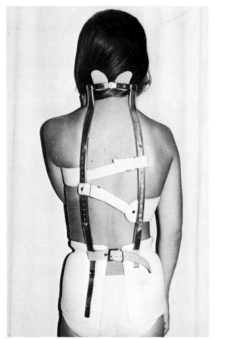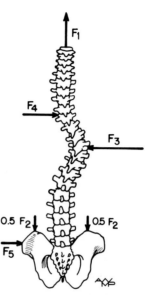

Fig. 7-16. Here the forces exerted by the Milwaukee brace for correction of a scoliotic deformity are analyzed. The spine is subjected to stretch by equal forces, F_1 and F_2, applied by way of the occipital-mandibular pads and the pelvic girdle, respectively. Forces F_3 (thoracic pad), F_4 (axillary sling), and F_5 (pelvic girdle) are all basically horizontal forces. They form a three-point system. The maximum bending moment for correction to the spine is applied at the level of the force F_3.

In order to obtain good fixation on the pelvis with additional support to the lower spine, the cast for the mold is carefully fitted to the pelvis with special attention to the iliac crests. When the final mold is made, the abdominal portion of the mold is carved out considerably before the actual pelvic girdle is fitted to it. This is done in order to assure significant compression and better fixation. This process is demonstrated in Figure 7-18.

Erect uprights perpendicular to a level pelvis are then constructed. These uprights support an occipital head piece and throat mold. A plastic throat mold has been employed in recent years as a substitute for the chin piece used in the past. The throat mold is shown in Figure 7-19. This has been quite effective in reducing the amount of dental changes associated with previous methods. The throat mold and the occipital piece, in conjunction with the uprights, all work together to provide a distracting force on the spine. Thus, they resist settling into the more deformed position. They resist gravity and the deforming forces intrinsic to a scoliotic spine. In addition, these components of the brace serve as reminders and reference points away from which the patient may actively move, employing his or her own muscles and actively correcting the deformity.

Localizer pads are used on this brace to provide the valuable function of both active and passive correction. The brace may employ any combination of three basic types of localizing pads. One is the typical thoracic pad, which is applied posterolaterally over the ribs. The pad is applied slightly posteriorly in order to have its force also serve to correct the rotational aspect of the scoliotic deformity by providing an axial torque. There is also a lumbar pad, which is generally

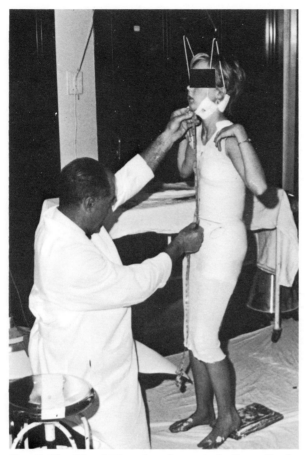

Fig. 7-17. The Milwaukee brace is built to fit the expected normal body mold for the particular patient. Moderate axial traction is applied. The foot is elevated to attain a level pelvis, upon which perpendicular uprights of the proper length may be measured and constructed. In addition, both knees are flexed to rotate the hips and pelvis in order to minimize lumbar lordosis.

smaller and more heavily padded. This is attached to the posterior uprights and presses posterolaterally on the erector spinae muscles at the apex of the lumbar curve. On occasion in scoliosis, a sternal pad may be employed. This pad fits on the anterior upright and it also is generally quite well cushioned. These localizer pads have a function similar to the distracting function of the uprights. In effect, they apply correctional loads and serve as a check mechanism to prevent progression of the deformity. At the same time, they serve as a reminder or a reference

point away from which the patient may voluntarily move, using his own intrinsic muscles, and thereby actively correct the deformity. The axillary sling is employed on the opposite side of the convexity of the curve. This is to offer a counterforce against the thoracic pad, which contributes effectively to a three-point fixation loading system and also prevents the patients from being pushed to that side by the thoracic pad. A detailed analysis of the force system and placement of lateral pads follows.

Placement of the Lateral Pads. Although there have been studies on the measurement of the forces applied by the occipital-mandibular pads to the spine under different activities, unfortunately very little objective information is available regarding force vectors of the lateral pads. Mulcahy and colleagues report that the average longitudinal force in the Milwaukee brace increases significantly on removal of the thoracic pad.[11] They believe that the forces extended through the chest cage play a major role in passive correction. There are three lateral pads, axillary, thoracic, and lumbar. For a particular patient, how many of them should be

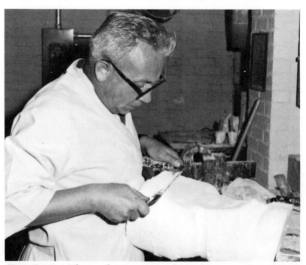

Fig. 7-18. The orthotist is working here on the plaster mold upon which the Milwaukee brace will be constructed. An important aspect of the fit, support, and foundation of the brace is the effectiveness of the abdominal compression. In order to assure a snug fit the abdominal portion of the mold is skived out, as shown here.

used, and in what combination? Where should they be located, and how much pressure should be applied through each pad for optimum results? Which way should the forces be directed from the pads so that there is some improvement of axial (y-axis) rotation of the vertebrae? These are all crucial questions which merit consideration.

At present all the answers are not available. However, the problem may be analyzed biomechanically and some practical recommendations offered. One of the most popular concepts regarding the lateral pads is to assume that the axillary pad, the thoracic pad, and the pelvic support form a three-point force system. In discussing the concept of balanced horizontal forces (see p. 353), one of the conclusions reached was that the maximum bending moment occurs just under the middle force (i.e., the thoracic pad). The question arises concerning the location of the thoracic pad with respect to the apex of the scoliotic curve. Orthopaedic opinion seems to be divided on this question. However, a majority of physicians prefer that the thoracic pad be placed against the ribs *attached* to the apex of the curve and not *at the level* of the apex of the curve. However, simple biomechanical analysis, based upon the three-point force system, reveals that the optimum placement of the thoracic pad is midway between the pelvic support and the axillary pad.[B] Additional investigation is required to clarify these considerations more definitely.

The concept of dynamic bracing is employed with the Milwaukee brace in two basic manners. One has already been discussed, the active movement away from the localizer pads. In addition, an integral part of the basic Milwaukee brace prescription includes a series of well conceived specific exercises to be followed under the supervision of a physical therapist. These consist of breathing exercises and activities to counteract a tendency for the development of an excessive lumbar lordosis. The routines include breathing, pelvic tilt, abdominal, back, hip, shoulder, and arm strengthening exercises.

Experimental studies have shown that the Milwaukee brace is an effective appliance for applying corrective and immobilizing forces to the spine. The brace has been shown to function in

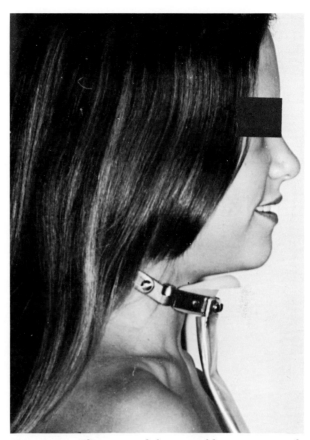

Fig. 7-19. This type of throat mold now commonly used appears to be therapeutically just as effective as its predecessor, the chin piece, yet it is much less likely to cause disruptions of the teeth.

these two ways in both the supine and the prone positions. It has been shown that the removal of the thoracic localizer pad, the occipital piece, or the head piece significantly impairs the effectiveness of the brace in applying correctional forces to the spine.[4,12]

Orthoses for Scoliosis with Pelvic Obliquity

There is an implementation of the halo apparatus that makes it the most effective orthosis for applying distractive correctional loads to the deformed spine. This instrument can effectively apply forces resulting in +y-axis translation and immobilization of the spine. The halo-hoop should be considered in the treatment of scoliosis with severe pelvic obliquities. Skeletal fixation is obtained in the outer table of the skull with the halo, and in addition fixation to the pelvis is achieved with the use of large pins applied through holes, in a circular hoop apparatus. The pins are applied through the upper and outer portion of the wings of the iliac crests. With a series of turnbuckle screw mechanisms, the desired amount of distraction is applied to the spine. A picture of this apparatus is shown in Figure 7-15. This devise is also useful in situations in which there is clinical instability in a portion of the spine that is yet to be stabilized surgically.

This device applies forces and controls to any area of the spine better than other currently available spine orthoses. Strain gauges can and probably should be incorporated in the apparatus so that the forces involved can be precisely controlled and monitored.

Milwaukee Brace in the Treatment of Kyphosis

This brace is used in essentially the same fashion, embodying identical principles in the treatment of this disease as with scoliosis. The basic difference is that the deformity and the curvature are in the saggital plane and without a significant element of axial rotation. The scoliotic deformity is largely in the frontal plane and embodies a significant element of axial rotation. Both diseases involve deformities within particular vertebra. This analogy is employed for descriptive reasons alone and does not imply similarities in etiologic or other aspects of the two diseases. The corrective forces are applied through the use of distraction between the well molded pelvic band and the occipital throat or chin piece. There are two localizer pads employed. One is a sternal pad and the other is a dorsal pad that is applied to the apex of the kyphotic deformity. An analysis of this orthosis in the saggital plane demonstrates three-point fixation systems (Fig. 7-20).

The correctional effects produced by the Milwaukee brace in treating kyphosis are based on the same biomechanical principles as are those for scoliosis. Figure 7-20 shows a patient using the Milwaukee brace for kyphotic correction. The spine and the correcting forces applied to it through the various pads are also shown. The five forces, F_1 through F_5, work in the sagittal plane in a manner similar to the five forces in the frontal plane shown for scoliotic correction in Figure 7-16. The sternal pad replaces the axillary sling, and the thoracic pad is replaced by the posterior pad. Figure 7-21 shows the therapeutic effectiveness of this orthosis. *Biomechanical adaptation* as a long-term therapeutic response to the appropriate use of an orthosis is further demonstrated in Figure 7-22. In Figure 7-22A the thoracic vertebrae are wedged shaped. In Figure 7-22B they are noted to be more rectangular.

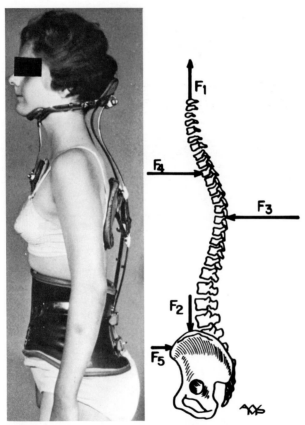

Fig. 7-20. Here the forces exerted by the Milwaukee brace for correction of a kyphotic deformity are analyzed. The spine is stretched by the two equal axial forces, F_1 and F_2, applied to the spine by way of the occipital-mandibular pads and the pelvic girdle, respectively. The other three forces, F_3, F_4, and F_5, are basically transverse to the spine axis and are applied by way of the posterior pad, sternal pad, and the pelvic girdle. These three forces form a three-point force system producing maximum bending moment and hence the correction potential at the posterior pad level.

Lumbar Region

Most of the long and sometimes confusing list of eponyms for spine orthoses are associated with this region of the spine. The number of appliances and their proliferation mirrors the confusion and complexity inherent in treatment of "low back pain." The "brace" represents a valiant effort among the many attempts to treat a formidable clinical problem.

Lumbar spine braces are most often used to reduce pain. They may be employed for giving support and/or immobilization following spine fusion or trauma to the spine. Mechanically, the braces generally seek to achieve increased abdominal support, to reduce the forces on the spine, and to achieve a straighter lumbar spine. Forces are applied to the normal or accentuated lumbar lordosis in order to hold it in a straighter position. It is commonly observed clinically that the less lordotic spine is more comfortable.

Experimental Studies. Although there are few investigative studies on the mechanics of braces, there is at least one important study, and it is probably the most objective scientific study of the effects of bracing on the lumbar spine. Norton and Brown investigated movement of the spine in braces using radiographs and the insertion of K-wires in the spinous processes for measurement.

Standing, sitting, and bending in flexion and extension was then studied, with a number of braces. The braces include an experimental brace created by the investigators, a chairback brace, a Goldwaith brace, a Williams brace, the Arnold Albert brace, a flexion Taylor brace, a rigid Taylor brace, a reinforced Taylor brace, a Jewett brace, and a plaster jacket.[14]

Although the investigators considered their extensive work preliminary, it provided interesting and worthwhile information. The pertinent findings are reviewed. Sitting with a brace, even when erect, was associated with substantial flexion of the lower two lumbar interspaces. Thus, if one of the goals is to immobilize the lower lumbar or lumbosacral spine, the patient should either avoid sitting or should wear some apparatus for immobilization that will be effective when sitting. The long back supports, such as the Taylor

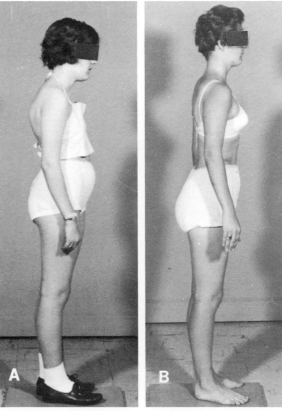

Fig. 7-21. These show the clinical effectiveness of the Milwaukee brace in the treatment of adolescent kyphosis. The brace was worn for 3.5 years. (*A*) Before treatment. (*B*) After treatment. This change may be thought of as *biomechanical adaptation.*

brace, concentrated their immobilizing effect in the region of thoracolumbar junction, which is much too high to immobilize the lower lumbar segments. Paradoxically, it was observed that lumbosacral flexion was actually greater when the long brace was employed. Presumably, this is due to the increased lever arm created by a relatively more rigid upper spine and a concentration of the movement in that lower relatively free portion of the spine. Thus, if it is desirable to thoroughly immobilize the lumbosacral joint as, for example, with spondylolysis, spondylolisthesis, or following lumbosacral spine fusion, the cast or brace must include at least one thigh. If it is desirable to allow the patient the alternative of occasional hip joint flexion for sitting, a drop-lock mechanism at the hip can be included.

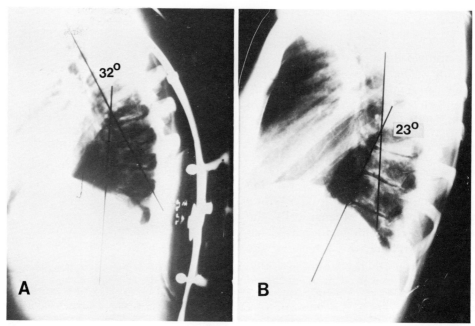

Fig. 7-22. This shows changes in the shape of thoracic vertebra associated with Milwaukee brace correction of adolescent kyphosis in the patient shown in Figures 7-20 and 7-21. (*A*) The deformity measures approximately 32 degrees and the vertebrae are wedge-shaped. (*B*) The spine after wearing the brace for 3.5 years. Note the new vertebral configuration as a result of *biomechanical adaptation*.

Actually, immobilization of the spine did not occur in any of the braces studied by Norton and Brown. In some instances, it was possible to limit movement in the interspaces. It is interesting that the effectiveness of the supports with respect to immobilization seemed to be related more to the discomfort they produce than to the actual magnitudes of the force transmitted from the apparatus to the body. The desirability of a paraspinal brace to immobilize the lumbosacral spine was questioned. They felt that these had limitations in two realms: the force was not localized low enough in the lumbar area; and these uprights did not produce the necessary discomfort. The investigators developed an experimental brace designed to utilize this information. The paraspinal uprights were replaced with lateral uprights which extended downward to the greater trochanters. The brace also applied a force to the lumbosacral region by means of a single crossbar. This component exerts a force over the bony prominance so that pressure and discomfort ac-

company the early ranges of movement. This is all mediated through an abdominal pad with its low attachment straps. Good counterpressure is offered, without impending sitting in the erect posture. In addition, side bending is effectively blocked by the lateral uprights.[14]

Increases in intraabdominal pressure provide additional support to the lumbar spine (see Chapter 1). This is important in the use of abdominal corsets and also in the use of the lumbosacral corsets and the chairback brace. Walters and Morris carried out studies of the electromyographic (EMG) response of the paraspinous and abdominal muscles with and without either a lumbosacral corset or chairback brace. These investigators found a decrease in the activity of the abdominal muscles with both the lumbosacral corset and the chairback brace.[23] This implies that these braces take over some of the function of the abdominal muscles by compressing and supporting the spine. Subjects wearing braces in the resting position showed either no effect or some decrease in the abdominal muscle activity. With ambulation, however, the wearing of the chairback brace was associated with an *increase* in muscle activity. This is presumably due to an attempt on the part of the muscles to overcome the immobilizing effect of the brace. If the use of the brace is based on resting paraspinous muscles, presumed to be causing pain through their spasmodic contractions, the desirability of using such a brace should be examined critically. This is because the study showed that with the two braces involved there is a *greater* paraspinous muscle activity. In other words, the brace could worsen the patient's condition.

The functions of a lumbar orthosis are as follows: to serve as a reminder and an irritant to the patient for restriction of movements and activity in the lumbar spine; to act as a support and a vehicle for application of abdominal pressure (which should somewhat alleviate the loads imposed on the lumbar spine); to provide some immobilizing efficiency of the upper portion of the lumbar spine and the thoracolumbar area; to maintain a straighter and comfortable back by employing the principle of three-point fixation.

Rather than review the extensive list of conditions of the lumbar spine that may be treated, the authors submit the following type of stepwise analysis for consideration. First, the clinician decides what goals he is attempting to achieve with the orthosis; what are the mechanical factors involved, the motions that are to be restricted, or the structures that are to be corrected or supported? When maximum immobilization is needed, a more rigid structure such as a cast or brace is required. For less rigid immobilization, a corset or a pelvic belt may be considered. If the goal is primarily to limit anterior or posterior movement (flexion and extension), then pelvic and thoracic bands connected to posterior uprights are probably the most effective. If lateral motion is also to be limited, then lateral uprights are desirable along with the consideration of the trochanteric pads of Norton and Brown's experimental brace. When axial rotation is to be diminished, then a well molded body plaster is applied. If rotation is to be controlled, perhaps a longer brace may be necessary with good pelvic fixation and fixation on the upper portion

of the thorax. If support is a major consideration, then the abdominal pad becomes a useful adjunct.

Minimum Control. This group is constituted by the various corsets that are available for the lumbar spine. They differ in the controls they apply, depending on the quality of the fit and the quality, quantity, and distribution of the staves.

Intermediate Control. Braces in this category include the low or short lumbar spine brace (Williams type), the slightly longer Knight, MacAusland, or chairback brace, and the long lumbar spine brace, which is actually a Taylor brace. These orthoses are used most commonly as a "crutch" for the patient with the chronically disabled back. Since they make the patient feel better and it is not certain that they cause disabling loss of intrinsic muscle function, it is reasonable to use them. Figure 7-23 shows back and side views of the basic designs of lumbar orthoses. The Norton and Brown experimental brace should be included in this group and is probably its most effective member. However, as a group, these braces provide little or no control of rotation; flexion/extension is not well controlled in the lower lumbar and lumbosacral area; and lateral bending is controlled to some degree (see Table 7-4.).

Most Effective Control. Based on our analysis, the appliances that most effectively control the lumbar spine are listed in their ascending order of control: Taylor brace with thigh attachment; molded plaster body jacket (lower lumbosacral area not immobilized); molded plaster body jack with thigh included; and the halo pelvic skeletal apparatus.

Braces from this category are used when control must be maximal. However, a broad range of control is represented in this group. The halo pelvic apparatus is the most effective external device now available for controlling all six degrees of freedom. The plaster casts are effective in reducing axial rotation due to pelvic and thoracic molding. Because of their compression of the abdomen and their rigidity, they are also effective against flexion/extension and lateral bending. This does not apply to the L4–S1 area, however, and the thigh is best included when maximum control of this area is important. Axial

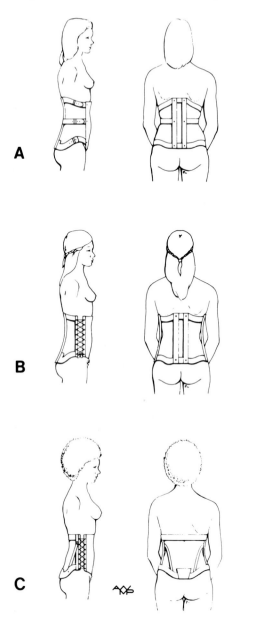

rotation, as well as flexion/extension, is better controlled by this maneuver. The Taylor and Norton and Brown braces are more effective controls than those of the intermediate group, but they are not nearly as effective as the halo pelvic apparatus or the plaster jacket with the thigh included.

CONCLUSION

Mechanical and psychologic factors can sometimes interact and become a major consideration in the prescription for an orthosis. For example, patients with severe neurologic deficits who do not have control of the trunk and pelvic musculature may not make use of a rigid spinal brace and attached lower extremity braces. In the hospital setting, the apparatus may seem to be helpful to some extent, but there is considerable psychologic support from physicians, nurses, and therapists. The same type of situation rarely works out well at home, and frequently such orthoses are discarded, and the patient simply uses a wheelchair.[7] Thus, it is important to be as realistic as possible about what can be expected of an orthosis from a practical as well as a mechanical view point.

With all the foregoing considerations, a clinical biomechanical approach to the use of orthotics may be taken through answers to the following questions. What are the pathologic conditions that are involved in the spine? What are the therapeutic mechanical goals? In what way should the mechanics of the spine be changed? Is the goal to protect the spine, to rest it, or to correct it? What kinds of forces are necessary in order to achieve the therapeutic aims?

The type of forces necessary can be determined by a review of the basic kinematics of the spine in the region where the forces are to be applied. Then it is possible to decide which orthotic devices are able to apply the needed loads so as to best achieve the desired mechanical result. There are limitations in the extent to which forces may be applied to the spine; these involve psychological, physiological, and mechanical factors.

Fig. 7-23. (A) MacAusland (chairback brace). This orthosis offers *intermediate control* for the upper lumbar spine in flexion and extension. It is less effective in lateral bending (no lateral uprights) and least effective in controlling axial rotation. (B) Knight brace. This orthosis offers *intermediate control* for the upper lumbar spine in flexion/extension and lateral bending (note lateral uprights). It is not an effective control of axial rotation. (C) Williams brace. This exerts *intermediate control* against flexion/extension, lateral bending, but not axial rotation. All the three braces provide general support and stability through compression with the abdominal supports.

Table 7-4. Functional Analysis of Spinal Braces

Orthosis	Spine Region	Degrees of Freedom Controlled	Effectiveness of Control
Soft cervical collar	Cervical	FE, LB	Min.
Hard plastic collar (Thomas)	Cervical	FE, LB, (AR)	Int.
Philadelphia	Cervical	FE, LB, (AR)	Int.
Four-poster	Cervical	FE, LB, AR	Int.
Long two-poster (Guilford, Duke)	Cervical	FE, LB, AR	Int. (high)
Minerva cast	Cervical	FE, LB, AR	Most
Halo device	Cervical	FE, LB, AR	Most (high)
Long thoracic corsets	Thoracic	FE, LB	Min.
Three-point (Jewett, Griswold)	Thoracic	FE	Int.
Taylor	Thoracic, thoracolumbar	FE	Int.
Taylor (with lateral uprights)	Thoracic	FE, LB, AR	Int.
Use of clavicle pads	Thoracic	AR	Int.
Milwaukee brace (tightly worn)	Thoracic, thoracolumbar	FE, LB, (AR) Kyphosis correction	Most
Risser plaster jacket	Thoracic, thoracolumbar	FE, LB, AR	Most
Milwaukee brace (loosely worn)	Thoracic, thoracolumbar	Scoliosis correction	Most
Halo pelvic device	Thoracic, thoracolumbar	FE, LB, AR	Most (high)
Corsets	Lumbar	FE, LB	Min.
Williams	Lumbar (except L4 to L5)	FE, LB	Int.
Knight	Lumbar (except L4 to L5)	FE (LB)	Int.
MacAusland	Lumbar (except L4 to L5)	FE (LB)	Int.
Taylor	Lumbar (except L4 to L5)	FE, LB, AR	Int.
Norton and Brown (exp. brace)	Lumbar (except L4 to L5)	FE, LB	Int. (high)
Taylor (with thigh attachment)	Lumbar	FE, LB, AR	Most
Molded plaster jacket	Lumbar (except L4 to L5)	FE, LB, AR	Most
Molded plaster jacket (thigh included)	Lumbar	FE, LB, AR	Most
Halo pelvic device	Lumbar	FE, LB, AR	Most (high)

FE: Flexion/extension (x-axis rotation)　　　Min.: Minimal
LB: Lateral bending (z-axis rotation　　　　Int.: Intermediate
AR: Axial rotation (y-axis rotation)　　　　Most: Most effective
( ) Slightly less controlled

In general, the corsets and collars and relatively flexible supports apply the least amount of control to the spine. Short models of the braces that employ rigid uprights and molds provide better control, followed by the longer braces. They have greater leverage, which offers additional mechanical advantage in the application of forces. Mechanical devices may be added to these braces to deliver additional therapeutic support. Examples include devices to limit axial rotation and a number of pads and supports that apply more discrete, localized loads for explicit purposes. This is effectively employed in the treatment of scoliosis or kyphosis. Spinal orthoses that incorporate the thigh or add some special extension, as in the Norton and Brown experimental brace to augment immobilizing efficiency, may also be used. Increased fixation where desired can sometimes be achieved through the use of more rigid material such as plaster.

Finally, the level of maximum immobilization is achieved through the use of external skeletal fixation with the halo apparatus in conjunction with a short or a long, well molded body cast. The long body cast offers a greater efficiency of immobilization due to greater purchase and leverage. The most effective device at present for immobilizing the entire spine is the halo pelvic apparatus.

CLINICAL BIOMECHANICS

The clinical problem is to apply forces to the spine in a manner that will somehow be therapeutic to the patient. The magnitude and resultant effects of these forces depend upon the biomechanics of the complex system.

Forces applicable to the spine from the outside are limited by skin discomfort and the stiffness of the structures through which they must be transmitted.

In a three-point fixation system, the middle force should be applied where the clinician wishes to obtain maximum correction or immobilization.

Selective discomfort imposed by the orthosis is one of the mechanisms through which motion is controlled.

For the most effective control of the degrees of freedom, the halo pelvic skeletal fixation should be employed.

A well molded plaster cast offers the best non-skeletal fixation against axial rotation of the spine.

In each case, consider the movement (i.e., flexion or extension) that must be prevented; then choose the orthosis accordingly.

Shoulder and thoracic support fixation adds to the unloading and general effectiveness of a cervical orthosis when standing but loses some of its effectiveness when the patient is recumbent.

In attempts to immobilize the upper cervical spine with the use of a cast or a brace, it should be remembered that complete immobilization is not possible. The patient's ability to talk and chew, is inversely related to the effectiveness of the immobilization.

The Jewett hyperextension brace probably has some ability to shift weight from the anterior to the posterior elements of the thoracic vertebrae.

The use of an abdominal corset with the chairback brace is valuable in diminishing the loads applied to the lumbar spine.

A cast or orthosis that seeks to immobilize the lumbosacral joint should include at least one thigh as part of the fixation.

NOTES

[A] *The forces.* The law of equilibrium states that (a) the sum of the forces be equal to zero, and (b) the sum of the moments be equal to zero. Therefore:

$$\text{(a)} \quad F_A - F_B - F_C = 0 \tag{1}$$
$$\text{(b)} \quad F_B D_B - F_C D_C = 0 \tag{2}$$

Solving these, we obtain:

$$F_B = \frac{F_A \cdot D_C}{D_B + D_C} \quad \text{and} \tag{3}$$

$$F_C = \frac{F_A \cdot D_B}{D_B + D_C} \tag{4}$$

Putting in the values of the example shown in Figure 7-7A gives

$$F_B = \frac{2F_A}{3} \tag{5}$$

$$F_C = \frac{F_A}{3} \tag{6}$$

Bending Moment Diagram. The bending moment diagram for the three-point force system is shown in Figure 7-7B. It is triangular in shape, and the maximum bending moment is equal to:

$$\text{Mmax} = F_A \cdot \frac{D_B \cdot D_C}{D_B + D_C} \tag{7}$$

$$= F_A \frac{1}{\dfrac{1}{D_B} + \dfrac{1}{D_C}} \tag{8}$$

Equation (8) clearly shows that maximum bending moment is maximized by largest values of D_B and D_C.

[B] Location of the thoracic pad. The goal of applying horizontal forces to the spine is to obtain maximum overall correction. Thus, for the three-point force system, the criterium for maximum angular correction is the angle change for the two vertebrae at the level of the two end forces. The engineering principles applicable here have to do with the deflection of a beam, subjected to bending moments from applied forces. The principle states that the resulting angulation between the two points on a beam is proportional to the area of the bending moment diagram between those two points. Applying this principle and maximizing the area as a function of the location of the middle force, it is shown below that the optimum place for this force is midway between the two end forces.

Referring to Figure 7-7B, the three-point principle and its bending moment diagram, an equation for the area of the bending moment diagram can be written:

$$\text{Area} = (D_B + D_C) \, \text{Mmax}/2 \tag{9}$$

Inserting the value for Mmax from equation (7) results in:

$$\text{Area} = \frac{F_A \cdot D_B \cdot D_C}{2} \tag{10}$$

Further, assuming that points B and C are given and that point A is varied to obtain the most efficient loading, it is possible to substitute for D_C:

$$D_C = D - D_B \tag{11}$$

Where D equals $D_B + D_C$. Putting equation (11) in (10), differentiating Area with respect to D_B, and equating the expression to zero, the value of D_B for which Area is maximum is obtained:

$$D - 2D_B = 0 \qquad (12)$$
$$D_B = D/2 \qquad (13)$$

Therefore, for maximum angular change between the two end vertebrae, the point A should be located midway between B and C.

In the above analysis, the Milwaukee brace and the patient are modeled as a pure three-point force system. If the pelvic support is allowed to take up bending moments (which it always does to a degree) the above assumption and the conclusion are no longer true. For example, if the axillary sling is absent, the three-point force system degenerates into a cantilever system where the bending moment created by the thoracic pad is balanced solely by the pelvic support. It all depends upon the brace configuration (presence of the various pads), fit of the brace, and the patient activity. In order to optimize these factors and thoroughly understand the mechanism that makes the Milwaukee brace so effective, additional biomechanical measurements on patients using the brace are required.

CLASSIFICATION OF REFERENCES

Basic spinal orthotics 2, 6, 10, 16, 20
Experimental studies, 4, 5, 6a, 12, 14, 23
Clinical descriptions 7, 11, 13, 15, 17, 21
Advanced reading 1, 3

REFERENCES

1. Andriacchi, T., Schultz, A., Belytschco, T., and Galante, J.: A model for studies of mechanical interactions between the human spine and rib cage. J. Biomech., 7:497, 1974. (*Analysis of the contribution of the rib cage to biomechanical behavior of the spine.*)
2. Bloomberg, M. H.: Orthopaedic Braces. Philadelphia, J. B. Lippincott, 1964. (*Catalogue and clear concise analysis of components.*)
3. Clark, J. A., and Kesterton, L.: Halo pelvic traction appliance for spinal deformities. J. Biomech., 4:589, 1971. (*A novel feature of the halo hoop described here is the force monitoring springs in the uprights which apply optimum distraction force to the spine.*)
4. Galante, J., Schultz, A., and DeWald, R.: Forces acting in the Milwaukee brace on patients undergoing treatment for idiopathic scoliosis. J. Bone Joint Surg., 52A:498, 1970. (*A valuable investigation with useful information.*)
5. Hartmann, J. T., Palumbo, F., and Hill, B. J.: Cineradiography of the braced normal cervical spine. Clin. Orthop., 109:97, 1975.
6. Jordan, H. H.: Orthopaedic Appliances. Springfield, Ill., Charles C Thomas, 1963. (*Description of some biomechanical considerations involved in brace construction.*)
6a. Johnson, R. M., et al.: Cervical orthoses. A study comparing their effectiveness in restricting cervical motion in normal subjects. J. Bone Joint Surg., 59A:332, 1977.
7. Kaplan, L. I., et al.: A reappraisal of braces and other mechanical aids in patients with spinal cord dysfunction: Results of a follow-up study. Arch. Phys. Med. Rehabil., 47:393, 1965.
8. Levine, D. B., and Hankin, S.: The halo yoke: A simplified device for attachment of the halo to a body cast. J. Bone Joint Surg., 54A:881, 1972. (*Recommend for any clinician using the halo.*)
9. Lysell, E.: Motion in the cervical spine. Thesis. Acta Orthop. Scand., 123 [Suppl.], 1969. (*One of the most accurate descriptions of the kinematics of the cervical spine.*)
10. Morris, J. M., and Lucas, D. B.: Biomechanics of spinal bracing. Ariz. Med., 21:170, 1974.
11. Mulcahy, T., et al.: A follow-up study of forces acting on the Milwaukee brace on patients undergoing treatment for idiopathic scoliosis. Clin. Orthop., 93:53, 1973.
12. Nachemson, A., and Elfstrom, G.: Intravital wireless telemetry of axial forces in Harrington distraction rods in patients with idiopathic scoliosis. J. Bone Joint Surg., 53A:445, 1971. (*An excellent in vivo biomechanical study with readily applicable clinical information.*)
13. Nickel, V. L., Perry, J., Garrett, A., and Heppenstall, M.: The halo, a spinal skeletal traction fixation device. J. Bone Joint Surg., 58A:1400, 1968. (*Recommend for careful study by anyone using the halo apparatus.*)
14. Norton, P. L., and Brown, T.: The immobilizing efficiency of back braces. J. Bone Joint Surg., 39A:111, 1957. (*A most significant work on this topic—worth no less than one hour of careful study.*)
15. O'Brien, J. P., Yau, A. C. M. C., Smith, T. K., and Hodgson, A. R.: Halo-pelvic traction. J. Bone Joint Surg., 53B:217, 1971.
16. Orthopaedic Appliances Atlas. vol. 1. American Academy of Orthopaedic Surgeons, Ann Arbor, J. W. Edwards, 1952. (*An excellent historical and comprehensive reference.*)
17. Perry, J.: The halo in spinal abnormalities. Orthop. Clin. North Am., 3:69, 1972. (*Recommended for any clinician using the halo.*)
18. Rolander, S. D.: Motion of the lumbar spine with special reference to the stabilizing effect of posterior fusion. Thesis. Acta Orthop. Scand., 90 [Suppl.], 1966. (*One of the most accurate descriptions of lumbar spine kinematics—an excellent bibliography.*)
19. Sharp, J., and Purser, D. W.: Spontaneous alanto-axial dislocation and ankylosing spondylitis in rheumatoid arthritis. Ann. Rheum. Dis., 20:47, 1961.
20. Spinal Orthotics Course Manual. New York University Post-Graduate Medical School, Prosthetic and Orthotics. Revision, 1972. (*Contains an operational classification of braces avoiding the traditional eponyms. There are analyses of various brace components, and information on prescription writing and checkout procedures.*)
21. Thompson, H.: The "Halo" traction apparatus—A method of external splinting of the cervical spine after injury. J. Bone Joint Surg., 44B:655, 1962.
22. Victor, D., Bresnan, M., and Keller, R.: Brain abcess complicating the use of halo traction. J. Bone Joint Surg., 55A:635, 1973.
23. Walters, R., and Morris, J.: Effects of spinal supports on the electrical activity of muscles of the trunk. J. Bone Joint Surg., 52A:51, 1970.

8 Biomechanical Considerations in the Surgical Management of the Spine

It is now, as it was then, and as it may ever be, conceptions
from the past blind us to facts which almost slap us in the face.
William S. Halsted, 1924

This chapter presents the major surgical procedures for the spine and discusses relevant biomechanical considerations. Biomechanical facts, theory, and data are reviewed.

Part 1: Surgical Decompressions

The indications for surgical decompression of the spinal cord are still in need of improvement. The guidelines that are generally followed are discussed here. Decompression is indicated in the presence of an incomplete or progressive neurologic deficit in which there is clinical evidence of pressure or encroachment on the spinal cord, associated with tumor, trauma, infection, and a variety of other disease states. It is desirable to recognize as accurately as possible the patient who has suffered damage to the cord from impact without physical residual impingement on the cord that can be relieved by surgical decompression.

The goal of decompression is to effectively remove abnormal spinal cord or nerve root pressure with the least possible surgical risk and the least disruption of the structural integrity of the spinal column. The first consideration is to localize the site of the abnormal pressure. The compression may be anterior, posterior or both; midline, lateral or both; at the interspace, behind the vertebral body, or both. Obviously, there are any number of possible combinations. The sources of compression may also be mixed or poorly localized. There are a number of accepted surgical procedures that may be employed to decompress the spinal cord and/or nerve roots. Each case should be carefully evaluated and the proper surgical procedure chosen.

Clinical evaluation is carried out to locate the source of abnormal pressure as accurately as possible. The history and neurologic examination are helpful; however, the determination of location is mainly based on radiographic studies. All of the following studies need not and can not always be carried out; however, using several in each case aids in localizing the source of pressure: plain anteroposterior and lateral and oblique radiographs; laminograms; radiopaque myelography; air contrast myelography; and computerized axial tomography. Clinical judgment and the equipment available dictate the combinations of studies that are used for a particular patient.

Generally, when the pressure is anterior, the decompression of choice should be anterior. Similarly, posterior decompression is generally best for relieving posterior pressure. If the surgeon decompresses the spinal cord anteriorly when the pressure is posterior, or vice versa, some significant liabilities result. Not only has an inappropriate, ineffectual procedure been carried out, but if normal structures have been violated in order to achieve the decompression, the procedure may have caused or added to already existing clinical instability. When the offending structure is between the vertebral body and the spinal cord, all or part of the vertebral body must be removed to decompress the lesion. Posterior decompression of the spinal canal, even with dentate ligament transection, may not relieve anterior impingement. This observation was made by Verbiest in post-traumatic situations,[115] and it applies to most anterior encroachments.[128]

The only situation in which a posterior decompression is helpful in the presence of anterior pressure (or vice versa) is when there is contrecoup compression. In such cases, there is both anterior and posterior pressure. The primary pressure is due to some abnormal lesion that is pressing directly on the spinal cord. On the opposite side, there is contrecoup compression, which is due to the displacement of the spinal cord from the primary lesion. The displacement causes contrecoup compression from impingement against a

normal structure. When the primary compression is relieved, contrecoup compression is also relieved. In these situations, decompression that is not at the site of the *primary* source of pressure is definitely not the procedure of choice. There are two examples shown in Figure 8-1. Clearly, anterior decompression though helpful is not adequate for primary posterior pressure. Conversely, posterior decompression is not adequate for primary anterior pressure. Although removal of the secondary pressure is helpful, the problem is not solved. The cord is not free to simply "float away" from the primary pressure source just because space for the release of contrecoup pressure is provided. The cord is under some tension normally,[12] and that tension is increased by a direct physical impingement. It was thought that sectioning of the dentate ligament could relieve this tension. This procedure was believed to allow a posterior laminectomy to be carried out to relieve anterior pressure by providing space and then permitting the spinal cord to move posteriorly and away from the offending

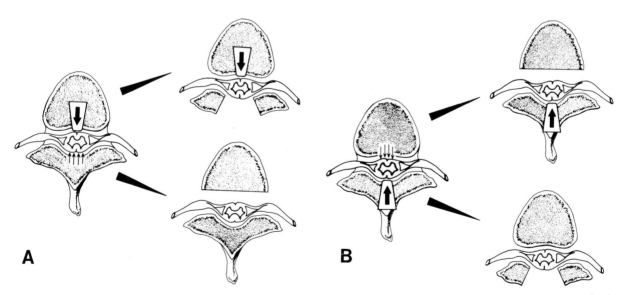

A **B**

Fig. 8-1. An illustration of the concept of contrecoup compression of the spinal cord and the possible methods of decompression. *(A)* Here the primary compression is anterior, and the contrecoup compression is posterior. Posterior decompression solves only the secondary source of pathology. Anterior decompression resolves both sources of compression on the spinal cord. *(B)* This is the converse situation. Removal of the anterior secondary compression does not solve the problem, but removal of the primary lesion posterior to the spinal cord permits full decompression. These concepts point out the importance of preoperative localization of the primary lesion causing compression whenever possible. This is greatly facilitated with the use of computerized axial tomography.

structure. This is no longer a tenable hypothesis. Because of the significance of the anterior spinal artery and the blood supply to the cord (Fig. 4-36), there is an additional reason for concern about unrelieved primary anterior spinal cord pressure in the cervical spine. Posterior laminectomy alone in the presence of primary anterior compression is not likely to give the best results.

Although some still advocate laminectomies at multiple levels and facet fusion for spondylitic myelopathy, it may not be the procedure of choice, for the same reasons described above. Posterior decompression for anterior osteophytes may offer some relief in many situations, but the best result may be shown with an anterior trough decompression, especially when the osteophytes are midline.

Sometimes, there is primary pressure anteriorly and posteriorly, or it is not possible to determine clinically where the primary source of pressure is located. In these situations, combined anterior and posterior decompression may be required. We suggest posterior decompression and facet fusion providing maximum immediate clinical stability, followed by anterior decompression and reconstruction if the recovery from the posterior decompression fails to meet reasonable expectations.

DECOMPRESSION IN THE CERVICAL REGION

Some of the most dire neurologic consequences occur from spinal cord injuries in this region. Most of the cervical spine is readily accessible surgically, either anteriorly or posteriorly.

Anteriorly Located Compression

There are a number of sites in which the spinal cord may be compressed anteriorly. Generally, some appropriate *anterior* decompression should be employed.

Anterior Midline Compression. Pressure may be exerted on the anterior midline portion of the cord at the level of the interspace only. This may be caused by a "hard disc" (primarily an osteophyte), a "soft disc" (primarily the annulus fibro-

sus), tumor, trauma, or infection. We believe that the Smith Robinson procedure is the operation of choice for anterior midline pathology located at the level of the interspace because it gives adequate exposure and provides a sound surgical construct for postoperative stabilization (Fig. 8-2:2A).[100] The surgical constructs for fusion are analyzed on page 400. The Bailey-Badgley procedure is also effective in these cases, although we believe that it is perhaps somewhat more extensive than is necessary for anterior midline pathology limited to the region of interspace.[5] The modified Bailey-Badgley, long trough decompression and fusion is a very appropriate procedure for multilevel cervical myelopathy secondary to midline osteophyte and/or disc protrusion. The operation provides decompression and offers a convenient effective construct for arthrodesis. The same comment applies to the Cloward and the Keystone graft procedures, except that the Cloward procedure is not such a stable construct (Fig. 8-2:2C).[57] A modification of the last three procedures is required for anterior decompression of the spinal cord. The vertebral body must be resected all the way back to the posterior longitudinal ligament and dura mater for full visualization and decompression.

When the lesion causing the pressure is cephalad or caudad to the level of the interspace, then additional considerations become important. Such a lesion may result from the same pathologic conditions mentioned above or, in addition, from ossification of the posterior longitudinal ligament. The procedure of choice in this situation is a modification of the Bailey-Badgley procedure. A cephalocaudal longitudinal trough through the vertebral body is extended through the posterior longitudinal ligament, which is then removed. This has the advantage of providing adequate exposure at the interspace and removal at the midline of as much cephalocaudal vertebral body as is required. This is a sound surgical construct which maintains considerable stability if one elects the option of leaving some part of the lateral portions of the annulus and the vertebral bodies intact (Fig. 8-25C). The Cloward and the Keystone procedures are also useful when only limited access to the space behind the vertebral bodies is needed (Fig. 8-2:2C). Another proce-

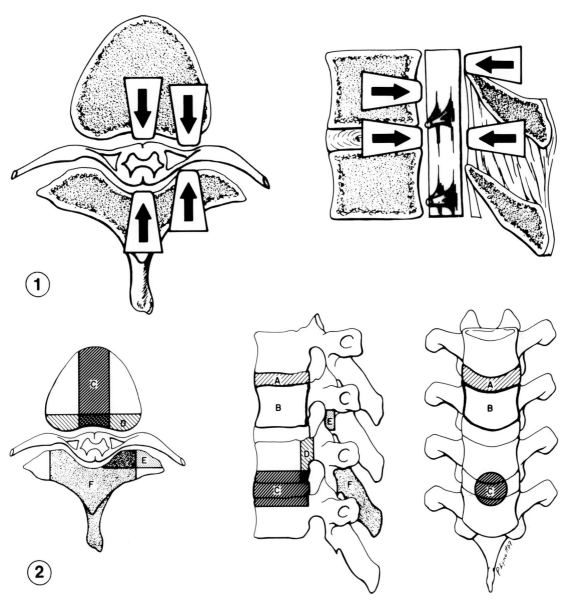

Fig. 8-2. Part 1. Compression sites. This illustrates the basic sites of spinal cord and nerve root compressions. The anterior compressions may be at the interspace level or up behind the vertebral body. They may also be midline or lateral. The same is the case for the posterior compressions. In selecting the surgical technique for decompression it is useful to first determine as accurately as possible the site of the compression. *Part 2.* Multiple decompressions. *(A)* The Smith-Robinson approach, removal of the intervertebral disc, decompresses the anterior cord and nerve root at the interspace level (Fig. 8-24). *(B)* Vertebral body resection decompresses the anterior cord and nerve roots (Fig. 8-32). The disc above and below is included, which provides even wider exposure and decompression. *(C)* The Cloward or dowel resection, when carried back through the posterior longitudinal ligament by careful dissection exposes the central portion of the cord behind the vertebral body. The lateral areas are exposed at the interspace by removal of remaining disc material. *(D)* An anterior decompression that begins at the neural foramen and removes only the posterior most portion of the vertebral body. This leaves as much of the anterior structures as possible to maintain clinical stability (Fig. 8-36). *(E)* This is the keyhole laminotomy and/or the facetectomy or posterior nerve root decompression (Fig. 8-3). Keyhole laminotomy is suggested only for a soft, anterolateral cervical disc that can be removed by the cephalad or caudad retraction of the nerve root. *(F)* Bilateral laminectomy (total laminectomy) for posterior decompression of the cord.

377

dure that can be useful in this situation is vertebral body resection, especially when extensive exposure and good visualization of the cord is important.[56] This is also shown in Figure 8-2:2B.

One *definitely suboptimal* choice should also be mentioned. If for some *unavoidable* reason an anterior approach is not possible, then two or more posterior laminectomies at two or more contiguous levels may be helpful. This may be justified because it alleviates any posterior contrecoup compression.

Anterolateral Compression.   Anterolateral pressure limited to the interspace can be caused by protruding joints of Luschka, a hard and soft disc, tumor, trauma, or infection. The Smith-Robinson procedure is the one we recommend

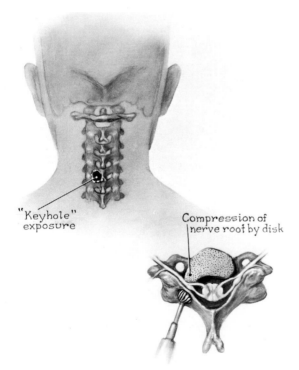

"Keyhole" exposure

Compression of nerve root by disk

Fig. 8-3. This limited laminotomy is adequate for removal of a herniated annulus fibrosus. In the cervical spine the roots pass through the intervertebral foramen approximately at right angles to the spinal cord. Thus, the roots should be carefully retracted cephalad or caudad, rather than medially as in the lumbar spine. (Robinson, R. A., and Southwick, W. O.: Surgical approaches to the cervical spine. *In* American Academy of Orthopaedic Surgeons: Instructional Course Lectures, vol. 17. St. Louis, C. V. Mosby, 1960.)

in this situation. We believe that for a well documented "soft disc," the keyhole laminotomy is also a useful operation (Fig. 8-2:2E; 8-3).

Sometimes, an anterolateral lesion may extend or be entirely located behind the vertebral body. This may be caused by the same diseases described above. In these situations, we suggest a vertebral body resection. If the clinical problem is such that a somewhat limited exposure would suffice, then the previously described modification of the Bailey-Badgley, the Cloward, or the Keystone procedure is a good choice.

Anterior Midline and Lateral Compression. When the lesion is at only the interspace, the Smith-Robinson procedure is the treatment of choice. If there is extensive disease behind the vertebral body, then vertebral body resection is the treatment of choice. Laminectomy at multiple levels is a secondary choice when the anterior approach is not possible.

Posteriorly Located Compression

Posterior pressure on the cervical spinal cord may come from a variety of conditions. There are the standard causes, tumor, trauma, and infection. Additional conditions include yellow ligament encroachment, spinal stenosis, and laminectomy membranes. When the offending disease is posterior, the decompression should be posterior. When the source of compression is posterior, its relationship to the interspace (along the y-axis) is not surgically important. This is because of the relative ease of adjustment of the level of laminectomy and its extension cephalocaudally. However, with the anterior approach there is a significant difference between cutting through the disc space and cutting through the vertebral body. It is also important to remember that multiple laminectomies[A] in the cervical spine, even in the presence of intact facet articulations, may jeopardize clinical stability, especially in children.[18] In other words, the surgeon should not decompress any more extensively than is necessary (see Chapter 5).

Posterior Midline Compression. This may be adequately decompressed with a single or multiple level bilateral laminectomy, as needed (Fig. 8-2:2F).

Posterolateral Compression. Compression

here may be relieved by a keyhole laminotomy, a unilateral laminectomy, or a laminectomy with facetectomy or nerve root decompression.

Posterior Midline and Lateral Compression. For this condition, we recommend the bilateral laminectomy or multiple bilateral laminectomies.

Anteriorly and Posteriorly Located Compression

There are situations in which the cord is compressed at or near the same level, both anteriorly and posteriorly. In addition to tumor, trauma, and infection, there are the so-called pincer mechanisms,[84] as well as combinations of hard and soft discs associated with yellow ligament encroachment.

Anterior and Posterior Compression, Limited to Interspace. This may be caused by either the pincer mechanism or combined yellow ligament and disc encroachment. For osteophytes impinging on the anterior or anterolateral portion of the cord and nerve roots associated with a yellow ligament impinging posteriorly, the Smith-Robinson procedure is an effective construct. The technique permits removal of anterior spinal cord impingement, and by spreading the interspace, it reduces the yellow ligament encroachment and increases the longitudinal (y-axis) diameter of the neural foramen.

The pincer phenomenon occurs as a primarily translatory displacement in the sagittal plane.[84] This is shown in Figure 8-4. In some instances, there has been extensive displacement, and the cord damage is due to the initial impact at the time of injury rather than the residual canal encroachment. In this type of situation correction of the encroachment is unlikely to be helpful with regard to spinal cord recovery. However, with reduction and/or decompression, there may be some nerve root recovery. If the trauma is not acute, or if there is reason to assume that the neurologic problem results from the residual encroachment rather than the initial impact, then one solution to the problem is to reduce the displacement and thus regain the original spinal canal diameter. This may be done through axial traction or open reduction in the case of fixed facet dislocation. If there is evidence that a displaced disc or bony fragment causes compression anteriorly or a bony fragment causes compres-

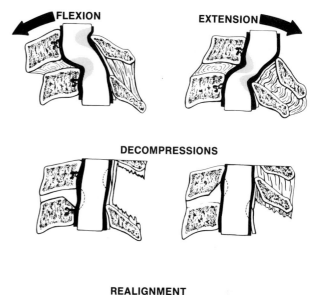

Fig. 8-4. The pincer phenomenon may be associated with different patterns of cord encroachment, depending upon whether the displacement at the level of disruption is in a flexion or an extension mode. Although the indications for decompression are controversial, this figure is intended to point out some of the mechanical factors that are important. When indicated, adequate decompression of a pincer problem may require a posterior approach, possibly in conjunction with an anterior procedure. Realignment may also be as satisfactory in some situations.

sion posteriorly, an appropriate decompression should be carried out. If the situation is such that the pincer mechanism is thought to be the only pressure-exerting pathology in an irreducible injury, we suggest a posterior decompression, which provides the opportunity for open reduction, if necessary. This could then be followed by anterior decompression should it be necessary. Eyring and colleagues reported a case in which anterior and posterior decompressions and fusions were done under the same anesthesia with the patient in a sitting position.[28] The decision to decompress and the surgical technique chosen should follow the guidelines presented in this chapter. A study of the evaluation of clinical stability in Chapter 5 shows that in all probability, a pincer phenomenon requiring decompression is more likely than not to fit the indications of a clinically unstable situation, which should be managed accordingly.

Compression Behind a Vertebral Body, Which May or May not Be at the Level of the Interspace. The possible causes include tumor, trauma, infection, and spinal stenosis.[77] The reasonable options are vertebral body resection, multiple bilateral laminectomies, or combined anterior and posterior decompressions.

Mixed or Poorly Localized Compression

This condition may occur as a result of any combination of the entities mentioned previously. If the indications for decompression are present but can not be well localized, we suggest vertebral body resection or combined anterior and posterior decompression. If the situation is associated with fracture, reduction and realignment may be useful.

DECOMPRESSION IN THE THORACIC REGION

Anterior Compression. The considerations involved are basically the same as those for the cervical region. Even though the thoracic spine is stiffer, the potential for clinical instability is greater and the effectiveness of laminectomy for decompression and exploration is considerably lessened. These factors are mainly due to the relative lack of free space for the spinal cord and its precarious blood supply (see Fig. 6-16). For the treatment of the possible combinations of anterior compression, we suggest either *partial* (Fig. 8-2:2D) or total vertebral body resection (Fig. 8-2:2B). Wherever possible, partial resection is preferable, since this leaves more structural integrity to maintain clinical stability and simplifies the necessary reconstruction.

Posterior Compression. For midline as well as combined midline and lateral problems, we recommend bilateral laminectomy at a single or at multiple levels, depending upon the cephalocaudal extent of the lesion. For posterolateral compression, the recommendation is unilateral laminectomy or laminectomy and facetectomy.

Anterior and Posterior Compression. Here, we suggest vertebral body resection or a combined anterior and posterior decompression. In some fractures and/or dislocations, reduction and realignment may be helpful. If the pincer phenomenon is present, reduction and realignment should be considered, followed by bilateral laminectomy if the preceding is impossible or not effective.

Mixed or Poorly Localized Compression. In these cases one may employ vertebral body resection, a combined anterior and posterior approach, and/or reduction and realignment.

DECOMPRESSION IN THE LUMBAR REGION

In the lumbar spine the problem of compression is less common and less severe. The cauda equina starts below L2 and there is relatively more free space for the cauda equina than there is for the cord in other regions of the spine. Another unique factor about this region is that in the large majority of situations, the neural elements can be decompressed through a posterior approach. It is usually possible to carefully retract the dura and cauda equina far enough laterally to expose and remove anterior compressing structures. Anterior decompressions are sometimes necessary and can usually be achieved through a posterior approach. Although an anterior or anterolateral approach makes the vertebral body readily accessible, in this region it has some serious complications.[54,97]

Anteriorly Located Compression

Anterior Midline Compression. Anterior midline lesions at the intervertebral disc only, as well as those behind the vertebral body, may be decompressed with bilateral laminectomy or multiple posterior laminectomies. Usually, the anterior structures may be exposed by side to side retraction of the dura and the cauda equina. In some instances it is necessary to include a partial or total vertebral body resection for the purpose of decompression or excision.

Anterolateral Compression. This condition may require one of several different procedures, depending upon the nature, size and location of the lesions. When they are at the interspace, a keyhole laminotomy may suffice. In most cases those compression sources at the interspace or at the level of the vertebral body require unilateral laminectomy, laminectomy with facetectomy, or in some instances partial vertebral body resection.

Anterior Midline and Lateral Compression. Such lesions at the interspace or elsewhere may be decompressed by bilateral laminectomy, multiple bilateral laminectomy, or when necessary, partial vertebral body resection.

Posteriorly Located Compression

Posterior Midline Compression. In addition to the common causes (tumor, trauma, and infection), spinal stenosis, laminectomy membrane, and yellow ligament encroachment may cause compression of the neural elements in this location. The problem can be solved by a bilateral laminectomy.

Posterolateral Compression. Tumor, trauma, and infection may be responsible. The procedure of choice is a unilateral laminectomy or a laminectomy and facetectomy (foramenotomy) if there is also compression in the root canal.

Posterior Midline and Lateral Compression. The causes are the same as those for posterior midline compression. The surgical procedure for decompression is bilateral laminectomy or multiple bilateral laminectomies, depending on the extent of the compressed area.

Anterior and Posterior Compression

When this occurs at the interspace only, the cause may be a combination of hard or soft disc disease with yellow ligament encroachment, spinal stenosis, or a pincer mechanism. Because of the space available in the lumbar spine, combined anterior and posterior encroachment at the interspace level is unusual. In most instances, bilateral laminectomy alone would be expected to be sufficient for decompression. In some instances, a partial vertebral body resection may also be necessary. If the lesion is also at the level of the vertebral body, multiple bilateral laminectomies may be required.

Mixed or Poorly Localized Compression Sites

In these unusual circumstances, discrete localization eludes a thorough clinical study. Bilateral laminectomy, multiple bilateral laminectomies, partial vertebral body resection, combined anterior and posterior decompression, or reduction and realignment are all the procedures that may be useful. These very difficult cases require a good deal of experience, excellent surgical judgment, and maybe even a bit of luck for successful management. There does not appear to be evidence for any more precise recommendations for surgical treatment in these situations.

GUIDELINES FOR SELECTING A SURGICAL PROCEDURE

The general guidelines for selecting a surgical procedure for decompression are summarized in Table 8-1. The basic approach is to accurately localize the site of the compression and then choose the appropriate surgical procedure to relieve it. The constraints are the risks and limitations of the various exposures and the liabilities created by the structural damage to the spinal column that is required to achieve decompression. The different regions of the spine vary in the accessibility and the necessity of the different approaches and decompression procedures.

Table 8-1 is also a guideline for the surgeon in training. It should be useful in emphasizing the importance of careful thought and evaluation to localize as accurately as possible the site of compression. Then, an *appropriate* rather than a *routine* procedure may be selected to effectively decompress the spinal cord and/or nerve root.

Table 8-1.
Recommended Guidelines for the Precise Selection of Surgical Procedures for Decompression of the Spine

COMPRESSION SITES	EXAMPLES	DECOMPRESSION SURGERY		
		Lower Cervical	Thoracic and Thoracolumbar	Lumbar and Sacral
ANTERIOR				
Midline At interspace only	Hard disc, soft disc, tumor, trauma, infection	SR, BB, C	VBR (P)	BL
Behind vertebral body ±interspace*	Hard disc, soft disc, tumor, trauma, infection / Ossification of the posterior longitudinal ligament	BB, C, KS, VBR, MBL	VBR (P)	BL, MBL, VBR (P)
Lateral At interspace only	Hard disc, soft disc, tumor, trauma, infection	SR, KH	VBR (P)	KH, UL, LF
Behind vertebral body ±interspace*	Hard disc, soft, disc, tumor, trauma, infection	BB, C, KS, VBR	VBR (P)	UL, LF, VBR (P)
Midline and lateral At interspace only	Hard disc, soft disc, tumor, trauma, infection	SR	VBR (P)	BL
Behind vertebral body ± interspace*	Hard disc, soft disc, tumor, trauma, infection / Ossification of the posterior longitudinal ligament	VBR, MBL	VBR, VBR (P)	BL, MBL, VBR (P)
POSTERIOR				
Midline	Tumor, trauma, infection, yellow ligament, laminectomy membrane, spinal stenosis	BL, MBL	BL, MBL	BL
Lateral		KH, UL, LF	UL, LF	UL, LF
Midline and lateral		BL, MBL	BL, MBL	BL, MBL
ANTERIOR AND POSTERIOR				
At interspace only	Pincer mechanism with anterior or posterior displacement	SR, VBR, BL, CAPD, RR	VBR, BL, CAPD, RR	BL, VBR (P)
Behind vertebral body ±interspace	Hard or soft disc with yellow ligament encroachment, spinal stenosis / Tumor, trauma, infection, spinal stenosis	VBR, MBL, CAPD	VBR, MBL, CAPD	BL, MBL
MIXED OR POORLY LOCALIZED				
	Tumor, trauma, infection, other	VBR, CAPD, RR	VBR, CAPD, RR	VBR, CAPD BL, MBL, RR

* The site of compression may or may not be at the level of the interspace.

SR: Smith-Robinson, disc removal, and anterior interbody fusion
BB: Bailey-Badgley trough decompression and fusion
C: Cloward anterior decompression and dowel graft fusion
KS: Keystone interbody resection and fusion
VBR (P): Vertebral body or bodies resected totally or (P) partially, replacement and graft

KH: Keyhole—small laminotomy
UL: Unilateral laminectomy or laminotomy
BL: Bilateral laminectomy or laminotomy
MBL: Multiple bilateral laminectomies
LF: Laminectomy and facetectomy (nerve root decompression)
CAPD: Combined anterior and posterior decompression
RR: Reduction and realignment

Part 2: Spine Fusions

Since the procedure was first introduced by Hibbs and Albee in 1911,[2,53] arthrodesis has been one of the most important and frequently employed operations of the spine. This part of the chapter discusses the mechanical aspects of the various techniques of spine fusion. Theoretical and experimental background information is provided along with relevant clinical data. We do not comprehensively catalogue all fusion operations. References for many of the procedures may be found in the work of Wu.[130]

Surgical fusions are recommended at various levels of sophistication. A physician may state, "The patient should have surgery," or "That patient needs a fusion," or "That patient needs a posterior C1–C2 Brooks fusion in order to provide for some immediate stability against anterior translation and restrict axial rotation while the union matures." Appropriate, detailed recommendations, such as the latter, require a sound mechanical understanding of the available surgical procedures.

Basic Goals of Spine Fusion

Spine fusions are used for one or more of the purposes listed below.

The ideal is to achieve one or more of the selected goals above with the minimal effective decrease in motion and minimal disruption of normal structure and function of the spinal column.

BIOMECHANICAL FACTORS IMPORTANT IN SPINE FUSION SURGERY

Surgical constructs (operations) should be chosen on the basis of suitability. In other words, for any given surgical problem, there are one or more constructs that effectively achieve the desired therapeutic goal. The various surgical procedures have their own unique structural and biomechanical characteristics. The surgeon's goal is to accurately understand the biological and mechanical aspects of the problem and select the appropriate surgical construct to solve it.

Clinical descriptions of surgical procedures in the literature devote ample attention to the indications for surgery, the anatomic aspects of procedures and postoperative care. A good deal less emphasis is placed on choosing the surgical construct. Factors that are not generally discussed are the mechanics of the surgical construct and the relationship of the mechanics to the clinical requirements and goals of the procedure.

Graft Materials

There are several important considerations concerning the choice of graft material and its use in surgical constructs. The graft may be used in several different manners. For example, it may serve as a structure to contribute to immediate postoperative stability, as a scaffold, a spacer, or as a bridge to span a particular spinal column defect. The basic biologic use of graft material is to induce, establish, or assist in osteogenesis. It has not been determined how this occurs or even if it does occur. The main effect may be limited to the provision of a lattice work or some structure for the ingrowth of new bone.

Cortical bone, except for a small portion of its osteocytes, dies after transplantation. The bone is more rapidly revascularized if its periosteum is removed. During the process of remodelling and revascularization, there is a relative osteoporosis and weakening of the graft. As creeping substitution progresses, the new bone takes on the mechanical characteristics that are dictated by the regional biomechanical environment. These are the three phases that have been well docu-

---

Reasons for Spine Arthrodesis

To support the spine when its structural integrity has been severely compromised (to reestablish clinical stability).

To maintain correction, following mechanical straightening of the spine in scoliosis or kyphosis or following osteotomy of the spine.

To prevent progression of deformity of the spine, as in scoliosis, kyphosis, and spondylolisthesis.

To alleviate or eliminate pain by stiffening a region of the spine (e.g., diminishing movement between various spine segments).

mented,[109] and they apply to cortical and cancellous grafts. Although the three phases have been given several names the following seem to adequately identify the process: (1) creeping substitution; (2) osteogenic regeneration; and (3) functional adaptation. As would be expected, there is considerable overlap among the three phases.

The fate of a cancellous bone graft is somewhat different from that of cortical bone. The cancellous bone, especially the red marrow of the ilium, will have a large number of surviving osteogenic cells in its deeper areas. In addition, revascularization is facilitated by the open spongy structure of cancellous bone. For a more detailed discussion and presentation of this material, the work of Burwell, Enneking and colleagues, and Stringa and Mignani are recommended.[15,16,27,109]

Iliac Crests.   Nature has thoughtfully and generously anticipated the needs of surgeons and provided the iliac bones. This ready source of bone has a number of advantages. It is expendable; it can be harvested with the patient in either the prone or supine position; there is ample cortical or cancellous bone; the structure lends itself to the removal and carpentering of a variety of useful shapes and sizes. Moreover, the cancellous bone can be impacted and molded to fit the irregular contours of the irregular bony structures to which it must be apposed. A careful study of a freely dissected ilium will easily familiarize the surgeon with the numerous varieties of natural shapes and combinations of cortical and cancellous grafts that are available (Fig. 8-5). Clinical observations show that use of iliac bone is preferable to tibia in lumbar spine fusions.[47] The disadvantages of the ilium as a donor site include its not uncommon source of complications, including severe pain, hematoma, numbness, myralgia paresthetica, infection, and bony overgrowth that sometimes has to be resected.[123]

Experimental studies that provide useful information about the relative strengths of some of the different configurations of iliac bone grafts have been carried out on fresh cadaveric ilia.[122] Relative compression strengths of different grafts are related to the postoperative stability of the surgical constructs. The results of the study were as follows. The small horseshoe config-

uration of bone (Smith-Robinson procedure) was the strongest, followed by the large horseshoe configuration (modified Bailey-Badgley procedure), and the weakest of the three was the dowel configuration (Cloward procedure). It was found that *all* three configurations sustained high loads. All specimens withstood loads approximately 2.5 times the average body weight. The calculations based on the publications of Ruff and Henzel report about 10 percent of total body weight is above T1 and about 50 percent is above T12.[50,92] The loads may be of greater magnitude if the joint reaction forces associated with functional, in vivo loading from muscle forces are considered. In the lumbar spine the lever mechanisms derived from the muscle forces impart loads to the spine comparable to as much as three to four times body weight (see Chapter 1). This information has significant implications. In the immediate postoperative period, with the muscles relaxed or the head supported, the load bearing capacity of the grafts are adequate. However, with the introduction of such variables as dynamic loading, physiologic muscle forces, creeping substitution of the bone graft, especially in the thoracic and lumbar region, the probability of the load bearing capacity of the grafts being exceeded increases significantly. Also, their *relative* strengths become more crucial.

Fibula.   A fibula graft is probably the strongest in resisting compression because of the relatively large amount of cortical bone. The weaker grafts from the ilium are probably strong enough in the immediate postoperative period. The fibula is reabsorbed slowly, and therefore can be depended upon for a longer period of time for its structural support against compressive loading. The disadvantages are the small amount of cancellous bone and the potential for functional compromise of the mechanics of the donor site. It has been shown that the fibula bears approximately one-sixth of body weight.[64] This liability can be virtually eliminated by the use of hemicylindrical fibular grafts.

Ribs.   Ribs are good bone graft material, especially for arthrodesis of the anterior thoracic spine, because they are so readily available.[29] Due to its structure, which consists of a modest cortex and porous cancellous bone, it has the ad-

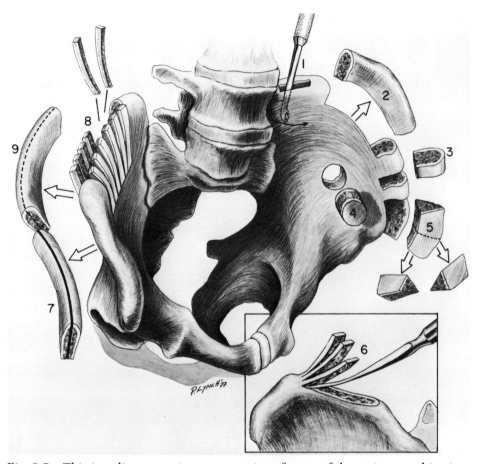

Fig. 8-5. This is a diagrammatic representation of some of the various combinations and configurations of bone grafts available from the ilium. *(1)* Cancellous bone may be curetted from any portion of the iliac crest. *(2)* Various lengths of horseshoe-shaped cortical cancellous graft may be taken for trough grafts and vertebral body replacements. *(3)* The smaller horseshoe configuration used in the Smith-Robinson fusion. *(4)* The dowel configuration. *(5)* A part of the ilium of variable sizes may be taken and fashioned for the Brooks C1-C2 fusion. *(6)* A technique for obtaining multiple onlay grafts with generous portions of cancellous bone. *(7)* A large horseshoe may be split longitudinally and employed in a variety of constructs, to fit a kyphosis or a lordosis with cancellous bone facing up or down. These may also be cut from the ilium so that they are C-shaped, or a mirror image of the same. *(8)* A convenient source of multiple corticocancellous strips. *(9)* Instead the portion labeled 8, this portion of the ilium, with a different natural shape, may be cut to provide additional uses, similar to those described for 7. When initial strength of bone graft is important, the anterior portion of the ilium may be preferable.[122]

vantage of reasonable strength without having a good deal of dense cortical bone which must be incorporated. Furthermore, its slight curvature gives it a certain resiliency and permits it to conform to a cervical or a lumbar lordosis or a thoracic kyphosis (Fig. 8-6).

Tibia. Tibial grafts are occasionally used in spinal arthrodesis. Although this provides a strong graft, we do not think that the liability incurred justifies its use. When the structure of the tibia is changed from a closed section and transformed into an open one, it is considerably

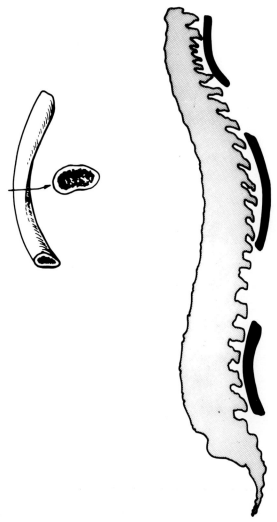

Fig. 8-6. This shows how the anatomy of the rib provides strength, with less dense bone to be reabsorbed. The variety of natural conformities to the normal curves of the spine are also illustrated. Strength is provided through its tubular structure. The cross-section shows the distribution of the cortical bone about the centroid, which gives it a large moment of inertia and good strength for torsional and bending loads.

weakened. The structure is much less able to resist both torsional and bending loads.[32] Chrisman and Snook estimated a refracture rate in skiers at 3 per cent.[20] This was due to a persistent cortical defect. Therefore, if at all possible, physicians should avoid weakening the tibia in this manner.

Allograft Bone. The physical properties of allografts may be presumed to be similar enough to those of autografts for the former to be used as a substitute, at least with respect to the immediate postoperative mechanics. If the immunologic factors could be eliminated or were shown to be insignificant, then the use of bank bone could be very advantageous. Besides eliminating all the donor site complications, the variety and availability of donor material could be enhanced. There is a study which suggests that the fusion rate for anterior cervical spine surgery is as good with freeze-dried allografts as it is with autografts.[94] On the other hand, Bosworth carried out a study and found autograft bone to be three times as good as frozen allograft bone.[8] The final answer is yet to be determined; however, it may well be that the freeze-dried bone allograft should be used more frequently.

Summary. Present knowledge suggests that the patient's own ilium is the best source of graft material. With surgery in the thoracic region, the rib provides an excellent bone graft. The fibula is preferable to the tibia, but both of these sources have some disadvantages. Allografts are useful in many situations and have the advantage of no complications at the donor site; a good bone bank can offer a variety of shapes and sizes. The disadvantages of allografts are related to storage problems and immunologic reactions.

Positioning of the Bone Graft

The relevant biomechanical considerations of the placement of bone grafts focus primarily upon sagittal plane mechanics, and frontal and horizontal plane mechanics in some instances.

The placement of a small fusion mass at the maximum distance from the instantaneous axes of rotation will be more effective in preventing movement around those axes. In preventing sagittal plane rotation of the upper vertebra in relation to the lower one, a fusion mass located on the tips of the spinous process is more effective than one that is placed closer to the instantaneous axes of rotation. This concept, which relates to leverage and area moment of inertia, is exemplified in Figure 8-7. Thus, in terms of discouraging motion of an entire motion segment, the further away from the instantaneous axes of rotation the graft is placed, the more effective it will be. This principle also applies to axial rotation and lateral bending. Looking at this point alone, the posterior fusion established some distance from the instantaneous axis of rotation is better than one that is placed closer to it.

The concept of leverage is also important with respect to the instantaneous axes of rotation and placement of a fusion mass. During flexion, assuming that the axes of rotation are located in the middle or slightly anterior portion of the disc, the leverage situation is as shown in Figure 8-7:2. It is readily apparent that an anterior bone graft has relatively less leverage than a posterior one with regard to its efficacy in preventing rotation of the upper vertebra in flexion or extension. Go a step further and assume that the instantaneous axes for axial rotation bear the same relationship to grafts A and B in Figure 8-7:2. If this were the case, then graft B would also have more leverage in preventing axial rotation.

This is not the first introduction of the biomechanical concept of leverage into the literature on spine surgery. The following points were made in 1911 by Albee in a discussion of the importance of splitting the spinous processes and inserting a bone graft between the two parts during a spine arthrodesis: "This method is be-

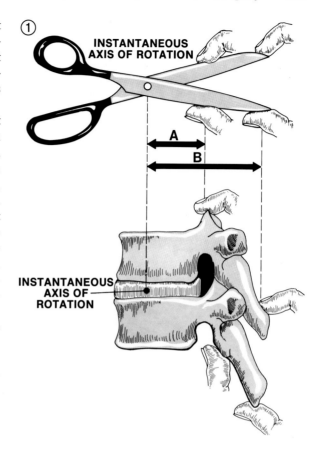

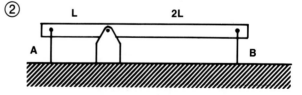

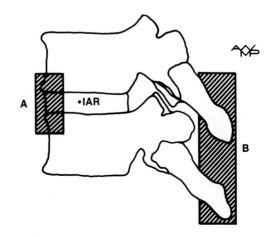

Fig. 8-7. *(1)* To prevent the opening of the blades of the scissors by holding them together, it is distinctly easier to pinch the blades together at the tips *(distance B)* rather than at the midpoint of the blade *(distance A).* Because distance B is further away from the instantaneous axis of rotation, there is greater leverage. The same concepts apply to the vertebral motion segment. Flexion, separation or opening of the spinous processes, is more readily prevented by placing the fingers at the tips of the spinous processes *(distance B)* than at the facet joints *(distance A).* Thus, with regard to a flexion movement, a healed bone graft at distance B, at the tips of the spinous processes, is more effective than one closer to the instantaneous axis of rotation, other factors being constant. These concepts partially explain the efficacy of the rather delicate interspinous and supraspinous ligaments. *(2)* The concept of leverage is shown again here. The anterior bone graft *A* is a short distance (analogous to *L*) from the instantaneous axis of rotation and therefore provides less leverage than bone graft *B*, which is a greater distance (analogous to *2L*) from the instantaneous axis of rotation.

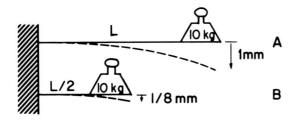

Fig. 8-8. The concept of rigidity as applied to spine fusions is illustrated here. The top figure shows a movement of 1 mm with a 10-kg mass placed at a distance L meters away from the attachment of the beam. If that same 10-kg mass is only one-half the distance away, the motion is reduced to ⅛ mm. In the second example (with a shorter distance), there is more rigidity. The analogous placement of a fusion mass in relation to sources of motion in a vertebra shows that fusion mass B will provide much more rigidity than fusion mass A.

B   INCREASES   RIGIDITY

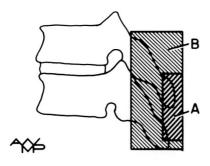

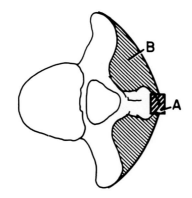

lieved to be preferable to any where breaking or cutting of the spinous processes destroys entirely or for the time being . . . the desired leverage of the spinous processes . . ."

There are other relevant mechanical considerations. The concept of rigidity is a crucial mechanical factor with regard to fusion. This concept is important from the viewpoint of the normal elasticity of the vertebral structure and the relative efficiency of the fusion mass in preventing deformation of the vertebra with various physiologic loads. The principle of rigidity and its application to the vertebral motion segment is shown diagrammatically in Figure 8-8. The practical significance of this concept is the fact that a fusion mass that involves the spinous processes, lamina, and transverse processes is more rigid and immobilizes more effectively than one which involves only the spinous processes.

Rolander demonstrated experimentally that the normal elastic properties of the bone are such that motion may still take place with physiologic forces applied to the motion segment after an adequate posterior fusion.[87] During in vitro experimental studies, he actually fixed *all* posterior elements except the pedicles with *cement* and found significant motion at the interspace with physiologic loading (Fig. 8-9). In the clinical situation a bone graft is a more elastic structure than the cement used in the experiment; therefore even more motion is permitted. Such a posterior fusion would be sufficient if its purpose were to substitute for the stabilizing role of destroyed ligaments. However, it would be sorely lacking if its goal were to totally eradicate motion at the disc interspace as a requirement for eliminating discogenic pain. Obviously, in the latter situation the principle of placing a fusion mass away from the instantaneous axes of rotation should be abandoned and an interbody fusion should be carried out. The interbody technique provides high rigidity by eliminating interbody motion (Fig. 8-10). This procedure when feasible not only eliminates movement between vertebrae to the maximum degree that is possible with bone, but it also removes all or part of the intervertebral disc.

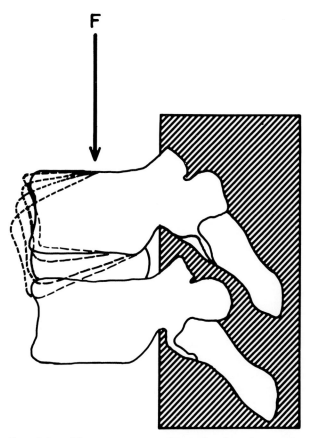

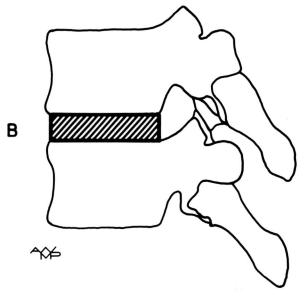

Fig. 8-10. This illustration shows the position of a bone graft B, which can provide maximum rigidity by eliminating interbody motion.

Fig. 8-9. This experiment by Rolander shows the mechanism through which a force F can cause motion between vertebral bodies in the presence of a solid posterior arthrodesis. The motion is permitted by the elastic properties of the free osseous structures. Since it is not known how much motion causes pain or if motion is responsible for pain, it is readily understandable that spine fusion for pain in the lumbar region has not been a particularly good procedure. (White A. A., et al.: The practical biomechanics of the spine for the orthopaedic surgeon. *In* American Academy of Orthopaedic Surgeons: Instructional Course Lectures. St. Louis, C. V. Mosby, 1974.)

Kyphotic Deformity and Bone Graft Positioning

Positioning of the graft is important in another context. This has to do with the use of a bone graft to prevent deformity, maintain correction, or substitute for damaged or absent structures in the presence of a curve. The mechanical principle involves the relationship of the bone graft material to the neutral axis. If the spine is thought

of as being analogous to a beam which is bent and loaded as shown in Figure 8-11A, there are compression stresses (−) on the concave side and tensile stresses (+) on the convex side. Somewhere in the middle at the neutral axis, there is neither compression nor tension. Furthermore, these stresses vary, with a maximum stress on the surface and no stress along the neutral axis (Fig. 8-11A). When an anterior bone graft is to be used as a spacer or to resist compressive forces, it should be placed at a more anterior location in the vertebral body. The closer the graft material is to the neutral axis, the less effective it will be. This applies to the role of the graft in resisting tensile as well as compressive forces. A graft placed at this anterior position offers more effective immediate postoperative stability against axial rotation and flexion or anterior collapse because it is placed further away from the respective axes of rotation. The more posterior of the two anterior interbody graft locations shown in Figure 8-11 is less effective in resisting the two motions than is the more anteriorly placed graft. These points are important in the treatment of kyphotic deformities.

Sometimes long, anterior strut graft fusions are required in the thoracic spine to maintain stabil-

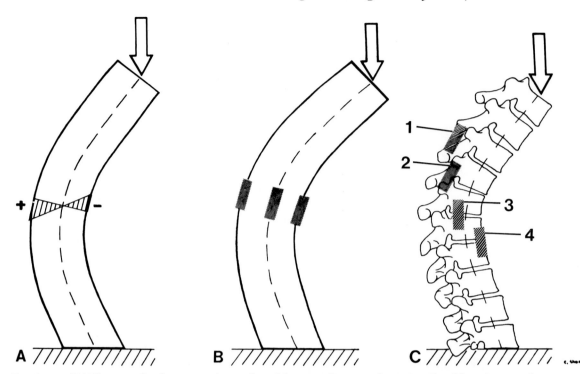

Fig. 8-11. *(A)* The spinal column may be analyzed by regarding it to be somewhat like a beam. There is tension on the convex side of the curve and compression on the concave side. The dashed line is the neutral axis, and there is neither tension nor compression at that point. *(B)* Bone grafts inserted at the various points tend to behave as follows. The graft on the convex side of the curve is mainly under tension and can not resist deforming forces until fully attached at both interfaces. The graft at the dashed line (neutral axis) experiences little or no resistance to bending in the plane of the page. *(C)* In the spine, the graft at position 1 is well away from the neutral axis and when biologically fused at both interfaces can offer effective tensile resistance against progressive kyphosis. The graft at position 2 can do the same, but is less effective because it is closer to the neutral axis. The graft at position 3 is not likely to be as effective as 1 or 2 in preventing progression of deformity because it is even closer to the neutral axis. Graft 4 is effective because it immediately begins to resist compressive forces, which tends to prevent additional deformity and angulation at that point. The graft is also some distance away from the neutral axis giving it mechanical advantage. (White, A. A., Panjabi, M. M., and Thomas, C. L.: The clinical biomechanics of kyphotic deformities. Clin. Orthop. *128*:8, 1977.)

ity against progressive kyphotic deformity.[11,128] Two questions are posed in relation to this problem. How many struts should be placed, and where should they be placed in order to be most effective? Sometimes, major portions of the vertebral bodies have been destroyed or removed, and this factor largely determines where the grafts should be placed. These questions are addressed below through an analysis of the three anterior bone graft locations shown in Figure 8-12.

Graft A is some distance away from the neutral axis but offers support only at the motion segment in which it is implanted. This can be effective if there is a sharply angulated kyphosis located at one motion segment, which may occur in some cases of trauma. There is a surgical construct in which graft A is not employed but B and C are used together. When this is employed, we must assume that only one of them, either B or C, is bearing the major portion of the compressive load. This is due to the fact that in the immediate postoperative period, the surgical construct is unlikely to be designed and erected precisely enough to have both grafts participate equally in the load bearing. However, at later stages when biomechanical adaptation occurs, both columns of graft would be expected to bear an appropriate share of the loads.

The surgeon may choose one of three alternatives. The construct may consist of B, of C, or of B and C, shown in Figure 8-12. The further the graft is located away from the neutral axis, the greater the lever arm with which the graft is working, and the more effective is the support. Thus, if only one is to be used, graft C may appear to be the most attractive alternative. However, there are other considerations. The *longer*, more anteriorly placed graft is more likely to fail from buckling. Its length is critical with regard to this situation. (A more detailed analysis of the concept of buckling is presented in Chapter 1.) It may also interfere with neighboring anatomic structures and is more difficult to revascularize because of its size and position. For these reasons, the more closely placed graft B is probably preferable, if only one is used. The best solution is to use both B and C and to place the anterior most graft as far from the neutral axis as is surgically feasible, recognizing that with biomechanical adaption they will in the long range *both* bear some of the loads.

Clinical experience suggests that for severe kyphosis, posterior fusion alone is likely to fail. Bradford and colleagues, Winter and colleagues, O'Brien, Amed and colleagues, and Hall have recommended in cases of severe kyphosis with tuberculosis that the patient have an anterior decompression followed by an anterior and a posterior fusion.[4,11,40,80,128]

Wolff's Law and Spine Fusions. Physicians frequently hear the following orthopaedic banality—"Don't put that bone graft under tension, it will be absorbed because of Wolff's law." Admittedly, most banalities are allowed to become such because they carry a certain element of truth or at least apparent truth. Wolff's law must be critically examined and put into some biomechanical perspective before we accept the above as true.

Wolff's law is considered to state that bone is laid down where stresses require its presence and bone is absorbed where stresses do not require it. Somehow, the law has been miscon-

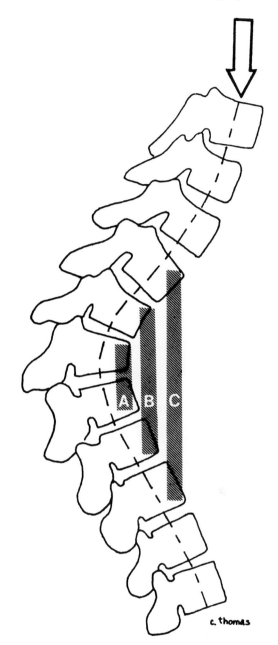

Fig. 8-12. This is an illustration of the various locations of anterior bone graphs for kyphotic deformity. The biomechanical considerations involved in choosing graft A, B, or C are discussed in the text. (White, A. A., Panjabi, M. M., and Thomas, C. L.: The clinical biomechanics of kyphotic deformities. Clinical Orthopaedics, *128*:8, 1977.)

trued to mean that bone is laid down or built up where it is loaded in *compression* and absorbed where it is loaded in *tension*. This is wrong. Bone is also built up or laid down where it is undergoing tensile stress. There is plenty of good strong bone on the anterolateral aspect of the femur. This area is under considerable tension. Experimental studies have actually used tensile loading to effectively stimulate osteogenesis.[52,69] Thus, it should not be assumed that bone on the convex side of a scoliotic or a kyphotic deformity will be absorbed just because it is under tensile loading. However, this does not relate to the relative effectiveness of this bone to perform various biomechanical functions; it simply means that because bone is loaded in tension, one need not assume that it must be reabsorbed.

Extent of Fusion

Stabilization of One Motion Segment. When trauma or disease has disrupted the stability of one motion segment, a simple posterior fusion fixing the vertebra of that motion segment can be completely satisfactory, provided certain conditions are present. There must be adequate posterior osseous structures to which the vertebra can be fused, and the anterior and posterior bony structures that remain in each vertebra must be in continuity with the rest of that vertebra. Obviously, stability can not be achieved if there is an ununited fracture of the pedicles of one vertebra and its posterior elements are fused to the adjacent lower vertebra.

Fusions Involving Two or More Vertebrae. When one or more vertebrae are structurally destroyed, partially or totally absent, or unable to provide clinical stability, then it is necessary to construct the fusion so as to attach it to one normal motion segment above or below the pathology. Examples include fusions for vertebral body resection, spondylolisthesis, or ununited fracture of the ring of C1 (requiring ocp-C2 fusion). The basic idea of this construct is to include in the fusion normal spine segments above and below the pathology. The abnormal segment(s) are included in the fusion to an extent that is possible, and they are bridged over when this is not possible.

We disagree in most situations with the recommendation to include more than one normal vertebra above and below the pathology. One normal motion segment should be as good as its adjacent normal one in withstanding loads. Moreover, there is an unnecessary restriction of motion when additional normal motion segments are included. Finally, it is well documented that the motion segment above a fusion may sometimes develop abnormal motion to the point of clinical instability, so that fusion is required. To fuse it before this is required eliminates an option unnecessarily and shifts the risk one motion segment higher or lower. There are two exceptions to the principle of fusion to just the first normal adjacent vertebra on either side of the pathology. Firstly, in patients with tumors, an adequate margin of resection is not always certain. There are cases in which a portion of destructive tumor must be left behind, and additional progression or recurrence is expected. Secondly, in some patients maximum postoperative stability is required. In these situations two adjacent normal vertebrae are incorporated into the fusion mass, for additional purchase and stability and a margin of safety.

In the special situation of fusion for the arrest of progression or the preservation of correction in kyphosis, other biomechanical principles are operative. We believe that posterior fusions for kyphosis should include *all* the vertebrae in the deformity. A short fusion has to work against a large moment arm created by the weight of the trunk above. The larger fusion is probably superior due to its greater mass and the reduction of the effective moment arm acting on it.

By including all the vertebrae in the kyphotic curve in the fusion and reducing the effective moment arm operating at the end of the fusion mass, the probability that additional vertebrae will become part of the deformity is reduced. In addition, the forces which contribute to abnormal motion at the end of the curve (Fig. 8-13) are also reduced. Attention to this principle tends to decrease the incidence of the type of problems reported by Wagner and colleagues.[117] These investigators noted that when an inadequate number of vertebrae were included in the fusion, kyphotic deformities developed above and below the fusion mass.

This same principle applies to fusion of a scoliotic curve. We believe that it is adequate to include the transitional vertebrae at either end of the curve. The possible exception is fusion of a rapidly progressing curve in a young person. In fusions at multiple levels, the fusion should include the first adjacent vertebra above and below the pathology that is part of a normal motion segment. To fuse beyond these limits is unnecessary and disadvantageous.

Spine Fusions in Children

Several questions are frequently raised about spine fusion in children. Will early fusion disrupt growth patterns and cause deformity or neural damage through an inability of the fused spine to accommodate the maturing neural elements? Another question relates to the feasibility of a therapeutic asymmetrical fusion in the correction of a deformity in the growing child. Will fusion on the convexity of a deformity (scoliosis or kyphosis) result in correction through subsequent symmetrical growth?

Children as young as 2 years of age may have cervical spine fusion without any of the problems of deformity or neurologic complications from relative hypoplasia of the fused section of the spine.[91] This is based on a report of 13 patients, aged 2 to 15 years. These observations are supported by the experience of Hallock, who also noted that surgeons should not generally anticipate any correction of kyphotic deformity from any asymmetrical growth associated with posterior arthrodesis.[41] With posterior fusion, there was continued growth. However, the anterior elements grew 37 per cent less than would have been expected without the fusion, and the posterior elements grew 47 per cent less than would have been expected. The vertebral and disc space heights in the fused segments were both less than the expected normal.

Bridge Constructs, Spacers, and Prophylactic Fusions

Rules without exceptions are unique, yet boring. In some special situations and constructs, for maximum immediate or long-range stability it is necessary to include more than one normal motion segment above and/or below the usual

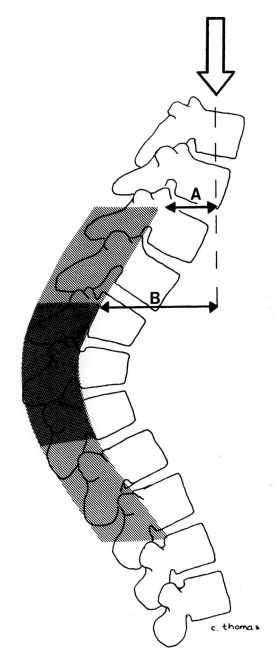

Fig. 8-13. This shows the mechanical advantage of a longer posterior fusion *(light and dark stipple)* over a shorter fusion *(dark stipple)*. With the short fusion alone, there is the possibility of an effectively longer moment arm *B* as opposed to the relatively shorter moment arm *A*. Also, the longer fusion, when mature, provides a more effective internal splint. (White, A. A., Panjabi, M. M., and Thomas, C. L.: The clinical biomechanics of kyphotic deformities. Clin. Orthop., *128:*8, 1977.)

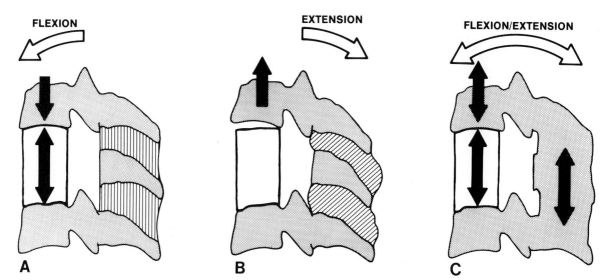

Fig. 8-14. (A) In the *immediate* postoperative period an anterior bone graft can serve as a spacer and can resist *compression,* provided the posterior elements are intact. Therefore, the construct is stable in *flexion. (B)* The construct cannot resist *tensile* loading and is therefore unstable in *extension. (C)* A construct that will resist *compression* and *tension* even if the posterior ligaments are destroyed. After incorporation of the graft this construct offers stability in both flexion and extension. The posterior bone block fusion mass and the anterior cement or bone spacer together provide stability in flexion and extension.

first vertebra in a normal motion segment. With massive resection of all or part of one or more vertebrae, a bone graft is sometimes used as a spacer or a bridge to span a defect (Fig. 8-14). It may be necessary to include more than one normal vertebra at one or both ends of the fusion mass in order to obtain some immediate postoperative stability. This is the case when the surgical construct is relatively weak as a result of loss of structure and/or anticipated exposure to large loads.

The concept of a prophylactic fusion also involves a spacer or a bridge construct, but in addition the process must anticipate damage by an aggressive metastatic tumor that would otherwise cause spinal cord or nerve root damage or irritation secondary to structural failure. Here, too, fusion to normal vertebrae in addition to adjacent vertebrae is employed. An example of this is discussed in more detail on page 418.

Immediate Postoperative Stability

Immediate postoperative stability is an important concept and involves the ability of the surgical construct to prevent subsequent neuro-

logic deficit, deformity, or disruption of the spine construct under physiologic loads, prior to the contribution of any biologic processes of healing or bony union to resist potentially damaging loads. The biologic processes involved in the maturation of bone grafts may significantly alter the structure of the spinal column through changes in the mass and the distribution of the osseous material.

Anterior versus Posterior Fusion

This question is frequently discussed and debated. There are a number of complicated factors involved. It is certainly important that the surgeon develop skills in both anterior and posterior fusions at all levels of the spine. The salient consideration is to determine why the fusion is being done and what one expects to achieve. Many biomechanical principles are applicable in this decision. When fusion is intended to establish clinical stability, generally the site of the major instability is considered. This is analogous to the admittedly facetious situation depicted in Figure 8-15. The fusion is done at the site where the structural damage has rendered the spine clinically unstable. This is usually the site of the major structural damage. When there is disruption of the anterior ligaments or excessive vertebral body destruction, or vertebral body resection, the fusion is best done anteriorly. When there is destruction or inability of the posterior elements to function, a posterior fusion is the procedure of choice. If a decompression is required and it becomes a source of clinical instability, here too, fusion should be carried out at the site of the destruction necessitated by decompression. There are a number of instances in which there is a need for both an anterior and a posterior arthrodesis. The following provides an analysis of a number of surgical constructs for anterior or posterior spine fusions, along with comments about their biomechanical characteristics.

EVALUATION OF CONSTRUCTS IN THE OCCIPITOCERVICAL REGION

Anterior Constructs

Anterior Ocp-C1 Fusion. The surgical approach and construct for this procedure has been described by De Andrade and MacNab.[24] The exposure is essentially a cephalad extension of the Southwick-Robinson exposure of the lower cervical spine.[56] This procedure must be avoided in a person who sings high notes. There is little to discuss concerning the biomechanics of the surgical construct. The anterior surface of the occiput and the ring of C1 are roughened, and cancellous bone chips are applied in the hollow above the anterior portion of C1 and then covered over with longitudinal strips of cortical bone (Fig. 8-16). Postoperative immobilization is achieved and maintained with a halo apparatus.

The procedure is indicated when posterior stabilization is not feasible. It is important to be aware that fusion of occiput to C1 alone in the absence of an intact transverse ligament will fail to establish clinical stability. If the transverse ligament is not intact, the fusion should include C2. There is a significant biomechanical advantage in not including C2 in the fusion either anteriorly or posteriorly. Leaving the C1-C2 articulation unfused preserves a considerable amount of axial rotation (see Chapter 2).

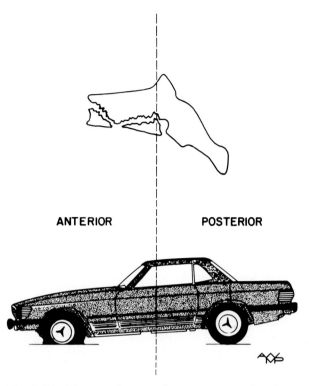

ANTERIOR　　　**POSTERIOR**

Fig. 8-15. This emphasizes the importance of evaluating the site of major clinical instability and selecting the proper surgical construct and approach to correct it (provided that the physician decides upon surgical treatment). If the front tire is damaged the back tire should not be repaired, and vice versa. If the posterior structures of the spine are disrupted, surgery should not be performed on the anterior elements. This is the general rule of thumb in the surgical treatment of the clinically unstable spines; the surgeon should work at the site of the instability. However, there are exceptions. Also, there are situations in which anterior and posterior clinical instability can be solved by anterior or posterior surgery alone.

Posterior Constructs

Simple Onlay Construct. This surgical construct for the posterior fusion of ocp-C1 and C2 is uncomplicated.[78] The base of the occiput, the middle one-half to two-thirds of the posterior ring of C1, and the posterior elements of C2 are exposed. These structures are all decorticated and cancellous chips are placed over the three decorticated structures. The patient is kept in a previously prepared plaster cast for 6 weeks. There is little to criticize about this surgical construct.

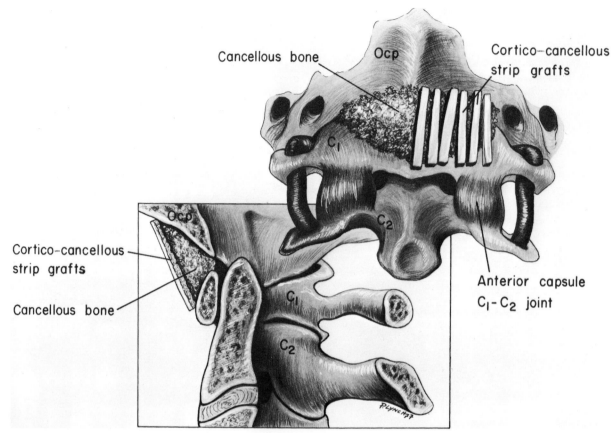

Fig. 8-16. A useful construct for anterior ocp-Cl fusion when a posterior approach or construct is not feasible. The construct has good osteogenic potential but it offers no immediate postoperative stability. If there is clinical instability, some form of halo fixation is desirable.

It obviously provides no immediate postoperative stability and thus alone it is not adequate when such stability is required, unless halo fixation is used. The value of this technique lies in its simplicity and accessibility. We consider this to be the procedure of choice for a routine case and would advise the use of a halo device for postoperative immobilization.

Construct With Wire Fixation. When fusion of the occiput to the cervical spine is required, the construct shown in Figure 8-17 provides an effective design.[42,86] The wiring and the bone graft provide some immediate postoperative stability. Both columns of the construct are able to effectively resist tensile and compressive loading during flexion and extension, respectively. Similarly, they can resist lateral bending in either direction by alternately taking up the tensile and compressive forces. Axial rotation is restrained by the anchoring effect of the posterior elements on each other as a result of their attachment to the graft. There is ample cancellous bone in the graft recipient bed interface. We suggest that in most instances, it is satisfactory to fuse distally only as far as C2, leaving C3 out of the fusion mass. This should be completely adequate and preserves precious motion, especially axial rotation.

Placing holes in the occiput involves the serious risk of bleeding from the sagittal sinus. Certainly, this procedure should not be used when a posterior C1-C2 fusion would suffice. This extensive construct is indicated when the occipital axial joint or the C1-C2 joint must be

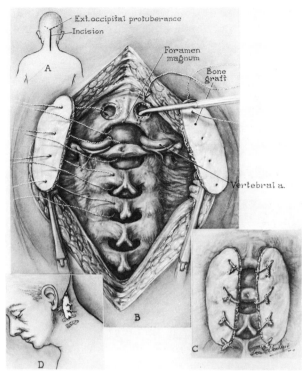

Fig. 8-17. A biomechanically stable construct for arthrodesis of the occiput to the cervical spine. The advantages are its stability against all modes of motion and the option for stable facet fusion should the posterior vertebral elements be absent. The disadvantage is the necessity of placing two holes so close to the sagittal sinus. (Robinson, R. A., and Southwick, W. O.: Surgical approaches to the cervical spine. *In* American Academy of Orthopaedic Surgeons: Instructional Course Lectures. Vol. 17. St. Louis, C. V. Mosby, 1960.)

stabilized and it is not useful or possible to employ the posterior ring of C1 in the fusion mass. This construct or some modification of it is also indicated when a massive fusion is required to bridge a grossly unstable, structurally impoverished cervical spine.

EVALUATION OF SURGICAL CONSTRUCTS IN THE UPPER CERVICAL SPINE

Anterior Constructs

Bilateral Screw Fixation. This technique was designed as a method for internal fixation of a fractured odontoid process.[7] The surgeon, dis-

satisfied with other methods of managing this fracture, devised this technique of *bilateral* screw fixation of the lateral mass of C1 to the body of C2 (Fig. 8-18). The proximal portion of the anterolateral approach described by Henry may be employed for exposure.[48] A 2.5 cm (1 in) screw is inserted through the lateral mass of C1 into the body of C2. The angle of the screw is determined by placing the drill at the anterior surface of the mastoid process and through the tip of the transverse process of C1, with the head in neutral rotation. The described landmarks keep the drilling and screw tract anterior and lateral to the vertebral artery. A guide to assure safe and proper orientation of the screw has been devised by E. H. Simmons in Toronto. A neck splint is worn for 6 weeks as a precaution until the time that flexion/extension films show a stable, healed arthrodesis requiring no further treatment.

We believe that this technique offers a secure fixation of C1 to C2. Axial rotation and flexion/ex-

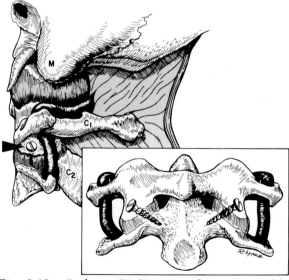

Fig. 8-18. Barbour C1-C2 screw fixation, a stable construct for the anterior arthrodesis. It required two operations through surgically challenging anatomic regions. The two articulations are denuded of cartilage; the joint space is filled with cancellous bone chips. The advantage is that it provides immediate postoperative stability and can be used when there is an absent, diseased, or structurally useless posterior ring of either C1 or C2. Operating on only one side does not suffice.

tension are solidly fixed. Although it may be a bit aggressive as treatment for a fractured odontoid, it has appeal as a fusion technique in situations where the posterior ring of C1 is not available for arthrodesis (e.g., the posterior ring has been removed, is congenitally absent, hypoplastic, necrotic, detached from the anterior portion of C1). For atlanto-axial joint arthrodesis the technique shown is supplemented by some bone graft in a trough along the anterolateral aspect of the trough between the C1-C2 articulations. This construct can be expected to offer good immediate postoperative stability.

The disadvantage of this procedure is that it requires two operations through a surgically rather difficult anatomic approach that is close to several important structures.

Fang Construct.   The anterior approach to C1-C2 through the mouth described by Fang may be useful in some cases for drainage of abscess, excision, or biopsy of tumor or removal of the odontoid (Fig. 8-19).[29] However, for fusion this

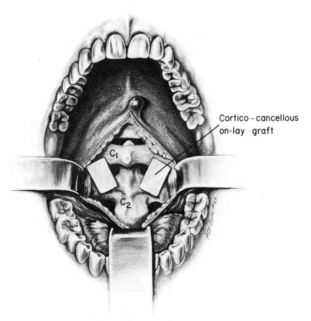

Fig. 8-19. This construct is not stable. In addition, the surgeon must proceed through the oral cavity. We believe that the potential for infection must be greater than with other approaches. The procedure is useful for drainage of infection, biopsy of tumor, and excision of the odontoid.

is not one of the more biomechanically sound constructs. It is better to have more of an interface between the vertebrae to be fused and the graft material. There is not a secure fixation of the bone graft to the recipient site. Therefore, if this procedure is used, we recommend a halo fixation. Finally, there is an increased risk of osteomyelitis involved in the transoral approach.

Posterior Constructs

Brooks Construct.   The success rate of posterior fusions of C1-C2 in general is not considered to be especially good.[33] There are a variety of techniques described.[14,31,35,65] We believe that the Brooks fusion is biomechanically sound, and it has been shown to be effective with clinical trials.[14,37] The surgical construct is shown in Figure 8-20.

Axial rotation is the major motion that occurs at the C1-C2 level. This rotation, along with flexion/extension that includes anteroposterior translation, is the movement that is clinically the most important one to control in order to achieve immediate postoperative stability. The bone grafts wedged and fixed circumferentially create a "friction block" effect and efficiently prevent axial rotation (Fig. 8-21). There is controversy about the amount of lateral bending at this level. If, however, there is lateral bending, the construct is effectively designed to prevent it. Tension is resisted on one side by the circumferential wires and compression is resisted on the other side by the bone graft. There is one additional aspect of this design that is mechanically useful. The two wedge-shaped configurations of graft allow a snug approximation of recipient site and graft and a control of the amount of flexion/extension between C1 and C2 without bringing the posterior elements of C1 and C2 too close together. A direct approximation of the rings of the atlas and the axis could cause too much extension and could aggravate pathologic aspects of a lesion in the neural canal or the anterior elements. To assure proper separation between the posterior elements of C1 and C2 the verticle dimension of the graft when in place should be 1 cm.[14] The wedges of bone are removed from the ilium and fashioned so as to place

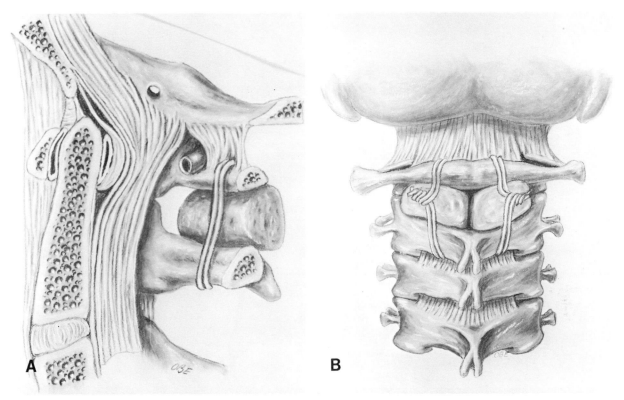

Fig. 8-20. (A) A posterior, sagittal plane view of the Brooks fusion construct. The wedge of corticocancellous bone, in conjunction with the wire that incorporates it with the lamina of C1 and C2, is the essence of the construct. (B) A posterior view showing the two doubled wires, one on each side. (Brooks, A. L., and Jenkins, E. G.: Atlanto-axial arthrodesis by the wedge compression methods. J. Bone Joint Surg., *60A:279*, 1978.)

cancellous bone at both interfaces of the fusion construct (Fig. 8-5:5). The wedged configuration also prevents graft migration toward the spinal cord. The relative mechanical advantages of the Brooks construct as compared with fusions involving simple midline wiring[35] and bone grafting are illustrated in Figure 8-21. Although there is the slight mechanical advantage of using two wires on each side, we suggest that the major practical biomechanical goals may be achieved with only one doubled or twisted wire around the middle of each of the interfaces of the bone graft recipient site, as described by Brooks, who reported a success rate of 11 out of 12 fusions (Fig. 8-22).[14] Thus, only two rather than four wires need be passed under the laminae of C1 and C2. This reduces risk of neural damage and also shortens

the operating time without any significant loss of mechanical advantage. The principle of the Brooks construct provides excellent immediate postoperative stability. The construct requires an orthosis of only minimal or intermediate postoperative control. We recommend a cervical brace with a thoracic support worn for 6 weeks.

Several other techniques for successful posterior fusion of C1 to C2 have been reported.[30,31,70] Several of these constructs are technically less dangerous because they have the advantage of only having to pass one doubled wire under *one* lamina. This is probably an important and valuable aspect, especially for the surgeon who has not had extensive experience operating in this region. One of the constructs described by Fielding is shown in Figure 8-23.

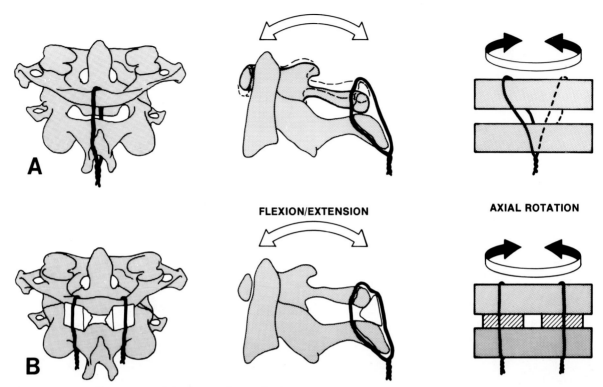

FLEXION/EXTENSION   **AXIAL ROTATION**

Fig. 8-21. An illustration of the biomechanical advantages of the Brooks construct. (*A*) A single midline wiring. This construct would be relatively stable in flexion; however, in extension there would be little stability, since the two rings would readily approximate. In axial rotation there is nothing to resist the relative horizontal displacement between the ring of C1 and that of C2. (*B*) With the Brooks construct, there is stability in both flexion and extension. The flexion is restrained by tension in the circumferential wires and extension is restrained by the bone graft, which serves as a buttressing block. Rotation is resisted by some combination of wire tension and bone block, but this time the mechanism is one of friction. The bone grafts compressed between the two posterior rings serve as friction blocks and offer stability against axial rotation.

EVALUATION OF SURGICAL CONSTRUCTS IN THE LOWER CERVICAL SPINE

There are several techniques for anterior cervical spine fusions. Only the most important and frequently used ones are discussed here.

Anterior Constructs

The Smith-Robinson Construct. This construct has several biomechanical advantages (Fig. 8-24).[100] The preparation of the graft bed removes the intervertebral disc and provides ample exposure for midline and lateral decompression of the anterior cord and nerve roots. The graft itself provides adequate support against vertical compression. The cancellous portion in contact with the vertebral end-plates readily permits revascularization and incorporation. The construct allows all or most of the vertebral end-plates to be left intact. The interspace is usually spread 7 mm, which opens the intervertebral foramen and reduces invagination of the yellow ligament. This procedure is best suited for the treatment of cervical spondylosis. Even though some surgeons think that for cervical spondylosis with neck, shoulder, and arm pain only annulus removal is necessary, we believe that the bone graft has some advantages. It provides immediate interspace opening, relieves nerve root compression, and the subsequent arthrodesis is believed to be helpful in the relief of pain from any associated arthritis. Since the disc is cleaned out and the

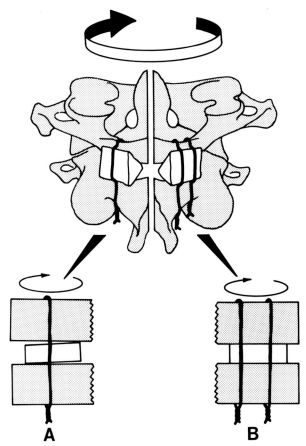

A   **B**

Fig. 8-22. Biomechanical considerations in the use of a single or a double wire for each side of the Brooks fusion construct. (A) When there is axial rotation with a single wire, the friction may cause the graft to tilt. (B) This is less likely to happen with a double wire because the two wires at either end of the graft more effectively prevent tilting. This is more of a theoretical than a practical point, and its advantage must be balanced against that of passing two wires rather than four under the posterior elements of the two vertebrae. A construct with one wire on each side of the midline is thought to be strong enough to resist displacement with flexion/extension.

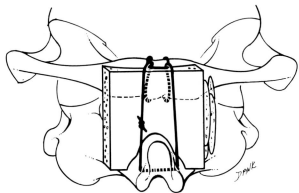

Fig. 8-23. This is another sound construct for posterior C1–C2 fusion. It is a simple design that requires only the passage of one loop of wire around the ring of the atlas. The construct is most effective in preventing flexion. (Fielding, J. W., Hawkins, R. J., and Sanford, A. R.: Spine fusion for atlanto-axial instability. J. Bone Joint Surg., 58A:400, 1976.)

interspace opened, it seems reasonable to offer the patient the additional benefits of a bone graft.

The disadvantages of this procedure include relatively limited exposure to the spinal cord. When more than two interspaces are to be fused, a construct that uses a trough is preferable. Such a procedure is more convenient, and there are fewer interfaceds between bone graft and recipient bed that must be incorporated. There is less probability of successful fusion when more than two interspaces are required.[124]

The Bailey-Badgley Construct and Modifications. This construct has some useful biomechanical advantages.[5] Figure 8-25 shows the Bailey-Badgley technique for fusing 1 and 3 motion segments. Also, a modification of the construct is shown which can be used in a similar manner. The modification is thought to supply additional mechanical support by providing more cortical bone and increasing the anteroposterior length of the bone graft. There is the possibility of conveniently fusing several interspaces. If exposure of the anterior midline portion of the spinal cord behind the vertebral body is necessary, it is readily achieved with this technique. The strength in the immediate postoperative period is adequate and there is the biologic advantage of cancellous to cancellous bone contact across the fusion interfaces.

One of the very important mechanical advantages of this technique is that the trough bed allows the surgeon the option of leaving some anterior stability through the annular fibers on both sides of the trough. This can be useful in a situation where there is instability posteriorly and there is a necessity to fuse anteriorly (e.g.,

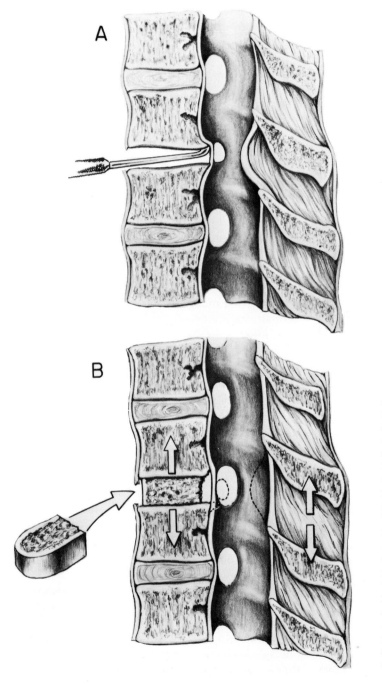

Fig. 8-24. (A) A narrowed intervertebral foramen, invaginated yellow ligament, and a curette removing an osteophyte. This procedure can also be done with a neurosurgical burr. (B) The horseshoe graft is being inserted where the disc has been removed, exposing the posterior longitudinal ligament, or the spinal cord if the surgeon desires. The graft should be approximately 7 mm high and cut with a double-blade saw if possible, such that its top and bottom surfaces are parallel. If there is any tendency for it to be wedge shaped extrusion may occur. The graft immediately separates the interspace, opens the neural foramen, reduces the yellow ligament invagination, and subsequently with successful arthrodesis the osteophyte reabsorbs.[123] This is the procedure we employ as the construct of choice when surgery is indicated for cervical spondylosis.

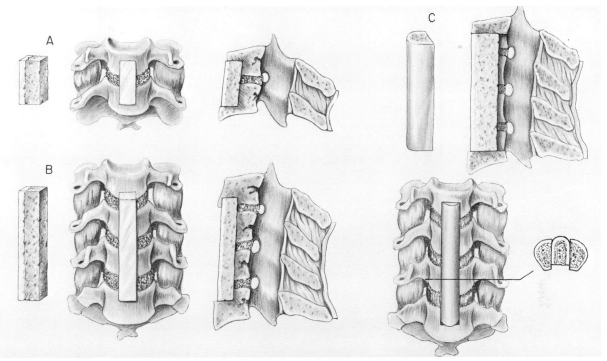

Fig. 8-25. (*A*) This is a diagram of the construct described by Bailey and Badgley, as used for anterior fusion at one level. The interspace is packed with cancellous bone. (*B*) A modification of the procedure in which the graft is tunneled into the upper most vertebral body and slotted into the lower most one. That portion of the disc not removed for placement of the bone graft (as shown in *C*) may be left intact to provide some degree of clinical stability. (*C*) Another modification, which employes a horseshoe-shaped configuration of iliac bone that is stronger in resisting axial compression. This also shows how the procedure may be used to decompress certain anterior areas of the cord. The option of leaving a portion of the disc for purposes of clinical stability is seen.

following multilevel extensive posterior element removal). Cattell and Clark found the construct useful in this situation.[18] If the entire annulus has to be removed to insert a horseshoe graft, then in the immediate postoperative period the patient with posterior element injury is not only unstable posteriorly but also anteriorly. It is certainly possible for a graft to slip in such an unstable situation. If the peripheral annular fibers (which are the strongest due to Sharpey's fibers) can be left intact, there is some preservation of intrinsic stability. Stauffer and colleagues have pointed out the liabilities of anterior interbody fusions in the presence of post-traumatic posterior instability.[103]

The Bailey-Badgley technique has been modified by using iliac bone with three surfaces of cortex, as shown in Figure 8-25C. In addition to this, we have found the trough construct to be useful in situations of clinical instability in which there is significant displacement between vertebrae that can not or need not be reduced. With significant anterior displacement, there is no good location in which the graft can be placed. However, with an anterolateral or a lateral interbody placement of an iliac graft in a trough, a useful construct is developed (Fig. 8-26). The bone block immediately locks the motion segment so as to resist further displacement. The lateral positioning allows for the construction of a smooth trough of uniform depth in both vertebrae, without the step-off that is inevitable with anterior placement. Furthermore, by taking only a portion of the annulus, any residual stabilizing influence is preserved. We have used this construct in the cervical spine as well as in other regions under similar circumstances (Fig. 8-32).

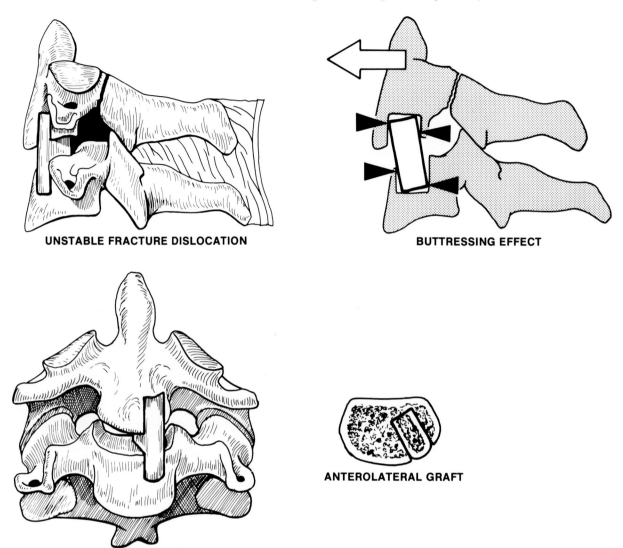

UNSTABLE FRACTURE DISLOCATION

BUTTRESSING EFFECT

ANTEROLATERAL GRAFT

Fig. 8-26. An illustration of the principle involved and the construct employed for the placement of a trough graft anterolaterally across an interspace in order to provide immediate postoperative resistance against sagittal plane translation. The mechanics are such that when there is either anterior or posterior sagittal plane motion, a portion of the graft buttresses against the osseous structures of the two vertebrae.

Cattell and Clark have employed another modification of the basic Bailey-Badgley anterior trough construct. They use a tibial graft which is tunneled into the body of the upper vertebra through its inferior end-plate and wired into the lower most vertebral body in the fusion (Fig. 8-25B). We expect that this modification offers little in the way of significant immediate postoperative stability. However, it is relatively more stable than the standard Bailey-Badgley construct

with regard to the probability of displacement of the bone graft.

The disadvantages of the Bailey-Badgley technique and its modifications are minimal. There is considerable bleeding when it is necessary to violate the central cancellous portion of a vertebral body.

The Cloward Construct. This construct is well instrumented, convenient, and provides good visualization of the midline anterior portion of the spinal cord at the interspace and for about 1 cm on either side of it.[22] The construct has been reported to collapse in a significant number of instances.[57] This is probably due to the fact that although the graft configuration itself is of adequate strength,[122] the total construct may be lacking after a period of time, possibly during the early phases of creeping substitution, when the graft is relatively more osteoporotic. Experimental vertical compressive loading of the construct suggests that failure may be caused when the two, coin-like cortical edges cut into the adjacent cancellous bone (Fig. 8-27). The Cloward construct, like the Bailey-Badgley construct, has the advantage of preserving some degree of stability by leaving a portion of the intact annulus fibrosus attached to the vertebral bodies. However, we see no reason to use this instead of the Bailey-Badgley construct when clinical stability is important.

Biomechanical Comparison of Constructs. The immediate, vertical compressive load bearing capacity of three surgical constructs designated as Smith-Robinson, Cloward, and modified Bailey-Badgley procedures were tested experi-mentally.[124] The results are given in Figure 8-28. The immediate postoperative load bearing capacity of the three constructs are listed in order of decreasing strength as follows: Type I, Smith-Robinson; Type II, Cloward; and Type III, Bailey Badgley (modified). The failure loads were greater than the expected range of physiologic loads in these static tests. It would be more useful to know the relative load bearing capacity of these constructs as they undergo creeping substitution. It is known that they will become mechanically weaker during the phase of creeping substitution. In dogs, experimental studies show that transplanted bone is greatly weakened between 6 months and 1 year after the transplant. It is reasonable to assume that the grafts continue to have the same relative strengths. The relative load bearing capacities of the three constructs, therefore, with regard to mechanical function becomes quite important.

The Keystone Graft Construct. This construct, described by Simmons and Ballah, has some biomechanical advantages (Fig. 8-29).[99] Mechanical studies comparing the keystone graft with the dowel (Cloward) graft revealed some useful in-

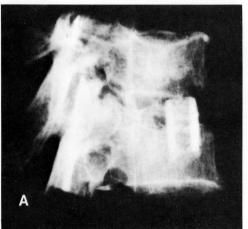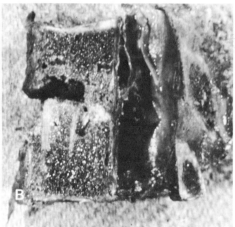

Fig. 8-27. (A) A lateral radiograph of an experimental dowel construct, loaded to failure. (B) A sagittal section of the actual specimen oriented as a mirror image of the radiograph. In both pictures, it is apparent that the dowel graft migrates into the cancellous bone of the vertebral body as a result of the verticle compression loading of the vertebra. This is at least part of the mechanism of collapse that is so commonly seen clinically with this construct. We do not consider it to be sound biomechanically. (White, A. A., Jupier, J., Southwick, W. O., and Panjabi, M. M.: An experimental study of the immediate load bearing capacity of three surgical constructs for anterior spine fusions. Clin. Orthop., 91:21, 1973).

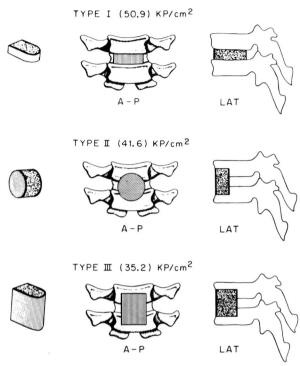

TYPE I (50.9) KP/cm^2

A-P   LAT

TYPE II (41.6) KP/cm^2

A-P   LAT

TYPE III (35.2) KP/cm^2

A-P   LAT

Fig. 8-28. Graft configuration: how the graft fits into vertebrae, and how the vertebrae are altered to receive it. The numbers are mean values for the load bearing capacity of each of the three surgical constructions. (White, A. A., Jupiter J., Southwick, W. O., and Panjabi, M. M.: An experimental study of the immediate load bearing capacity of three surgical constructs for anterior spine fusions. Clin. Orthop., *91*:21, 1973.

formation. Studies of surface area, an important consideration in bone graft surgery with respect to fusion and incorporation, showed that for fusion of one interspace the rectangular (keystone-shaped) graft had approximately 30 per cent more surface area than the cylindrical graft of comparable size. For a fusion of two interspaces, the surface contact area was 70 per cent greater in the rectangle than would be the case with two separate cylindrical grafts.

The immediate postoperative stability of these grafts was also studied. In autopsy specimens in which the two surgical constructs were created, experiments were carried out to test flexion/extension and lateral bending. The flexion/extension studies were carried out with a constant ejection force applied to both types of grafts. The

dowel grafts were extruded with 20 to 25 degrees of extension, but the keystone grafts were not extruded before there was fracture and complete disruption of the spine. The two constructs were compared in the lateral bending mode by measuring the relative motion between the graft material and the recipient vertebral body. The keystone construct required four times more lateral bending force to produce such motion than did the dowel construct.[99] The investigators pointed out one additional mechanical point. If there is concern about extrusion, the graft should be placed as close as possible to the posterior portion of the vertebral body.

The investigators reported a clinical series of keystone and Cloward constructs in which there was greater fusion rate and relief of pain with the keystone construct.[99] This occurred despite the fact that the series of keystone constructs included a higher incidence of multilevel fusions. We believe that the keystone technique has some important advantages with respect to sound biologic and mechanical principles. The configuration and position are effective in providing excellent immediate stability against extrusion and motion in lateral bending. The large surface area of cancellous to cancellous bone contact should provide sound arthrodesis. If a trough construct is indicated and the surgeon is able to build a keystone construct, we recommend this as the procedure of choice.

The use of wedge-shaped configurations of bone grafts have been employed in anterior cervical constructs to compensate for wedging of vertebral bodies secondary to trauma.[115,116] We advise against the use of any *unsecured* configuration of bone graft in which there is a wedge. If such a configuration is used with the base of the wedge facing anteriorly extrusion is a risk; when the base is facing posteriorly, spinal cord impingement is a risk if there is nothing to block migration of the bone graft. The keystone graft, a trough graft, and a graft with carefully carpentered parallel surfaces are mechanically more sound, being less likely to become displaced anteriorly. The keystone construct, followed by the Bailey-Badgley construct, is the construct of choice for patients with multilevel anterior arthrodesis.

The Notched Fibula Construct. This technique, described by Whitecloud and LaRocca,[125] is similar in principle and indication to the Bailey-Badgley trough graft, except for the graft material. The construct is shown in Figure 8-30 and was designed to prevent collapse and avoid extrusion, both of which would improve the success rate for arthrodesis. It is recommended for multilevel fusions. The initial experience shows more success with prevention of collapse than with extrusion. There have been problems with extrusion in three of 20 cases. This is at least in part due to the procedure, which is analagons to putting a square peg in a round hole, or more accurately, a straight fibula in a semicircular (lordotic) cervial spine. We believe that the construct has the advantage of preventing collapse. The notching technique is ingenious but somewhat counteracted by placing the straight graft in the lordotic cervical spine. It should be reiterated that the iliac crest is more expendable than a segment of fibula. Collapse of grafts using full thickness of the ilium (Fig. 8-5:2) have not been a problem in our clinical experience.

Plate and Screw Fixation.   The radiograph shown in Figure 8-31 demonstrates a form of fixation that we have not used, but perhaps it should not be condemned hastily. One surgeon has reported the successful use of this construct in 38 patients.[89] The objections about screw loosening, migration, and damage to vital structures may have been overemphasized. Moreover, it is possible with proper radiographic monitoring to recognize this in time to prevent any catastrophe. We are not recommending this construct; rather, we are saying that it is not by definition bad and it may be a reasonable option in a situation where immediate anterior postoperative stability is crucial.

Vertebral Body Replacement.   Replacement of one or more vertebral bodies is sometimes indicated for wide decompression, visualization of the cord, excision of an infected, tumerous, or grossly destroyed vertebral body.[56] The construct for the replacement of a vertebral body is shown in Figure 8-32, which may be used in any region of the spine for vertebral body replacement. With some of the very large vertebrae, it is necessary to use several ribs or two or more pieces of ilium. This construct provides a spacer

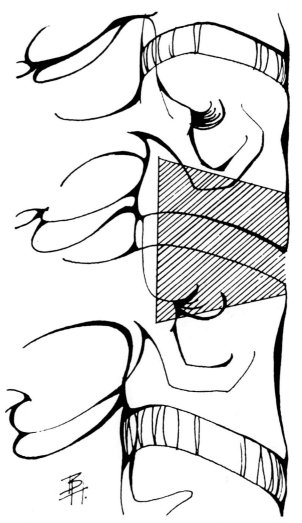

Fig. 8-29.   This construct has been shown by biomechanical studies to be stable, and the graft is very unlikely to extrude. We recommend it as one of the better surgical constructs. The "keystone" features are the posterior placement of the graft and the construction of an adequately beveled bone graft and recipient bed. The angles at the posterior portion of the keystone should be about 75 degrees. (Simmons, E. H., and Bahalla, S. K.: Anterior cervical discectomy and fusion. A clinical and biomechanical study with eight-year follow-up. J. Bone Joint Surg., *51B:*225, 1969.)

as a substitute support in the immediate postoperative period. Graft extrusion during extension is resisted by the spikes at either end (Fig. 8-32B, C). Its resistance against vertical compression comes from the strong, horseshoe-shaped

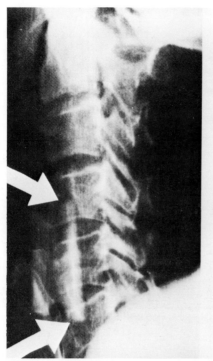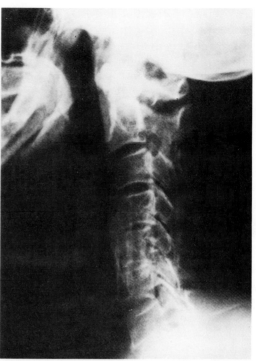

Fig. 8-30. The use of a strong fibular graft and notching to straddle the anterior cortex of the vertebral body shell are the main features of this construct. Although it has these advantages, we consider the disruption of a normal fibula and the long period of time required for incorporation of this type of graft to be disadvantages. (Whitecloud, T. S., and LaRocca, H.: Fibula strut graft in reconstructive surgery of the spine. Spine, *1*:33, 1976.)

configuration of uiac bone, with cortex on three sides (Fig. 8-32B, C, D). The resistance against axial rotation and lateral bending is modest. An excised vertebra can also be advantageously replaced by a keystone construct in this situation. The keystone construct has the advantage of greater stability, but because the dissection violates the intact cortical shell and extends into the central cancellous bone, there is more hemorrhage. Because the graft is seated in cancellous bone in the lower regions of the spine, the limits of its vertical load bearing capacity of the construct may reach its limits. Therefore, we do not recommend its use below the cervical spine unless it is reinforced by some additional support.

Posterior Constructs

Posterior Fusion and Wiring. The following technique is recommended for use in wiring around spinous processes. Rather than pass the wire through a hole in each spinous process, we suggest that the wire be passed around the caudal border of the spinous processes, which are generally at an angle that will not allow it to slip off. This is stronger because the wire is exerting forces on an intact cortex. For the cephalad process, we suggest a hole close to the anterior surface at the base of the spinous process. This will be the weaker point, but it provides the maximum margin of safety against pullout in the caudal direction (Fig. 8-33).

The surgical constructs for various extents of arthrodesis are demonstrated in Figure 8-33. One motion segment can be wired as shown. This provides some restriction of motion. Strips of bone are added to achieve fusion. When it is necessary to fuse more than one motion segment, each vertebra can be wired to the adjacent one and the entire group encircled by another wire (Fig. 8-33B). The posterior wiring supplies some immediate postoperative stability, provided the anterior elements are structurally intact or only minimally disrupted. If immediate postoperative stability is a major goal, one of the stronger bone grafts materials should be used, such as rib, fibula, or tibia, instead of ilium or bone strips. Increasing the number of wirings between the vertebrae in the fusion mass and wiring the graft to the vertebral elements both contribute to the *immediate* postoperative stability. Immediate stability can be further improved by including more intact motion segments in the fusion mass. This has the liability of decreasing motion and increasing loads upon the motion segment above the fusion mass. However, it offers more structure upon which to securely anchor the surgical construct. The greater and more effective the purchase, the stronger is the construct.

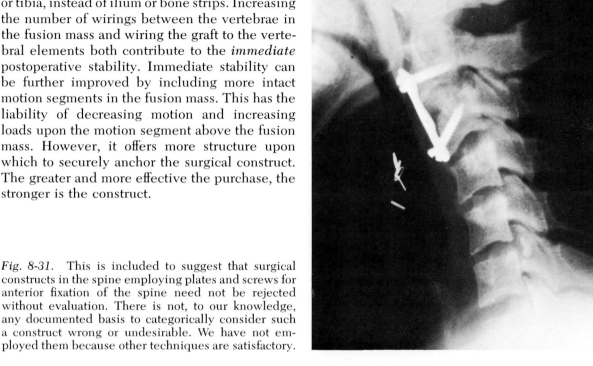

Fig. 8-31. This is included to suggest that surgical constructs in the spine employing plates and screws for anterior fixation of the spine need not be rejected without evaluation. There is not, to our knowledge, any documented basis to categorically consider such a construct wrong or undesirable. We have not employed them because other techniques are satisfactory.

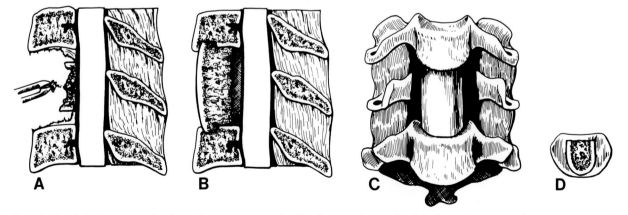

Fig. 8-32. (A) Excision of infected, tumorous, or badly damaged vertebral body and anterior decompression of the spinal cord. (B) Sagittal section of the construct, showing the use of iliac bone graft as a spacer. This construct is clinically unstable in the immediate postoperative period. (C) An anterior view of the construct, with the bone graft notched in place to prevent extrusion or posterior displacement into the spinal cord. The construct is relatively stable postoperatively during flexion if the posterior elements are intact, but it is clinically unstable in both flexion and extension if they are not intact. (D) A cross-section to show how the cortical bone purchase on the intact portion of the end-plate offers resistance to vertical compressive loading.

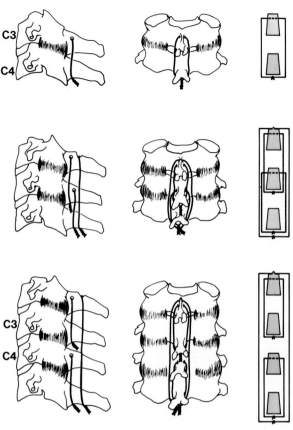

Fig. 8-33. Recommended placement of the wire about the base of the spinous process. When the angle of inclination of the spinous process permits it, on the caudad side it is better to leave the cortex intact and go around the structure. The cephalad side should be secured in a transverse tunnel so what it will not slide off. Additional stability may be provided when the construct involves four vertebrae by adding wire fixation of C3–C4, of the type shown in the top construct between C3 and C4. The technique of wiring the spinous processes provides some immediate postoperative stability by restricting flexion.

Facet Fusion and Wiring. Experiments by Haas on dogs supported the idea that it is desirable to destroy the intervertebral articulations when a posterior spine fusion is performed.[39] The construct described here makes use of these facet articulations in a different manner. Instability in the presence of a unilevel laminectomy may be satisfactorily treated using posterior fusion and wiring. However, when the surgeon is faced with the problem of stabilizing a spine that

lacks laminae at two or more levels, we recommend the construct shown in Figures 8-34 and 8-35.[86,17a] The facet fusion construct offers considerable immediate postoperative stability with variations in effectiveness that are associated with choice of graft material. This construct provides stability against several patterns of motion, particularly flexion/extension and lateral bending. Motion in the sagittal and frontal planes specifically is effectively restrained. Most of the mechanical advantages result from the principle of bridging and the bilateral wiring of the lateral masses to a strong bone graft. We recommend the rib for this procedure. It has several mechanical advantages. Its natural curvature fits the cervical lordosis. It has relatively good strength compared to iliac bone configurations because of its higher moment of inertia, which is due to the closed section created by the tube of cortical bone. It has a flexibility which allows it to bend rather than break. There is also a biologic advantage; the loose cancellous bone in the medullary canal allows it to be relatively more readily absorbed. This procedure has an additional clinical advantage; in the event of a condition requiring reexploration of the spinal cord, the cord is not covered by bone graft.

EVALUATION OF SURGICAL CONSTRUCTS IN THE THORACIC SPINE

Most of the principles and techniques of surgical constructs in the cervical spine also apply to the thoracic spine. The thoracic spine is discussed to some extent in the treatment of kyphosis (see p. 389). Here, biomechanical considerations that are unique to the thoracic spine are discussed with respect to arthrodesis. It should be emphasized that the loads in this region are much higher than in the cervical spine (about five-fold) and that there is a normal kyphotic angulation. The relative advantages of different locations for placement of the grafts are discussed.

Anterior Constructs

Of the previously described anterior constructs, the trough construct, employing either a modified Bailey-Badgley construct or the key-

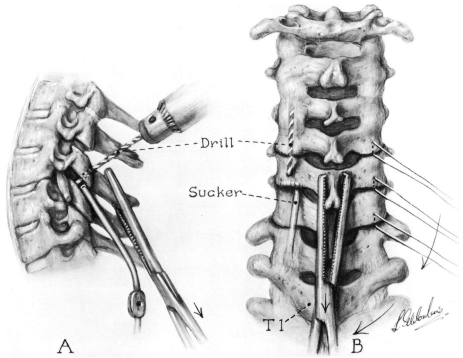

Fig. 8-34. (*A*) A technique for constructing a tunnel for wire to be passed through a facet joint. Usually, there is not a spinous process to grasp, so an elevator is worked into the joint where the sucker is shown. The drill hole should be perpendicular to the plane of the joint. (*B*) The posterior view of three wires in place. (Robinson, R. A., and Southwick, W. O.: Surgical approaches to the cervical spine. *In* American Academy of Orthopaedic Surgeons: Instructional Course Lectures. vol. 17. St. Louis, C. V. Mosby, 1960.)

stone principle, is the most useful construct applied to the thoracic spine. Because of the great vessels and the relative ease of exposure, the anterolateral and lateral aspects of the vertebral bodies are more readily accessible than the midline, anterior aspect.

Decompression and Anteior Fusion. In some instances, it is desirable to decompress the thoracic spine anteriorly. When at least the anterior portion of the vertebral body or bodies involved are intact, we suggest the construct shown in Figure 8-36. This is essentially the same procedure described by Hodgson.[29] It provides adequate decompression and exposure of the anterior portion of the thoracic cord and leaves the supporting structures of the anterior vertebral bodies intact. This may be done laterally and is very useful for removal of a herniated thoracic disc. The two segments of rib are embedded in the cancellous portions of previously intact vertebral bodies above and below. The ribs ultimately provide stability when incorporated. Initially, the postoperative stability depends upon the remaining portion of intact vertebral body anteriorly and tensile supporting structures posteriorly. If the posterior elements are not intact, we recommend a Milwaukee brace if the surgery is above T6 and a Jewett brace if it is below that level.

The following is a unique construct. In the treatment of kyphotic deformity, a rib with blood supply maintained is used. This functions as a living pedicle graft to the anterior portion of the thoracic spine.[88] Investigators report that although the graft is not effective in the correction of deformity, it does prevent progression. The graft is also reported to hypertrophy with growth.

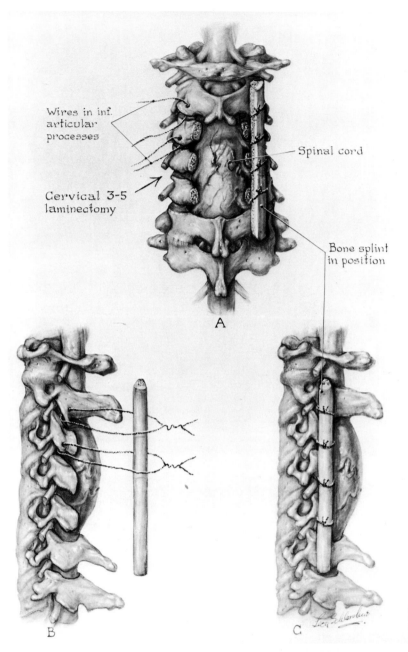

Wires in inf. articular processes

Cervical 3-5 laminectomy

Spinal cord

Bone splint in position

A

B

C

Fig. 8-35. (A) The appearance of the exposed cord, with one strut of the tibia graft wired into place. (B) The wires are passed through the facet articulations and around the bone graft. (C) Here the second tibial graft is fixed in place. A rib or a selectively removed segment of ilium that has a natural curvature that fits the cervical lordosis and also forms an oval around the exposed portion of spinal cord may be used. (Robinson, R. A., and Southwick, W. O.: Surgical approaches to the cervical spine. *In* American Academy of Orthopaedic Surgeons: Instructional Course Lectures. vol. 17. St. Louis, C. V. Mosby, 1960.)

Posterior Constructs

Location and Extent of Posterior Fusions. A posteriorly placed fusion is perfectly adequate for substitution of disrupted ligamentous structures (Fig. 8-33). More leverage and greater contact area for interface adhesion are provided by including all the posterior elements. The technique and principles described for the cervical spine apply equally well to the thoracic spine. This includes wiring techniques, the selection of graft material, and the proper instruments to enhance immediate postoperative stability. The experience with arthrodesis in the treatment of scoliosis suggests that decortication of the posterior elements and disruption of the facet articulations are essential.

Facet Fusion and Wiring. The principles, indications, and technique of facet fusions in the thoracic spine are the same as those of the cervical spine (see p. 410). The rib grafts may be placed with their convexity posteriorly to fit the normal lordosis of the thoracic spine.

When immediate postoperative stability is not important, simple fusion of the facets and transverse processes alone may be employed.

EVALUATION OF SURGICAL CONSTRUCTS IN THE LUMBAR AND SACRAL SPINE

Anterior Constructs

Interbody Fusions. There are a number of techniques for anterior interbody fusion of the lumbar spine. Most are performed through an anterior approach,[17,44,54,55,97,104] but a posterior approach is possible.[127] Interbody fusions are advantageous when all the posterior elements are destroyed or in cases where repeated posterior endeavors have failed, or when the posterior approach is not accessible for clinical reasons. The technique was initially and is currently employed in the treatment of spondylolisthesis. Collapse in this region is not catastrophic, so that constructs that have ample quantities of cancellous bone at the graft bed interspace are preferred. The major disadvantages of anterior lumbar approaches and fusions are the associated complications, death, venous thrombosis, and im-

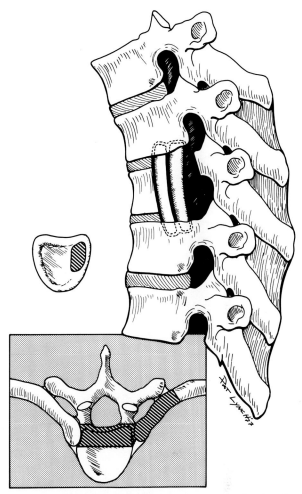

Fig. 8-36. A construct for decompression and arthrodesis. The decompresion is designed to effectively relieve anterior spinal cord pressure and leave some of the vertebra for structural support. A bone graft of two segments of ribs or a portion of iliac crest is implanted into the vertebral bodies above and below. In situations where the anterior portion of the remaining disc and vertebral body are intact, this construct has a moderate amount of immediate postoperative stability.

potence.[54,97] Based on the risks involved and the adequacy of posterolateral constructs, we find that these procedures are rearly indicated.

Trough Graft Technique. This technique is valuable when the posterior elements are not available for fusion, or when the posterior approach is not possible. Also, it is useful as a spacer when all or part of a vertebral body must be removed. This type of construct offers considerable immediate postoperative stability, especially against sagittal plane translation, which can be the most devastating to the neural elements. A clinical example follows.

Patient I.L. is also discussed on page 259, in relation to clinical instability. Pain, neurologic deficit, and progressive posterior translation of L2 and L3 were present. By employing an anterolateral graft of a large piece of iliac bone wedged into the trough, immediate postoperative stability was attained (Fig. 8-37).

Peg Graft for the L5-S1 Joint. The relative inaccessibility of the anterolateral approach to the lumbosacral joint is dictated by the wings of the ilia, the common iliac veins, and their associated branches. Therefore a direct anterior approach to the L5-S1 joint with the use of a peg graft to gain immediate stability is used (Fig. 8-38).[97] Fibula, rib, or ilium may be employed; the last is generally the most readily accessible. This construct has the added advantage of fusion and some moderate degree of fixation of a progressive or irreducible spondylolisthesis.

Interbody Fusion, Posterior Approach. This technique, described by Wiltberger,[127] is a sound construct and is demonstrated in Figure 8-39.

The specifics of the technique are important, and, of course, should be reviewed in detail before using the procedure.

This construct may be useful when the surgeon is limited to a posterior exposure or when the posterior elements are inadequate for fusion. Such a situation might exist after failed attempts at fusion by more conventional procedures, either anteriorly or posteriorly. There may be a need for extensive removal of the posterior elements or the necessity of good visualization of the cauda equina. This technique is also advantageous because it does not expose the sacral symphathetic fibers, and therefore there is no risk of impotence in the male. It also avoids the complex plexus of viens which can sometimes obviate an easy anterior exposure of the lumbosacral joint. Biomechanically, the procedure is sound in that the bone graft is under some variable compressive force; it consists of ample cortical bone (although we do not encourage the use of the tibia), as well as some cancellous bone, and the construct is precisely carpentered for adequate immediate postoperative stability. The graft is in a position to provide both leverage and rigidity.

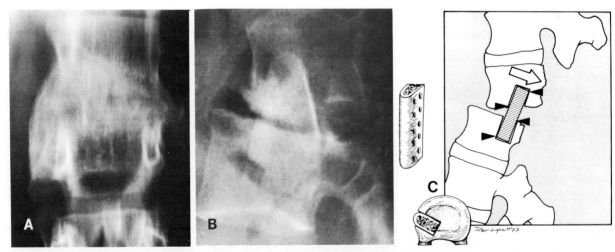

Fig. 8-37. *(A)* An anteroposterior and *(B)* a lateral radiograph of patient I.L. following an anterolateral trough graft to prevent additional posterior translation of L2 on L3. *(C)* This diagrammatic representation shows the construct more clearly. The bone graft is placed in the region of the remaining overlap of the two vertebral bodies in the sagittal plane. Force arrows indicate the mechanism of locking, which provides immediate postoperative stability against posterior translation. The cortical sides of the graft have several drill holes to facilitate revascularization. The forces associated with the subluxation tend to lock the graft in place.

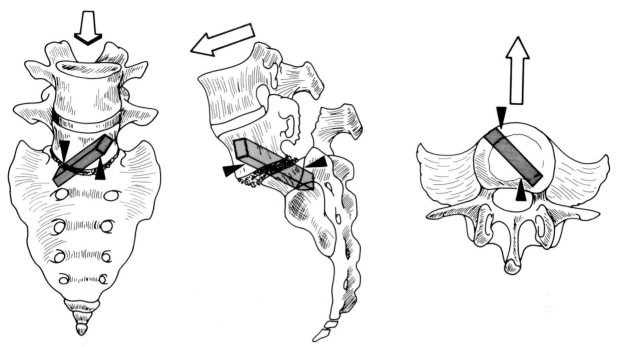

Fig. 8-38. Fusion construct for spondylolisthesis. The disc between L5 and S1 is resected and replaced by spongiosa chips; a tibial graft, 5 cm long and 1 cm wide, is inserted into the sacrum through the vertebral body of L5. Placing the bone graft peg in the spatial orientation shown offers resistance to some extent against translation in the sagittal, frontal, and the horizontal planes. The real disadvantage of this construct is that when the annulus fibrosus is removed to implant the bone chips, virtually all remaining anterior stability is eradicated. This is a serious liability.

The major disadvantage with this procedure is the possibility of posterior protrusion of graft material and the necessity for ample nerve root retraction. The probability of posterior protrusion of graft material is reduced by good carpentry and adequate protection in the postoperative period (body jacket including one thigh, worn for 6 weeks); ample nerve root retraction is achieved by careful surgical technique. During surgery the patient should be positioned with hips and knees flexed. This so-called tuck position has its own liabilities, which should be weighed against the advantages of allowing more generous retraction of the cauda equina.[3]

Posterior Constructs

The various posterior spine fusions that include the spinous processes and lamina are satisfactory for arthrodesis designed to reestablish clinical stability.[8,105,111,112,118] Wires may be employed to provide some element of immediate postoperative stability and are especially needed when clinical stability has been lost. The basic constructs for posterior element fusions are shown in Figure 8-40. The variations on these basic surgical constructs are numerous.

The "H" Graft. The "H" or clothespin graft of Bosworth has received a good deal of attention.[8] This construct does not appear to have any particularly significant biomechanical advantage over the number of other constructs for posterior lumbar spine fusion. It is extremely unlikely that the motion segment, placed in a position of flexion such that there is pressure on the "H" graft from tensile loading of the ligamentous structures, offers any technical or therapeutic advantage. Furthermore, the pressure cannot be expected to remain. The relaxation associated with the viscoelastic properties of the disc and other ligamentous structures, as well as that of the donor and

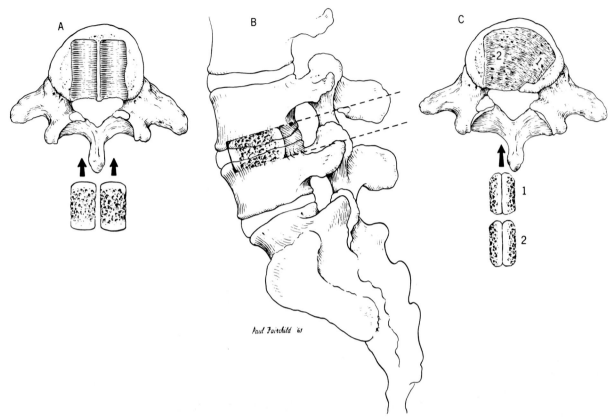

Fig. 8-39.   (*A*) Bilateral insertion of iliac bone dowels. (*B*) A lateral view of inserted dowels. (*C*) The insertion of two cortical bone dowels by a unilateral, partial laminectomy. This construct is useful if the physician wishes to do an interbody fusion at the time of posterior exposure or if an anterior approach is not feasible. The disadvantages are technical difficulties of adequate exposure and possible extrusion of bone graft. (Wiltberger, B. R.: Intervertebral body fusion by the use of posterior bone dowel. Clin. Orthop., 35:69, 1964.)

recipient bone, all contribute toward reducing any pressure within 2 or 3 hours following insertion. The compressive fixation aspect of this construct is only short-lived. The clinical results have been good; however, this is more likely related to other aspects of the surgical technique, such as the meticulous debridement, decortication of all the posterior graft elements and placement of ample cancellous graft material.

Posterolateral Arthrodesis.   There is also the option of performing a posterolateral fusion. This involves the outer portion of the facet joints, the pedicles, the transverse processes, and the gutters between them. This type of construct may be used in addition to, or in the case of spondylolisthesis or multiple laminectomies, instead of those which involve just the

spinous processes and lamina. The bilateral posterolateral fusion technique described by Watkins,[118] and modified by Truckly and Thompson[118] has been suggested for use instead of just an adjunct to fusion involving only the spinous processes and laminae. The modifications suggested by Truckly and Thompson were very successful (92% union). They consist of the following: no screw fixation; use of slivers rather than large blocks of bone graft; two separate posterolateral incisions; no attempt at facet articulation disruption. Truckely and Thompson report continued success in an additional 125 cases with essentially the same percentage of successful arthrodesis.[113]

Posterolateral fusion has the advantage of not obstructing the dura, which makes the area more readily accessible to subsequent surgery. The dura is protected from migrating bone fragments in the short-term postoperative period. It has also been suggested that the lateral gutters and recesses are more vascular.[118] Biomechanically, this construct (Fig. 8-40C) is superior to the posterior construct (Fig. 8-40B); it considerably increases the area moment of inertia, so that greater stability is obtained in axial rotation and lateral bending. We recommend this construct as the procedure of choice for posterior lumbar spine fusion.

Clinical reports in the literature suggest that the inclusion of the posterolateral structures (facets, pedicles, and transverse processes) significantly increases the incidence of solid fusions (see Table 8-2).[105,112,118] Hensinger and colleagues

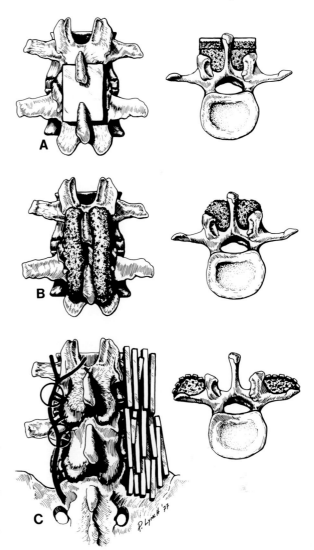

Fig. 8-40. (A) The basic construct of the "H" graft. The added technique of constructing the "H" graft for distraction of the posterior elements and compression of the graft offers no real biomechanical advantage. (B) The midline (Hibbs) construct is a standard, acceptable one. (C) Fusion of the lateral elements, in our opinion, is the construct of choice. It has shown the best reported results with clinical experience; the fusion bed is in an area of good blood supply; there is less risk of lamina hypertrophy and spinal stenosis; posterior decompression of the cord may be easier during initial surgery or subsequently; and the location of the fusion mass is biomechanically at the best site, without performing an interbody fusion, for maximum immobilization in all parameters. Note the two circles in *C*. These indicate points recommended by MacNab and Dall[73] for cauterization to control bleeding in this procedure.

Table 8-2. Results of Lumbosacral Fusion (L4 to S1)

Author	No. of Operations	Technique	Incidence of Nonunion (%)
Cleveland, Bosworth, and Thompson (1948)	357	"H" graft	17.4
Thompson and Ralston (1949)	169	Hibbs	23.6
	49	Transfacet screws	55.1
Straub (1949)	80	Wilson's plate and cortical graft	14.
McBride and Shorbe (1958)	77	Facet block	36.
Shaw and Taylor (1956)	55	Onlay cortical	36.
Watkins (1953)	10	Posterolateral, block	20.
Truckly and Thompson (1961)	41	Posterolateral, slivers	7.3

(Truckly, G., and Thompson, W. A. L.: Posterior lateral fusion of the lumbosacral spine. J. Bone Joint Surg., *44A*:505, 1962.)

reported 100 per cent fusion using this technique to treat spondylolisthesis in 20 patients, averaging age 14.5 years of age.[49] These are thought to be more effective constructs than the simple, midline spinous process and lamina fusions and also preferable to the anterior interbody fusions.[107]

MacNab and Dall reviewed a series of comparable reports in an attempt to compare different techniques of lumbar spine fusion. They found that for fusions of L4 to S1, the results were as follows. The pseudarthrosis rate for anterior fusions was 30 per cent, for posterior midline fusion, 17 per cent and for posterolateral fusion, 7 per cent. The advantages of posterolateral fusions were also pointed out: The graft bed is larger and uninterrupted (i.e., the yellow ligament in midline fusions); the zygapophyseal joints are included in the fusion mass; by including the transverse process and the pars interarticularis of the cephalad most vertebra, it is more firmly incorporated into the fusion mass; by avoiding decortication of the lamina, the syndrome of spinal stenosis from thickening of the lamina ventrally as well as dorsally is avoided. The work of these investigators includes some illuminating anatomy, describing the blood supply to this region. They suggest that hemorrhage can be greatly reduced by the use of a modified, flexed hip and knee position, relieving abdominal pressure. Secondly, there is cauterization of vessels at the base of the transverse process on the caudal side and at the dorsal edge of the superior articular facet.[73]

Fusion should not be performed only to relieve pain from intervertebral disc pathology, since it is not reasonable to anticipate success. It is known from the biomechanical studies of Rolander that even with all the posterior elements fused, there may still be motion between vertebral bodies. This is due to the normal elasticity of the bone that comprises the pedicles (Fig. 8-9). No particular technique of posterior lumbar fusion has been shown to be clinically superior in eliminating pain. The crucial consideration is to understand the reason for arthrodesis and then to design the construct so that the appropriate posterior elements of the vertebrae in question are incorporated into a fusion mass.

Lumbar spine fusions for low back pain in the absence of clinical instability or spondylolisthesis are not well justified by clinical experience. In June, 1974, the International Society for the Study of the Lumbar Spine held its inaugural meeting in Montreal, Canada. The results and the techniques of several methods of spine fusion were discussed. We would like to share with the reader the comments of two distinguished surgeons who helped to place these numerous techniques in some perspective.

We are all probably aware of the rather poor results that have recently been reported for these patients regardless of whether the fusion was performed from the front the back or laterally. . . . In my own mind and also in the minds of many colleagues there is no doubt that for the majority of our patients suffering from low back pain, the treatment is not fusion, no matter what type of approach [construct] is used. [Alf Nachemson, M.D.[76]]

. . . Clearly the essential issue is not developing a better technique [construct] for obtaining spinal fusion but rather more clearly defining those instances in which spinal fusion is truly necessary and will yield a high degree of relief of symptoms. . . . For these reasons I feel a more restrictive role is indicated for the operation of spinal fusion in light of our present knowledge. [Richard Rothmann, M.D., Ph.D.[90]]

EVALUATION OF UNCOMMON SURGICAL CONSTRUCTS

Massive Fusion for Low Grade Malignancy

The basic concept here involves the use of biomechanical principles to develop a surgical construct that will preserve cord function as long as possible in the presence of a low grade malignancy. In such a situation the tumor is locally recurrent and not thought to be resectable.

The patient was a 53-year-old man with a metastatic salivary gland tumor, reported by Friedlaender and colleagues.[34] Despite treatment with resection and radiation, the tumor recurred locally and progressed. First, there was a posterior fusion of the occiput through C5 using iliac bone graft. Because of the destruction of the anterior elements, there was an iliac graft after excision of the bodies of C2 and C3. The fusion went from the ring of C1 to the body of C5. The remaining vertebrae were destroyed by the tumor. Following minor trauma, the posterior iliac graft fractured. The patient was subsequently stabilized with a fibula graft extending from occiput to C7. The patient never had any neurologic deficit but died from respiratory failure more than 3 years following the last bone graft operation. The radiograph of the final construct is shown in Figure 8-41.

This case shows how repeated bone graft procedures in juxtaposition to the site of a malignant condition can stabilize the spine. As the structure of the spinal column was destroyed by tumor, support was effectively provided by the bone grafts. In this situation, acrylic cement alone would not have sufficed. It does not provide an adequate interface with bone posteriorly to withstand the tensile loads that the fused bone graft is able to resist. In such cases, the physician should attempt to stay ahead of the destructive malignancy and protect the cord by establishing columns of support with bone graft fused to normal osseous structures.

The final surgical construct used in the patient, a fibula graft, deserves review (Fig. 8-42). The construct is essentially that of a large rectangle built around the tumor. Massive bone grafts are secured anteriorly and posteriorly to available normal structures in hopes of providing enough material to maintain stability even after subsequent local invasion of the malignancy. The massive graft includes as much as possible of the normal structure above or below. This gives more purchase and some margin of safety despite tumor invasion of previously normal structures and bone graft.

Reconstruction following Total Spondylectomy

Complete vertebral body removal and subsequent reconstruction and fusion in the patient discussed below exemplifies sound biomechanical principles.

The patient, a 49-year-old farmer, was afflicted with a chondrosarcoma arising from the body of the seventh thoracic vertebra.[108] The tumor extended into the mediastinum and the spinal canal where it displaced the spinal cord. All of the seventh thoracic vertebra and parts of the sixth and eighth were removed along with the tumor. The thoracic spine was reconstructed as shown

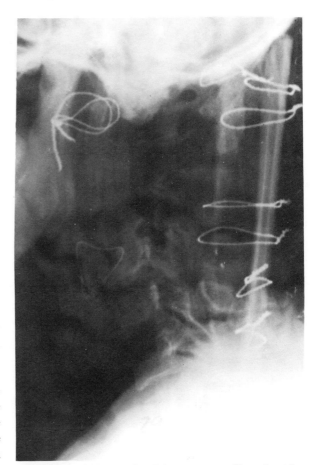

Fig. 8-41. Radiograph of the patient, afflicted with a slowly aggressive salivary gland tumor. This surgical construct shows the principle involving repetitive anterior and posterior bone grafts in order to stay ahead of the tumor and provide support to the severely eroded spinal column. Anteriorly, there is a large column of iliac bone graft. Posteriorly, support comes from a column of iliac bone graft which fractured after 2 years and was subsequently reinforced by a fibula graft. (Friedlaender, G. E., Johnson, R. M., Brand, R. A., and Southwick, W. O.: Treatment of pathological fractures. Conn. Med., 39:765, 1975.)

in Figure 8-43. Fifteen months after surgery, the patient was well and walking. There were no signs of metastasis. Radiographs showed that the bone graft was completely incorporated and fused to the partially resected vertebrae above and below.

This construct uses two portions of iliac bone, with their cortices intact on three sides. This pro-

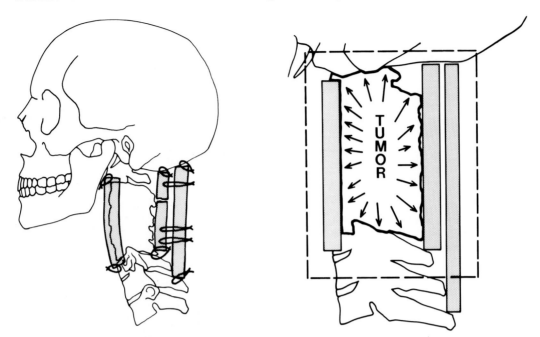

Fig. 8-42. The mechanical principles of the construct described in Figure 8-41. The basic design is to build pillars or columns anterior and posterior to the invading tumor. This makes a rectangle, with the two short sides being composed of normal anatomic structures and the two long sides being composed of bone graft. The columns must alternately resist compression and tensile loading as the patient flexes or extends the head. Axial rotation is effectively resisted by the grafts and because the graft location is a good distance away from the instantaneous axes of rotation, they provide an effective polar moment of inertia. Although the desirability of using cement in this type of situation is worth considering, we beleive that use of bone has two advantages. The first is the potential for a secure osseous union between bone graft and recipient site, so as to resist tensile loading effectively. The second is the well documented capacity of bone to be effective for a long period of time. However, an important advantage of cement is that it is not destroyed by tumor.

vides good resistance to vertical compressive loading, an excellent spacer, and good cancellous to cancellous bone contact at the graft bed interfaces. In order to resect the tumor with adequate margin, a modification of the keystone principle is used, and the graft is wedge-shaped, with the apex of the wedge pointing posteriorly instead of anteriorly as in the keystone graft described by Simmons and Ballah. The keystone is reversed here to prevent migration of graft material back into the spinal cord. The construct effectively compensates for the tendency to anterior displacement, caused by the passage of two cerclage wires in the horizontal plane around the grafts

and through the two plates posteriorly. In addition, there are two wires in the frontal plane, at the caudal and cephalad ends of the graft, which go through the respective adjacent intact vertebral bodies, T5 and T9. These fixations also offer some resistance against anterior protrusion of the grafts. The patient in this case was kept in bed in a plaster shell for 3.5 months.

The primary, immediate postoperative stability of the construct is provided by two posterior stainless steel plates, which are bent to conform to the normal thoracic kyphosis and wired to the transverse processes of the two partially resected vertebrae. They are also wired to *three* intact

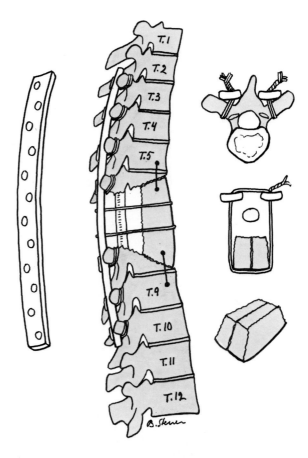

Fig. 8-43. Reconstruction of the spine. The antero-inferior half of the body, the inferior articular processes, the spinous process of the sixth thoracic vertebra, all of the seventh, and the anterosuperior half of the body, and the superior articular processes of the eighth have been removed along with the tumor. Two plates have been fastened with double steel wires to the transverse processes of the third to the sixth and the eighth to the tenth vertebrae (*middle and top right*). Two iliac bone-blocks with obliquely cut ends have been put together (*bottom right*) and inserted between the obliquely cut bodies of the sixth and eighth vertebrae (*middle*). The blocks have been fastened to the spine with silk threads passed through holes in the blocks and the vertebrae. Further fixation has been provided by two steel wires fastened to the plates and gripping the bone-blocks (*middle and middle right*). (Stener, B., and Johnsen, O. E.: Complete removal of three vertebrae for giant-cell tumor. J. Bone Joint Surg., 53B:278, 1971.)

vertebrae above and *two* intact vertebrae below. This fixation and purchase on several normal vertebrae provides stability against both tensile and compressive loads. Thus, there is good stability against flexion and extension, and with the laterally placed attachments to the transverse processes, there is stability against lateral bending. Axial rotation may be resisted reasonably well through the fixation of the transverse process to the plate, which impinges against the lamina and the base of the spinous processes when axial rotation is attempted. Some degree of additional stability can be expected from the relative intrinsic stiffness and modest motion in the thoracic spine, as well as the stiffness and support supplied by the rib cage. Figure 8-44 shows a radiograph of the construct almost 5 years after surgery. These constructs demonstrate the sound judgment and ingenuity of the surgeons, as well as good clinical biomechanics.

SOME GUIDELINES ON THE BIOMECHANICS OF POSTOPERATIVE MANAGEMENT OF PATIENTS UNDERGOING SPINAL FUSIONS

To discuss as much material as we have about biomechanics of spine fusions and not tackle the very cogent mechanical problem of the postoperative management would be nothing other than intellectual cowardice. How long should the patient be kept in bed after undergoing a spinal fusion? Should some type of orthosis be used afterward, and if so, for how long? The literature recommends almost every conceivable type of

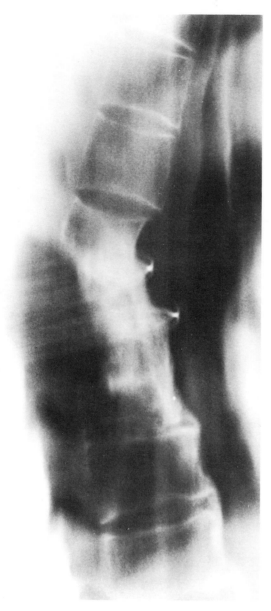

Fig. 8-44. Radiograph of a patient 4.75 years following surgery. The iliac bone grafts now form a block-vertebra in conjunction with the partially resected adjacent vertebral bodies of T6 and T8. The patient is able to walk 30 m in 50 seconds and 400 m without rest. There are no signs of recurrence or metastases. The surgical construct is stable and completely successful from a biomechanics standpoint. Note the osteophyte between T9 and the bone graft. The patient subsequently complained of some pain in the back that did not require medication. (Stener, B.: Acta Orthop. Latinoamericana, 7:189, 1974.)

osseous healing; IV, mature osseous healing. During Stage I, maximum protection should be provided, along with rest with or without some protective orthosis. In Stage II, there is a need for relative protection either by some type of orthosis or through major restrictions in activity. In Stage III, the patient is allowed normal, nonvigorous activity with progression of rehabilitative exercises. In Stage IV, the patient has reached maximum healing and may undergo a program of vigorous rehabilitative activities and exercises, within reasonable limits that are determined for each patient.

The first three stages consist roughly of 5 weeks each, and Stage IV may be prolonged. The total time allowed for arthrodesis maturation may be increased or decreased, on any given patient, depending on a variety of considerations. The cervical, thoracic, and lumbar spines, in that order, tend to require progressively more time for healing. The greater is the extent of fusion (e.g., the number of motion segments), the more time is necessary for healing. As a corollary to this, the larger are the size of the bone grafts, the longer it takes for complete fusion. We must assume that wound infections, loosening of hardware, or one or more previous operations, tend to slow the rate of arthrodesis. Patients in poor health also require relatively more time for completion of arthrodesis.

Clinically *unstable* patients require more time, especially in Stages I and II. The above considerations also apply to these patients. Precise schedules are difficult to generate because the number of variables and problems of evaluation of fusions in mechanical situations make it virtually impossible for an investigation to generate the

management, depending upon which mechanical variables are considered ideal, the age and condition of the patient, the region of the spine, and the type of operation.

The management of these patients is basically contingent upon the presence or absence of clinical stability. Management of clinically stable patients is simpler. There are four stages of maturation of the arthrodesis: I, fibrous healing; II, mixed fibrous and osseous healing; III immature necessary data. We occasionally offer specific schedules for the postoperative management of various conditions. However, our recommendations for basic general guidelines for postoperative management of patients with spine arthrodesis are summarized and presented in Table 8-3 and the following list. If factors in this list strongly favor the patient, or if the opposite is true, the time intervals for the different stages are adjusted accordingly.

Factors That Tend to Prolong Healing Time
in Spinal Arthrodesis

Extensive fusion
Large bone grafts
Wound infections
Loosening hardware
Previous surgery in the same area
Aged patients
Debilitated patients
Clinically unstable spine

Table 8–3. Clinical Biomechanical Stages of Spine Arthrodesis and Their Management

	STAGE	APPROXIMATE TIME REQUIRED (weeks)		MANAGEMENT
I	Fibrous healing	5	Maximum protection	Bed rest, restricted activity Protective orthosis
II	Mixed fibrous and osseous healing	5	Relative protection	Less restricted activity No protection Protective orthosis with less control than above
III	Immature osseous healing	5	Sedentary, nonvigorous activity	Minimal or no orthosis All but vigorous activity Regular or light duty if job permits
IV	Mature osseous healing	5 or more	Maximum convalescence and activity	Maximum allowable activity

Part 3: Surgical Constructs Employing Methylmethacrylate

The use of methylmethacrylate as an adjunct to or instead of spine arthrodesis is becoming more widespread.*[26,35,58,59,81,95,102] There does not appear at this time to be any definitive data which demonstrates an increased incidence of infection over comparable surgery without methylmethacrylate. Studies indicate that there is probably no direct toxic effect, no detrimental exothermic reaction, and no chemical reaction at nearby bone.[68,85] This section presents the available biomechanical information that will be helpful to the surgeon in decisions about the use of methylmethacrylate for spine fixations.

---

* Personal communication, K. Ono.

BIOMECHANICAL FACTORS

Cement Bone Interface

The material is a cement and not a glue. The bonding between methylmethacrylate and bone is not one of adhesion but is based on the interdigitation of cement particles and bone trabeculae, with the two being separated by a thin layer of fibrous tissue.[19,36] This bonding is obviously most effective at the cement *cancellous* bone interface. The tensile, compressive, and shear strength of methylmethacrylate is greater than that of cancellous bone. Thus, the strength of the interface bonding depends upon the strength of the interdigitated cancellous bone spicules. This factor is important with regard to surgical constructs using methylmethacrylate. Attention must be paid to the development of improved bonding between bone and cement in the design of an effective construct with this material.

This material is likely to be most effective in resisting compressive loads. We should remember, however, that for most compressive loading situations human bone itself can be expected to be strong enough for adequate support.[122] Methylmethacrylate, compared to its ability to withstand compression, is less effective in resisting tensile loading. Therefore, it will also be relatively weaker in bending. It has been shown, however, that as is the case with concrete, its tensile load bearing capabilities may be significantly enhanced through the incorporation of wire or wire mesh that has a high tensile resistance.[93] The additional advantage provided by the mesh is the great opportunity for interdigitation interface bonding between surgical wire, mesh, and methylmethacrylate. It is known that abnormal motion can develop at a motion segment next to a fusion mass. Presumably, the high stiffness materials such as methylmethacrylate may accentuate this problem.

Mechanical Functions of Methylmethacrylate in Surgical Constructs

The material is used in spinal surgical constructs in several fashions. It may be employed as a spacer,[21,43,81] an internal splint,[58,95,102] and/or as a fixation device (Fig. 8-45). It is apparent that the spacer basically supports compression loading. This provides more than adequate immediate postoperative stability against flexion, with some clinical stability against lateral bending and axial rotation. Stability against extension is not provided in the spacer construct; therefore, the construct should be protected by an appropriate orthosis. The use of methylmethacrylate for splint and fixation requires adequate bonding of the cement to the bone. When the cement is to withstand bending (tensile) loads, adequate reinforcement is required. The use of the splint here may be somewhat analogous to the plate described by Stener (Fig. 8-43.)[108] While the stainless steel plate is a well known

entity of proven worth with great tensile strength, methylmethacrylate does offer the advantage of a highly individualized configuration, since it can be poured, molded, and packed into various anatomic caverns and crevices.

Postmortem Mechanical Test of Surgical Construct Involving Methylmethacrylate

M.A. is a 53-year-old male who was hit by a truck and sustained a fracture dislocation of C6 on C7 associated with paraplegia. Neurosurgical and orthopaedic evaluation resulted in a decision to carry out open reduction, decompressive laminectomy, and stabilization. Total laminectomies and foraminotomies were carried out at C6 and C7. The following surgical construct was established.

Wires were passed through the spinous processes of C4 and T2, and C5 and T1. These wires formed ellipses around the C6–7 laminectomy. Stainless steel mesh was cut to size and placed over the laminectomy site.[c] Methylmethacrylate was then mixed and applied in one piece as an ellipse, the center of which was the laminectomy, and pressed down over the wires, C7, and posterior elements of T1 and T2. The central aperture was designed to allow flow of blood out of the spinal canal, in case of epidural bleeding and subsequent hematoma. Unfortunately, the patient developed gastrointestinal bleeding which was not controllable and on the 18th postoperative day, after several cardiac arrests and resuscitations, he died.

Radiographs of the surgical specimen are shown in Figure 8-46. The specimen was set up in an Instron testing machine to be tested to failure in a manner that simulates flexion.[83] The results are shown in Figure 8-47. The first audible crack occurred when the upper wire pulled out of the spinous process of C4 (Fig. 8-48A). The specimen reached its maximum energy absorption capacity (strength) when the wire pulled out of the spinous process of T2 (Fig. 8-48B).

Although no firm conclusions can be drawn from the study of one specimen, there are some points that merit discussion. Methylmethacrylate significantly increased the stiffness of the spine between C4 and T2. Consequently, there is con-

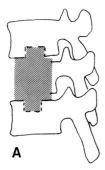
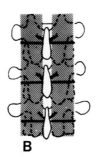
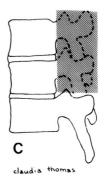

A B C

claudia thomas

Fig. 8-45. The uses of methylmethacrylate in surgical constructs. (A) As a *spacer*, methylmethacrylate is most effective in resisting compressive forces during flexion. During extension, tension is applied to the cement bone interface and may cause failure. (B) When the cement is used as a *fixation splint*, it is subjected to bending loads. The key biomechanical factors in this situation are reinforcement of the cement and an effective attachment of the cement to the posterior elements. (C) When the cement is used as a *fixation clamp*, the effectiveness of the interface with the posterior elements depends solely upon their anatomic configuration and the placement of the methylmethacrylate.

siderable stress concentration at C3–4 and T2–3. These are the obvious points at which failure is likely to occur and, in fact, did occur. The failure of the constructs due to the wires pulling out shows that, at least for this particular construct, the point of attachment of the wires was the weakest link in the chain. This is important in regard to the value of the construct in contributing to postoperative stability. The first crack (pullout of the wire from the spinous process of C4) occurred at 70 N (16 lbf) (see point 3 in Fig. 8-47). This is in the range of 10 per cent of body weight, which is about the weight of the head. In other words, the weak link of the construct without the assistance of active muscle forces or braces is alarmingly close to expected physiologic loads. This constitutes a tolerance limit or margin of safety that is not particularly generous.

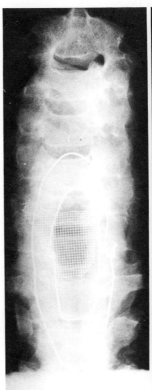
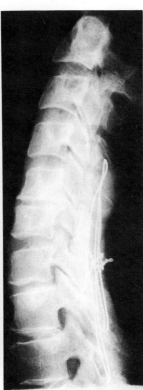

Fig. 8-46. Anteroposterior and lateral radiographs of the specimen to be tested. The construct consists of oval wiring through the spinous process of C4 and T2. The stainless steel mesh was used to cover the exposed dura. (Panjabi, M. M., Hopper, W., White, A. A., and Keggi, K. J.: Posterior spine stabilization with methylmethacrylate. Biomechanical testing of a surgical specimen. Spine, 2:241, 1977.)

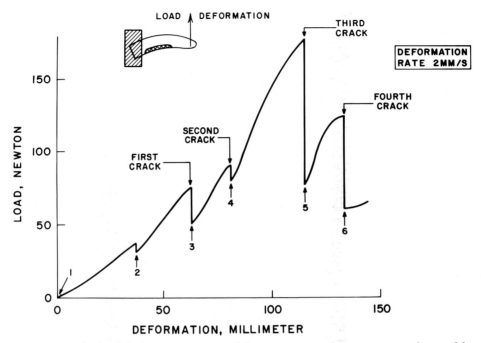

Fig. 8-47. The load-deformation curve of the specimen. This curve was obtained by loading the specimen in the transverse direction at C2. The deformation was measured at the point of loading. Numbers 1 through 6 are the points in time when the testing machine was stopped in order to take a lateral radiograph and a photograph. The vertical drops of the curve· are the relaxations of the load that occurred when the machine was stopped. The failure is described and shown in Figure 8-48. (Panjabi, M. M., Hopper, W., White, A. A., and Keggi, K. J.: Posterior spine stabilization with methylmethacrylate. Biomechanical testing of a surgical specimen. Spine, *2:*241, 1977.)

PRINCIPLES AND INDICATIONS FOR THE USE OF METHYLMETHACRYLATE

A conservative approach to the use of this material is suggested. This is recommended because of the problems and risks associated with the use of this material. Although it is not known whether the material itself potentiates infection, infection in a wound involving methylmethacrylate is very difficult to treat. Because of this we suggest that orthopaedists should not do with glue (cement) that which can be done with bone. If the various principles and indications provided are followed and if the physician is convinced that bone alone will not suffice, then the cement should be employed. If methylmethacrylate is used with a clear understanding of the precise role that it is to play in the construct, then clinical success is likely. Is it to be used as a spacer, a splint, or a fixation device? The surgeon should also determine the absolute or relative importance of immediate postoperative and long-range clinical stability. This consideration is crucial in deciding whether or not to include bone graft arthrodesis in the surgical construct. If long-range stability is needed, then an arthrodesis should be included. The surgeon must also have a basic understanding of the biomechanics of spine stability, surgical constructs, and methylmethacrylate. Finally, it is necessary to have the technical knowledge and surgical ability to achieve the biomechanical goals. These and other principles are listed on the following page.

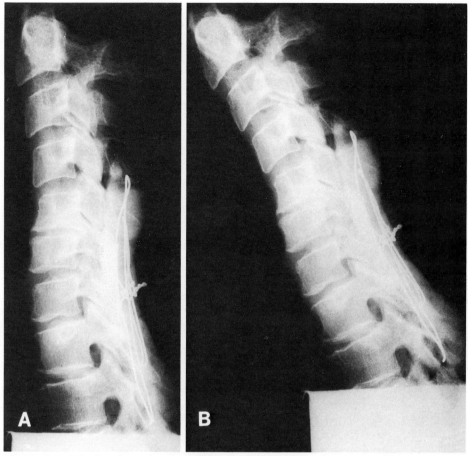

Fig. 8-48. (A) This lateral radiograph was taken when the first audible crack was heard. It corresponds to the time marked 3 on the graph of Figure 8-47. The transverse load had a value of 70 N (16 lbf). Note that the spine segment C2–C4 has displaced anteriorly as compared to the rest of the specimen. This is due to the pulling out of the wire from the spinous process of C4. (B) The maximum load of 175 N (39 lbf) was reached with a loud audible crack. This is the lateral radiograph of the specimen taken at this time, which corresponds to the time marked 5 on the graph of Figure 8-47. Note the failure, wire pullout, at the spinous process of T2. (Panjabi, M. M., Hopper, W., White, A. A., and Keggi, K. J.: Posterior spine stabilization with methylmethacrylate. Biomechanical testing of a surgical specimen. Spine, 2:241, 1977.)

Some Principles in the Use of Methylmethacrylate in Spine Surgery

(1) Consider the use of bone before cement.

(2) Determine what is expected of the cement.

(3) Determine immediate and long-range need of clinical stability. Fuse if necessary.

(4) Analyze biomechanics of clinical stability and surgical constructs.

(5) Develop technical knowledge and ability to design and develop a construct.

(6) Reinforce the cement with stainless steel; mesh if the construct must resist tension.

(7) Provide vertebra with holes, pins, screws, and wires for as much interdigitation as possible between bone and cement.

Below we suggest indications for the use of methylmethacrylate in surgical constructs. At least one of the conditions should be present. One may anticipate that recommended indications may become less stringent in the future provided the clinical experience with the techniques are shown to have a low ratio of risks to benefits.

Some Indications for the Use of Methylmethacrylate in Spine Surgery

Maximum immediate postoperative clinical stability is crucial to the survival of the patient.
There is no source for bone autograft or allograft.
The patient is extremely ill requiring stabilization.

The value of methylmethacrylate in the extremely ill patient should not be underestimated. Its use can readily reduce anesthesia time and blood loss by 50 per cent or more. Pain and complications from a bone graft donor site are also eliminated.

ANALYSIS OF SOME SPECIFIC CONSTRUCTS

Construct for Maximum Immediate Clinical Stability

Given present knowledge and our interpretation of spine biomechanics, we suggest the construct shown in Figure 8-49 for achieving the *maximal* immediate postoperative clinical stability. The important features are as follows: firm fixation of the cement to the spine; reinforcement of the cement by a stainless steel mesh; fixation of the spine by wires and mesh, which is effectively fixed with the cement, into which both are incorporated; the use of two normal vertebrae above and below the pathology for stable anchoring of the construct and for more site of purchase and interfaces between cement metal and bone; curettage of the facet articulations in order to attain some biologic arthrodesis; tapered and rounded structure of the cement ends.

The same basic construct may be employed in patients with multiple laminectomies. In such patients, there are two normal vertebrae above and below the upper most total laminectomy, and the rolled wire mesh is wired to the facets, just as the bone graft is attached as shown in Figure 8-49. If there are facetectomies, the stainless steel mesh and cement filler are used to bridge the defect.

One possible advantage of the basic construction presented here is the relative ease of removal. If the facets are not wired, the entire wire cement complex can be removed by resection of the spinous process near its base.

Cement as a Temporary or Permanent Spacer

In cases of extensive anterior element destruction by tumor or resections of one or more vertebral bodies, cement may be useful. Methylmethacrylate may be used in this situation as a spacer or a filler (Fig. 8-50). The cement provides a good purchase in the cancellous bone. If necessary, a notch, a trough, or some undermining procedure may be useful. Several examples of the use of methylmethacrylate as a spacer are given in Figure 8-50. Various techniques for preventing extrusion of the cement block and resisting tensile loading during bending (as in extension) are shown. It is difficult to compare the relative effectiveness of the three constructs without any experimental data. They all look as though they would be stable in flexion. The crucial factor is stability in extension. The construct with the cement packed into the mushroom-shaped space should be the strongest. We believe that screw-fixed cement is more secure than cement fixed by K wires.

Ono and Tada have employed a simple but ingenious device to be used as an anterior spacer to replace a vertebral body.[81] The device and the surgical construct are shown in Figures 8-51 and 8-52. The quadrilateral cylinder controls the placement of methylmethacrylate and prevents it from overheating the spinal cord. Ono has suggested that the construct be employed in those patients who have primary cancer localized in the spine or metastatic cancer in the spine without

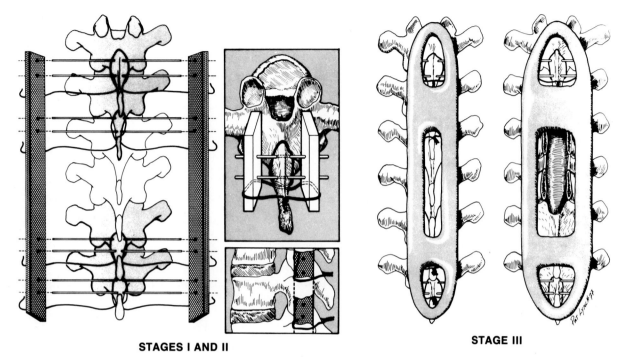

STAGES I AND II   **STAGE III**

Fig. 8-49. Based on our analysis and appreciation of the clinical biomechanics involved, we recommend the surgical construct illustrated here as the procedure of choice to provide the maximum immediate postoperative stability with methylmethacrylate. *Stage I* exposes two *normal* vertebrae above and below the level of the pathology. This is to provide adequate purchase for the fixation splint (methylmethacrylate). Place two parallel transverse 5/64-in K wires at the base of the 4 normal spinous processes. Anterior to the transverse K wires, wrap a no. 24 twisted stainless steel wire around the base of the spinous process and twist it 5 to 10 times. (The twisted wire forms a more stable interface with the methylmethacrylate.) Let these wires extend out laterally in both directions. *Stage II.* Take two strips of stainless steel mesh of the appropriate length, 1 cm in width. This should be punctured with an awl, making holes large enough and in the proper position to admit the four transversely placed K wires. The ends of the twisted wires are then crossed and brought around the strips of wire mesh and twisted together so as to hold them in place. *Stage III.* Methylmethacrylate is then prepared and while it is still soft, the oval shape with the tapered ends and transverse bars is fashioned in and around the previously implanted stainless steel. Stages I to III are also carried out on the abnormal vertebrae if the posterior elements are intact. In a patient who has undergone laminectomies, a modification *(far right)* should be used. The implantation of too much methylmethacrylate can make wound closure difficult. The construct may be used regardless of the status of the posterior elements of the involved vertebra. If both lamina and facets are absent, the region is bridged; if the facets are present the facet wiring (see Figs. 8-34, 8-35) is done with the methylmethacrylate being treated as bone graft. This construct provides secure splint fixation by attachment to two normal vertebra above and below, secure methylmethacrylate-bone interface through stable wiring, wire mesh reinforcement of the methylmethacrylate, and minimization of stress concentration by decreasing the mass of material and thus the stiffness at each end of the oval.

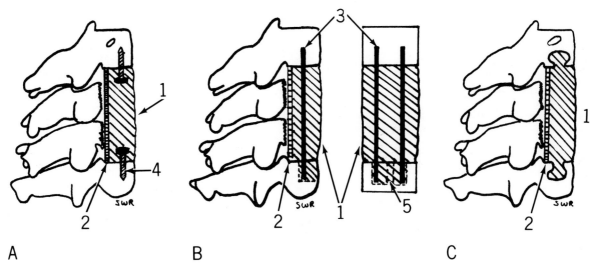

Fig. 8-50. Some of the different constructs for securing the methylmethacrylate-bone interface when methylmethacrylate (*1*) is used as a spacer. (*A*) The use of screws (*4*) in cancellous bone. The construct can be expected to be more stable if a cancellous bone screw is used. This constitutes a sound construct against extrusion and against tensile loading. (*B*) Here K wires (*3*) are employed. This construct is reasonably effective in resisting extrusion but not very effective against tensile loading. (*C*) This undermining technique, when well done, is effective against extrusion and tensile loading. (*2*) This represents a bone plate positioned to protect the dura and its contents. Experiments are required to determine assuredly the relative effectiveness of the three constructs. We favor the construct shown in *C* followed, by *A*, and then *B*. (Dunn, E. J.: The role of methylmethacrylate in the stabilization and replacement of tumors of the cervical spine. Spine, 2:15, 1977.)

pulmonary metastasis. He warns that if the patient has a tracheostomy, this cement-metal construct is prone to serious infection.* We have suggested a modification of the Ono device, one which provides some immediate postoperative clinical stability against extension. The modification involves the use of a screw transfixing the prosthesis to the remaining anterior lip of the vertebra and to the methylmethacrylate inside the vertebra. This modification of the Ono device is shown in Figure 8-51E.

Another technique for insuring clinical stability in these situations is to supplement the construct with posterior fusion immediately or later, when the patient's condition permits. The spacer resists compressive forces very effectively. However, there is no good resistance against tensile

forces, either by the cement or the interdigitation interface. However, a posterior bone graft provides stability by acting as a band to resist tension in flexion (as do intact posterior ligaments), and in extension it resists compressive loads well. The posterior bone graft, to augment the anterior spacer, is therefore an advisable adjunct when feasible. If the posterior elements are destroyed or unable to function, use of the anterior spacer alone is very likely to leave a clinically unstable situation.

Since several complications of structural failure have been reported in patients with constructs using methymethacrylate, it is suggested that some attention be paid to the technical aspects of the use of this material. A review and analysis of the purposes for which the material is being used is helpful. If the surgeon is conversant with the information concerning general prin-

---

* Personal communication, K. Ono., M.D.

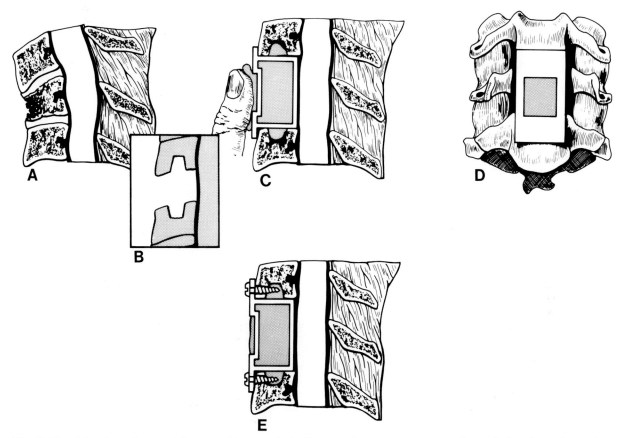

Fig. 8-51. The Ono device. This stainless steel shell is used in conjunction with methylmethacrylate when the latter is used as a spacer. (*A*) The diseased vertebra is shown. (*B*) The vertebral body is resected and a rectangular tunnel of bone is made in the two adjacent vertebrae. (*C*) The device is put in place and the methylmethacrylate is packed in. (*D*) An anterior view of the construct with the cement in place. The device protects the neural structures from the cement and is designed so that the cement can be thoroughly packed. On the lateral view (*C*), one can observe bone wedged between the methylmethacrylate and the outside rim of the shell. The locking of this little segment of bone tends to resist extension and make the construct more stable. (*E*) We suggest the following modification of this construct, which will offer additional immediate postoperative stability against extension. The rectangular steel device is altered so that two screws can be placed through the stainless steel shell, into the anterior portion of the vertebral body and into the methylmethacrylate.

ciples and analysis of the constructs presented here, he may be better equipped to use this material successfully as a spine implant.

It is of interest to note that methylmethacrylate has been used as a spacer for the intervertebral disc,[21] despite the striking paucity of biomechanical similarity between the two substances. The procedure consists of laminotomy, removal of the herniated disc fragment or the entire disc, and insertion of soft, freshly prepared methylmethacrylate into the interspace. Cleveland reports having performed this on 126 patients with "extremely satisfactory results."[21] We view this with respectful skepticism and look forward to a more detailed documentation of the effectiveness of this procedure.

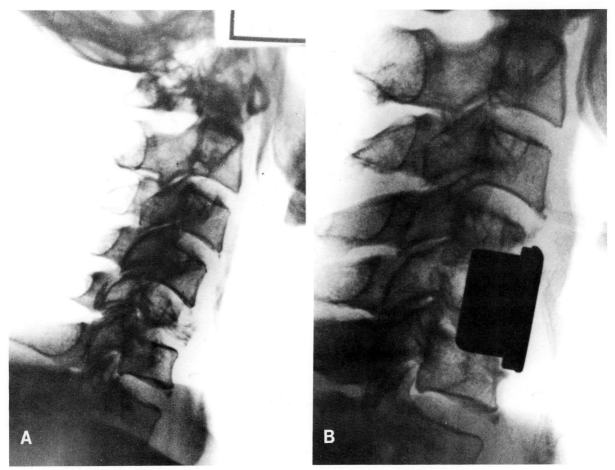

Fig. 8-52. (*A, B*) Radiographs of a patient before and after the insertion of the Ono device. (Dunn, E. J.: The role of methylmethacrylate in the stabilization and replacement of tumors of the cervical spine. Spine, 2:15, 1977.)

Part 4: Biomechanical Considerations in the Art and Science of Spine Instrumentation

This section presents some mechanical information, concepts, and ideas about the types of instrumentation that are used in spine surgery. Chapter 3 provides some additional information.

WIRES, MESH, AND SCREWS

The use of stainless steel wire posteriorly in surgical spine fusion has been very useful. It may serve a large variety of functions, most fre-quently being used as a tension band to coapt and fix posterior elements. It is also employed to attach, immobilize, and secure bone graft to the recipient site.

Twisted versus Nontwisted Wire

This is largely a matter of individual preference. The most important factor is that the wire be large enough to carry the anticipated loads and that it be used in a most effective manner in the surgical construct. The major considerations, pro and con, for the use of twisted wire are presented below. It is assumed that the cross-sectional area of the units compared are the same, and the hole for twisted wire is 40 per cent larger than that for single wire. A convenient method for twisting the wire is shown in Figure 8-53.

Mesh

Stainless steel wire mesh is available in several different sizes. We recommend that it be used whenever possible to reinforce methylmethacrylate that will be subjected to significant tensile and bending loads. The size suggested is the stiffest one that is compatible with a reasonable ease of handling. This mesh should also permit ease of penetration with an awl so that it can accept wires and pins of various sizes.

Screws

A technique involving the use of screws has been described for C1–C2 fusion. Screws have also been recommended in the lumbar spine.[10,61] With regard to their role in preventing displacement, screws can be presumed to be effective in the cervical spine in view of the magnitude of the physiologic loads exerted there. However, in the lumbar spine, either across a spondylolisthesis defect or across the facet joints, it is unlikely that screw fixation is an effective method of immobilization.[6,10,51] We do not believe that the screw techniques described for the lumbar spine have been shown to be beneficial enough to expose the patient to the possible complications of hardware failure, or neural or vascular irritation.

When a screw is intended to be anchored in cancellous bone a cancellous bone screw should be employed, using the appropriate technique. If the screw is to be anchored in cortical bone, the screw should be properly tapped.

Comparison of Single and Twisted Wires

Single Wires
   Less chances of fatigue
   Less chances of corrosion
Twisted Wires
   Bigger purchase area in bone
   More flexible
   Stronger due to coldworking
   Smooth tip; less risk of damaging soft tissues
   More secure with methylmethacrylate[93]

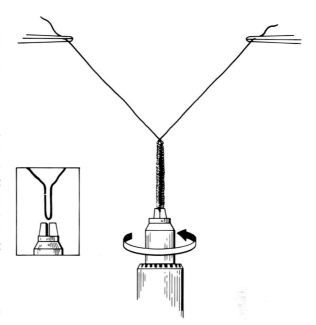

Fig. 8-53. Technique for the preparation of a twisted wire. *Step I.* Take a no. 24 stainless steel wire, at least 2.5 times the length desired for the twisted wire. Blend it on itself at the middle, as shown in the insert. *Step II.* Place about 1 cm of a 0.5-in portion of the wire that is bent on itself into the chuck of a hand drill. A Kelly clamp is applied to each of the two free ends of the wire. *Step III.* The two clamps are held with slight tension such that an angle of 90 degrees is formed at the tip of the chuck. The drill is then turned at a steady rate, which twists the wire as shown.

GRUCA-WEISS SPRINGS, HARRINGTON COMPRESSION, AND DISTRACTION RODS

Gruca-Weiss Springs

This device was first developed by Gruca in 1956 for the correction of scoliosis.[38] In 1975 Weiss described its use for stabilization of the lumbar spine.[120] The instrument system consists of two heavy springs with hooks on both ends. The springs are under tension and are applied over the section of the diseased spine to be corrected or stabilized. The hooks are inserted in the transverse processes or the laminae at the top and the bottom of the curve that is to be corrected. When treating kyphosis, they should be inserted in the lamina. The two springs lie over the intervening laminae separated by the spinous processes. When scoliosis is being treated, the hooks are better placed over the transverse processes on the convex side of the curve to create a greater moment arm for correction of abnormal rotation in the frontal plane.

Figure 8-54A shows the combined forces applied to the spine by a pair of springs. The forces on the end vertebra are equal in magnitude to the tension in the two springs. Due to the curvature of the spine, the springs also apply small, radially directed forces on each of the vertebrae within the curve.

These forces produce two different kinds of bending moments on the spine. The two large forces produce bending moments that tend to correct the angular deformity, while the small radial forces have an opposite effect. The net

effect is such that a modest correction occurs. In addition to the bending moments, there is also a large compression produced between the vertebrae.

Harrington Compression Rod

This instrument system is designed to apply compression to the spine at the points where the hooks are inserted. Figure 8-54B shows the characteristic forces that are applied to the spine with these devices. As a result of the bending of the compression rods in the sagittal plane, there are modest transverse forces which tend to pull the hooks posteriorly and push the apex of the kyphotic deformity anteriorly.[82] This combination of forces (a pull at the ends and push at the center) constitutes a three-point bending system. As this system operates in the sagittal

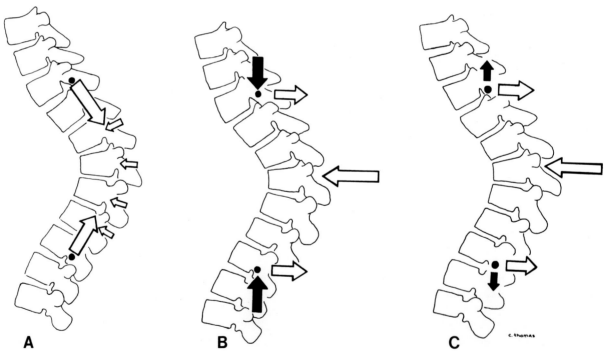

Fig. 8-54. A simplified diagram showing the forces operating on the spine due to the three instrumentations. (A) Gruca-Weiss springs. The large arrows represent the forces equal to the tension in the springs, while the small arrows indicate the pressure of the springs against the spine. (B) Harrington compression rods. The three light arrows represent the forces due to the three-point bending of the spine as the Harrington rod is inserted between the two hooks. The black arrows are the compressive forces applied by tightening the nuts. (C) Harrington distraction rods. The three-point bending forces are similar to those shown in B but larger in magnitude. The smaller black arrows represent the distraction forces, which are probably of lesser magnitude than the compression forces created by compression rods. (White, A. A., Panjabi, M. M., and Thomas, C. L.: The clinical biomechanics of kyphotic deformities. Clin. Orthop., *128*:8, 1977.)

plane, it tends to correct the kyphotic deformity. The action of the *compression* force, however, is to *increase* the angulation of the deformity. The mechanics are the same whether the deformity is due to tumor, trauma, or surgery.

Harrington Distraction Rod

When the Harrington rod is used in the distraction mode, tension is applied to the spine in addition to the three-point bending previously described.[B] The tensile forces produce bending moments, so that the distraction rods are more efficient than the compression rods in correcting the deformity. These forces are illustrated in Figure 8-54C. It has been shown that a *combination* of axial distraction and transverse loading provides the most effective correction, regardless of the degree of the curve (see page 102). This produces bending moments in addition to those produced by the three-point bending system. In other words, the angular correction is improved over that offered by the compression rod system. This, then, can be presumed to be useful instrumentation for correction of clinically stable kyphotic deformities. These considerations apply much more to post-traumatic conditions than to Scheuermann's kyphosis. In developmental kyphosis, the forces which must be resisted are significantly large. Bradford and colleagues operated on over 50 patients for this disease.[11] They found the deformity was very resistant to correction. This is probably related to the observed hypertrophy of the anterior longitudinal ligaments, which increases the tensile resistance to the correctional forces. In addition, the basic deformity itself is considerably stiff. Bradford and colleagues found that these resting forces often required considerable bending of the distraction rod prior to correction. It is important to emphasize that in the correction of kyphosis the Harrington distraction rods *are not used primarily as distractors. They are used to produce bending moments* that apply correcting couples and then serve as internal splints. The distraction mechanism is then employed to lock the rods into place. The hook is fixed on the rod by the tension produced in the soft tissue, which locks the hook into the riveting mechanism of the rod. If there is gross disruption of the ligaments of a motion segment, the distraction system may have certain limitations or even dangers. This may be an indication for the use of a combined system described on page 436.

Comparison of Clinical Biomechanics of the Three Systems

Although we do not know the quantity of forces applied in the three systems, a simple mechanical analysis generates some useful information. Measurements were made of the three-point bending stiffness of the compression and distraction Harrington rods.[82] The Harrington distraction rod was found to be 4.7 times as stiff as the compression rod of the same length. This implies that the three-point bending in the two procedures is approximately five times more effective with the Harrington distraction rod. The distraction rod has the additional advantage of producing a distraction force, which further increases its effectiveness by providing corrective bending moments. In summary then, the distraction rods are clearly more efficient in correcting deformity, and the compression rods may be useful through their ability to provide some immediate clinical stability by means of impaction. We believe that the functioning of both of these instruments is most effective in the presence of an intact anterior longitudinal ligament.

The Gruca-Weiss spring has a different mode of action and is difficult to compare with the Harrington systems. We do not recommend the Gruca-Weiss spring for the corrective instrumentation of kyphotic deformity.

Can these methods by applied without any consideration of the clinical stability of the spine? Bending moments in the sagittal plane, which tend to correct kyphotic deformity, produce tension in the anterior and compression in the posterior elements of the spine. Therefore, the efficiency of the surgical instrumentation in the correction of kyphosis is directly related to the ability of the anterior elements of the spine to withstand tensile loads. When the anterior elements are known to be disrupted, the Gruca-Weiss springs and the Harrington compression rods that are able to apply some anterior compressive force are relatively more attractive. This is due to the fact that the compressive forces can provide some stability. Additional details of this analysis are available.[82,124a]

An experiment was performed by Stauffer and colleagues on cadaver spines to study the relative stability provided by the three fixation procedures described above. The disruptive bending load applied to the spine to test its stability was a combination of flexion moment and axial torque. They found that Harrington compression rods provided the maximum stability of the three, followed by Harrington distraction rods, and the Gruca-Weiss Springs.[106] The compression rods provide stability through the vectors of force that impact or provide an element of compression between the upper and lower portions of the spine (Fig. 8-54B). Similar studies by Meyer and colleagues confirmed this work.[75] These investigators also showed that the best instrument fixation of the disrupted spine sustained loads that

were only 50 per cent of the loads that the normal spine could bear.[75] We believe that when a clinically unstable spine is to be corrected, one or two Harrington compression rods should be considered.

Combined Use of Harrington Distraction and Compression Rods

We have shown previously that the bending moments created by the distraction rod are the most effective in correction of the traumatized spine. It has also been shown that in situations in which clinical stability is a factor, especially with a nonfunctional anterior longitudinal ligament, the compression rods can be expected to contribute significantly to clinical stability through impaction at the disrupted spine segments. Therefore, it is reasonable that in situations in which strong correctional forces are needed in addition

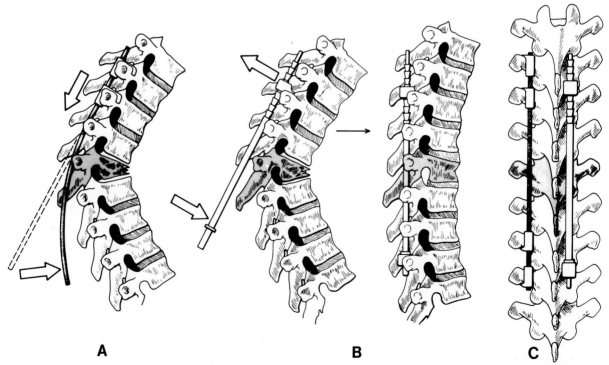

A   **B**   **C**

Fig. 8-55. Rationale and biomechanics for the combined use of Harrington compression and distraction rods. (*A*) The compression rod has a relatively low stiffness and may not be helpful in correcting deformity. (*B*) The distraction rod is about five times as stiff as the compression rod. It applies a strong couple to the deformity and is likely to correct it. The rod is then attached and serves as a splint to maintain correction. It is not employed as a distractor. (*C*) The compression rod is then applied to stabilize the two parts of the kyphos in their corrected position. Frontal plane rotation is small because of the short distance between the two rods and is restricted by the buttressing of the spinous processes against the stiff Harrington distraction rod.

to compression for clinical stability, combined compression and distraction rods may be the treatment of choice (Fig. 8-55). Although one might be concerned about frontal plane rotation in this system, it is not significant for two reasons. Firstly, the couple formed by the distraction and compression forces has a short lever arm, resulting in a small frontal plane bending moment. Secondly, this moment is adequately resisted by numerous anatomic constraints, particularly the spinous processes, which immediately buttress against the rod to prevent frontal plane rotation.

A New Technique for Application of Harrington Rods

Concommitant with our analysis of the mechanics of corrective forces, we developed a new technique for the application of dual Harrington rods in the treatment of kyphosis. Two Harrington rods may be attached to *opposite* ends of a kyphotic deformity of any type and *simultaneously* reduced and implanted in order to efficiently apply couples to *both* ends of the deformity (Fig. 8-56). This is a sound, efficient and effective way to apply Harrington rods to a kyphotic deformity.

The Hinge Principal in the Correction of Kyphosis

In the correction of a kyphotic deformity, when the angle between the two arms of the kyphos is increased by corrective displacement, a hinge of some sort is necessary. This was pointed out by O'Brien in the correction of tuberculous kyphosis.[80] His recommendation was that a portion of bone be left posteriorly as a hinge. The principle is analogous to aligning the position of a door in relation to the wall. If there is a *hinge* it works beautifully. The door is closed and the 180-degree angle with the wall is readily achieved. If there is no hinge, the door simply pulls away from the wall. The two analogous situations are shown in Figure 8-57. The hinge does not have to be comprised of posterior bone. Other tissues, such as the intertransverse ligaments, the facet capsules, or the anterior longitudinal ligament, can also serve that function. It is suggested that the surgeon be aware of situations in which there is no hinge and take this important factor into consideration when correctional force

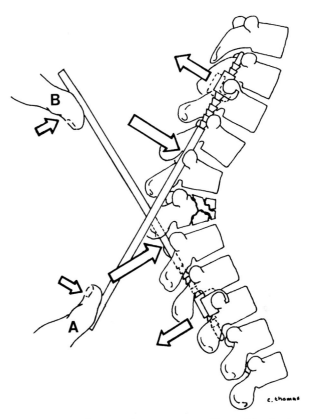

Fig. 8-56. The simultaneous use of two Harrington distraction rods to correct kyphotic deformity. These rods, which are about five times as stiff as the compression rods, can be employed to create two effective correcting couples to *each* end of a kyphotic deformity. This is actually a four-point bending system. One rod is placed in the traditional manner with the upper hook in place, as for correction of scoliosis. This rod exerts a couple on the upper segment of the spine through a force applied by the lower finger *(A)*. The second rod is placed on the other side in the "upside down" position. It exerts a correcting couple to the lower portion of the spine through a force applied by the upper finger *(B)*. This technique has the practical advantage of providing good control and corrective forces (couples) to *both* portions of the deformity. (White, A. A., Panjabi, M. M., and Thomas, C. L.: The clinical biomechanics of kyphotic deformities. Clin. Orthop. *128*:8, 1977.)

vectors are applied. In addition to the correctional moments, there will be a need to apply some loads which will approximate and align the two limbs of the kyphotic deformity. Consequently, when there is no hinge one should be provided by the appropriate instrumentation. We suggest a Har-

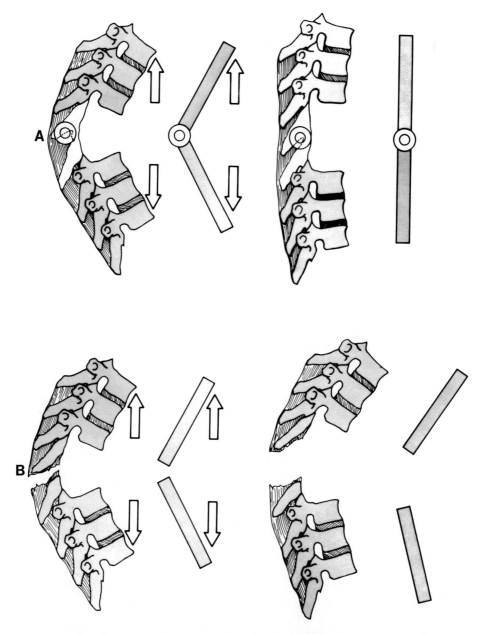

Fig. 8-57. This illustrates the necessity for some type of hinge in order to correct a deformity. *(A)* The anterior longitudinal ligament, the intertransverse ligaments, bone, or posterior ligamentous structures may serve as a hinge. For obvious reasons, the spinal cord should not be the hinge. *(B)* With no hinge, it is not possible with an axial force to change the angle between the limbs of the deformity. The two portions tend to separate.

rington compression rod or wiring of the posterior elements or Gruca-Weiss springs, in that order of preference, but depending upon the particular clinical problem.

Scoliosis Instrumentation

The mechanics of the Harrington instrumentation for scoliosis has certain similarities to that of kyphosis. This is reviewed in Chapter 3, along with an analysis of the Dwyer instrumentation.

LUMBAR AND LUMBOSACRAL FIXATION DEVICES

Lumbosacral Spring Fixation

A construct has been described by Hastings and Reynolds in which a coiled spring with an outside diameter of 4.3 mm is employed in conjunction with a hook in lumbosacral spine fusions.[45] Small hooks that can be screwed into the coiled spring are inserted into or hooked over the lamina. The bone grafts lie between the spring and the host bed. The investigators present a chart which allows the determination of tension in the spring for various elongations. This careful kind of measurement of forces applied to the body is a commendable principle. The tensed spring probably holds the bone graft in place effectively. However, we doubt that the tensile loads of 60 to 80N (13–18 lbf) are very significant in fixing the motion segments against the large magnitude of forces, three to four times body weight, exerted at the lower lumbar spine.

Wilson Plates

These plates are for use in the lumbar and lumbosacral spine.[126] The plate is designed to be attached to the spinous processes on one side, with a matching bone graft on the other side. The plate was intended primarily to be an effective form of internal fixation of the vertebrae to be fused. This device may create a construct that is too rigid, resulting in loosening of the plate and ultimate failure of effective immobilization. We believe that the same considerations apply to the Meurig-Williams plates.

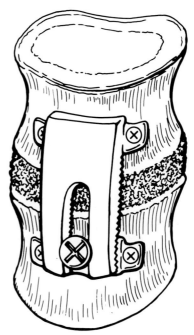

Fig. 8-58. This is an illustration of a slotted plate which is designed to fix and apply compression across an interbody fusion. The compressive force is applied and maintained by a clamp while the screws are inserted.

Knodt Rods

These devices were designed for internal fixation of the spine, the theory being that it is somehow beneficial to fuse the motion segment in some degree of flexion. A report showing a 60 per cent failure rate suggests that they are not particularly helpful.[25]

Slotted Compression Plate

Humphries, Hawk, and Berndt reported on the use of a compression plate for anterior lumbar spine surgery (Fig. 8-58).[55] They designed plates for arthrodesis of one or two motion segments. Compression was applied with a clamp and a slotted mechanism, which was then subsequently tightened. The clamp was held in place by two non-cancellous bone screws. The disc was removed and the space was packed with cancellous bone chips. The patient was permitted out of bed with no orthosis when he so desired. The mechanical weakness of this construct is due to the fact that cancellous bone chips in the disc space can not support the large loads of three to four times body weight. The plate screw system, with its purchase in the cancellous bone of the vertebral bodies, should not be expected to hold. The screws are likely to pull or cut out of the cancellous bone of the vertebral body. Despite the above analysis, Humphries, Hawk, and Berndt reported no failures of the construct in 14 cases. It would seem desirable to study a larger series before using this construct.

The Table Staple Construct

This construct is discussed because it is unique, clever, and reported to give 97 per cent excellent results.[121] The surgical construct, its preparation, and the Mario-Stone table staple are shown in Figure 8-59.

There are certain aspects of the construct which should be discussed. It fixes the vertebra in the flexed position, although this has not been proven to be desirable (see Chapter 6). Wertlick, however, suggests that this may be helpful in relieving posterior bulging of a disc onto the nerve root.[121] There is good blood supply, cancellous to cancellous bone contact, and some element of immobilization with initial compression. The desirability of compression for arthrodesis also awaits proof. Wertlick points out that the staple is held firmly in the vertebral body by the serrations of the legs. The major forces acting on the legs are at right angles to the long axes of the legs and are not parallel to them. Forces acting parallel to the legs would tend to pull them out. The patients were helped out of bed in 12 to 36 hours after surgery with no orthotic device.

The patients in this series had "progressive" low back pain or lumbosacral instability, with severe continuous low back sprain and/or disability. Based on the fact that 127 of 131 patients were able to return to their original employment (time after surgery not given) with a stable *asymptomatic* lumbosacral spine, 97 per cent were reported to show excellent results. This is truly phenomenal. It is difficult to explain in view of the experience of most other surgeons. Surely, the construct alone would not be expected to make such a difference. Although we are skeptical and there are aspects of the report that can be criticized, we believe that this construct merits further evaluation.

Just as the surgical construct is not the crucial

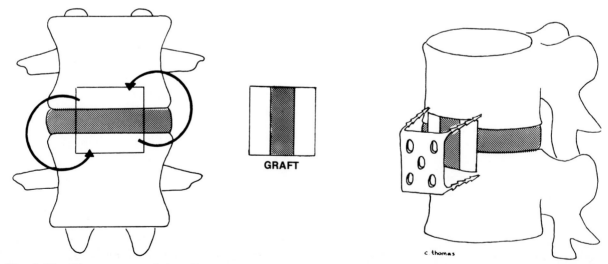

GRAFT

c thomas

Fig. 8-59. The purpose of this illustration is to show the Mario-Stone table plate. Each bone graft measures ¾ × ¾ × ¼ in. After they are rotated 90 degrees as shown, the placement is marrow to marrow. The individual dowels are separated either by remaining annulus fibrosus or silicone rubber spacers. The Mario-Stone table staple is 1 in long, ¾ in wide and has legs 1 in long, which are serrated. This appears to be a sound and stable fixation device and surgical construct. We do not believe, however, that it accounts for the astonishingly high figure of 97 per cent excellent results reported in 131 patients.

factor in lumbar spine fusion, the instrumentation implanted is not crucial. The main consideration is to determine the proper indications for arthrodesis and demonstrate the benefits. Evaluation of fixation devices, as with that of constructs, is obscured by the cloud of confusion about the advantages of and indications for arthrodesis. We find little indication that any of the systems of fixation consistently withstand the high magnitude of forces that are active in this region. There may be situations, however, when there is a need for some immediate postoperative stability. Depending upon the unique considerations for the patient involved, one may select one of the devices presented here or consider the use of methylmethacrylate.

TONGS AND TRACTION

The history of the use and development of tongs for the application of skeletal traction to the spine is interesting. The stimulus apparently was created in 1932, when a 22-year-old woman was in an automobile accident. She sustained, along with a number of other injuries, a compound fracture of the mandible and an open fracture dislocation of C2 on C3. The jaw injury obviated the usual head halter treatment of the dislocation. A consulting physician, Dr. Coleman, suggested to the attending physician, Dr. Crutchfield, that extension tongs be applied to the skull. The sharp points were removed from the extension tongs and they were inserted into the skull, held together by a heavy elastic band. The treatment was successful and the case was reported in 1933.[22a,23] The apparatus was subsequently modified for clinical use and came to be known as Crutchfield tongs.

Crutchfield Tongs

These are probably still the most commonly used tongs. They are simple, effective and easy to use. However, even in the hands of the experienced user they not infrequently slip out. There are two mechanical factors that may be helpful in preventing slippage. The first relates to the magnitude of the axial load. The location of the tongs and their mechanism of attachment is such that they simply should not be employed when large loads are to be applied. If the physician wishes to use up to a 20- or 25-kg (40–50-lb) weight to reduce a facet dislocation or to do a stretch test, it is better to use the Vinke tongs. The second factor involves the relationship of the axial force vector to the cranium at the site of implant of each of the pins (Fig. 8-60). This is best achieved by using the following guidelines: (1) Spread the tongs about 10 to 12 cm (4–5 in) apart for determining sites of insertion. Also use the approximation of the rope ring to the skull as a guideline, as shown in Figure 8-60B. (2) Since the preceding guideline may be affected by the shape of the cranium, we suggest these additional guidelines. Try to position the tongs such that the implanting pins are as close as possible to an angle of 90 degrees to the table of bones of the skull and the line of pull of the traction. The skull pin angle is the more important. (3) Check the tongs daily and tighten them only when they loosen.

In the sagittal plane it is recommended that the tongs be placed in line with the external auditory meatus. The ability to attain a flexed or extended position of the cervical spine through the choice of placement of the tongs in the sagittal plane is at best limited. First of all, there is a limitation of the possible points at which the tongs may be placed. Secondly, it is unlikely that the influence of this placement on flexion/extension would be very significant, and in the most optimal conditions, the influence would be limited to the upper cervical spine. We suggest that the direction of pull of the traction and the positioning of the shoulders are much more important factors in determining the flexion/extension position of the neck than is the site of tong insertion.

Vinke Tongs

These are the tongs of choice. They are more versatile, and they are safer. The versatility results from the fact that very large loads of 20 to 25 kg (40–50 lb) may be applied with much less risk of the tongs pulling out. Vinke tongs are safe because they are less likely to penetrate the skull or to pull out than are other tongs. They are an improvement over the Crutchfield tongs in

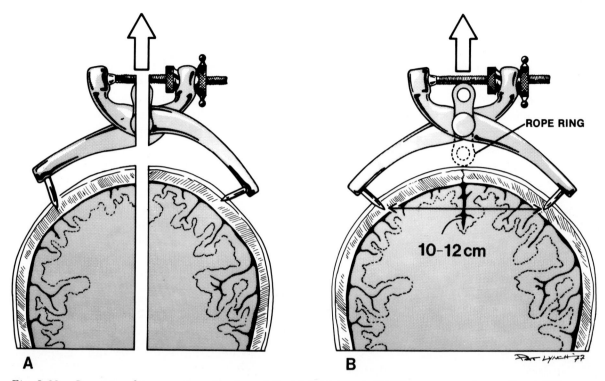

Fig. 8-60. Correct and incorrect positioning of Crutchfield tongs. *(A)* The tongs tend to pull out if they are placed such that either pin is aligned parallel to the line of pull *(left side)* or too close to the vertex of the skull; or, if they form an angle that approximates a 180-degree angle with the skull at the point of attachment *(right side)*. *(B)* The tongs should be spread 10 to 12 cm apart and the rope ring distance is used as a guideline. This tends to place the pin approximately perpendicular to the skull and avoids a parallel orientation with the major traction vector.

biomechanical design and instrumentation. The value of the design is shown in Figure 8-61. The pin attachments are both automatically placed at about 90 degrees to the line of pull and the table of the cranium at the site of implant. There is the added insurance against pullout, which comes from the flange mechanism that spreads out between the two tables of the skull. This gives added protection against penetration through the inner table and makes it impossible to pull the pin out without tearing through the outer table of the skull or twisting the flange mechanism back to its original position. This feature alone justifies our strong preference for this instrument over the Crutchfield tongs, which have been associated with death from brain abscess due to skull penetration by the pins.[119]

The Halo Apparatus

This device is responsible for a number of significant advancements in the surgical management of the spine.[79,80] It consists of a stainless steel ring with holes through which pins may be passed, implanted into the outer table of bones of the skull, and then fixed to the circumferential rim (halo). The device has numerous clinical advantages and uses. A discussion of prominent biomechanical characteristics follows.

Through its multiple attachment points, it is possible to gain excellent fixation of the cranium. This permits the application of large loads over a long period of time because alternate pin sites may be employed. We have found that it is useful in children who need rigid skull fixation because the bone of a child's skull is relatively softer and more elastic and therefore pin fixation of the skull is very difficult. The multiple points of attachment permitted with the halo apparatus reduces the stress at any one point (Fig. 8-62B). The multiple fixations allow for more precise control of the head in all three planes. This provides excellent indirect control of the cervical spine, which can be particularly helpful in a grossly unstable situation. With this apparatus, forces and moments can be applied to the spine to control flexion/extension, lateral bending, and axial rotation. The halo is a useful technique when one wishes to place the head and neck in the desired position with the patient awake. With this device, there are the options of simple skeletal traction, attachment to a plaster body jacket, to a fabricated plastic body jacket, or to a pelvic ring attached to the iliac bones.

In order to guard against penetration of the pins into the skull, the pins are inserted with a torque wrench, and the torque should not exceed 62.5 N cm (5 in lb) in children or 65 N cm (5.5 in lb) in adults.[62,79]

How Much Traction?

This is an extremely difficult problem which requires excellent clinical judgment and careful radiographic monitoring. Traction for pain and for diagnostic evaluation is discussed in Chapters 6 and 5, respectively.

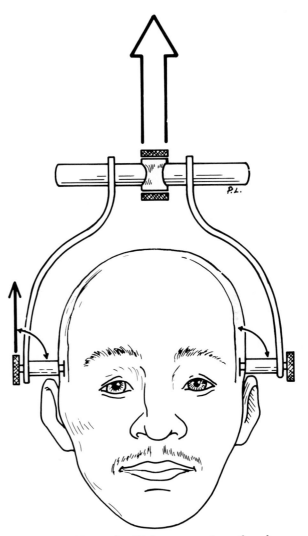

Fig. 8-61. We prefer Vinke tongs, since they have a superior design. The pins are inserted at an angle of 90 degrees to the major traction vector and 90 degrees to the surface of the cranium. The flange mechanism prevents the tongs from coming out from between the tables of the skull.

Here, traction is discussed with respect to immobilization of the spine and correction of a local or regional deformity.

Crutchfield suggested the guidelines shown in Table 8-4. His concern was that excessive distraction should not occur.

Table 8-4. Cervical Traction Weights for Treatment of Fractures and Dislocations at Various Levels in the Cervical Spine

Level of Injury	Minimum Weight kg (lb)	Maximum Weight kg (lb)
C1	2.3 (5)	4.5(10)
C2	2.7 (6)	5.4(12)
C3	3.6 (8)	6.8(15)
C4	4.5(10)	9.0(20)
C5	5.4(12)	11.3(25)
C6	6.8(15)	13.6(30)
C7	8.2(18)	15.9(35)

(Crutchfield, W. G.: Skeletal traction in the treatment of injuries to the cervical spine. J.A.M.A., *155*:129, 1954. Copyright © 1954, American Medical Association.)

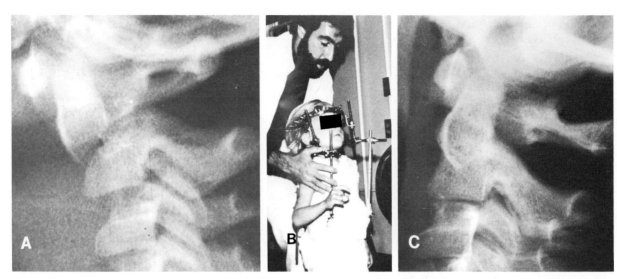

Fig. 8-62. The use of the Halo apparatus, employing multiple pin fixation to diminish individual pin stress in the relatively soft bone of a 4-year-old boy with a fractured odontoid. *(A)* The initial displaced fracture of the odontoid is shown. *(B)* Application of the halo apparatus with extra pin fixation. *(C)* Fracture after 10 weeks of immobilization.

Traction is sometimes used for fixation and not distraction, essentially as an anchor. This is the situation in which a patient has an injury that is not clinically unstable, but the patient needs to be held quiet with the spine protected from intrinsic muscles, loads imposed by gravity, movement, or low magnitude forces that might be applied from the outside.

The next level is that in which alignment must be attained or maintained against moderate physiologic or deforming forces. This requires more of a force and the amount of that force increases as the lesion moves caudally.

When a recalcitrant deformity must be overcome, as with scoliosis, kyphosis, or a fracture that is difficult to reduce, the ranges increase considerably. For the unique situation of a unilateral facet dislocation which is difficult to reduce, we suggest traction of up to one-third body weight, but not to exceed 32 kg (65 lb). For a summary of the traction guidelines, see Table 8-5. These figures are only guidelines. They should all be reduced by about 20 or 30 per cent if an antifriction device is placed under the patient. These figures are our recommendations based on various data sources in the literature and our own research and clinical experience. For any given clinical situation, the guidelines may be employed initially. Then, the traction is adjusted to fit the unique requirements of the individual patient. The adjustments are made with careful monitoring of the situation through checks for pain, neurologic status, and radiographic analysis.

Table 8–5. Suggested Guidelines for the Amount of Traction to Achieve Various Clinical Goals

REGION	ANCHOR	PHYSIOLOGIC ALIGNMENT	CORRECTION OF A DEFORMITY†
Cervical	4–8 kg (8–18 lb)	8–10 kg (18–22 lb)	10–28 kg (22–62 lb)
Upper thoracic	8–10 kg (18–22 lb)	10–15 kg (22–30 lb)	15–28 kg (30–62 lb)
Mid- and lower thoracic	10–15 kg (22–30 lb)	15–20 kg (30–44 lb)	15–28 kg (30–62 lb)
Lumbar*	10–15 kg (22–30 lb)	18–27 kg (40–60 lb)	23–36 kg (50–80 lb)

* Values were calculated for the lumbar region under the assumption that no antifriction device is employed.
† Reduction of difficult dislocation or fracture dislocation.

Part 5: An Analysis of the Mechanics of Spine Osteotomies

BASIC OSTEOTOMY

The basic goals in the use of osteotomy are to gain correction, to achieve and maintain clinical stability, and to avoid damage to vital structures. The ideal site for osteotomy from the geometrical and mechanical standpoint is at the apex of the curve of the deformity.

The basic design of spinal osteotomies has been that of a wedge cut through the posterior elements. The base of the wedge of the osteotomy should be in the direction in which the apex of the curve is pointing. The apex of the wedge should reach at least as far anteriorly as the center of motion about which the correction is to take place. Thus, the apex of the wedge should be at or close to the posterior longitudinal ligament (Fig. 8-63).

The size of the angle of the wedge is the same as the angular correction that will be achieved and usually is in the range of 40 to 60 degrees.[72] The structure that is the greatest distance away from the center of motion opposite the osteotomy on the concavity of the curve must be cut, broken, or deformed. Care should be taken to construct the osteotomy so that the centers of motion or the fulcrum about which the correction takes place is *not* behind the spinal canal, since the correctional rotation about the axes could cause excessive stretch and damage to the neural elements.[1] The literature shows that circumstances in which there is difficulty in rupturing the anterior ligamentous structures rarely occur. Some of the variations of the basic osteotomy and some of the relevant biomechanical factors are discussed.

CERVICAL AND CERVICOTHORACIC OSTEOTOMY

The actual site of deformity is generally in the cervicothoracic region. In terms of the pure mechanics, this is the most logical place to carry out the corrective osteotomy. This site, at the lower cervical spine below C6, is used to avoid the vertebral artery area. Operating in this area carries the high risk of spinal cord damage. When all the posterior elements are transected and the anterior elements are ruptured, a clinically unstable situation is produced.[51] Posterior wedge osteotomy and section of vertebral body from the posterior exposure with alternate side to side retraction of the spinal cord has been reported.[74] There is relatively little extra space for the neural elements in this region; therefore, the risk of damage either from displacement or surgical encroachment is high. For these reasons, in cervical osteotomies we suggest a halo device[98] or some method of obtaining immediate postoperative stability, such as internal wiring. It is also advantageous to design the osteotomy so that there is room for the unobstructed posterior displacement of the spinal cord (Fig. 8-64).[51,99,114] Thoracic spine osteotomies have also been carried out.[51] The considerations are essentially the same as for the cervical spine.

LUMBAR SPINE OSTEOTOMIES

In this region also there are problems of clinical instability and neural damage associated with osteotomy and the subsequent displacement of the spine. However, the risks are reduced because of the increased space for the neural elements and the relative clinical stability of the lumbar region. However, here too post-osteotomy instability has been reported.[51] With the exception of Briggs and Keates, who used Wilson plates,[13] most surgeons have used casts, traction, or recumbency rather than internal fixation for lumbar spine osteotomies. There have been a number of variations on the basic constructs described by Smith-Petersen.[101]

In the frontal plane, the osteotomy may be transverse or V-shaped. The latter design, originally suggested by Smith-Petersen, is preferable.

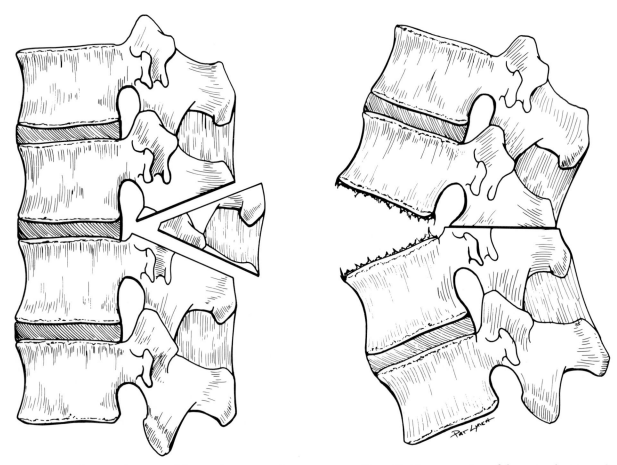

Fig. 8-63.   This is a diagram of the configuration of an osteotomy. It applies to any region of the spine but is probably safest in the lumbar region. The apex of the wedge is in the region of the posterior longitudinal ligament, and the angle at the apex is the same as the angle of the correction.

It provides good potential for correction and some post-osteotomy stability against anterior posterior translation and axial rotation.

Anterior surgery to release the anterior longitudinal ligament and the annulus in addition to the posterior osteotomy has been suggested.[63] The purpose is to control the correction and avoid any damage that may come from the relatively imprecise, directive, "bend until there is a resounding snap." Osteotomies at two or more levels have also been recommended to reduce the stress at one level and/or to gain additional correction.[72] There have also been modest variations relevant to the exact configuration of the osteotomy.

Some of the more significant variations are discussed here. Briggs and Keates emphasized the importance of foramenotomy of the posterior portion of the intervertebral foramen in addition to a portion of the pedicle to avoid nerve root encroachment at the time of correction following osteotomy. Adams recognized the advantages of doing the procedure with the patient in the lateral position (see the list below).[1] He also designed an apparatus with which to correct the deformity on the operating table with gradual, controlled application of three-point bending. This device is described in his publication and would be useful to any operating theater doing more than an occasional spinal osteotomy.

Advantages of the Lateral Position for Corrective Spinal Osteotomies*

Facilitates positioning of the grossly flexed patient
Facilitates administration of anaesthesia
Blood flows out rather than welling up
Eliminates injury risk to ankylosed cervical spine
Provides sturdier and more comfortable position for the surgeon

---

* As most patients who are treated for spinal osteotomy have severe ankylosing spondylitis, it is important to keep in mind the fact that they are primarily abdominal breathers, since their costovertebral joints are generally ankylosed. The value of protecting the cervical spine from injury in these patients is not theoretical, as one death has been reported from fracture dislocation in this region associated with lumbar spine osteotomy in the prone position.[1]

The overall mortality from spinal osteomoties is about 10 per cent.[51,66] The complications are listed below.

Complications from Spinal Osteotomy

Ruptured aorta or inferior vena cava
Paralytic ileus (superior mesenteric artery syndrome)
Cervical fracture or fracture dislocation
Nerve compression from vertebral subluxation
Death from postoperative cervical instability

There are other situations in which spinal osteotomies are indicated for kyphosis. Sharrard has described a procedure for congenital kyphosis in meningomyelocele.[96] Osteotomies have also been carried out in adolescents and adults with partial or complete paralysis associated with severe kyphosis. A variety of osteotomies have been performed for scoliosis associated with unilateral vertebral bars and hemivertebra. Sometimes in severe scoliosis, it is necessary to perform an osteotomy on a iatrogenic or spontaneously fused segment to gain correction with either halo pelvic or halo femoral distraction.* The basic principles previously discussed apply in virtually any corrective osteotomies. They are resection at the location of maximal deformity, protection and preservation of neural structures, and the establishment of adequate postoperative clinical stability, with internal or external fixation as needed.

---

* Personal communication, J. P. Kostuik, M.D.

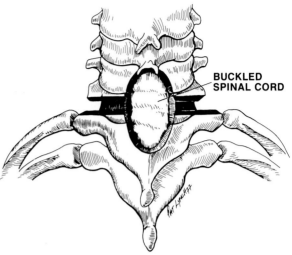

BUCKLED SPINAL CORD

Fig. 8-64. The Simmons construct for cervical osteotomy, in which there is also adequate laminectomy above and below to allow for any buckling or displacement of the cervical spine that may occur with the correction. The lateral resections are beveled toward each other so that opposing surfaces will be parallel and in apposition following extension osteotomy. (Modified from Simmons, E. H.: The surgical correction of flexion deformity of the cervical spine in ankylosing spondylitis. Clin. Orthop., 86:132, 1972).

CLINICAL BIOMECHANICS

Decompressions

It is essential to use all available clinical and radiographic information to localize the site of the offending pressure as accurately as possible.

The site of pressure must be identified in relation to the spinal cord, the vertebral body, and the midline. The most appropriate operation and surgical construct can then be selected.

There may be encroachment both anteriorly and posteriorly due to a contrecoup situation, in which there is primary pressure or encroachment on one side, which pushes the cord through the remaining free space and then against normal anatomic structures on the opposite side. Removal of the primary pressure initially is the best choice of surgical construct.

Anterior exposure is recommended for anterior structures, with the selection of the appropriate procedure to cover situations in which the offending pressure is behind the vertebral body.

The multilevel laminectomy is not the best choice for anterior pressure. It should be employed when the anterior approach is not possible. Laminectomy is the procedure of choice for primary posterior compression problems.

The considerations of decompression in the thoracic region are essentially the same for the other regions, except that posterior decompressions are less effective and more frequently show complications.

In the lumbar spine the majority of neural encroachments may be thoroughly decompressed from the posterior approach.

Spine Fusions

Spine arthrodesis is generally employed to reestablish strength, maintain correction, prevent progression of deformity, and alleviate or eliminate pain by altering the regional mechanics.

The choice of bone graft material for a particular surgical construct involves some biomechanical considerations. The ilium is generally preferable and probably the most versatile. However, the ribs offer some appealing advantages. The use of the fibula and tibia have some liabilities. In some situations, allografts may be equally as effective, with some practical advantages.

Positioning of bone grafts is important. If fusion is performed to provide clinical stability, then posterior positions with maximum leverage is important. If movement between the vertebral bodies is expected to affect the disc, then interbody placement of the graft is preferable.

The placement of a bone graft on the compression side *away* from the neutral axes is most effective in a surgical construct used to treat kyphosis. However, the longer the bone graft is, the more likely it is to succumb to buckling failure.

The extent of fusion depends upon the clinical goals that the surgical construct is designed to achieve. Generally, it is best to fuse to the first adjacent normal motion segment. With special

constructs in the treatment of major deformities, additional normal motion segments should be included. In kyphosis, all vertebrae in the deformity should be included.

As a first approximation, a reconstructive spine arthrodesis is carried out at the site of major destruction. If it is anterior, the reconstruction should be anterior; if it is posterior, the reconstruction should be posterior. There are exceptions.

Anterior occiput to C1 fusion is useful when the posterior route is not available. The transverse ligament should be intact to insure clinical stability.

Posterior ocp-C1 or C2 fusion may be achieved by a simple technique which can be clinically stabilized with a halo apparatus. A more complex and difficult wiring procedure is also available. The latter is useful when posterior elements are missing and immediate maximum stability is required.

Bilateral anterior screw fixation of the lateral masses provides good fixation of the atlanto-axial joint for arthrodesis.

Circumferential wiring of an iliac bone graft between the posterior elements of C1 and C2 (Brooks construct) provides a stable construct for atlanto-axial fusion. We suggest that this is the construct of choice when posterior fusion of C1-C2 is indicated.

Anterior cervical interbody fusion with the horseshoe graft (Smith-Robinson construct) removes the disc, exposes the medial and lateral aspects of the interspace, enlarges the neural foramen, elongates the yellow ligament, and resists collapse. We suggest this operation as the procedure of choice for cervical spondylosis.

Anterior cervical trough fusion (Bailey-Badgley construct) removes all or part of the intervertebral disc, exposes midline portions of the cord behind the vertebral body, can enlarge the interspace and elongate the yellow ligament, resists collapse, provides immediate postoperative stability even in some difficult situations, and conveniently fuses one or more motion segments.

Anterior dowel interbody fusion (Cloward construct) removes all or part of the intervertebral disc, exposes midline posterior cord, has risk of collapse.

Anterior keystone interbody fusion removes all or part of the intervertebral disc, exposes the midline portion of cord behind the vertebral body, can enlarge the neural foramen and elongate the yellow ligament, and provides a large surface area for contact. This construct in biomechanical tests did not extrude its graft before fracture and complete disruption of the spine. We suggest this procedure followed by the modified Bailey-Badgley construct as the surgical constructs of choice for multilevel anterior fusions.

The notched fibula graft construct is designed to prevent extrusion and collapse. It is useful for multilevel fusions. The spiked horseshoe or keystone construct may be effectively utilized to replace an excised vertebral body.

Posterior cervical spine fusion may have its immediate postoperative stability augmented by posterior wiring and the use of rib, fibula, or tibia bone graft.

Posterior facet fusion is a very useful construct for situations in which immediate stability is important and the laminae have been removed.

The use of rib grafts in an anterolateral or lateral trough provides a biomechanically sound construct for thoracic spine fusions associated with decompressions.

Anterior interbody fusion of the lumbar spine is rarely required. The benefits overshadow the liabilities only when the clinical goals cannot be achieved with a posterior arthrodesis.

The anterolateral trough graft technique is a useful procedure for gaining considerable immediate postoperative stability, especially in resisting sagittal plane translation.

The interbody fusion can also be carried out from the posterior approach.

With regards to lumbar spine fusions, there do not appear to be any significant biomechanical advantages to the so-called "H" graft. Posterolateral fusion (transverse processes) is probably the most advantageous, and we recommend it as the construct of choice. Lumbar spine fusion for pain, other than in patients with a diagnosis of spondylolisthesis, is not generally recommended regardless of the surgical construct employed.

Spinal cord function and clinical stability can be maintained in the face of a slow-growing tumor through the use of multiple, massive fusions around the lesion.

With the use of sound biomechanical principles in conjunction with the proper implants and bone graft configurations, the vertebral column may be reconstructed following total spondylectomy.

The progress of a fusion mass following surgery may be divided into four stages, which may be correlated with patient management and adjusted according to the unique considerations of each patient.

Surgical Constructs Employing Methylmethacrylate

Methylmethacrylate has no adhesive qualities but forms its attachment to bone through interdigitation with regional bone spicules.

Methylmethacrylate is most effective in resisting compressive loads. Its ability to resist tensile loads is improved by the incorporation of wire or wire mesh.

Methylmethacrylate is used surgically in the spine as a spacer, an internal splint, or as a fixation device.

Biomechanical study of a methylmethacrylate surgical construct suggests that the weak link is the attachment of the cement to the bone.

A conservative approach to the use of methylmethacrylate is recommended.

A posterior construct is suggested for the achievement of maximum immediate clinical stability using methylmethacrylate. A modification for long range stability is also described.

Biomechanical Considerations in the Art and Science of Spine Instrumentation

Using wires of adequate tensile strength is the most important factor. There are some advantages in using twisted wire.

Stainless steel mesh wire is recommended for use with methylmethacrylate that will undergo tensile loading.

Screw fixation appears to work in upper cervical spine fixations; however, in the lumbar spine the loads are likely to be too great for screws to be effective.

The Gruca-Weiss springs have a modest correcting effect on a kyphotic curve and apply a significant amount of compression between the vertebrae that are spanned.

The Harrington compression rods have a net correctional influence on a kyphotic deformity through a three-point bending mechanism. This device is useful in the treatment of a clinically unstable kyphotic deformity.

Distraction Harrington rods, because of their relative stiffness, are the most effective method of *correcting* post-traumatic kyphotic deformity when clinical stability is present.

An analytical comparison of the two Harrington systems suggests that the distraction rod is the system of choice to correct a traumatic kyphotic deformity. However, in the presence of gross instability the compression system provides some stability and is therefore preferable.

It is sometimes advantageous to use a Harrington distraction rod in combination with a Harrington compression rod.

A new technique using paired Harrington distraction rods was shown to provide a mechanical advantage in kyphotic deformities that are difficult to correct.

Internal fixation devices in the lumbar spine are likely to fail because of the large forces active in this region. In some special circumstances, it may be necessary to provide crucial, immediate postoperative stability.

Crutchfield tongs are simple and easy to insert. They may pull out, especially if large traction forces of 20 kg or more must be applied.

Vinke tongs are preferable from both the surgical and biomechanical standpoint.

The halo apparatus provides the best available mechanical control of the spine by external means.

Axial traction is used in the spine to anchor, to gain alignment resisted by physiologic forces, or to correct resistant deformity. Guidelines for starting traction loads in different regions of the spine are provided.

Spine Osteotomies

The basic spine osteotomy consists of removal of a wedge taken from the posterior elements; the apex of the wedge is at or near the posterior longitudinal ligament. In the frontal plane, the wedge is V-shaped.

In the cervical region, the osteotomy should include prophylactic decompression and postoperative halo fixation.

There are significant advantages in the use of the side lying position for lumbar spine osteotomy.

NOTES

[A] There is some confusion and disagreement about terminology with regard to laminectomy. We use laminotomy to indicate the removal of a portion of a given lamina. Complete laminectomy or bilateral laminectomy indicates removal of the spinous process and the entire lamina on each side of it. Hemilaminectomy or unilateral laminectomy indicates removal of the lamina on one side of the spinous process only.

[B] The biomechanical analyses are based upon the assumptions that the Harrington rods are not *permanently* bent during the operation, and the compression rods do not have multiple hooks. The clinical studies, in which rods have been bent to accommodate a stiff curve or compression rods are used with multiple hooks, may significantly differ from the conclusions of our analysis.

[C] This is a good construct designed by K. J. Keggi; however, the authors now recommend something more similar to the construct shown in Figure 8-49, without steel mesh placed over the laminectomy site.

CLASSIFICATION OF REFERENCES

Decompressions 3, 12, 18, 28, 65
Spine fusions
  Clinical
    Occipitocervical 24, 42, 78
    Atlanto-axial 7, 14, 29, 31, 33, 35, 37, 48, 56, 57, 60, 70, 130
    Lower cervical 5, 18, 22, 28, 34, 86, 89, 99, 100, 103, 115, 116, 123, 125, 130, 48, 56
    Thoracic 4, 9, 11, 29, 40, 56, 60, 88, 107, 108, 117, 128, 130
    Lumbar 2, 6, 8, 9, 10, 17, 29, 40, 44, 47, 49, 53, 54, 55, 56, 60, 61, 71, 73, 76, 77, 90, 97, 104, 105, 111, 112, 113, 118, 127, 130
  Bone grafts 9, 15, 16, 27, 39, 52, 69, 94, 109, 122, 129
  Biomechanics 41, 87, 99, 122, 124
Methylmethacrylate stabilization
  Clinical 21, 26, 43, 58, 59, 81, 95, 102
  Biomechanics 19, 36, 68, 83, 85, 93

REFERENCES

1. Adams, J. C.: Technique, dangers and safeguards in osteotomy of the spine. J. Bone Joint Surg., *34B*:226, 1952. (*This work is highly recommended for any one undertaking this procedure. The principles of the operation are well presented and the technique clearly illustrated.*)

2. Albee, F. H.: Transplantation of a portion of the tibia into the spine for Pott's disease. A preliminary report. J.A.M.A., 57:885, 1911.

3. Alexander, J.: Problems associated with the use of the knee–chest position for operations on the lumbar intervertebral discs. J. Bone Joint Surg., *55B*:279, 1973.

4. Amed, K. B., et al.: Anterior spine surgery in the treatment of kyphotic spine deformity. Scoliosis Res. Soc., Ottawa, 1976.

5. Bailey, R. W., and Badgley, C. E.: Stabilization of the cervical spine by anterior fusion. J. Bone Joint Surg., *42A*:565, 1960. (*The original description of the classic Bailey-Badgley operation.*)

6. Baker, L. D., and Hoyt, W. A.: The use of interfacet vitallium screws in the Hibbs fusion. South. Med. J., *41*:419, 1948.

7. Barbour, J. R.: Screw fixation in fracture of the odontoid process. South Aust. Clin., 5:20, 1971. (*Brief description of a unique construct with little clinical information about patients' complications and follow-up.*)

8. Bosworth, D. M.: Technique of spinal fusion in the lumbosacral region by the double clothespin graft (distraction graft: "H" graft) and results. *In* American Acad. of Orthopaedic Surgeons: Instructional Course Lectures, vol. 9. Ann Arbor, J. W. Edwards, 1952.

9. Bosworth, D. M., Wright, H. A., Fielding, J. W., and Goodrich, E. R.: A study in the use of bank bone for spine fusion in tuberculosis. J. Bone Joint Surg., *35A*:329, 1953.

10. Boucher, H. H.: A method of spinal fusion. J. Bone Joint Surg., *41B*:248, 1959.

11. Bradford, D. S., Moe, J. H., Montalvo, F. J., and Winter, R. B.: Scheuermann's kyphosis. Results of surgical treatment by posterior spine arthrodesis in twenty-two patients. J. Bone Joint Surg., *57A*:439, 1975.

12. Brieg, A.: Biomechanics of the Central Nervous System: Some Basic Normal and Pathological Phenomena. Stockholm, Almquist & Wiksell, 1960. (*An important, thorough and very well illustrated presentation of the biomechanical anatomy of the spinal cord and nerve roots.*)

13. Briggs, H., Keates, S., and Schlesinger, P. T.: Wedge osteotomy of spine with bilateral intervertebral foraminotomy: Correction of flexion deformity in five cases of ankylosing arthritis of spine. J. Bone Joint Surg., 29:1075, 1947.

14. Brooks, A. L. and Jenkins, E. G.: Atlanto-axial arthrodesis by the wedge compression method. J. Bone Joint Surg., *60A*:279, 1978.

15. Burwell, R. G.: The fate of bone grafts. *In* Apley, A. G. (ed.): Recent Advances in Orthopaedics. London, J & A Churchill, 1969. (*A thorough and comprehensive review of the important information on bone grafts.*)

16. ————: The fate of freeze-dried bone allografts. Transplant. Proc. [Suppl.], *1*:95, 1976.

17. Calandruccio, R. A., and Benton, B. F.: Anterior lumbar fusion. Clin. Orthop., *35*:63, 1964.

17a. Callahan, R. A., et al.: Cervical facet fusion for control of instability following laminectomy. J. Bone Joint Surg., *59A*:991, 1977.

18. Cattell, H. S., and Clark, G. L.: Cervical kyphosis and instability following multiple laminectomies in children. J. Bone Joint Surg., *49A*:713, 1967. (*A useful modification of the Bailey-Badgley construct.*)

19. Charnley, J.: The bonding of prosthesis to bone by cement. J. Bone Joint Surg., *46B*:518, 1964.

20. Chrisman, O. D., and Snook, G. A.: The problem of refracture of the tibia. Clin. Orthop., *60*:217, 1968.

21. Cleveland, D.: Interspace reconstruction and spinal stabilization after disc removal. Lancet., *76*:327, 1956. (*Describes placement of cement between vertebral bodies at the time of laminectomy and disc excision.*)

22. Cloward, R. B.: New method of diagnosis and treatment of cervical disc disease. Clin. Neurosurg., 8:93, 1962.

22a. Crutchfield, W. A.: Skeletal traction for dislocation of cervical spine. Report of a case. South. Surg., 2:156, 1933.

23. Crutchfield, W. G.: Skeletal traction in the treatment of injuries to the cervical spine. J.A.M.A., *155*:29, 1954.

24. DeAndrade, J. R., and MacNab, I.: Anterior occipitocervical fusion using an extra-pharyngeal exposure. J. Bone Joint Surg., *51A*:1621, 1969.

25. Dubuc, F.: Knodt rod grafting. Orthop. Clin. North Am., 6:283, 1975.

26. Dunn, E. J.: The role of methylmethacrylate in the stabilization and replacement of tumors of the cervical spine. Spine, 2:15, 1977. (*An informative resume of the current uses, advantages and problems.*)

27. Enneking, W. F., Burchardt, H., Puhl, J., and Piotrowski, G.: Physical and biological aspects of repair in dog cortical-bone transplants. J. Bone Joint Surg., *57A*:237, 1975.

28. Eyring, E. J., Murry, W. R., Inman, V. T., and Boldrey, E.: Simultaneous anterior and posterior approach to the cervical spine. Reduction and fixation of an old fracture-dislocation with cord compromise. J. Bone Joint Surg., *46A*:33, 1964.

29. Fang, H. S. Y., Ong, G. B., and Hodgson, A. R.: Anterior spinal fusion. The operative approaches. Clin. Orthop., *35*:16, 1964.

30. Fielding, J. W., and Griffin, P. P.: Os odontoideum: An acquired lesion. J. Bone Joint Surg., *56A*:187, 1974.

31. Fielding, J. W., Hawkins, R. J., and Ratzan, S. A.: Spine fusion for atlanto-axial instability. J. Bone Joint Surg., *58A*:400, 1976. (*A useful review of the indications and results of arthrodesis of C1 to C2.*)

32. Frankel, V. H., and Burstein, A. H.: Load capacity of tubular bone. *In* Biomechanics and Related Bioengineering Topics. Proc. Glasgow Symposium, Sept., 1964. Oxford, Pergamon Press, 1965.

33. Fried, L. C.: Atlanto-axial fracture-dislocations failure of posterior C1 to C2 fusion. J. Bone Joint Surg., *55B*:490, 1973.

34. Friedlaender, G. E., Johnson, R. M., Brand, R. M., and Southwick, W. O.: Treatment of pathological fractures. Conn. Med., *39*:765, 1975.

35. Gallie, W. E.: Fractures and dislocations of the cervical spine. Am. J. Surg., *46*:495, 1939.

36. Greenwald, S. A., and Wilde, A. H.: Some observations on the interface strength of bone cement. Biomech. Lab. Res. Rep. 002-74. Cleveland, The Cleveland Clinic Foundation, 1974.

37. Griswold, D. M., et al.: Atlanto-axial fusion for instability. J. Bone Joint Surg., *60A*:285, 1978.

38. Gruca, A.: Protocol of the 41st Congress of Indian Orthopaedics and Traumatology. Bologna, 1956.

39. Haas, S. L.: Study of fusion of the spine with particular reference to articular facets. J. Bone Joint Surg., *18*:717, 1936.

40. Hall, J.: The Anterior Approach to Spinal Deformities. A symposium on current pediatric problems. Orthop. Clin. North Am., *3*:8, 1972.

41. Hallock, H., Francis, K. C., and Jones, J. B.: Spine fusion in young children. J. Bone Joint Surg., *39A*:481, 1957. *(A carefully executed and well documented study of the effects of posterior spine fusion on vertebral growth in children.)*

42. Hamblen, D. L.: Occipital-cervical fusion, indications, technique and results. J. Bone Joint Surg., *49B*:33, 1967.

43. Hamby, W. B., and Glaser, H. J.: Replacement of spinal intervertebral discs with locally polymerizing methylmethacrylate: Experimental study of effects upon tissues and report of a small clinical series. Journal of Neurosurgery, *16*:311, 1959. *(Of historical interest.)*

44. Harmon, P. H.: End results from lower lumbar-spine vertebral body fusions for the disc syndromes. Carried out by an abdominal extraperitoneal approach. J. Bone Joint Surg., *41A*:1355, 1959.

45. Hastings, C. G. A., and Reynolds, M. T.: Lumbo-sacral fusion with spring fixation. J. Bone Joint Surg., *57B*:283, 1975.

46. Helfet, A. J.: Spinal osteotomy. S. Afr. Med. J., *26*:773, 1952.

47. Henderson, E.: Results of the surgical treatment of spondylolis. Thesis. J. Bone Joint Surg., *48A*:619, 1966. *(A good historical and etiological review of the problem and its surgical management.)*

48. Henry, A. K.: Extensile Exposure. Baltimore, Williams & Wilkins, 1963.

49. Hensinger, R. N., Lang, J. R., and MacEwen, G. D.: Surgical management of spondylolisthesis in children and adolescents. Spine, *1*:207, 1976. *(A useful and comprehensive review of the treatment of spondylolisthesis in this age group.)*

50. Henzel, J. H., Mohr, G. C., and vonGierke, H. E.: Reappraisal of biodynamic implications of human ejections. Aerospace Med., *39*:231, 1968.

51. Herbert, J. J.: Vertebral osteotomy for kyphosis, especially in Marie-Strumpell arthritis. A report on fifty cases. J. Bone Joint Surg., *41A*:291, 1959.

52. Hert, J., Pribylova, E., and Liskova, M.: Reaction of bone to mechanical stimuli. Part 3: Microstructure of

compact bone of rabbit tibia after intermittent loading. Acta Anat., *82*:211, 1972.

53. Hibbs, R. A.: An operation for progressive spinal deformities. A preliminary report of three cases from the service of the Orthopaedic Hospital. New York State Med. J., *93*:1013, 1911. *(The original.)*

54. Hodgson, A. R., and Wong, S. K.: A description of a technique and evaluation of results in anterior spinal fusion for deranged intervertebral disc and spondylolisthesis. Clin. Orthop., *56*:133, 1968. *(A detailed account of an extensive experience with the procedure.)*

55. Humphries, A. W., Hawk, W. A., and Berndt, A. L.: Anterior interbody fusion of lumbar vertebrae: A surgical technique. Surg. Clin. North Am., *41*:1685, 1961.

56. Johnson, R. M., and Southwick, W. O.: Surgical approaches to the spine. Rothmann, R. H., and Simeone, F. A. (eds.): The Spine. Philadelphia, Saunders, 1975. *(Detailed clinical instructions for a number of surgical techniques to be used on the spine.)*

57. Kebish, P. A., and Keggi, K. J.: Mechanical problems of the dowel graft in anterior cervical fusion. J. Bone Joint Surg., *49A*:198, 1967.

58. Keggi, K. J., Southwick, W. O., and Keller, D. J.: Stabilization of the spine using methylmethacrylate. J. Bone Joint Surg., *58A*:738, 1976.

59. Kelley, D. L., Alexander, E., Davis, C. H., and Smith, J. M.: Acrylic fixation of atlanto-axial dislocations. Technical note. J. Neurosurg., *36*:366, 1972. *(This paper describes the use of cement essentially as an internal splint wired to the vertebra.)*

60. Kemp, H. B. S., Jackson, J. D., Jeremiah, J. D., and Cook, J.: Anterior fusion of the spine for infective lesions in adults. J. Bone Joint Surg., *55B*:715, 1973.

61. King, D.: Internal fixation for lumbosacral fusion. J. Bone Joint Surg., *30A*:560, 1948.

62. Kopits, S. E., and Steingass, M. H.: Experience with the "halo-cast" in small children. Surg. Clin. North Am., *50*:935, 1970. *(Helpful reference for those using the halo apparatus for children.)*

63. LaChapelle, E. H.: Osteotomy of the lumbar spine for correction of kyphosis in a case of ankylosing spondylitis. J. Bone Joint Surg., *28*:851, 1946.

64. Lambert, K. L.: The weight-bearing function of the fibula. A strain gauge study. J. Bone Joint Surg., *53A*:507, 1971. *(A neat and convincing study.)*

65. LaRocca, H.: The Laminectomy membrane. Studies in its evolution, characteristics, effects and prophylaxis in dogs. J. Bone Joint Surg., *56B*:545, 1974.

66. Law, W. A.: Surgical treatment of rheumatic disease. J. Bone Joint Surg., *34B*:215, 1952.

67. Leidholdt, J. D., et al.: Evaluation of late spinal deformities with fracture-dislocations of the dorsal and lumbar spine in paraplegics. Paraplegia, 7:16, 1969.

68. Linder, L.: Reaction of bone to the acute chemical trauma of cement. J. Bone Joint Surg., *59A*:82, 1977.

69. Liskova, M., and Hert, J.: Reaction of bone to mechanical stimuli. Part 2. Periosteal and endosteal reaction of tibial diaphysis in rabbits to intermittent loading. Folia Morphol., *19*:301, 1971.

70. McGraw, R. W., and Rusch, R. M.: Atlanto-axial arthrodesis. J. Bone Joint Surg., *55B*:482, 1973.

71. MacKenzie, A. B.: Fusion in flexion. Orthop. Clin. North Am., 6:289, 1975.

72. McMaster, P. E.: Osteotomy of the spine for fixed flexion

deformity. J. Bone Joint Surg., *44A*:1207, 1962. (*A well presented overview of the problem summarizing the not very extensive experience up to that time.*)

73. MacNab, I., and Dall, D.: The blood supply of the lumbar spine and its application to the technique of intertransverse lumbar fusion. J. Bone Joint Surg., *53B*:628, 1971. (*A very informative study important to any surgeon operating in this region.*)

74. Mason, C., Cozen, L., and Adelstein, L.: Surgical correction of flexion deformity of cervical spine. Calif. Med., 79:244, 1953.

75. Meyer, P. R., Pinzur, M., Lautenschlasger, E., and Dobozi, W. R.: Measurement of internal fixation device support—Thoracic lumbar spine. Scientific Exhibit. Am. Acad. Orthop. Surg., Las Vegas, 1977.

76. Nachemson, A. L.: Comment. Orthop. Clin. North Am., 6:290, 1975.

77. Newman, P. H.: Surgical treatment for derangement of the lumbar spine. J. Bone Joint Surg., *55B*:7, 1973. (*A comprehensive and concise review of this topic, recommended reading.*)

78. Newman, P. H., and Sweetnam, R.: Occipito-cervical fusion. An operative technique and its indications. J. Bone Joint Surg., *51B*:423, 1969. (*This work includes a discussion of the pros and cons of ocp-C1-C2 vs. C1-C2 and also some expectations about probable changes in range of motion.*)

79. Nickel, V. L., Perry, J., and Garrett, A.: The halo. J. Bone Joint Surg., *50A*:1400, 1968 (*A comprehensive review of the technique and use of this apparatus.*)

80. O'Brien, J. P.: The halo-pelvic apparatus; A clinical, bioengineering anatomical study. Acta Orthop. Scand. 163 [Suppl.], 1975. (*A most informative work, highly recommended for anyone using the halo pelvic apparatus.*)

81. Ono, K., and Tada, K.: Metal prosthesis of the cervical vertebrae. J. Neurosurg., 42:562, 1975. (*An ingenious device to increase the safety, ease, and effectiveness of the use of methylmethacrylate.*)

82. Panjabi, M. M., and White, A. A.: Biomechanical analysis of Gruca-Weiss and Harrington instrumentation in the treatment of kyphosis. To be published.

83. Panjabi, M M., Hopper, W., White, A. A., and Keggi, K. J.: Posterior spine stabilization with methylmethacrylate. Biomechanical testing of a surgical specimen. Spine, 2:241, 1977.

84. Penning, L.: Functional pathology of the cervical spine. Amsterdam, N. Y., Excerpta Medical Foundation, 1968. (*A highly recommended monograph for the basic clinical radiography of the cervical spine.*)

85. Reckling, F. W., and Dillon, W. L.: The bone-cement interface temperature during total joint replacement. J. Bone Joint Surg., 59A:80, 1977.

86. Robinson, R. A., and Southwick, W. O.: Surgical approaches to the cervical spine. *In* American Academy of Orthopaedic Surgeons: Instructional Course Lectures, vol. 17. St. Louis, C. V. Mosby, 1960.

87. Rolander, S. D.: Motion of the lumbar spine with special reference to stabilizing effect of posterior fusion. Acta Orthop. Scand. Suppl., 90:1966.

88. Rose, G. K., Owen, R., and Saunderson, J. M.: Transplantation of rib with blood supply for the stabilization of a spinal kyphos. J. Bone Joint Surg., *57B*:1112, 1975.

89. Rosenweig, N.: "The get up and go" treatment of acute

unstable injuries of the middle and lower cervical spine. J. Bone Joint Surg., *56B*:392, 1974.

90. Rothmann, R. H.: Comment. Orthop. Clin. North Am., 6:297, 1975.

91. Roy, L., and Gibson, D. A.: Cervical spine fusions in children. Clin. Orthop., 73:146, 1970. (*Good documentation of the absence of growth problems associated with arthrodesis in children.*)

92. Ruff, S.: Brief acceleration: Less than one second. German aviation medicine World War I. *1*:584, 1950. Department of the Air Force, Washington.

93. Saha, S., Taitsman, J. P., Johnson, T. R., and Albright, J. A.: Metal reinforced bone cement I: tensile behavior. Proceedings of the Fourth New England Bioengineering Conference. Pergamon Press, New York, 1976.

94. Schneider, J. R., and Bright, R. W.: Anterior cervical fusion using preserved bone allografts. Transplant. Proc. [Suppl.] *1*:73, 1976.

95. Scoville, W. B., Palmer, A. H., Samra, K., and Chong, G.: The use of acrylic plastic for vertebral replacement on fixation in metastatic disease of the spine. Technical note. J. Neurosurg., 27:274, 1969.

96. Sharrard, W. J. W.: Spinal osteotomy for congenital kyphosis in myelomeningocele. J. Bone Joint Surg., *50B*:466, 1968.

97. Sijbrandij, S.: The value of anterior interbody vertebral fusion in the treatment of lumbosacral insufficiency with special reference to spondylolisthesis. Acta Chir. Neerland., 14:37, 1962. (*This is an informative and well presented review of the major considerations in the treatment of spondylolisthesis. The study also includes a precise exposition of the surgical construct.*)

98. Simmons, E. H.: The surgical correction of flexion deformity of the cervical spine in ankylosing spondylitis. Clin. Orthop., 86:132, 1972. (*Explanation of technique carried out under local anesthesia in the sitting position.*)

99. Simmons, E. H., and Bhalla, S. K.: Anterior cervical discectomy and fusion. A clinical and biomechanical study with eight-year follow-up. J. Bone Joint Surg., *51B*:225, 1969. (*An informative clinical biomechanical analysis of this surgical procedure.*)

100. Smith, G. W., and Robinson, R. A.: The treatment of certain cervical spine disorders by anterior removal of the intervertebral disc and interbody fusion. J. Bone Joint Surg., *40A*:607, 1958.

101. Smith-Petersen, M. N., Larson, C. B., and Aufranc, O. E.: Osteotomy of the spine for correction of flexion deformity in rheumatoid arthritis. J. Bone Joint Surg., 27:1, 1945. (*The introductory description offers some useful technical suggestions.*)

102. Spence, W. T.: Internal plastic splint and fusion for stabilization of the spine (letter to the editor). Clin. Orthop., 92:325, 1973. (*This work describes the use of splint with attachment through horizontal plastic bar through base of spinous process.*)

103. Stauffer, E. S.: Fracture-dislocations of the cervical spine instability and recurrent deformity following treatment by anterior interbody fusion. J. Bone Joint Surg., 59A:45, 1977.

104. Stauffer, R. N., and Coventry, M. B.: Anterior interbody lumbar spine fusion: Analysis of Mayo Clinic Series. J. Bone Joint Surg., *54A*:756, 1972. (*A thorough infor-*

mative, well documented clinical review with little resultant enthusiasm for the procedure.)

105. ———: Posterolateral lumbar-spine fusion: Analysis of Mayo Clinic Series. J. Bone Joint Surg., *54A:*1195, 1972. (*A detailed account of a broad experience with this particular method of arthrodesis.*)

106. Stauffer, E. S., and Neil, J. L.: Biomechanical analysis of structural stability of internal fixation in fractures of the thoracolumbar spine. Clin. Orthop., *112:*159, 1975. (*A useful biomechanical analysis.*)

107. Stener, B.: Complete removal of three vertebrae for gaint-cell tumor. J. Bone Joint Surg., *53B:*278, 1971.

108. ———: Total spondylectomy in chondrosarcoma arising from the seventh thoracic vertebra. J. Bone Joint Surg., *53B:*288, 1971. (*A clearly described surgical resection and reconstruction. Useful reading for the surgeon who plans extensive vertebral resection.*)

109. Stringa, G., and Mignani, G.: Microradiographic investigation of bone grafts in man. Acta Orthop. Scand. Suppl., *99:*1, 1967. (*An excellent documentation of the physical and biological processes involved in the fate of bone grafts in a variety of clinical settings.*)

110. Thompson, W. A. L., and Ralston, E. L.: Pseudoarthrosis following spine fusion. J. Bone Joint Surg., *31A:*400, 1949.

111. Thompson, W. A. L., Gristina, A. G., and Healy, W. A.: Lumbosacral spine fusion. A method of bilateral posterolateral fusion combined with a Hibbs fusion. J. Bone Joint Surg., *56A:*1643, 1974.

112. Truckly, G., and Thompson, A. L.: Posterior lateral fusion of the lumbosacral spine. J. Bone Joint Surg., *44A:*505, 1962.

113. ———: Posteriorlateral fusions 14 years' experience with a salvage procedure for failures of spine fusion. To be published.

114. Urist, M. R.: Osteotomy of the cervical spine. Report of case of ankylosing rheumatoid spondylitis. J. Bone Joint Surg., *40A:*833, 1958. (*Initial description of procedure in sitting position with local anesthesia.*)

115. Verbiest, H.: Anterolateral operations for fractures and dislocations in the middle and lower parts of the cervical spine. J. Bone Joint Surg., *51A:*1489, 1969. (*A comprehensive clinical documentation of the management of 47 patients.*)

116. ———: Anterolateral operations for fractures or dislocations of the cervical spine due to injuries or previous surgical interventions. Clin. Neurosurg., *20:*334, 1973.

117. Wagner, D., et al.: Surgical management of Scheuermann's kyphosis. Scoliosis Res. Soc., Ottawa, 1976.

118. Watkins, M. B.: Posterior lateral fusion in pseudathrosis and posterior element defects of the lumbosacral spine. Clin. Orthop., *35:*80, 1964.

119. Weisl, H.: Unusual complications of skull caliper traction. J. Bone Joint Surg., *54B:*143, 1972.

120. Weiss, M.: Dynamic spine alloplasty (spring loading corrective device) after fracture and spinal cord injury. Clin. Orthop., *112:*150, 1975.

121. Werlinich, M.: Anterior interbody fusion and stabilization with metal fixation. Int. Surg., *57:*269, 1974. (*An optimistic, intriguing report of a promising surgical construct and fixation device.*)

122. White, A. A., and Hirsch, C.: An experimental study of the immediate load bearing capacity of some commonly used iliac bone grafts. Acta Orthop. Scand., *42:*482, 1971.

123. White, A. A., et al.: Relief of pain by anterior cervical spine fusion for spondylosis. J. Bone Joint Surg., *55A:*525, 1973.

124. White, A. A., Jupiter, J., Southwick, W. O., and Panjabi, M. M.: An experimental study of the immediate load bearing capacity of three surgical constructions for anterior spine fusions. Clinical Orthopaedics, *91:*21, 1973.

124a. White, A. A., Panjabi, M. M., and Thomas, C. L.: The clinical biomechanics of kyphotic deformities. Clin. Orthop., *128:*8, 1977.

125. Whitecloud, T. S., and LaRocca, H.: Fibula strut graft in reconstructive surgery of the spine. Spine, *1:*33, 1976. (*A well illustrated and candid exposition and review.*)

126. Wilson, P. D., and Straub, L. R.: Lumbosacral fusion with metallic-plate fixation. *In* American Academy of Orthopaedic Surgeons: Instructional Course Lectures, vol. 9. Ann Arbor, J. W. Edwards, 1952.

127. Wiltberger, B. R.: Intervertebral body fusion by the use of posterior bone dowel. Clin. Orthop., *35:*69, 1964. (*An example of a precise description of a surgical construct.*)

128. Winter, R. B., Moe, J. H., and Wang, J. F.: Congenital kyphosis. Its natural history and treatment as observed in a study of one-hundred thirty patients. J. Bone Joint Surg., *55A:*223, 1973.

129. Wolff, J.: Das Gesetz der Transformation der Knochen. Berlin, Hirschwald, 1892.

130. Wu, K. K.: Surgical techniques for arthrodesis of two to four adjacent spinal vertebrae throughout the entire spinal column. Henry Ford Hosp. Med. J., *23:*39, 1975. (*A superb bibliography on virtually all the well known spine fusions.*)

Appendix: Glossary

Introduction

This glossary contains most of the terms and engineering concepts that are applicable to orthopaedic biomechanics. The authors feel that it provides a thorough understanding of the material presented in this book and of other literature on the subject.

The material here is presented in a way that is useful, understandable, and palatable to the clinician. The term is first defined in scientific prose, and units of measurement are given if applicable. This is followed by an explanation of the term, a familiar lay example, and an orthopaedic example in most cases. Mathematical formulas have been presented in the Explanatory Notes, along with an occasional discussion.

When units of measure are given, the new S.I. (Systeme International d'Unites) system has been adopted as a rule, while the presently used U.S.A. system is given in parentheses.

Acceleration

Definition. The rate of change of linear velocity. The unit of measure of its magnitude is meters per second per second (feet per second per second).

Examples. Since acceleration is a vector quantity, changes in magnitude or direction may occur. When the driver of an automobile presses the accelerator and accelerates from a speed of 0 to 5 to 20 to 100 km/h (60 mph), the car undergoes linear acceleration. When the driver brakes, the car undergoes linear deceleration or retardation. These ideas are depicted in Figure A-1A, and a mathematical derivation is given below.

Now, consider the rate of change of direction. A change in velocity direction with time without change in magnitude also produces acceleration. A passenger in a car taking a right turn is pushed to the left as the car negotiates the turn at a constant speed. This push is due to the change in the direction of the velocity vector. The concept is illustrated in Figure A-1B, and the mathematical derivation is given below.

Generally, the term acceleration is used to represent linear acceleration. Another kind of acceleration is angular acceleration.

Explanatory Notes. First consider changes in magnitude (speed). If a body (automobile), shown in Figure A-1A, at a certain point in time t_1 has speed V_1, and at another point in time t_2 has speed V_2, then the average acceleration is $(V_2 - V_1)/(t_2 - t_1)$. The instantaneous acceleration at time t is the average acceleration when the time interval $(t_2 - t_1)$ approaches zero. If the speed decreases during the time interval, there is negative acceleration or deceleration.

Referring to Figure A-1B where the car is turning, the only change within time interval $(t_2 - t_1)$ is the change in the direction of the velocity vector from V_1 to V_2, the speed being the same. The acceleration is (vector V_2 − vector V_1)/$(t_2 - t_1)$. The resulting acceleration vector (see *Vector*) is directed toward the center of the turning circle of the car. In other words, to turn the car from the direction of vector V_1 to that of V_2, an acceleration directed toward the center of the circle must be applied. This is called centripetal acceleration. Because of the body inertia, the passenger feels a push directed opposite to the

CHANGE IN VELOCITY MAGNITUDE

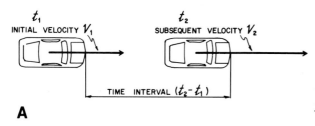

A

CHANGE IN VELOCITY DIRECTION

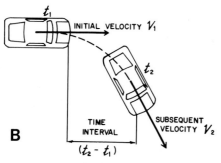

B

Fig. A-1. Linear acceleration (*A*) due to change in the magnitude (speed) of velocity and (*B*) due to change in the direction of velocity.

direction of car acceleration (i.e., away from the center). This push is called centrifugal force. The outward push in this case is similar to the backward push felt by a passenger sitting in a car that is accelerated forward.

Allowable Stress

Definition. A stress value that is higher than that due to the normal loads but is lower than the yield stress of the material. The unit of measure is newtons per square meter or pascals (psi).

Examples. In designing structures for carrying mechanical loads it is necessary, in addition to normal loads, to allow for dynamic loads, accidental overloads, inaccuracies in material and workmanship, and other unknown variables. For these reasons, a margin of safety is generally provided by choosing the design or allowable stress much below the yield point (see *Yield Stress*) so that no permanent deformation can take place as a result of these unwelcome loads.

Bridges are built with allowable stress. They are built to carry greater loads than those to which they are expected to be subjected.

The same is true of the human skeleton. Our bones tolerate a broad range of physiologic loading. The routine human activity of walking, running, and jumping may be thought of as being in the physiologic range. When the pole vaulter, ski jumper, or paratrooper has an imperfect fall and does not break or permanently deform his skeleton, the bones have been overloaded and have reached the range of allowable stress.

Angular Acceleration

Definition. The rate of change of angular velocity. Since acceleration is a vector quantity, changes in magnitude or direction may occur. The unit of measure of its magnitude is radians per second per second (degrees per second per second).

Examples. The change in the angular velocity with time constitutes angular acceleration. In whiplash injury, when an auto is hit from behind, the trunk is linearly accelerated forward in relation to the head which, because of its inertia, is slow to respond and is therefore angularly accelerated backward. Hence the mechanism of injury is dependent upon the angular acceleration of the head as well as its inertia (see *Inertia*).

Because the angular velocity is a vector, a change in its direction with time without a change in its magnitude also produces acceleration. A gyroscope, as shown in Figure A-2, consists of a heavy wheel rotating at a high speed. It is able to balance on the tip of a pen because, if it tilts, its angular velocity vector changes direction, thus producing angular acceleration. This, by Newton's second law of motion, develops a counterbalancing moment that tends to bring the gyroscope back to its original position. Through this mechanism a stable position is maintained as long as the gyroscope rotates. This gyroscopic "trick" intrigues the intuition because angular acceleration due to change in direction is not a part of the every-day experience. However, the gyroscope obeys the same laws of mechanics as does a car being hit from behind.

Explanatory Notes. A mathematical expression for the angular acceleration can be derived.

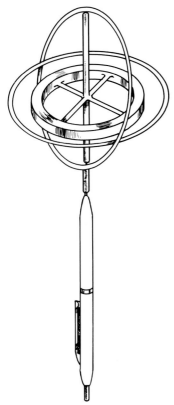

Fig. A-2. Angular acceleration. A gyroscope balances on the tip of the pen because of the high rotatory speed of its wheel.

Consider a body, at a certain point in time t_1, that has angular speed W_1, and at another point in time t_2 has angular speed W_2. Then the average angular acceleration is $(W_2 - W_1)/(t_2 - t_1)$. The instantaneous acceleration at time t is the average acceleration when the time interval $(t_2 - t_1)$ approaches zero. If angular speed decreases during the time interval, the acceleration is negative and is called angular deceleration.

Anisotropic Material

Definition. A material is anisotropic if its mechanical properties vary with different spatial orientations.

Examples. If one takes a test sample of an anisotropic material, its mechanical properties such as strength and elasticity will vary according to relative orientation within the material. Some examples of anisotropic materials are wood, bone, ligaments, and cartilage.

Take out a cubic specimen of cancellous bone from a vertebra (Fig. A-3). It is first loaded in an axial direction (A), and then in the transverse direction (B). If the specimen is shown to be stronger or weaker during axial loading than during transverse loading, the anisotropic quality of the bone has then been demonstrated.

Bending

Definition. When a load is applied to a long structure that is not directly supported at the point of application of the load, the structure deforms, and this deformation is called bending.

Examples. If a plastic ruler is bent as shown in Figures A-4A and A-4B, it is apparent that the same ruler is stronger when loaded as shown in Figure A-4B than when loaded in the manner shown in Figure A-4A. This is due to the fact that the material is further away from the center with respect to the bending mode in B (see *Sectional Moment of Inertia*).

The vertebral arch has a cross-section that is especially suitable for taking up bending loads in the sagittal plane. The moment of inertia of an elliptical cross-section is greatest for the bending loads in the direction parallel to its major axis, as shown in Figure A-4C. This is probably the reason that the pedicle cross-section is elliptical, with its long axis vertical as shown in Figure A-4D. In other words, the structural design of the vertebra is capable of best resisting bending loads in the direction in which those loads are likely to be greatest.

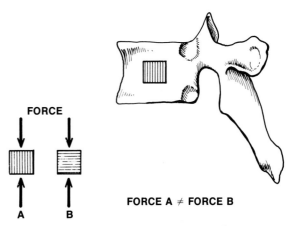

FORCE

FORCE A ≠ FORCE B

A   B

Fig. A-3. Anisotropic material.

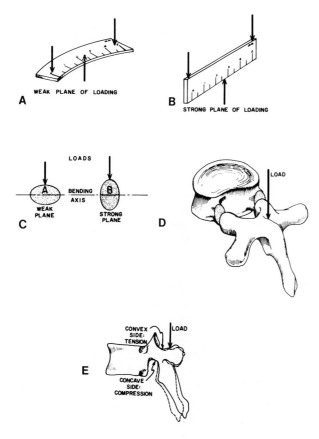

Bending Moment

Definition. A quantity at a point in a structure equal to the product of the force applied and the shortest distance from the point to the force direction. The unit of measure is newton meters (foot poundforce).

Examples. A monkey sitting on a tree branch is subjecting the various sections of the branch to bending moments (Fig. A-5). The bending moment changes in magnitude from zero under his seat to the maximum at the junction of the branch and the trunk of the tree. (The same concept applies to the weight of the branch itself.) The natural structure of the branch enables it to resist the progressively higher moments created at various sections from the tip to the base of the branch by the distribution of correspondingly more material with a larger sectional moment of inertia of the cross-sections.

It has been shown by in vivo disc pressure measurements that the disc pressure and the axial disc load in the lumbar region increase when a sitting subject lifts a telephone that is a fair distance away.[2] (In separate cadaver experiments, the disc pressure has been shown to be directly related to axial load.) The mechanism of the increase of the axial load is as follows. The small weight of the telephone applies a substantial

Explanatory Notes. Fibers on the concave side of the bent structure are compressed, while those on the convex side are elongated. Figure A-4E shows a vertebra being loaded just posterior to the facets. The amount of fiber stress σ (sigma) is given by the following formula:

$$\sigma = \frac{M \times Y}{I}$$

where M = bending moment
Y = fiber distance from the neutral axis
I = sectional moment of inertia

The radius of curvature R of the bent structure is given by another equation:

$$R = \frac{E \times I}{M}$$

where E = modulus of elasticity of the material.

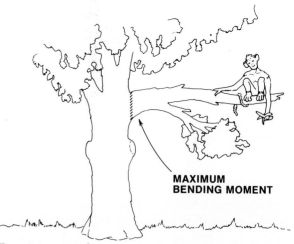

Fig. A-5. Bending moment. The thickness of the branch at any section is related to the bending moment at that section.

bending moment at the disc due to the large lever arm. This bending moment is counterbalanced by the bending moment provided by muscle and ligamentous forces, which have a much smaller lever arm and therefore must exert forces of very large magnitudes in order to maintain the equilibrium. It is this large muscle force that accounts for the large axial load and pressure in the disc.

Bending Moment Diagram

Definition. A diagram showing the amount of bending moment at various sections of a long structure subjected to bending loads.

Example. Knowing the bending moment diagram and the dimensions of the structure and its material properties, it is possible to compute the normal stress, the shear stress, angulation, and deflection at every point of the structure when it is subjected to a given set of loads.

Figure A-6A shows a portion of the spine in three-point bending. The three forces are F_1, F_2, and F_3. Figure A-6B is the bending moment diagram. The shape of the diagram shows that the maximum bending moment will occur under the force F_1. Assuming that the spine structure and its material have properties that are the same along its entire length, the point under F_1 will be the point of highest stress and failure.

A bending moment diagram for any given load situation can be obtained by a simple method described below.

Explanatory Notes. The shape of the bending moment diagram for a given set of loading situations may be determined by the following procedure. Referring to Figure A-6A, at a point X on the spine at distance A_x from the left support, the bending moment is:

$$M_x = \text{force} \times \text{lever arm}$$
$$= F_2 \times A_x$$

This is the height of the bending moment diagram under the point X (Fig. A-6B). The complete bending moment diagram is obtained by moving point X from the left support to the right support and taking moments of all the forces to the *left of point X*. For a three-point bending load, the bending moment diagram is a triangle with its apex under the middle force. For other kinds of loads the bending moment diagram would have other shapes.

The highest bending moment under the force F_1 is as follows:

$$M_{max} = \frac{F_1 \times A_2 \times A_3}{A_2 + A_3}$$

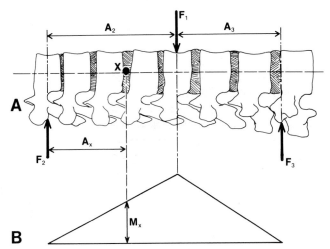

Fig. A-6. Bending moment diagram. The bending moment at any section of the spine equals the height of the diagram at that section.

Biomechanical Adaptation

Definition. Biologically mediated changes in the mechanical properties of tissues (material properties and/or structural changes) in association with the application of mechanical variables to those tissues.

Examples. A simple and fairly universal example of biomechanical adaptation is the common foot callous. When the feet are subjected to significant loads over normal or abnormal prominences, the skin and the subcutaneous tissues become harder and thicker, a material and a structural change, respectively.

Another example, demonstrating structural changes, is shown in Figure A-7. Part A shows the lateral view of a normal ankle joint. In Part B, observe the build-up of a large triangular segment of bone at the distal anterior tibial eminence. This is a biologically mediated change in the ankle, associated with the repeatedly applied forces and deformation in that area that are generated by the "push off" activities of the athlete.

Wolff's law describes a type of biomechanical adaptation.

Center of Motion

See *Instantaneous Axis of Rotation.*

Centroid

Definition. The centroid of an area is a point on which the total area may be centered.

Example. One way to approximate the centroid of a given area is to do the following experiment. Draw the area whose centroid is required on a piece of thick paper and cut it out. The center of gravity of this piece of paper is the centroid of the area. To find the center of gravity, choose a point on the paper, and hang the paper by a thread from this point. Orient the paper in an arbitrary plane and let it go. If it can maintain that orientation when hanging freely, then that point is the center of gravity for this particular piece of paper and the centroid for the section. Several trials may be required to find the right point. Results of this experiment can be obtained mathematically if the boundary can be described mathematically. The formulas are given below.

The centroid of a section is required, among other things, to determine bending strength of structures and other related items like the neutral axis and the sectional moment of inertia. The centroids of some simple cross-sections are shown in Figure A-8A.

Explanatory Notes. In mathematical terms, the centroid of an area may be obtained in the following manner. Choose a stainless steel fixation plate, as shown in Figure A-8B, as an example. The area to be analyzed is shown in an enlarged view in Figure A-8C. The area is given by the integral:

$$A = \int y \, dx$$

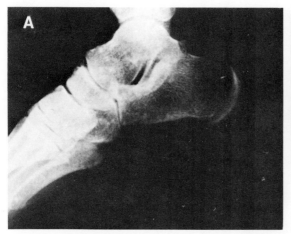
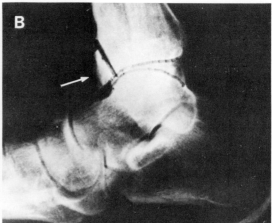

Fig. A-7. (*A, B*) Biomechanical adaptation. Notice the additional bone (*arrow*) in *B*. (Courtesy of James Nicholas, M.D., New York, N.Y.)

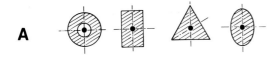

A

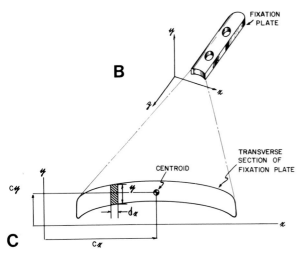

B

C

Fig. A-8. Centroid. (A) Centroid of some common sections. (B) A fracture fixation plate. (C) A close-up view of the plate section showing the method of computing the location of the centroid.

where y and dx refer to a small strip of the area as seen in Figure A-8C. The coordinates of the centroid of the area, C_x and C_y, are given by equations:

$$C_x = \int \frac{xy\,dx}{A}$$

$$C_y = \int \frac{xy\,dy}{A}$$

Center of Gravity

Definition. The point in a body where the body mass is centered.

Example. If the body were hanged from this point by a rope (Fig. A-9), the body could then be oriented in any direction whatsoever, and it would remain in that orientation hanging freely.

The center of gravity of the body lies in the midsagittal plane (due to anatomic symmetry) and somewhat anterior to the upper sacral spine.

It is reported to be 4 cm in front of the first sacral vertebra in the standing anatomic position. This probably is the reason for carrying a backpack on the back, which tends to bring the center of gravity more in line with the spine, thus reducing the bending stresses. It must be realized that the center of gravity is different for different body postures. The center of gravity refers to three-dimensional bodies, and the centroid to plane, two-dimensional areas. The principle behind the concept of the center of gravity is further explained below.

Explanatory Notes. At the center of gravity the sum of the moments due to weights of all the parts comprising the body are equal to zero. Therefore, when a body is hanged from its center of gravity, the moments due to the body parts on the right hand side of the center of gravity are exactly equal and opposite to those exerted by

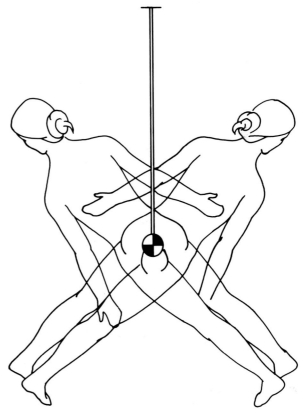

Fig. A-9. Center of gravity. A body suspended from its center of gravity may be oriented in any direction.

the body parts on the left hand side. Hence, there is zero moment at the point of hanging and therefore also zero rotation.

Clinical Stability

Definition. The ability of the spine under physiologic loads to limit patterns of displacement so as not to damage or irritate the spinal cord or nerve roots and, in addition, to prevent incapacitating deformity or pain due to structural changes.

Any disruption of the spine components (ligaments, disc, facets) holding the spine together will decrease the clinical stability of the spine.

When the spine loses enough of these components to prevent it from adequately providing the mechanical functions of protection, measures are taken to reestablish the stability.

Coefficient of Friction

Definition. The ratio of tangential force to the normal interbody compressive force required to initiate a sliding motion between two bodies. This ratio has no units of measure.

Example. A skater glides effortlessly on ice (Fig. A-10A). The ratio of her effort (tangential force) to her body weight (normal force) is very small, thus this interbody action has a rather low coefficient of friction. A boulder sitting on the road, on the contrary, requires considerable effort to move it, denoting a high coefficient of friction between it and the road (Fig. A-10B).

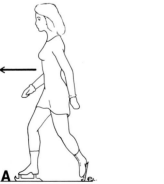
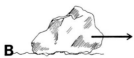

Fig. A-10. (*A*) A skater on ice has a low coefficient of friction. (*B*) In contrast, a boulder on the road has a high coefficient.

Some typical values of the coefficient of friction (static) for different contacting surfaces are as follows:

Stone on ground	0.75
Steel on ice	0.01
Bearing with lubrication	0.01
Animal ankle joint	0.005

For further discussion, see *Joint Reaction Force.*

Compression

Definition. The normal force that tends to push together material fibers. The unit of measure is newtons (poundforce).

Examples. The weight of a building applies compression to its foundation.

The intervertebral disc is the main compression-carrying component in the spine. It is subjected to direct compression, even when a person is not carrying any loads. This compression is due to several causes: direct weight of the trunk, initial tension in other ligaments (e.g., ligamentum flavum), and additional tension in ligaments and muscles required to balance the eccentric trunk weight.

Compressive Stress

See *Stress.*

Conversion Table

The following table gives conversion factors for entities specified in the presently used U.S.A. system and the new S.I. system (Systeme International d'Unites) proposed for use in the U.S.A.

To obtain the U.S.A. measurement when the S.I. unit is given, multiply the S.I. quantity by the factor X. Use the factor Y instead to convert from the U.S.A. to the S.I. system. Examples are given below. The symbols used in the table are as follows:

degree	= deg	newton	= N
foot	= ft	pascal	= Pa
inch	= in	pound	= lb
joule	= J	poundforce	= lbf
kilogram	= kg	radian	= rad
meter	= m	second	= s

Examples.

Moment: 100 ft lbf = 1.3557 × 100 = 135.57 N m

Pressure: 100 N/m² = 100 × 0.0209 = 2.09 lbf/ft²
            100 Pa = 100 × 0.000145
                   = 0.0145 lbf/in²

Coordinate Systems

Definition.   Reference systems that make it possible to define position and motion of rigid bodies in space or with respect to each other.

The motion of a body may be determined by knowing its position before and after a given time

Table A-1. Conversion Factors

ENTITY	S.I.	→ X ← ← Y ←	U.S.A.
Acceleration	m/s²	3.2808 0.3048	ft/s²
Angle	rad	57.296 0.0175	deg
Area	m²	10.763 0.0929	ft²
	m²	1550.0 0.000645	in²
Density	kg/m³	0.0624 16.018	lb/ft³
	kg/m³	0.0000361 27680.	lb/in³
Energy, work	N m = J*	0.7376 1.3558	ft lbf
Force	N	0.2248 4.4482	lbf
Length	m	3.2808 0.3048	ft
	m	39.370 0.0254	in
Mass	kg	2.2046 0.4536	lb
Mass moment of inertia	kg m²	23.730 0.0421	lb ft²
Moment, torque	N m	0.7376 1.3557	ft lbf
Polar moment of inertia, section moment of inertia	m⁴	115.86 0.0086	ft⁴
Pressure, stress	N/m² = Pa*	0.0209 47.870	lbf/ft²
	N/m² = Pa*	0.000145 6896.5	lbf/in²
Stiffness	N/m	5.667 0.177	lbf/in
Velocity	m/s	3.2808 0.3048	ft/s
Volume	m³	35.313 0.0283	ft³
	m³	61023. 0.0000164	in³

* Official recommended units of S.I.

interval. The three-dimensional description of motion of an object requires a three-dimensional coordinate system. There are many types of coordinate systems available, but the following three are probably the most widely used: the cylindrical, the spherical, and the rectangular systems. The choice of a particular coordinate system depends upon the convenience it offers.

Examples. The cylindrical coordinate system is used for objects or motions with some circular symmetry about an axis. An egg has an axis of revolution. Any point P on its surface may advantageously be represented by cylindrical coordinates: r, θ, y (Fig. A-11A).

The spherical system is preferable for situations where spherical symmetry may be present. To define a point on earth that resembles a sphere, the spherical system is most convenient. Radius, longitude, and latitude are the three required coordinates: r, θ ϕ (Fig. A-11B).

The musculoskeletal system has a plane of symmetry (the sagittal plane). The rectangular coordinate system is most convenient here. The right-handed Cartesian orthogonal coordinate system, the proper name for the rectangular system most preferred, is defined as a system consisting of three straight lines mutually perpendicular and intersecting. These lines, called the axes, may be named x, y, and z. The point of intersection is called the origin.

A vertebra with the origin of the Cartesian coordinate system placed at the center is shown in Figure A-11C. To define the mutual direction of the axes, imagine an ordinary (right-handed) screw placed along the z-axis with its tip pointing toward the +z-axis. Then rotation of the screw

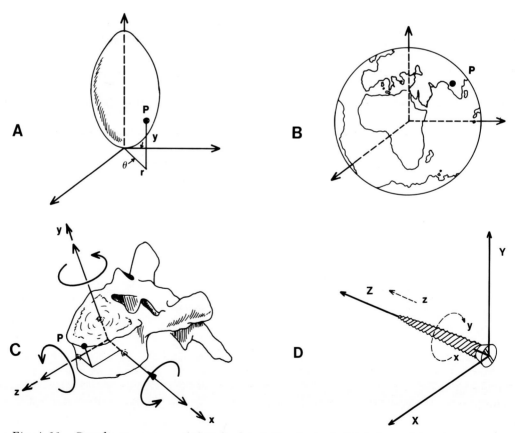

Fig. A-11. Coordinate systems. (*A*) Cylindrical, P = (r, θ, y). (*B*) Spherical, P = (r, θ, ϕ). (*C*) Cartesian, P = (x, y, z). (*D*) A screw, by its movement, defines the right-handed coordinate system.

head from the +x-axis to the +y-axis will produce screw translation in the positive direction of the z-axis (Fig. A-11D).

This right-handed system as opposed to the left-handed system is universally preferred by convention. Also, by convention, the senses of motion are defined. Figure A-11C shows positive translations and rotations about the three axes. Translatory motion along an axis toward its positive direction is called positive, while in the opposite direction it is called negative. A clockwise rotation about an axis, looking from the origin of the coordinate system toward the positive direction of the axis, is called positive rotation, while the counterclockwise rotation is termed negative.

Recommendations have been offered for a standard use of the Cartesian coordinate system in the human body.[11,22]

Couple

Definition. A pair of equal and opposite parallel forces acting on a body and separated by a distance. The moment or torque of a couple is defined as a quantity equal to the product of one of the forces and the perpendicular distance between the forces. The unit of measure for the torque is newton meters (foot poundforce).

Example. A couple (of forces) is applied to the steering wheel of a car when it is turned (Fig. A-12). This pair of equal and opposite forces creates a torque that turns the steering shaft.

Explanatory Notes. In the case of the steering wheel, the torque T is given by the following equation:

$$T = F \times D$$

where F is the force in newtons (poundforce) and D is the perpendicular distance in meters (feet).

Coupling

Definition. A phenomenon of consistent association of one motion (translation or rotation) about an axis with another motion about a second axis. One motion cannot be produced without the other.

Example. Vertebral motion, both in and out of the sagittal plane, produces other associated motions of translation and rotation.[9] Anterior

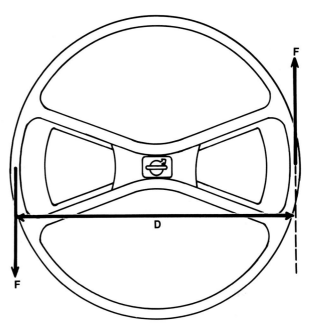

Fig. A-12. Couple. Two parallel forces F separated by distance D produce torque F × D.

translation of a vertebra produced by force F is always associated with flexion rotation (Fig. A-13A). Similarly, axial rotation produced by axial moment M is consistently associated with lateral bending (Fig. A-13B).

In scoliosis, lateral deformity is coupled with axial rotation, such that the posterior elements tend to rotate toward the concavity of the curve.[21]

Creep

Definition. A viscoelastic material deforms with time when it is subjected to a constant, suddenly applied load. The deformation-time curve approaches a steady state value asymptotically. This phenomenon is called creep.

Examples. When an individual's height is measured in the morning and again at night after standing all day, the second measurement is found to be less than the first. Some of this change is due to compression of the intervertebral discs. The change in height (deformation) is not due to additional weight the person has gained, but rather to creep. The same load over a period of time has caused a subsequent deformation and loss of height.

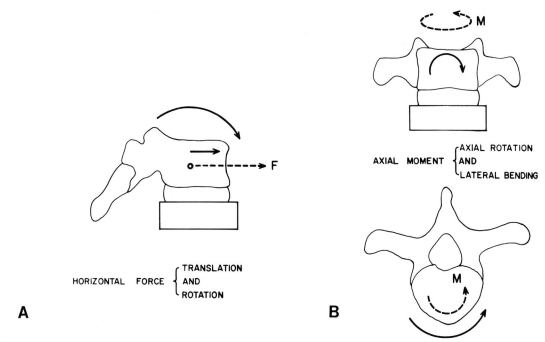

Fig. A-13. (*A*) Coupling. Anterior horizontal force F produces translation and rotation. (*B*) Axial torque or moment M produces axial and lateral rotations.

In Figure A-14, the creep test is performed on a spine motion segment. On the left, the motion segment is shown without load. In the middle, a sudden tensile load is applied, producing immediate deformation (see the deformation-time diagram). On the right, the same motion segment is shown 1 hour later. Additional deformation has taken place within this time. Results of the creep test are plotted as a deformation-time curve. This is an important mechanical characteristic of the spine and other biologic structures. The creep phenomenon in Figure A-14 is the result of tensile loading, whereas the previous example is the result of compressive loading. However, both demonstrate the viscoelastic creep.

Cylindrical Coordinates

See *Coordinate System.*

Damping

Definition. A material property that constitutes resistance to speed.

Examples. To visualize the damping effect, consider a syringe (Fig. A-15). A certain force applied to the plunger gives the plunger a certain speed. A slow movement of the plunger requires a smaller force, while a fast movement requires a considerable force. Figure A-15 also shows the force-speed curve for the syringe. The slope of the curve is called the damping coefficient.

The shock absorber in a car utilizes the damping effect of the "fluid in a syringe" to smooth out the sharp vibrations of the wheels on a rough road and provide a smooth ride.

In engineering, the phenomenon of damping is represented by a mathematical model called the dashpot (see *Dashpot-Mathematical Element*). All biologic materials, bone, ligaments, joints, and the spine, exhibit damping properties in the form of viscoelastic behaviour.

Explanatory Notes. When the resistance offered by damping is proportional to the speed, it is called viscous damping. If a force is applied to deform a structure, the ratio of force exerted to the deformation speed is the measure of damping and is called the damping coefficient. The units of measure are newton seconds per meter (pound-force seconds per foot) for translatory motion and

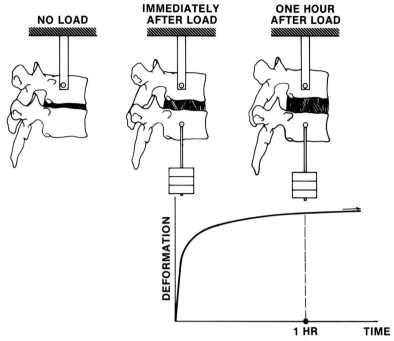

Fig. A-14. Creep. A deformation-time curve quantifies creep.

newton seconds per radian (poundforce seconds per degree) for rotatory motion.

Dashpot-Mathematical Element

Definition. A component used in building mathematical models of structures or materials that exhibit time-dependent behavior.

Examples. A boat on water symbolizes this element. The difficulty with which one must push or pull a boat across the surface of the water is dependent upon the speed of the movement. This phenomenon is due to the viscosity of the water.

The intervertebral disc has strong damping properties and is sometimes referred to as the shock absorber of the spine. Sudden motions of the lower part of the body are attenuated by viscera, skin, bones, discs, and vertebral bodies before reaching the head.

Most probably, the blood in the vertebral capillaries and sinusoids also offers resistance to deformation, thus acting as a dashpot. In rapid rates of loading, the blood cannot escape through the foramina rapidly enough and thus provides resistance. The system is viscoelastic. With lower loading rates, the blood offers much less resistance and the system is nearly elastic.

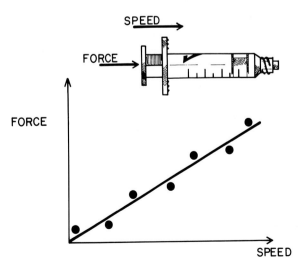

Fig. A-15. Damping. A force-speed curve quantifies damping.

Explanatory Notes. The damping properties of a tissue or a system represented by the dashpot-mathematical element can be quantified. The damping characteristics of the tissue are quantified by the relationship between the load applied and the speed produced (Fig. A-16). The slope of the load-speed curve is called the damping coefficient. The coefficient that varies with the load characterizes nonlinear damping. The area under the load-speed curve represents the rate of energy loss during the loading/unloading cycle. Also shown in Figure A-16 is the dashpot symbol: a piston pushing on the fluid contained in a cylinder.

Deceleration

See *Acceleration* and *Angular Acceleration*.

Deformation

Definition. The change in length or shape. Deformation is generally represented in the form of strain (see *Strain*).

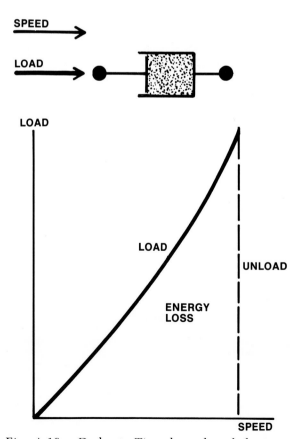

Fig. A-16. Dashpot. Time-dependent behavior is modeled by a dashpot.

Degrees of Freedom

Definition. The number of independent coordinates in a coordinate system required to completely specify the position of an object in space.

The term is loosely applied to specify the independent motion components that are involved in the characteristic movements of a given rigid body. The motion of a rigid body in space has six degrees of freedom; three translations (expressed by linear coordinates) and three rotations (expressed by angular coordinates). When bodies are interconnected in a system, certain constraints are placed on the possible motions, and the number of degrees of freedom decreases.

Example. A bead on tracks has a single degree of freedom, as shown in Figure A-17A. A body moving in a plane has three degrees of freedom, two translations along mutually perpendicular directions in the plane and one rotation around an axis perpendicular to that plane. An example of such a body movement is a "nickel" moving freely on a table (Fig. A-17B).

A body has six degrees of freedom if it is allowed to move freely in the three-dimensional space. The vertebra (Fig. A-17C) is capable of performing all the six motions in space as the trunk is manipulated with respect to the pelvis. Thus, it has six degrees of freedom.

Explanatory Notes. It should be pointed out that although only three coordinates are required to completely define a point in space (see *Coordinate System*) a minimum of six coordinates is needed to specify position of a rigid body.

Dry Friction-Mathematical Element

Definition. A component used in building mathematical models of structures or materials that exhibit plastic behaviour.

Examples. One cannot move a heavy anatomy book lying on a table by just blowing on it. If an increasing amount of force is applied, a threshold is reached, following which the book begins to move. It will continue to move without any subsequent increase in force. Upon removal of the force, the book will suddenly stop and will not go back to its original position. This is a characteristic of dry friction between bodies. There are other natural phenomena in which the relation between force and motion is similar. An example is the stretching of a ligament beyond its elastic limit, thus producing permanent deformation.

The ligament is said to be plastically deformed. To describe these phenomena quantitatively, a mathematical model may be constructed where a dry friction-mathematical element may represent the actual behaviour.

In Grade I spondylolisthesis, L5–S1, suppose the annulus and all the other supporting soft-tissue elements were removed. The patient then develops a moderately stable syndesmosis between the two vertebral bodies. Mild forces would not be strong enough to push L5 further forward with respect to S1. However, a large force could transcend the threshold of the dry friction offered by the syndesmosis, and L5 would slip indefinitely but for other clinical factors that create new dry friction thresholds and restrict further displacement.

The mathematical concept, as exemplified above, is utilized to represent those properties of a tissue that are characterized by a sudden displacement after a threshold load is reached and by permanent deformation at the removal of the load. In Figure A-18 the relationship between the load and the deformation is shown. It is characterized by the threshold load and permanent deformation. Also the dry friction symbol is shown: a block resting on a surface.

Ductility

Definition.   The property of a material to absorb relatively large amounts of plastic deformation energy before failure.

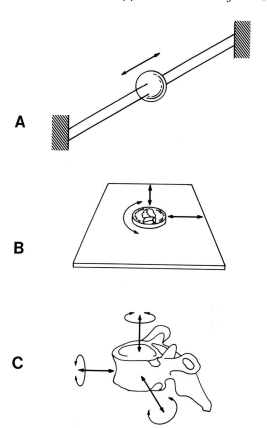

Fig. A-17.   (A) A bead on a track has one degree of freedom. (B) A nickel moving freely on a table has three degrees of freedom. (C) A vertebra is capable of all six degrees of freedom.

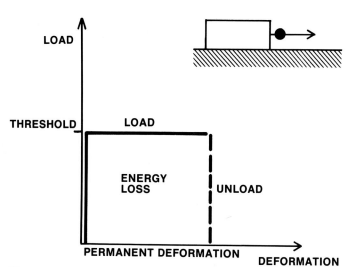

Fig. A-18.   Dry friction. The load deformation curve shows the motion of a block being pulled by a force.

Materials possessing large amounts of ductility are called ductile. In contrast, nonductile or brittle materials have a relatively small plastic energy absorbing capacity (Fig. A-19). Ductility of a material is quantified either by percentage elongation in length or by percentage decrease in cross-sectional area at the time of failure. Generally, materials that exhibit less than 5 per cent elongation are called brittle, while materials that exhibit more are called ductile.

Examples. Most metals are ductile, while ceramics, hard plastics, and cortical bone are brittle. Implants made of ductile materials can undergo large deformations and absorb substantial amounts of energy before failure. However, in general, they have lower ultimate tensile strength and therefore cannot take up overloads. Some examples of ductile and brittle materials are given in Table A-2.

A spine with Ehlers-Danlos syndrome is more ductile than one with Marie-Strumpell's disease.

Dynamic Load

Definition. A load applied to a specimen is called dynamic if it varies with time.

A dynamic load is the opposite of the static load. A dynamic load with a repetitive pattern of variation is called a cyclic load.

Examples. The lumbar spine of a pilot of a disabled high speed aircraft is subjected to tremendous dynamic loads as he is ejected out of the craft by a rocket attached to his seat.

During normal gait, all body parts are subjected to dynamic loads. The head of the femur (Fig. A-20) is stressed under varying degrees of dynamic compression as the load is transferred from one leg to the other.[13] This is a cyclic load since the loading pattern is repeated at each

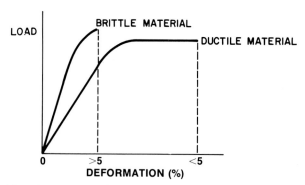

Fig. A-19. Ductility. A ductile material has greater deformation and absorbs larger amounts of energy before failure as compared to a brittle material.

cycle of gait. In contrast, a static load is applied when a person is standing still.

Dynamics

Definition. A branch of mechanics that consists of the study of the loads and the motions of interacting bodies.

Example. Gait analysis is a good example. Here the loads applied by the muscles to the bones, the ground reactions (as measured by the force plate), and the various body motions produced are studied.

Elasticity

Definition. The property of a material or a structure to return to its original form following the removal of the deforming load.

Energy is stored during loading and released completely during unloading. Thus, no energy is lost in the process, and there is no permanent deformation. Stress and strain curves of an elastic

Table A-2. *Physical Properties of Some Materials*

MATERIAL	ULTIMATE STRENGTH		ELONGATION	PROPERTY
	(MPa)	(lbf/in²)	(%)	
Stainless steel, annealed*	517	75 000	40	Ductile
Stainless steel, cold worked*	862	125 000	12	Ductile
Cortical bone, wet†	81	11 800	1.2	Brittle
Cortical bone, dry†	107	15 500	0.66	Brittle

* American Society for Testing and Materials. Standards for Surgical Implants. Philadelphia. Table 2, 1971.
† Evan, F. G.: Mechanical Properties of Bone. Charles C Thomas Publisher, Springfield, p. 51, 1973.

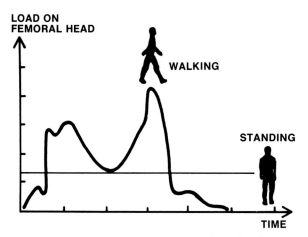

Fig. A-20. Dynamic load. The head of the femur is subjected to dynamic (varying) loads in walking and static (constant) loads in standing.

material may be linear or nonlinear, but the loading and unloading curves are always the same.

Example. All materials are elastic to a varying degree. A person jumping off a diving board utilizes the elastic properties of the board. He stores energy as he pushes the board downward by jumping on its unsupported end. The board in turn gives back the stored energy during the diver's push-off.

Elastic Range

Definition. A range of loading within which a specimen or a structure remains elastic.

Examples. When a specimen or a structure is subjected to a load, it deforms. If the deformation is such that upon release of the load the specimen or the structure returns to its preload shape, then the deformation is called elastic deformation. Figure A-21A shows the load-deformation curve for a specimen. The elastic range is represented by line OB in the figure. Within the elastic range, the deformation may be proportional to the load (proportional or linear range), line OA, or it may vary (nonlinear range), line AB.

A rubber band or the old comic book character "Plastic Man" (Fig. A-21B) demonstrates linear and nonlinear elasticity. Actually this name is a biomechanical misnomer, since "Plastic Man" never exhibited any plastic deformation, always being in the elastic range. He might never have sold, however, under the correct engineering appelation of "Elastic Man."

Implants are designed so that during normal physiologic activity, the maximum stress remains

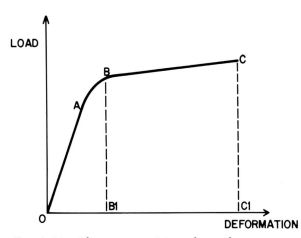

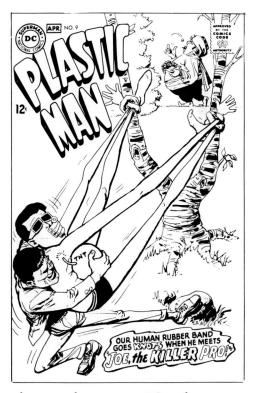

Fig. A-21. Elastic range. OA = elastic, linear range; AB = elastic, nonlinear range; BC = plastic range. (Carton reproduced from the cover of *Plastic Man*, April, 1968. © 1968 DC Comics Inc.)

within the elastic range. Although they can take up much greater loads before failure, the elastic range is the only useful range, for once there is loading beyond this range, permanent deformation and implant failure occur.

Elastic Stability

Definition.   The ability of a loaded structure, given an arbitrary small elastic deformation, to return to its original position.

Examples.   The stability of an elastic structure is a function of the geometry of the structure and the quantitative and qualitative characteristics of the applied load. The classic example of elastic instability is the axially loaded columns that were studied by Euler in the 18th century. A cylindrical bar with its lower end fixed in the ground and its upper end loaded with weights was investigated (Fig. A-22A). Euler applied increasing loads on the column until the column was no longer able to maintain its straight vertical position. He called this final load "the critical load." The mathematical formula for determining this load is given below.

It has been shown by cadaver experiments that a spine specimen, T1 to pelvis, relieved of its musculature and the rib cage, has a critical load of about 20 N (4.4 lb) under which it is unstable and buckles like an elastic column (Fig. A-22B).[8] This points out the importance of the spinal muscles and certain other anatomic structures in maintaining the elastic stability of the spine. Note that this elastic stability is distinctly different from what is referred to as clinical stability.

Explanatory Notes.   Euler's formula for calculating the maximum load W in newtons (pound-force), the so-called critical load, is as follows:

$$W = \frac{\pi^2 \, EI}{4 \, L^2}$$

where $\pi = 3.1416$

    E = modulus of elasticity in N/m^2 (lbf/ft^2)

    I = section moment of inertia in m^4 (ft^4)

    L = length in m (ft)

Energy

Definition.   The amount of work done by a load on a body. The unit of energy is newton meters (foot poundforce).

If the load deforms or displaces the body, the energy is called the strain or the potential energy, respectively. If the load imparts motion to the body, it is called the kinetic energy.

Example.   The strain or potential energy of a structure subjected to a load is represented by the area of its load-deformation diagram. Assume that the load-deformation diagram shown in Figure A-23 is for a spine segment. Then, if the spine has been elastically deformed to point B, the elastic energy stored is the area O-A-B-B1-O and is fully recoverable on removal of the load. Deformation from B to C is plastic (i.e., due to high load the

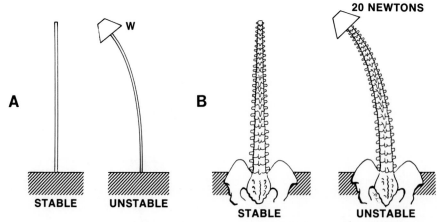

Fig. A-22.   Elastic stability. (*A*) The column does not remain straight when W reaches a critical value. (*B*) The critical load for the human cadaver spine is less than 20 N (4.5 lbf).

structure is breaking down on a microscopic scale). If a fracture takes place at C, then the areas B1-B-C-C1-B1 and O-A-B-C-C1-O represent the plastic and total energies, respectively. The total energy has been expanded in plastically deforming vertebrae and ligaments, creating fracture surfaces, and imparting kinetic energy to the fractured pieces. (For further discussion, see *Potential Energy* and *Kinetic Energy*.)

Explanatory Notes. Mathematical expressions for the two kinds of energy are as follows:

$$\text{potential energy} = F \times D$$
$$\text{kinetic energy} = \frac{m \times V^2}{2}$$

where F = force (constant magnitude) in N (lbf)

D = displacement of the point of force application in m (ft)

m = mass in kg (lb)

V = velocity (constant magnitude) in m/s (ft/s)

The above formulas take on integral forms if force and velocity are not constant.

Energy Absorption Capacity

Definition. The mechanical energy absorbed by a structure loaded to failure. The unit of measure is newton meters (foot poundforce).

This energy is expanded during plastic deformation, fracture surface generation, and in imparting motion to fractured fragments. It is conveniently given by the total area (O-A-B-C-C1-O) under the load-deformation curve shown in Figure A-23.

Examples. Higher energy absorption capacity is generally synonymous with high ductility of materials. A stainless steel fixation plate, although designed for loads under its yield stress may, in an accident, be subjected to high energy impact. If the plate has high energy absorption capacity it may help the patient in one of two ways. It may deform considerably without failure due to its ductility, thus maintaining some of the alignment and eliminating additional complications; or, it may deform and break by absorbing large amounts of impact energy, thus decreasing the amount of energy available to cause soft-tissue damage.

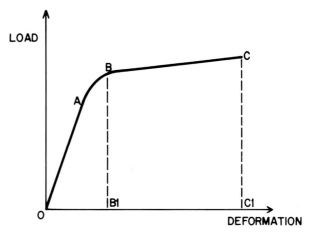

Fig. A-23. Energy (see Fig. A-21). The area under the load-deformation curve represents the energy. Area $OABB_1O$ represents the elastic energy. Area $B_1BCC_1B_1$ represents the plastic energy.

Equilibrium

Definition. A body is said to be in a state of equilibrium if it is at rest or in uniform motion under a given set of forces and moments.

The concept of equilibrium arises from Newton's second law of motion (see *Newton's Laws*). All forces and moments acting on a body must balance each other so that the body does not accelerate.

Examples. Figure A-24A shows part of a lumbar spine and a horizontal bar carrying weight, representing the weight of the upper body. Due to eccentricity of the weight, the lumbar spine is subjected to forces as well as bending moments. To estimate the loads acting on the L4 vertebra, when a person is lifting a weight, six equilibrium equations may be set up by the method of free body analysis (see below). The vertebra, with possible forces and moments acting on it, is shown in Figure A-24B. The solution to the equilibrium equations constitutes a calculation of the magnitude of forces and moments acting on the vertebra.

Explanatory Notes. For a body or a structure to be at rest, or in uniform motion, the two following conditions must be satisfied: (1) The sum of forces in all directions acting on it must be equal to zero; and (2) the sum of moments, taken at any

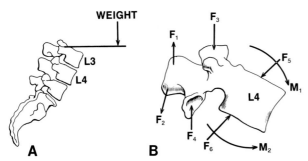

Fig. A-24. Equilibrium. Relationships between various forces and moments are given by equilibrium equations. F_1 and F_2 = muscle and ligamentous force; F_3 and F_4 = facet forces; F_5 and F_6 = disc forces; M_1 and M_2 = disc bending moments.

point of the body, around all axes, also must be equal to zero.

If the force and moment vectors are broken down into their components along the three axes of a coordinate system, then mathematically the following six equilibrium equations apply:

$$\Sigma F_x = 0, \ \Sigma F_y = 0, \ \Sigma F_z = 0$$
$$\Sigma M_x = 0, \ \Sigma M_y = 0, \ \Sigma M_z = 0$$

where F = forces at the point on the body
M = moments at the point on the body

Subscripts x, y, z refer to the axes of an orthogonal coordinate system at that point. The symbol Σ (sigma) stands for summation of all the forces and moments. The six equations of equilibrium, as given above, are probably one of the most important biomechanical tools for the mechanical analysis of the musculoskeletal system. They may be used in any situation: a single force or a complex combination of forces and moments in three-dimensional space acting at different points on a body. A simple graphical solution may be used for forces acting in one plane, such as forces exerted by various traction devices. For the three-dimensional loading situations the algebraic solution of the six equations above is probably the most efficient method.

Fatigue

Definition. A process of birth and growth of cracks in structures subjected to repetitive load cycles. The load is generally below the failure load of the structure.

Examples. When a fatigue crack reaches a certain size, the stress in the rest of the structure becomes so high that the structure fails. This is the fatigue failure. Another way to look at this phenomenon is to consider it as a summation effect. As soon as the structure is subjected to a repetitive load, however small, the "fatigue clock" starts ticking. The speed of the clock is in proportion to the magnitude of the load. The higher is the load, the faster runs the clock. The life of a given structure may then be measured by its "fatigue clock." When the structure has lived its full life, as measured by the "clock," it fails.

The magnitude of the cyclic load is generally in the elastic range and is far below the failure load of the structure. For steel, cyclic loads of magnitudes as low as 20 per cent of the failure load will cause fatigue failure in a reasonable time interval. A similar figure for a sample of cortical bone is 35 per cent. In implants and bone, it is the combination of somewhat higher physiologic loads and their cumulative repetition that brings about the failure. The method by which fatigue failure may be calculated is given below.

Most probably, in living bone, the fatigue limit is relatively higher than 35 per cent, since reparative biologic processes may compensate the propagation of cracks. However, fatigue fractures in bone do occur, indicating either that loads above the fatigue limit have been applied for a sufficient period of time, or that the bone healing process failed to repair the minute fatigue cracks at a sufficiently rapid rate. Fatigue fractures have been often called "stress fractures," which is a biomechanical misnomer. All fractures are created by excessive stress. What is special about fractures due to fatigue is the repetitive nature of the loads of relatively low magnitude applied over a certain period of time.

Explanatory Notes. The process of fatigue is documented by the Wohler or fatigue curves. The load is plotted on the ordinate, while the number of load cycles to failure, in the logarithmic scale, is plotted on the abscissa (Fig. A-25A). Ultimate load is the same as the static failure load. The fatigue limit, also called the endurance limit, is the lowest load that will cause fatigue failure. Any loads lower than the fatigue limit never cause a fatigue failure within a reasonable time

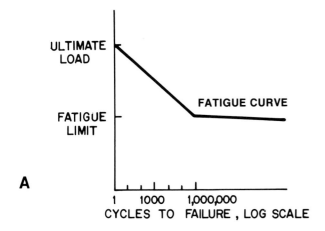

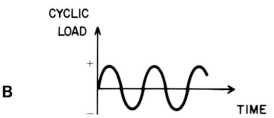

Fig. A-25. Fatigue. (*A*) The fatigue curve. (*B*) Cyclically varying loads are applied to the test specimens to determine the fatigue curve.

interval. For the purpose of standardization, the fatigue curve is generally obtained for cyclic loads that vary with time from a maximum in one direction to a maximum in the opposite direction, as shown in Figure A-25B.

Flexibility Coefficient

Definition. The flexibility coefficient of a structure is defined as the ratio of the amount of displacement produced to the load applied. It is a quantity that characterizes the responsiveness of a structure to the applied load. Units of measure are meters per newton (feet per poundforce) for linear displacement and radians per newton meter (degrees per foot poundforce) for angular displacement.

Examples. For a structure with a linear load-displacement curve, the flexibility coefficient is a constant and is the inverse slope of the curve. For more complex structures, the flexibility coefficient may vary with the magnitude of the load.

A supple scoliotic spine has a relatively high flexibility coefficient. In such a spine only small forces are required to produce large deformations. Thus, such a spine might be expected to respond well to treatment with a Milwaukee brace.

Explanatory Notes. Mathematically speaking, the flexibility coefficient f is related to the applied load F and the displacement D by the following formula:

$$f = \frac{D}{F}$$

The inverse of the flexibility coefficient is generally called the stiffness coefficient k:

$$k = \frac{1}{f}$$

It should be pointed out that, strictly speaking, in complex structures such as the human spine, with true three-dimensional motions that are coupled, the simple relationship of reciprocity between the flexibility and stiffness coefficients does not hold. In such instances, the two coefficients can be meaningfully related by means of matrix inversion only, a much more complex mathematical operation.

Force

Definition. Any action that tends to change the state of rest or of motion of a body to which it is applied. The unit of measure for the magnitude of force is newtons (poundforce).

Examples. A woman sitting in a chair is at rest under the action of two equal and opposite forces (Fig. A-26A). The earth's gravitational field is trying to accelerate her toward the center of the earth. The chair is applying an exactly equal force in the opposite direction, thus preventing her motion. If one suddenly removes the chair (Fig. A-26B), the gravitational force (mass times acceleration) will quickly change her position and attitude of rest.

Force is a vector quantity and is completely specified by its magnitude, direction, point of application, and sense. A hospital bed on wheels serves as an example. To specify the force that will be applied, the magnitude of force in newtons (poundforce) must be defined. The orientation of the direction of the force must be dis-

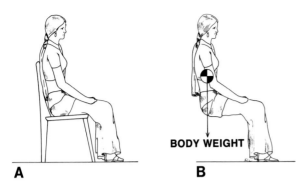

Fig. A-26. Force. (*A*) Balanced equal and opposite forces with the body in equilibrium. (*B*) Unopposed gravitational force with body accelerating toward the floor.

cerned (e.g., is the force applied in the vertical direction, or in a horizontal direction, or in any other direction in space?). The point at which the force is being applied must also be specified. Finally, the type of force, push or pull, must be determined. Once all four parameters are defined and the force is applied to the bed, it will move in a certain direction. A change in any of the parameters will produce a different motion of the bed.

Four-Point Bending

Definition. A long structure is loaded in four-point bending when two transverse forces are applied on one side and two on the other.

If all the forces are equal and arranged symmetrically (Fig. A-27A) a unique situation results, so that the structure between the inner pair of forces is subjected to a *constant* bending moment or stress. The mathematical derivation for this is given below. Since the bending moment is constant along the length B, a constant corrective effect is obtained along the corresponding region of the spine. This may be useful in certain clinical situations. Three-point bending, in contrast, has a varying bending moment with a peak just under the middle force.

Explanatory Notes. As shown by the bending moment diagram in Figure A-27B the equation for the maximum bending moment is as follows:

$$M = F \times C$$

It is interesting to note that dimensions D and B are not included in the above formula. The

reason is that the bending moment at a point of a long structure is the summation of all the moments on one side of the point. Above the point P_2 there is only force F located at P_1 a distance C away (Fig. A-27A). As one travels from P_2 to P_3 there are equal and opposite contributions toward the bending moment from the two F forces located at P_1 and P_2. Thus, the bending moment remains constant between P_2 and P_3.

Free-Body Analysis

Definition. A technique used for determining the internal stresses at a point in a structure subjected to external loads.

Examples. The part of the structure to be analyzed is isolated or cut away from the rest by an imaginary boundary. At the boundary internal stresses are represented by forces and moments as if they were the loads applied to the isolated portion of the structure by the rest of the structure. Equilibrium equations (see *Equilibrium*) are then applied to the isolated portion of the structure to evaluate the internal stresses at the boundary in terms of the external loads. This method is based on the fact that the isolated structure must be in complete balance with respect to all the forces and moments applied to it. This process is called free-body analysis and the isolated portion of the structure is referred to as the free-body diagram.

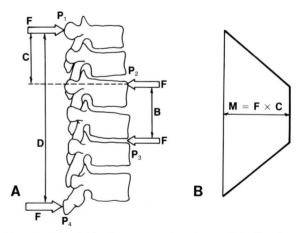

Fig. A-27. (*A*) Four-point bending. (*B*) Bending moment diagram with constant bending moment applied between points P_2 and P_3.

In studying the stresses in the C7–T1 disc when a person is bending forward, so that the cervical spine is in the horizontal plane (Fig. A-28A), the imaginary boundary is drawn between C7 and T1. The isolated structure consists of the head and the whole cervical spine. The external load is the weight of the head (Fig. A-28B). The internal forces and moments at the boundary are F_1, F_2, F_3 and M. They have replaced the interaction of the rest of the structure. By applying six equilibrium equations to the isolated structure, the disc force F_3 and disc bending moment M are obtained. Knowing the disc loads and the geometrical and material properties of the disc, the required stresses may be computed.

Friction

See *Coefficient of Friction*.

Helical Axis of Motion

Definition. A unique axis in space that completely defines a three-dimensional motion between two rigid bodies. It is analogous to the instantaneous axis of rotation for plane motion.

Examples. In three-dimensional motion, a rigid body is displaced from one position to another position in space. According to the laws of mechanics, a rigid body may always be moved from position one to position two by a rotation about a certain axis and a translation along the *same axis*. This constitutes helical motion. A total of six numbers are required to define the three-dimensional motion: four define the position and orientation of the helical axis, and two define the amount of rotation about and translation along it.

The helical axis of motion is one of the most precise ways to define the three-dimensional motion of a rigid body. This method of presentation is well suited for describing motion of irregular bodies, such as anatomic structures upon which it is difficult to consistently and accurately identify reference points. Because the helical axis of motion describes any kind of general motion, there are many illustrative examples.

If one throws a perfect "bullet" pass with an American football, as shown in Figure A-28C, then instantaneous motion of the ball is defined by a helical axis that runs through the center and

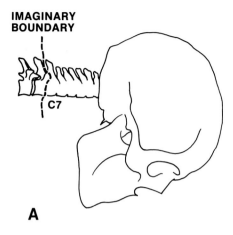

IMAGINARY
BOUNDARY

C7

A

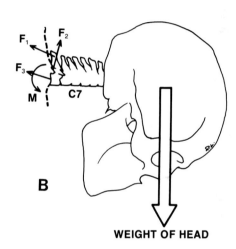

F_1 F_2

F_3

M   C7

B

WEIGHT OF HEAD

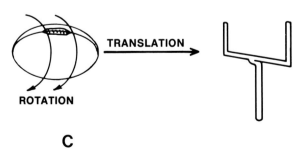

TRANSLATION

ROTATION

C

Fig. A-28. Free-body analysis. (*A*) A structure is isolated for analysis. (*B*) The external load and possible internal forces and moments are shown. (*C*) Helical axis of motion.

is oriented along the longitudinal axis. The ball is translating along that axis and is rotating about that same axis.

When a screw is driven into the bone to fix a fracture, the screw translates into the bone as its head is rotated. The motion of the screw is a helical motion, and the axis of the screw is the helical axis of motion. It is for this reason that the helical axis is sometimes called a screw axis of motion.

The helical axis has been used in two instances in orthopaedics, namely to define intervertebral motions in the thoracic spine,[20] and the motions of the metacarpophalangeal joint.[10] A potential use for the helical axis is to define precisely the movement that has taken place in the transition from a normal spine to a scoliotic spine for each vertebra.

Hysteresis

Definition. Hysteresis is a phenomenon associated with energy loss exhibited by viscoelastic materials when they are subjected to loading and unloading cycles.

Examples. It is known that the area under a loading curve in a load-deformation diagram represents the energy of deformation (see *Energy*). If the unloading curve is exactly the same as the loading curve, then the energy of deformation is completely regained during unloading. On the other hand, if the unloading curve is *below* the loading curve then the energy regained is less than the energy expended. The area enclosed between the two curves represents the energy lost and is called hysteresis.

Figure A-29 shows the results of a tension test experiment performed on a cruciate ligament of a rabbit.[19] Note that the load-deformation curve during the unloading cycle is below the curve for the loading cycle. Measurements from the diagram show that 17 per cent of the total energy is lost during a cycle.

Impulse

Definition. Linear impulse of a force is the product of the force and the time interval of force application. The unit of measure is newton seconds (poundforce seconds).

Angular impulse of a moment is defined as the product of the moment and the time interval of

moment application. The unit of measure is newton meter seconds (foot poundforce seconds).

Examples. When one pushes a stalled car on the road, it gains speed slowly. At any point in time the speed of the car is in direct proportion to the magnitude of the force, and the time interval for which it is applied. According to the definition, this is impulse. If larger impulse is applied to the same car or if the same impulse is applied to a smaller car, both cars will achieve higher speed.

In trauma, the destruction of the tissue (hard as well as soft) depends not only upon the magnitude of the force but also upon the time duration of force application. It has been shown in spinal cord trauma experiments, in which a weight is dropped from a certain height, that the amount of damage to the cord is directly related to the magnitude of impulse of the falling weight.[4]

Inertia

Definition. The property of all material bodies to resist change in the state of rest or of motion under the action of applied loads.

Examples. A bicycle has mass, and therefore inertia. One must apply forces to the pedals to get the bike moving from its state of rest. To slow down, it is necessary to apply braking forces to alter the state of motion to a slower one.

The concept of inertia is important in the analysis of trauma to the spine. When an acceleration

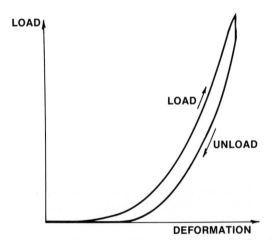

Fig. A-29. Hysteresis. The area between the two curves is the energy loss in one load/unload cycle.

is imparted to the lower portion of a resting spine in a rear end collision (whiplash) the inertia of the head and upper portion of the body resists the change. This resistance imparts potentially injuring forces to the spine and adjacent structures (see *Angular Acceleration*).

Instantaneous Axis of Rotation

Definition. When a rigid body moves in a plane, at every instant there is a point in the body or some hypothetical extension of it that does not move. An axis perpendicular to the plane of motion and passing through that point is the instantaneous axis (center) of rotation for that motion at that instant.

Examples. Plane motion is fully defined by the position of the instantaneous axis and the magnitude of rotation about it. Figure A-30 shows a graphical technique of determining the instantaneous axis of rotation when a body moves from position 1 to position 2. The axis is found to be at the intersection of the two perpendicular bisectors of translation vectors $A_1 A_2$ and $B_1 B_2$ of any two points A and B on the body.

Vertebrae undergo plane motion during flexion/extension of the spine. Each vertebra has instantaneous axes of rotation in relation to an outside frame of reference (e.g., the ground) as well as in reference to each of the other vertebrae. During motion from full flexion to full extension or vice versa, different anatomic components (ligaments, muscles, and portions of facet articulation) come into play as motion progresses. In other words, the structure of the spine motion segment changes. Since an instantaneous axis of rotation is related to a certain structure, it also changes as a function of the degree of bending.

The beauty of the concept of the instantaneous axis of rotation is that any kind of plane motion may be described: translation, rotation, or a combination of the two. For a detailed study of complex plane motion, one may regard the motion as being made up of smaller steps. Thus, a set of instantaneous axes of rotation (IAR) may be established to represent the total motion. This pattern of IAR has been successfully utilized in clinical evaluation of knee injuries.[7]

Instantaneous Velocity

Definition. The average velocity when the time interval approaches zero. The unit of measure is meters per second (feet per second).

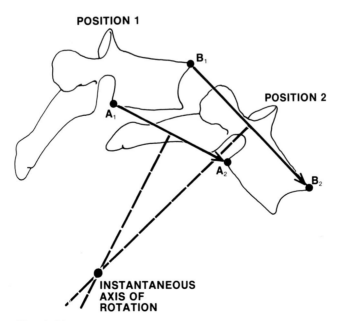

Fig. A-30. Instanteneous axis of rotation. A construction for determining the IAR is shown.

Velocity is linear when the motion is translation and angular when it is rotation. It is a vector quantity and therefore has magnitude (speed) and direction.

Examples. A car travelling from Yale to Harvard (Fig. A-31), for some unfathomable reason, has an average speed (velocity magnitude) of 100 km/h (60 mph). At a certain instant in time the speed is probably higher or lower than the average (i.e., the instantaneous speed varied). At another instant in time the direction of the speed probably differs from the direction of Yale to Harvard. A complete description of velocity of the car, therefore, requires full documentation of its instantaneous velocity vectors, which includes changes in both speed and direction throughout its journey from excellent toward good. On the straight portions of the road (Fig. A-31A), if the speed changes, the velocity vector varies. On the curved portions of the road (Fig. A-31B), the speed may remain constant, but the velocity vector will vary due to the continually changing direction.

Integration, Integral

Definition. An incremental summation process.

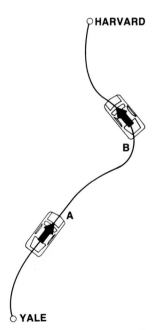

Fig. A-31. Instantaneous velocity.

Examples. Integration is used for finding lengths, areas, and volumes of complex objects by adding together all the small bits into which the object could be divided.

To find the volume of a whole tibia, cut it into transverse sections that are a millimeter (0.04 in) thick. By measuring the areas of all cross-sections and multiplying these by the thickness and adding them all together, the tibia volume is obtained. This physical process can be done mathematically if information regarding variation of the cross-sectional area as a function of axial length can be expressed mathematically. Then,

$$\text{tibia volume} = \int_{l_1}^{l_2} A\, dl$$

where $\int$ represents the concept of integration. The mathematical function that describes the variation of the cross-sectional area with length is denoted by letter A and dl is the symbol denoting that the integration (summation) is to be performed along the length. Quantities l_1 and l_2 are the boundaries of the length l.

The right-hand side of the expression above is the integral and the process of computation is called integration. It should be read as follows: "integral of A with respect to l between the limits l_1 and l_2." Sometimes the limits l_1 and l_2 may be missing from the expression, which implies that these are either understood or have not yet been defined.

Isotropic Material

Definition. A material is called isotropic if its mechanical properties are the same in all directions.

In other words, if one takes a sample of the isotropic material for testing, then the values of its mechanical properties (strength and modulus of elasticity) will be the same regardless of the orientations of the test samples.

Examples. Metals, hardened methylmethacrylate, and ice are examples of isotropic materials. Wood and bone, as a contrast, are not isotropic because they have fibers (collagen and cellulose, respectively) oriented in preferred directions. There is, to our knowledge, no isotropic tissue in the body because every tissue is highly specialized to resist loads optimally in a certain direction only. Therefore, a tennis ball is used here rather than an organ to demonstrate isotropic properties.

Wherever the surface of the tennis ball is hit, its mechanical properties are the same, provided that the force vector remains constant. When the ball is hit its subsequent motion depends upon the load-deformation characteristics in the direction of the force vector at the time of the ball-racket contact. This consistency of mechanical response is isotropy.

Experiments have shown that cortical bone is highly sensitive to the direction of force application and is therefore not isotropic.[16]

Joint Reaction Force

Definition. If a joint in the body is subjected to external forces in the form of external loads and/or muscle forces, the internal reaction forces acting at the contact surfaces are called the joint reaction forces. The unit of measure is newtons (poundforce).

Example. The contact surface of the metacarpal portion of a metacarpophalangeal joint (Fig. A-32A) has two components of joint reaction: one that is perpendicular to the contact surface, called the normal component, and the other parallel to the surface, called the tangential or frictional component (Fig. A-32B). The perpendicular component is always compressive. The tangential component in the healthy joints is generally very small, about 1 per cent of the normal component. This is due to very low joint friction. The direction of the tangential component is always opposite to the sliding motion. The ratio of the two components (tangential to normal) is the coefficient of friction of the joint.

Kilopond

Definition. A metric measure of force. It is equal to the gravitational force applied to one kilogram of mass at the earth's surface.

Example. If a 1-kg mass is held in the hand, a downward force of 1 kp is applied to the hand by the earth's gravity. Therefore, there is a one to one relation between mass in kilograms (or pounds) and its force in kiloponds (or poundforce). Unfortunately, this relationship is strictly earthbound. It does not apply to forces on the

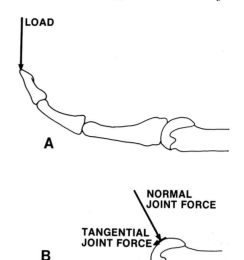

Fig. A-32. Joint reaction force.

moon, for example. Because the moon's gravity is only one-sixth of that of the earth, a 1-kg (1-lb) mass on the moon applies a downward force on the hand of only one-sixth of a kilopond (or poundforce). This is one of the reasons that in the newly adopted Systeme International d'Unites, the unit of force is newtons (see *Newton*).

The kilopond is abbreviated as kp and conversion factors to units of force are as follows:

1 kilopond (kp)	= 9.806	newtons
1 kilopond (kp)	= 2.205	poundforce
1 newton (N)	= 0.1020	kilopond
1 newton (N)	= 0.2249	poundforce
1 poundforce (1bf)	= 0.4536	kilopond
1 poundforce (1bf)	= 4.448	newtons

Kinematics

Definition. That division of mechanics (dynamics) that deals with the geometry of the motion of bodies: displacement, velocity, and acceleration, without taking into account the forces that produce the motion.

Examples. Range and pattern of motion of various anatomic joints are good examples of kinematic studies. When a scoliotic deformity, as measured by Cobb's method, is compared at different times, a kinematic study of the disease is being performed.

Kinetic Energy

Definition.   The energy that a body possesses due to its velocity. The unit of measure is newton meters or joules (foot poundforce).

Examples.   An automobile weighing 2500 kg (3290 lb) travelling at 50 km/h (30 mph) possesses a kinetic energy of 241,127 newton meters (167,000 foot poundforce; Fig. A-33A). Doubling the speed makes the kinetic energy four times greater (Fig. A-33B). Therefore, a collision at twice the speed is potentially four times more damaging because of the kinetic energy that must be dissipated at the time of collision.

Explanatory Notes.   Mathematically, the kinetic energy T in joules is expressed as follows:

$$T = \frac{m \times V^2}{2}$$

where n = mass of the body in kilogram (pound)
   V = velocity (speed) in meters per second (feet per second).

Kinetics

Definition.   A branch of mechanics (dynamics) that studies the relations between the force system acting on a body and the changes it produces in the body motion.

Examples.   Observe an athlete starting for the 100-meter dash. From a standstill, he reaches his cruising speed in a few seconds. His muscles apply forces at appropriate points on the bones to produce maximum acceleration of the whole body. A study involving relationships between the various muscle forces applied and the body acceleration produced is a kinetic study of the mechanics of short-distance running.

A study of the forces acting on a scoliotic spine to move it from a deformed position to a more corrected position is another example of kinetics.

Linear

See *Nonlinear.*

Load

Definitions.   A general term describing the application of a force and/or moment (torque) to a structure. The units of measure are newtons (poundforce) for the force and newton meters (foot poundforce) for the moment.

Because the force and moment are three-dimensional vectors each having three components, the load may be thought of as a six-component vector.

Examples.   When a person lifts a weight (Fig. A-34), the spine is loaded. The L5 vertebra is subjected to weights (forces) from the upper body and the lifted weight. It is also subjected to the bending moment caused by the forces because these forces are away from the center of the L5 vertebra. Thus, the load vector at L5 completely describes all the forces and moments acting on it.

Load-Deformation Curve

See *Stress-Strain Diagram.*

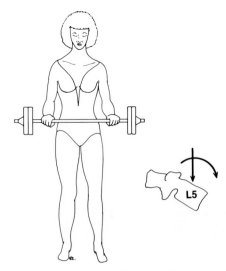

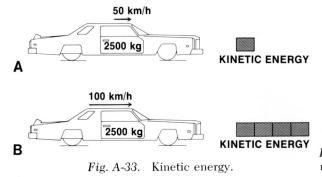

Fig. A-33.   Kinetic energy.

Fig. A-34.   Load is equivalent to forces and/or moments.

Mass

Definition. The quantitative measure of inertia for linear motion. The unit of measure is kilograms (pounds).

Example. Imagine a cart of mass M kilograms (pounds) on frictionless wheels on a table, as shown in Figure A-35. Apply a given force F newtons (poundforce) to the cart by means of a string. The cart will accelerate into motion. If the mass of the cart is doubled and the same force is applied again, the cart starts moving rather slowly, at precisely half the acceleration. The additional mass doubles the total inertia, thus reducing the acceleration.

The above phenomenon was first critically observed by Newton and forms the basis of Newton's second law of motion, which states that a body is accelerated in direct proportion to the amount of force applied. The constant of proportionality between the acceleration and the force is called mass (see also *Newton's Laws*).

Weight of a body is a term that is loosely used. However, it is defined as a measure of the *force* applied to the body by the earth's gravity. Therefore, when 1 kg of sugar is held in one's hand, the sugar is being pulled downward with a force of 1 kilogramforce (1 kilopond or 9.81 N).

Mass-Mathematical Element

Definition. In mathematical modelling, mass is used to represent the inertia of heavy bodies to linear motion.

Example. Consider a model of a passenger-automobile system involved in a collision. This is a dynamic situation. Relatively heavy parts of this system (e.g., the automobile, trunk, head, arms, and legs) offer considerable resistance to change in motion due to their mass. Representation of this behaviour in a mathematical model is done by the mass-mathematical elements.

Mass Moment of Inertia

Definition. The quantitative measure of inertia for change in angular velocity. The unit of measure is kilogram meter squared (pound foot squared).

Examples. A bicycle wheel off the ground, if given a certain speed, continues to rotate for a long time. It does this because of the mass mo-

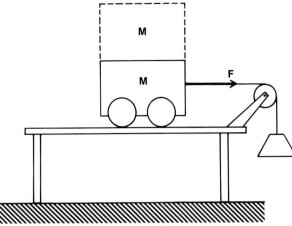

Fig. A-35. Mass. The same force F applied to twice the mass will produce half the acceleration.

ment of inertia of its rim. This inertia is equal to the mass of the rim times the square of the radius of the wheel. If the same rim mass is concentrated into a small disc around the wheel axle and is given the same speed, it slows down much faster because of its lower radius and the mass moment of inertia. It is this mass moment of inertia of the wheels that keeps a bicycle stable in its upright position when it is in motion.

Another example of this phenomenon is the figure skater who is spinning with both arms abducted out to the sides. Gradually bringing the arms in causes an increase in the spin (Fig. A-36).

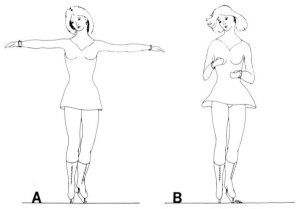

Fig. A-36. Mass moment of inertia. (A) In this position, the skater is spinning at a slow speed and has great inertia. (B) Bringing the arms toward the sides decreases the inertia and increases the speed of spinning.

This may be explained on the basis that the angular momentum (mass moment of inertia times the spin speed) of the body remains the same. As the arms are brought in there is a decrease in the radius of gyration and the mass moment of inertia. Because the angular momentum is constant, there is a corresponding increase in the spin speed.

Explanatory Notes. Mathematically, the mass moment of inertia, called I, is given by the following:

$$I = m \times R^2$$

where m = mass of the body in kilograms (pounds)
R = radius of gyration in meters (feet)

Mathematical Model

Definition. A set of mathematical equations that quantitatively describes the behavior of a given physical system.

Examples. There are situations that cannot be duplicated experimentally. Examples are human spine behavior during pilot ejection from disabled aircrafts, whiplash injury in automobile collision, and landing of the lunar module on the moon. However, these situations can be simulated by a computer using the technique of mathematical modelling.

Consider the simulation of the mechanism of whiplash injury (Fig. A-37A). The simplest model represents the human body-automobile system as consisting of three masses: the head (M_1), the trunk (M_2), and the automobile including the rest of the body (M_3), as shown in Figure A-37B. As a first approximation, the cervical spine and the hip joint may be represented as hinges and the seat belt as a spring. The rear end collision is simulated by a sudden acceleration applied to the mass M_3.

A simple idea of the mechanism may be obtained by building a physical model in wood. However, for more accurate and detailed studies, a complex mathematical simulation in a computer is required. In an analysis of this kind, the effects of such variables as design of the passenger seat, stiffness of the seat belt, body weight, viscoelastic properties of the cervical spine, and severity of the collision may easily be simulated. Complex

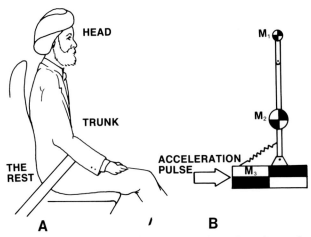

Fig. A-37. Mathematical model. (*A*) The physical system may be divided into three entities: the head, the trunk, and the rest (remaining body and all of the automobile). (*B*) A simple mathematical model consists of three masses, M_1, M_2, and M_3, representing the three entities and spring-like elements joining the masses.

simulations utilize the capacity of computers to deal with massive quantities of information at very high speed.

Modulus of Elasticity

Definition. The ratio of normal stress to normal strain in a material. The unit of measure for the modulus of elasticity (E) is newtons per square meter (poundforce per square foot).

Examples. The modulus of elasticity defines the mechanical behavior of the *material* of a structure. It is a measure of the stiffness of the material. Cortical bone has a high modulus of elasticity and subcutaneous fat, sometimes quite aesthetically, has a low modulus of elasticity. The higher the value, the stiffer the material.

To appreciate the biomechanical interaction between the components of an orthopaedic design, the moduli of elasticity of some relevant materials are given in Table A-3.

The modulus of elasticity is generally obtained by calculating the slope of the linear elastic part of the stress-strain diagram of a material.

Moment

See *Couple.*

Table A-3. Moduli of Elasticity

	× 10⁹ N/m²	× 10⁶ psi
Stainless steel*	200	29
Cortical bone†		
Longitudinal	8.9	1.3
Tangential	4.3	0.6
Radial	3.8	0.5
Methylmethacrylate	1.0	0.15
Cancellous bone†	0.14	0.02

* American Society for Testing and Materials. Standards for Surgical Implants, Tab.2. Philadelphia, 1971.
† Evans, F. G.: Mechanical Properties of Bone. Springfield, Charles C Thomas, 1973.

Moment of Inertia of an Area

Definition. A measure of the distribution of a material in a certain manner about its centroid. This distribution determines the strength in bending and torsion. The unit of measure is meters (feet) to the fourth power.

Examples. Consider an object with circular cross-section. How should its material be distributed to make it strong in bending and torsional loading? The concept of moment of inertia of an area is useful here in a comparison of a solid rod and a hollow rod, both with the same cross-section.

A rod 10 mm (0.394 in) in diameter, shown in Figure A-38A, has a moment of inertia about its diameter of 490 mm⁴. Redistributing this same material into a hollow tube of 1-mm (0.039-in) thickness results in an outer diameter of 26 mm (1.024 in) and moment of inertia of 3256 mm⁴ (0.0078 in⁴). Now the bending strength (the moment of inertia divided by the radius; see *Bending*) of the two rods may be calculated. The 26-mm, thin tube is 2.56 times as strong as the 10-mm rod. If similar calculations are made for the torsion loading (see *Torsion*), the mass distribution effect is even more dramatic. The corresponding strength ratio is 5.12 in torsion.

One of the best examples of the above concepts is the construction of human bones. They are hollow and cancellous on the inside and hard and cortical on the outside. This provides maximum "strength" for weight and also some neat space for making blood cells.

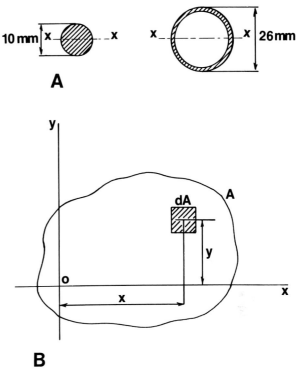

Fig. A-38. Area moment of inertia. (A) The hollow tube is 2.56 times stronger in bending and 5.12 times stronger in torsion than the solid tube. Both tubes have the same amount of material. (B) Mathematical interpretation.

Explanatory Notes. The moment of inertia for a given section of a long structure is calculated by the formulas given below. Figure A-38B shows a sectional area A. Its moments of inertia about x-axis and y-axis passing through point O are given by formulas:

$$I_{xx} = \int y^2 \, dA$$

$$I_{yy} = \int x^2 \, dA$$

where integration is done over the whole area A. For a circular section, as depicted in Figure A-39A the following applies:

$$I_{xx} = I_{yy} = \frac{\pi d^4}{64}$$

where $\pi \simeq 3.14$ and d is the diameter.

Momentum

Definition. Linear momentum of a particle or rigid body is the product of its mass and its velocity. The unit of measure is kilogram meters per second (pound feet per second).

Angular momentum of a particle or rigid body is defined as the product of its mass moment of inertia and its angular velocity. The unit of measure is kilogram meter squared per second (pound foot squared per second).

Motion

Definition. The relative displacement with time of a body in space, with respect to other bodies or some reference system.

Examples. A general displacement of a rigid body consists of rotation about a certain axis combined with translation along a certain direction. The body that is not constrained has six degrees of freedom. One method used to describe the general motion of a rigid body is to measure translation vectors of any three identifiable points on it. Another method is to break down the observed motion into its two natural components, namely a translation vector of a chosen point and rotation of the body about an axis through that point. Finally, the most elegant method is to determine the helical axis of motion, which does not require any points on the body (see *Helical Axis of Motion*).

A special case of general motion is motion in which the body moves in a plane and has only three degrees of freedom. This motion may be described by translation vectors of any two points on a rigid body. Alternately, a translation vector of a point and a rotation about that point are sufficient. More concisely, it is defined by its instantaneous axis of rotation and the angle of rotation (see *Instantaneous Axis of Rotation*).

Another simplified version of general motion is out-of-plane motion. Again, there are three degrees of freedom: two rotations about mutually perpendicular axes and a translation perpendicular to the plane formed by the axes.

Motion Segment

Definition. A unit of the spine representing inherent biomechanical characteristics of the ligamentous spine.

Physically, it consists of two adjacent vertebrae and the interconnecting soft tissue, devoid of musculature. In the thoracic region, two articulating heads of ribs with their connecting ligaments are also included.

Motion Segment is the most commonly used term that is used to explain this concept. However, it is grammatically incorrect. An acceptable alternative would be to use the hyphenated form motion-segment. The functional spinal unit, which is discussed in Chapter 1, is the term of choice, as it adequately describes the concept and is grammatically correct.

Neutral Axis

Definition. A longitudinal line in a long structure where normal axial stresses are zero when the structure is subjected to bending.

If a long structure with symmetrical cross-section is subjected to bending loads in its plane of symmetry, it develops a curvature. The fibers on the convex side of this curvature are then in tension, while those on the concave side undergo compressive stresses. Somewhere in between these two layers is a layer of fibers that has zero normal stress. This is the neutral plane.

When the bending takes place in the vertical (x, y) plane (Fig. A-39), the fibers in the horizontal (x, z) plane will be stress-free. This is the neutral plane for this loading. If bending loads were applied in the x, z plane, the x, y plane would be the neutral plane. The line of intersection of the two neutral planes is called the neutral axis. It should be noted that although the normal stress is zero at the neutral axis, there may be shear stresses present due to transverse forces.

If the long structure is subjected to torsion about the neutral axis, again the fibers at the neutral axis are unique, and the shear stress is zero.

From the above discussion, we conclude that the fibers at and around the neutral axis have very low stresses compared to the fibers at the periphery during bending and torsional loads. In human bones, the development of hollow structures, with cortical bone distributed toward the periphery where the stresses are highest, may be an example of biomechanical adaptation.

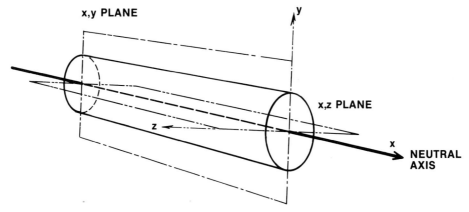

Fig. A-39. Neutral axis. The x, y and x, z planes shown here are the neutral planes. Their intersection is the neutral axis.

Newton

Definition. The unit of force in the Systeme International d'Unites. One newton is the amount of force required to give a 1-kg mass an acceleration of 1 meter per second per second.

A newton is the best unit of force because it is not dependent upon the earth's gravitational field for its definition, in contrast to the kilopond and poundforce. Thus, it is the universal measure of force. It is based upon Newton's second law of motion, which states that a force in newtons equals the mass in kilograms multiplied by acceleration in meters per second per second. The name has been chosen to honor the man who laid the foundation of modern mechanics.

The abbreviation is N and the conversion factors to other units of force are as follows:

1 newton (N)	= 0.2248 poundforce
1 poundforce (lbf)	= 4.48 newtons
1 newton (N)	= 0.1020 kilopond
1 kilopond (kp)	= 9.806 newtons
1 newton (N)	= 100,000 dynes

Newton's Laws

Definition. Isaac Newton (1642–1727) postulated three laws that form the basis of mechanical engineering science. These are based on his observations and since their inception they have been shown to be in agreement with other observations. The laws and their simple interpretations are as follows:

(1) A body remains in a state of rest or of uniform motion in a straight line until it is acted upon by a force to change that state. In other words, a book on the table will stay there forever and a golf ball once hit will keep travelling with constant velocity (assuming no air resistance or gravity) until some force interferes.

(2) The rate of change of momentum is equal to the force producing it. Stated differently, force equals mass times acceleration. For rotatory motion, moment equals mass moment of inertia times angular acceleration.

(3) To every action there is an equal and opposite reaction. A classical example is a rocket. The exhaust gases are pushed toward the rear (action) while the rocket is pushed forward (reaction).

Nonlinear

Definition. The concepts utilized in characterizing the relationship between two variable quantities.

If the ratio of one variable quantity to the other variable quantity is constant through a defined range of values, then the relationship is said to be linear within that range. Any deviation from linearity is defined as nonlinear behavior. If this relationship is plotted on graph paper, only the linear relation will be a straight line.

Examples. A tracing of an actual load-deformation curve* of a motion segment including two vertebrae subjected to compressive loading is shown in Figure A-40. The initial portion of the curve, 0–3 mm of deformation, is highly nonlinear, which may be demonstrated by drawing a straight line from the origin to the 3-mm point on the curve. If a similar line is drawn from the 3-mm point to the 5-mm deformation point on the curve, it is seen that the deviation from linearity of the actual curve is rather small. Therefore, for all practical purposes, the later portion of the curve is considered linear. For more precise quantification of nonlinearity see the explanation below.

Explanatory Notes. If one needs to be precise, the percentage of nonlinearity may be defined. This is the percentage ratio of maximum deviation from the straight line (f) to the highest range (F), as shown in Figure A-40. In this example, the 0- to 3-mm range has nonlinearity of 44 per cent, and the corresponding figure for the 3- to 5-mm range is 3.7 per cent.

Normal Stress

Definition. The intensity of force perpendicular to the surface on which it acts. The unit of measure of normal stress is newtons per square meter, also called pascals (poundforce per square foot).

Example. When a structure such as a long bone or an implant is subjected to tension, compression, and/or bending, the axial fibers of the structure are subjected to normal stress. Figure A-41A shows a bone being subjected to bending moments. Normal stresses act perpendicular to a surface. It can be either a positive normal stress as in tension, or a negative normal stress, as in compression. In bending, there is compressive stress on the concave side and tensile stress on the convex side of the neutral axis (Fig. A-41A, B). There is also a normal stress in fibers oriented 45 degrees to the longitudinal axis when a tubular structure is subjected to torsional loading. This is the mechanism involved in spiral ski frac-

---

* Unpublished data from the Engineering Laboratory for Musculoskeletal Diseases, Yale Medical Center, New Haven, Conn.

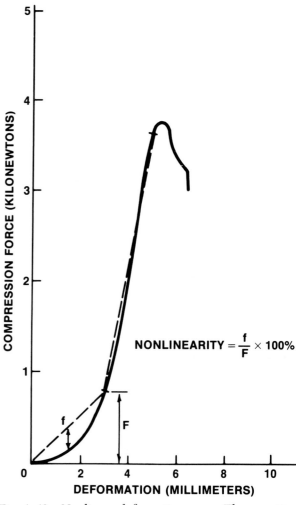

$$\text{NONLINEARITY} = \frac{f}{F} \times 100\%$$

Fig. A-40. Nonlinear deformation curve. The quantity *nonlinearity* specifies the amount of departure from a straight line.

tures. A simple equation for the normal stress is given below.

Explanatory Notes. The common symbol for denoting the normal stress is the Greek letter σ (sigma). Mathematically, the normal stress is given by the following formula:

$$\sigma = \frac{F}{A}$$

where F is the applied force in newtons (poundforce) and A is the area in square meters (square feet).

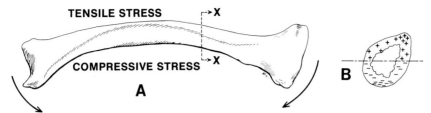

Fig. A-41. Normal stress. (*A*) A bone subjected to bending moments. (*B*) Cross-section at x-x. The tensile stresses (+) are on the convex side while compressive stresses (−) are on the concave side.

Out-of-Plane Motion

Definition. A motion of a rigid body in which the body does not move in a single plane.

Out-of-plane motion is a combination of translation and rotation. It has three degrees of freedom: rotation about two mutually perpendicular axes, forming a plane, and translation perpendicular to that plane.

Example. The lateral bending of the spine exemplifies this type of motion. A vertebra in the spine undergoing lateral bending is shown in Figure A-42. The vertebra rotates about a horizontal axis (z-axis) and translates out of the sagittal plane into the horizontal plane. It goes from Position 1 to 2 to 3, as shown in Figure A-42. (Because of the coupling there may also be axial rotation, which is not shown here.) In contrast to this motion, plane motion is depicted in Figure A-43.

Plane Motion

Definition. A motion in which all points of a rigid body move parallel to a fixed plane.

This motion is a combination of translation and rotation. It has three degrees of freedom: translations along two mutually perpendicular axes and rotation about an axis perpendicular to the other two axes.

Example. Flexion/extension of the spine (Fig. A-43) translates a vertebra in the horizontal and vertical directions. At the same time it rotates the vertebra about an axis perpendicular to the sagittal plane, from position 1 to 2 to 3. The motion takes place in a single plane. This is in contrast to out-of-plane motion (see *Instantaneous Axis of Rotation*).

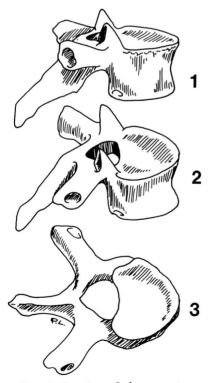

Fig. A-42. Out-of-plane motion.

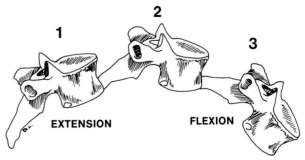

Fig. A-43. Plane motion.

Plasticity

Definition. The property of a material to permanently deform when it is loaded beyond its elastic range.

Examples. The stress-strain curve for a material is shown in Figure A-44. When the material is loaded beyond its elastic range (AB), it enters the plastic range (BE). Unloading within the plastic range, as shown by the line CD, always produces permanent deformation, shown as AD. On reloading, the material generally passes back into the plastic range as if unloading and reloading had not taken place.

To understand and visualize plastic behavior, engineers make use of a simple model consisting of a friction block connected in series with a spring, as shown in the lower portion of Figure A-44. The motion of the free end of the spring describes the behavior of the material subjected to a force.

The application of the force produces deformation of the spring, but no motion of the friction block. This corresponds to the elastic material behavior (AB). This behavior continues until the force reaches a value that is just sufficient to move the friction block. This corresponds to the

yield point B for the material. A small additional force produces motion of the entire model with no additional deformation of the spring. This behavior corresponds to the plastic behavior of the material (BC). On release of the load (at C) the spring recoils (CD), but the friction block does not go back to its original position, thus producing permanent deformation (AD). Reloading (DCE) duplicates the loading behavior (ABC).

The permanent deformation of a ligament after it has been subjected to greater than 40 per cent of its ultimate load is one of the examples of plastic behavior.[18] Under such high load, collagenous fibers glide over one another, in the manner of the friction block.

Plastic Range

Definition. If a specimen is loaded beyond its elastic range, it enters the plastic range.

Examples. In Figure A-44, AB is the elastic range, and BE is the plastic range. Modelling the elastic and plastic behavior by a friction block connected in series with a spring is a simple way to visualize what is happening. The larger the plastic range until failure, the higher is the ductility and energy absorption capacity of the material.

When Dizzy Gillespie first began playing his trumpet as a young man, the deformation of his cheeks was in the elastic range, and they returned to their normal size. In later years, with strong forces and perhaps some alterations in the tissues, his cheeks went into the *plastic range of deformation* (Fig. A-45).

Poisson's Ratio

Definition. The ratio of transverse to axial strain. It is generally represented by the Greek letter ν (nu). Since it is a ratio, there is no unit of measurement.

Examples. Take a rubber band and stretch it. A careful observation shows that it gets thinner when stretched. The reverse will happen if a piece of rubber such as a pencil eraser is compressed. In both instances the changes in the transverse dimensions take place because, in general, the material is incompressible (this is not true of gases). The volume remains constant. An increase or decrease in the length is accom-

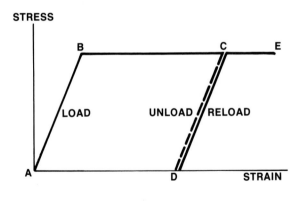

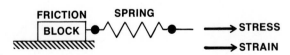

Fig. A-44. Plasticity. AB = elastic loading (spring); BC = plastic deformation (friction); CD = elastic unloading (spring); AD = permanent deformation (friction); DCE = reloading cycle; DCE ≡ ABC.

panied by corresponding decrease and increase, respectively, in the transverse dimensions. Poisson's ratio quantifies this material behavior.

When a screw is employed to fix a fracture, Poisson's ratio is in action. As the screw is tightened, the bone is compressed and the screw is lengthened. Because of Poisson's effect, the thread diameter in the bone expands and the screw diameter decreases. Therefore, a screw that is all right under no load may become loose when tightened. The chances of this happening are small if the standard hole is drilled for a given screw. (This phenomenon is different from the mechanism of a screw pullout, in which the bone between the threads is stripped by driving the screw too hard.)

This effect was first discovered by Poisson in the early 19th century. The theoretical upper limit for this ratio for any material is 0.5. Bone and steel have a Poisson's ratio of approximately 0.3.

Explanatory Notes. If a rubber eraser, cylindrical in shape, is subjected to compression, the axial strain is the change in unit length, $(L_1 - L_2)/L_1$, and the transverse strain is the change in unit diameter, $(D_2 - D_1)/D_1$. The ratio of the first to the second strain is Poisson's ratio.

Polar Moment of Inertia

Definition. A property of the cross-section of a long structure that gives a measure of the distribution of the material about its axis so as to maximize its torsional strength. The unit of measure is meter to the fourth power (foot to the fourth power).

Examples. When a long structure is subjected to torsion, the maximum shear stress and angle of rotation are functions of the torque applied, the material properties, and the geometry of the cross-sections. The last quantity is characterized by the polar moment of inertia of the section. The more distant the mass is with respect to the axis of torsion, the greater is the polar moment of inertia. The general expression for determining the polar moment of inertia for a given section is given below.

The juncture of the middle and distal thirds of the tibia fractures more frequently than any other area. This is the shaded area shown in Figure

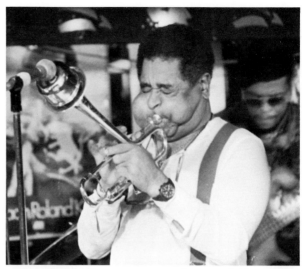

Fig. A-45. Plastic range. (Photograph by Ozier Muhammad. *In* JET Magazine, November 10, 1977. Copyright © 1977 by Johnson Publishing, Inc., Chicago.)

A-46B. Fracture is common largely because the polar moment of inertia at this distal section is minimal compared to the rest of the tibia. (In reality it is the polar moment of inertia divided by the radius that determines the sheer stress in the tibia; see *Torsion*.) The diagram shows the actual polar moment of inertia of a human tibia on the vertical axis (ordinate) and the distance from the distal end on the horizontal axis (abscissa).[15]

Explanatory Notes. Referring to Figure A-46A the mathematical expression for the polar moment of inertia is as follows:

$$J = \int r^2 \, dA$$

where J = polar moment of inertia of an area
  dA = small area away from axis
  r = radius to the center of dA
  $\int$ = integration over the whole section

Potential Energy

Definition. Energy that may be stored within a structure as a result of deformation or displacement of that structure. The unit of measure is newton meters or joules (foot poundforce).

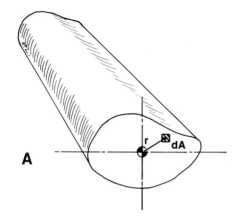

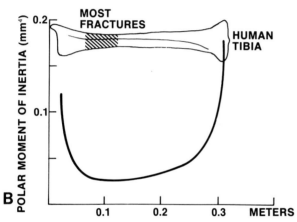

Fig. A-46. Polar moment of inertia. (*A*) Mathematical interpretation. (*B*) Experimentally determined values for the human tibia.

Explanatory Notes. Referring to Figure A-47A, the formula for the potential energy is as follows:

$$U = \frac{F \times D}{2}$$

where U = potential energy in N m or J (lbf ft)
F = force of deformation in N (lbf)
D = deformation in m (ft)

The above formula is valid for a force proportional to deformation, as shown in Figure A-47A. For other force-deformation relationships, the equation will be in an integral form.

Principal Planes

Definition. In a structure, those planes in which the shear stress is zero and only the normal stresses are present.

When a structure is subjected to loads, stresses are created within it. Looking at a single point in

Examples. By testing a spring in a testing machine, its load-deformation graph may be drawn as shown in Figure A-47A. The shaded area under the graph is the potential energy stored in the spring for the given deformation. This energy is recoverable in the form of useful work. A clock with a spring-wound motor works on this principle. Other mechanical clocks work by storing the potential energy in the form of displacement of the weights against gravity.

Pulling back a bow stores the potential energy of deformation of the bow (Fig. A-47B). On release of the arrow this energy is converted into the kinetic energy of the arrow (see *Kinetic Energy*).

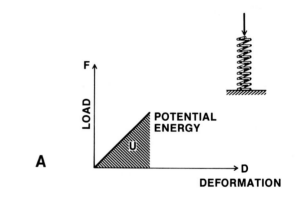

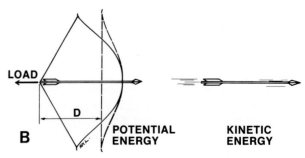

Fig. A-47. Potential energy. (*A*) The deformation of a spring stores potential energy. (*B*) Potential energy may be converted into kinetic energy.

the structure, innumerable planes may pass through that point in various directions. On each of these planes there are stresses perpendicular to the planes (normal stresses) and parallel to the planes (shear stresses). The proportion of normal to shear stresses varies with different planes. Those planes in which there are only normal stresses (i.e., no shear stresses) are called the principal planes (by definition). Because the material generally fails due to excessive tensile, normal stresses, determination of directions along which these stresses are highest (principal planes) is of great practical importance. At a given point in a structure subjected to a load, there are always three principal planes, and they are perpendicular to each other. One or two of these planes may not be of any interest in simple loading situations, but they are still there. A few examples are described below.

Examples. If a cylindrical test specimen were taken from a bone and were subjected to tension, there would be only one principal plane of interest, the plane perpendicular to the axis, as shown in Figure A-48A. The other two planes are in axial directions.

One of the mechanisms of ski fracture injuries in the tibia is that of torsional loading, applied by a transverse force to the tip of the ski (Fig. A-48B1). If one were to look for the principal planes in the tibia subjected to torsional loading, there would be two planes, mutually perpendicular to each other, and at 45 degrees and 135 degrees to the tibial axis (Fig. A-48B2). The third plane is in the axial direction.

A more complex loading situation is that of the disc when the spine undergoes lateral bending (Fig. A-48C). The disc carries at least a vertical load, a bending moment, and an axial torque. In such a complex situation all three principal planes are of interest. Mathematical techniques are available to determine these planes, given the structure and the loading situation.

Principal Stresses

Definition. The stresses normal to the principal planes are called the principal stresses. The unit of measure is newtons per square meter or pascals (poundforce per square foot).

Examples. At a point in a three-dimensional

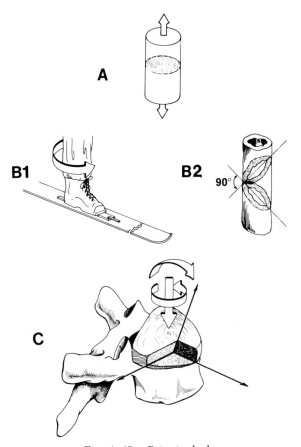

Fig. A-48. Principal planes.

body subjected to complex loads it is always possible to find three mutually perpendicular planes where shear stress is zero. Such is the case for a vertebra when the spine is subjected to bending. For a biaxial stress field (loading in one plane) there are two principal stresses of interest. An example is a ski fracture. In a uniaxial stress field (tension or compression applied to a bar) there is only one principal stress of interest. (For further explanation, see *Principal Planes.*)

Radius of Curvature

Definition. The radius of a circle that fits a given curve at a point as snugly as possible. The unit of measure is meters (feet).

The radius of curvature is a measure of smoothness or crookedness of a curve. The greater is the radius of curvature, the smoother or less crooked is the curve.

Examples. To find the amount of curvature at a point X of a curve (Fig. A-49A), mark two points A and B, one on each side at an equal distance from X. Draw a circle through the three points. (This is always possible and it will have a unique radius.) Now move the points A and B closer to X and draw a new circle. Keep repeating this procedure until the points A and B are practically the same as X. The radius of the circle at that moment, R, is the radius of curvature of the curve at that point X. The curvature is defined as the reciprocal or inverse of the radius of curvature.

Cobb's angle for measuring scoliotic spines does not give the most accurate quantification of the spinal curvature. Two scoliotic curves which are markedly different, as shown in Figure A-49B, have the same Cobb's angle measurement ($\theta_1 = \theta_2$). A more precise and descriptive quantification may be given by also measuring the radius of curvature at the apex of the curves (R_1 and R_2 in Fig. A-49B). If this method is adapted to a clinical situation, templates for measuring the radius of curvature could be used.

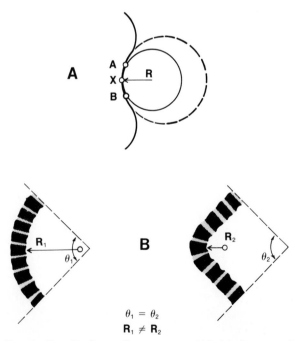

$$\theta_1 = \theta_2$$
$$R_1 \neq R_2$$

Fig. A-49. Radius of curvature. (*A*) Mathematical interpretation. (*B*) Two scoliotic spines may have the same Cobb's angle but different shapes. The latter may be defined by the radius of curvature.

Range of Motion

Definition. Quantities that indicate two points at the extremes of the physiologic range of translation and rotation of a joint for each of its six degrees of freedom. The units of measure are meters (feet) and degrees, respectively.

Example. In a motion segment of the cervical spine, one range of motion would be the number of degrees rotated or translated between the points of full active voluntary extension and full active voluntary flexion.

Rate of Deformation

See *Stress and Strain Rates.*

Rate of Loading

See *Stress and Strain Rates.*

Relative Motion

Definition. Between two moving objects, the motion of one object observed from the perspective of the second object.

Examples. Consider the following. A person sitting in a car speeding at 50 km/h (30 mph) in front of a camera set up on the ground with an open shutter holds out his arm through the car window and drops a ball from his hand. Now look closely at the relative motions of the ball with respect to the car and to the camera. Assuming that there is no air resistance to the falling ball, its motion outside the car is the same as if it were dropped inside the car. It is known that the ball inside the car will drop straight downward. Therefore the relative motion of the ball with respect to the car is a vertical, downward, straight-line motion. Now, consider the picture taken by the camera. The ball has traced a parabolic path on the picture. This is due to the fact that the ball has a horizontal velocity of 50 km/h with respect to the camera at the start of the fall. This motion is being supplemented by the increasing vertical velocity of the ball as it falls. The result is a parabolic motion, just like that of a projectile fired horizontally.

Therefore, the relative motion of an object is dependent upon the motion of the observer or the frame of reference.

The spine is a collection of vertebrae connected in a chain-like structure. When a person bends forward, the head moves with respect to the ground. This is sometimes termed an *absolute motion*. The motion of the head with respect to the C1 vertebra is the *relative motion*.

Relaxation

Definition. The decrease in stress in a deformed structure with time when the deformation is held constant.

Examples. Let a specimen of viscoelastic material be stressed and then its deformation fixed. The internal stresses decrease with time exponentially, reaching a lower value (zero at infinite time). This phenomenon is *relaxation*.

If one jumps up, grabs a branch of a nearby great tree, and pulls it so that the tip of the branch touches the ground but does not break, a certain force is required. The force necessary to hold the branch tip to the ground diminishes with time. This diminution of force is due to relaxation.

As another example, we may take a spine motion segment that has been instrumented with a force-measuring transducer (Fig. A-50A). The clamping vise is tightened to produce a certain deformation and internal stress in the motion segment. Let the deformation be kept constant (Fig. A-50B). The force transducer reading then indicates a decrease with time (Fig. A-50C). The curve of force versus time is called the relaxation curve. It is the manifestation of the viscoelastic properties of the motion segment.

Retardation

See *Acceleration* and *Angular Acceleration*.

Rigid Body

Definition. A collection of particles joined together rigidly.

Theoretically speaking, a rigid body when subjected to finite loads must not deform. However, for practical purposes the following definition is used: A body is said to be rigid if its deformation as compared to the other bodies (the so-called flexible bodies) in the system is small within a given range of the loads applied.

Examples. During flexion of the spine the motion of the head with respect to the pelvis can

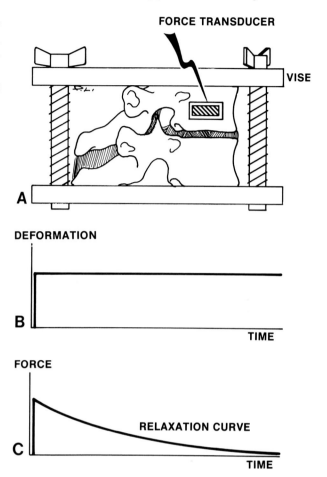

Fig. A-50. Relaxation. (*A*) Experimental set-up. (*B*) A constant deformation is applied. (*C*) The force in the specimen decreases with time.

be fully accounted for by the deformations of the discs, the vertebral arches, the spinous processes, and the ligaments. Deformation of the bodies of the vertebrae is negligible, comparatively. Thus, the vertebral bodies may be considered as rigid bodies in the spine system, under these loading conditions.

Rotation

Definition. Motion of a rigid body in which a certain straight line of the body or its rigid extension remains motionless. This line is the axis of rotation. The unit of measure is radians or degrees.

Examples. The spin of a tennis ball is a rotation about an axis through one of its major diameters. A bicycle wheel rotates about its hub axis.

All joints of the body have predominantly rotatory motions. The axis of motion, however, may vary during the complete range of motion. The variation may be in location as well as in orientation. Consider the knee. During the first 70 to 80 degrees of extension, the axis of rotation of the tibia with respect to the femur is approximately perpendicular to the femur axis. However, its position changes in a well-defined pattern as extension progresses. In the last 10 to 20 degrees of extension, it also undergoes axial rotation. This implies that near the end of extension, the axis of rotation lies at an angle different from 90 degrees to the femur axis.

Explanatory Notes. Rotation is not really a vector, since it does not obey the basic vector rules. However, small rotations (5°) may be approximated as vectors for ease of mathematical considerations. In such a case, the axis of rotation becomes the direction of the vector. The length of the vector then represents the magnitude of rotation.

Scalar

Definition. A quantity that is completely defined by its magnitude.

Examples. Room temperature is a scalar that may be measured and defined in centigrade or farhrenheit scales. Unlike vectors, scalars do not have direction, and therefore they are not dependent upon a coordinate system.

Other examples of scalar quantities are volume, density of a material, and the energy absorption capacity of bone and muscle mass.

Section Moment of Inertia

See *Moment of Inertia of an Area.*

Shear Modulus

Definition. The ratio of shear stress to the shear strain in a material. The unit of measure is newtons per square meter or pascals (poundforce per square foot).

Examples. Shear modulus is a material property. The relation of shear modulus to shear is analogous to the relation of modulus of elasticity

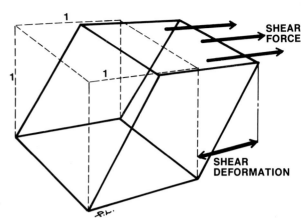

Fig. A-51. Shear modulus. Shear force deforms a cube into a parallelepiped. The ratio of shear force to deformation in a cube is a measure of the shear modulus of the material.

to tension and compression. As an example, take a cube of rubber of convenient measurements of 1 cm of length, width, and depth (Fig. A-51). Application of shear force (parallel to the upper surface) deforms the cube. Because the length and area of the chosen cube are unity, the shear force and deformation are also the shear stress and strain, respectively. The shear modulus is the ratio of the two (by definition). However, it is not an independent property of a material but is related to the modulus of elasticity and Poisson's ratio. Its exact relationship is described by a formula below.

Materials with a low modulus of elasticity (rubber, ligament) have a lower shear modulus, and those with a higher modulus of elasticity (steel, bone) have a higher shear modulus. The shear modulus is generally 37 to 40 per cent of the modulus of elasticity.

Explanatory Notes. The relationship between the shear modulus G and the other two material constants is given by the following formula:

$$G = \frac{E}{2(1 + v)}$$

where E = modulus of elasticity, N/m² (lbf/ft²)
    v = Poisson's ratio

Shear Stress

Definition. The intensity of force parallel to the surface on which it acts. The unit of measure

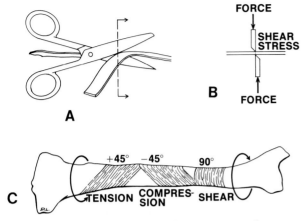

B

FORCE

SHEAR
STRESS

FORCE

A

C

+45° −45° 90°

TENSION COMPRES- SHEAR
SION

Fig. A-52. Shear stress. (*A, B*) Scissors cut the material by producing shear stresses. (*C*) Torsion produces different types of stresses in different directions.

is newtons per square meter or pascals (pound-force per square foot).

Examples. Scissors, sometimes called shears, are in fact just that, instruments that operate by producing shear stress (Fig. A-52A). They function effectively in cutting the material. Their mechanism consists of the utilization of equal and opposite forces applied to the material by means of the two blades to create nearly pure shear stress in the material (Fig. A-52B).

Shear stress is somewhat synonymous to torsion, but the failure mode in torsion may not be due to shear. An example to illustrate this point is the ski fracture. Torsion to the tibia is applied due to rotation of the foot with respect to the knee. The transverse and axial sections of the tibia are subjected to shear stresses, while sections +45° and −45° to the long axis are under normal stress (tension and compression; Fig. A-52C).

It can be shown theoretically that the magnitudes of the shear and the two normal stresses are the same. The observation that torsional loading generally produces spiral fractures implies that bone is weaker in tension than in shear.

S.I. Units

See *Conversion Table*.

Sine

See *Trigonometric Functions*.

Spherical Coordinates

See *Coordinate System*.

Spring-Mathematical Element

Definition. An elastic mathematical element. It is used in conjunction with other elements to mathematically represent observed phenomenon where elastic behaviour is present.

Examples. Elastic behaviour is depicted graphically in Figure A-53A. The loading and unloading curves for such a behaviour are exactly the same. The stiffness coefficient, the slope of the curve, quantifies the spring behaviour. If it is constant, the spring element is a linear spring and the load-deformation curve is a straight line. If the coefficient varies with load, it is a nonlinear spring and the curve is no longer a straight line (Fig. A-53A).

A model representing the action of shooting an arrow from an archer's bow basically consists of a spring. The spring, in this case, is most probably nonlinear and represents the combined properties of the bow and the string in the direction of the pull.

All biologic materials are viscoelastic in their mechanical behaviour. In order to mathematically simulate this, a combination of viscous and elastic elements are utilized. The load-deformation curve of a rabbit cruciate ligament is shown in Figure A-53B.[19] Note that the concavity of the curve is toward the load axis. This implies that the spring element is nonlinear, and its stiffness coefficient increases with load. In other words, the cruciate ligament of the rabbit becomes stiffer

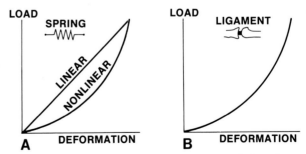

LOAD

SPRING

LINEAR

NONLINEAR

A DEFORMATION

LOAD

LIGAMENT

B DEFORMATION

Fig. A-53. Spring. (*A*) Representation of the elastic (spring-like) behavior of a material by load-deformation curve. (*B*) Such a curve can represent the behavior of a ligament.

with increasing load and thus provides greater stability as it tightens. The experiment was performed at a certain loading rate. For a different loading rate, there would be a different curve.

Stability

See *Elastic Stability* and *Clinical Stability*.

Statics

Definition. The branch of mechanics that deals with the equilibrium of bodies at rest or in motion with zero acceleration.

This is probably the most useful part of mechanics for solving day to day orthopaedic biomechanical problems. The tool most often used for solving the problem is free-body analysis, using equilibrium equations (see *Free-Body Analysis* and *Equilibrium*).

Example. To apply traction to the spine of a patient lying in bed, force is applied to the head on one side and to the femur on the opposite side (Fig. A-54). If 180 N (40.2 lbf) is applied to the head and 250 N (55.9 lbf) to the femur, how much of the force is being applied to the spine? Answers to such questions come from the science of statics. In this example, the friction forces are generated between the body and the bed as the traction is applied. The friction forces under the pelvis, back, and head are assumed to have values and directions as shown in Figure A-54. From the laws of statics, in this example the cervical spine is subjected to a traction of 170 N (38 lbf). Of course, if there were no friction forces, the two tractions and the spine force would all be equal.

Static Load

Definition. A load applied to a specimen is called static if it remains constant with respect to time. Its antonym is dynamic.

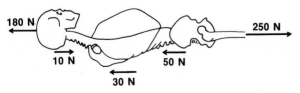

Fig. A-54. Statics. Various forces are generated between the body and the bed when the spine is subjected to traction.

Example. Imagine a person standing on a nice sunny beach. The depth of his footprints is an indication that he is applying a static load to the earth. If he jumps up and comes down on the sand, he is applying a dynamic load. The foot prints will be deeper, indicating higher loads. In most cases, dynamic loads are additions to static loads already present, and therefore they produce higher stresses.

A smooth recovery from anesthesia after a Harrington rod procedure for scoliotic correction is of great advantage in keeping the *static* distraction force low. However, if the recovery is violent due to coughing, additional *dynamic* forces are applied to the system. A distraction hook may penetrate through the bone as a result.

Stiffness

Definition. A measure of resistance offered to external loads by a specimen or structure as it deforms. This phenomenon is characterized by the stiffness coefficient.

Examples. Stiffness and elasticity are two similar but quite different concepts. The former represents mechanical behavior of a *structure* including the material, shape, and size, while the latter is a pure *material* property. For example, stainless steel has a higher modulus of elasticity as a material than cortical bone. This is indicated by the stress-strain curves in Figure A-55A. A hip nail has lower stiffness than the neck of the femur in the characteristic loading patterns, as shown in Figure A-55B. This discrepancy is explained by an analysis of the amount and distribution of the two materials. The nail has a smaller cross-section and its material is relatively near to its axis. In contrast, the femur neck has a bigger cross-sectional area and its material is distributed farther away from the axis, thus providing much more resistance to bending through the larger moment of inertia of its cross-section.

A spine with ankylosing spondylitis is a structure that has a high stiffness. The supple spine of a newborn has a low stiffness.

Stiffness Coefficient

Definition. The property of a structure defined by the ratio of force applied to the deformation produced. It quantifies the resistance that a structure offers to deformation.

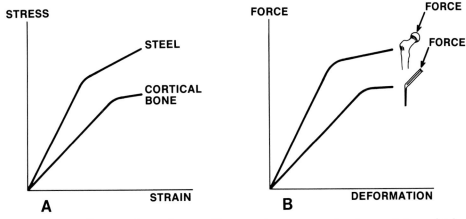

Fig. A-55. Stiffness. (A) Steel is a stiff material as compared to bone. It has a higher modulus of elasticity. (B) The femoral neck is stiffer than any hip nail. This is due to advantageous distribution of material in the femoral neck.

For a particular structure, the slope of its load-displacement curve is the stiffness coefficient. When the curve is linear the slope and therefore the stiffness coefficient is a constant. For a specimen with nonlinear stiffness behaviour, the stiffness coefficient varies with the magnitude of the load. The unit of measure is either newtons per meter (poundforce per foot) or newton meters per radian (foot poundforce per degree).

Examples. One may take a rubber band and hang a 100-g (0.22-lb) weight from its end. If the rubber band is stretched 1 cm (0.033 ft), then one may calculate the stiffness coefficient of the rubber band as 98.1 N/m (6.67 lbf/ft). (A 100-g (0.22-lb) weight applies 0.981 N (0.22 lb) of force.) If an additional 100 g (0.22 lb) produces another centimeter (0.033 ft) of stretch, the rubber band exhibits linear behavior; if not, the behavior is nonlinear.

Take an entire spine from a *patient with ankylosis spondylitis* and fix it at the sacrum. Then apply a pull by way of a spring balance at C7 until the spring balance registers a force F of 20 N (4.47 lbf; Fig. A-56A). Let the distance that the vertebra C7 moves be D_1. Now repeat the same experiment with a *supple spine of an agile adolescent.* Apply the same amount of force and measure the motion of C7 again. Its value is D_2 (Fig. A-56B). The ratio of the force to the displacement is the coefficient of stiffness. It is found that F/D_1 is greater than F/D_2 and therefore the stiff spine has a higher stiffness coefficient.

Explanatory Notes. Mathematically, the stiffness coefficient k is given by the following formula:

$$k = \frac{F}{D}$$

where F = load applied (force or moment), and
D = displacement produced (translation or rotation)

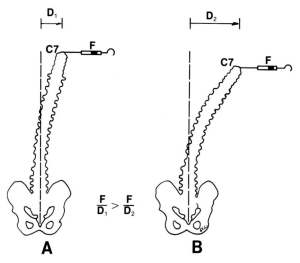

Fig. A-56. Stiffness coefficient. (A) Stiff spine, ankylosing spondylitis. (B) Supple spine in an agile adolescent.

Strain

Definition.   The change in unit length or angle in a material subjected to load.

There are two types of strain: normal, symbolized by the Greek letter ϵ (epsilon), and shear, symbolized by γ (gamma). The former is defined as the change in length divided by the original length. The latter is defined as the change in angle. There are no units of measure.

Examples.   Figure A-57A shows a long specimen, a bar made of rubber, being deformed. In Figure A-57A, A1 has become elongated by applying tension. It may be compressed by applying a compressive force, as shown by A2. The ratio of the change in length to the original length is the *normal* strain.

Figure A-57B shows a square specimen being deformed by a horizontal force. The shape of the specimen is changed from a square to a parallelogram. The upper right hand corner of the specimen has been displaced. The *shear* strain is defined as this displacement divided by the height. If this ratio is small, then the shear strain may be conveniently represented by the angle of the inclined face of the specimen, as shown. However, the angle must be measured in radians.

A tennis ball hit normally to the wall is compressed as it comes in contact with the wall producing normal strain. However, if the ball is hit nearly tangential to the wall, a large amount of shear strain is produced. The two cases are shown in Figure A-57C.

Strains and Sprains

Definition.   Clinical terms that characterize injury to capsular, ligamentous, or musculotendenous structures.

Examples.   In reality, they are often used in clinical situations when there is no possibility of determining exactly what has happened to the injured structure. The terms are not applied when a complete rupture or failure of the structure is clearly involved. Usually they are not used when there is a clinically demonstrable plastic deformation or laxity of the structure. With strains and sprains, the structures have been loaded and deformed to a point at which pain is produced, and this is about all that can be determined. What has happened biomechanically when these terms are used is not known.

Stress

Definition.   The force per unit area of a structure and a measurement of the intensity of the force.

There are two kinds of stress: normal, symbolized by the Greek letter σ (sigma), and shear, symbolied by τ (tau). The normal stress is perpendicular to the plane of a cross-section (Fig. A58A). Shear stress is parallel to the cross-section

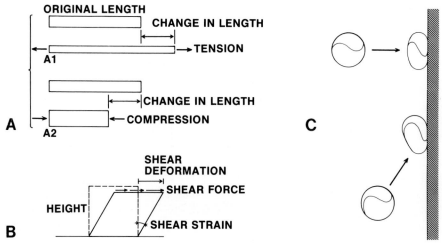

Fig. A-57.   (*A*) Normal strain. (*B*) Shear strain. (*C*) *Normal* and *shear* strains in a tennis ball.

(Fig. A-58B). The unit of measure is newtons per square meter or pascals (poundforce per square foot).

Examples. When a structure is loaded with forces or moments, stresses are created throughout within the body. How much of the normal and shear stresses are present at a given point in the body depends on the orientation of the plane to which the stresses are referred. Changes in orientation of the cross-sections through a point in a structure alter the ratio between the normal and shear components, although the total stress remains the same. As an example, take the case of ski fractures. The tibia is subjected to torsion and fails with a spiral fracture (Fig. A-58C). Torsion produces shear stress in a cross-section normal to the axis. At ±45 degrees to the axis, the stress is no longer composed of shear, but is pure tensile or compressive, depending upon the direction of torsion. At cross-sections between these two planes, there is a combination of shear and normal stresses.

Explanatory Notes. For torsional loading of a long structure the three principal planes are oriented at +45, −45, and 0 degrees to the long axis (the shear stresses are zero in those planes; see *Principal Planes*). Any other plane has a combination of normal as well as shear stresses. The transverse and axial planes are somewhat special. Here the normal stress is zero, and therefore only the shear stress is present. This can be checked out by applying the free-body analysis.

Stress-Strain Diagram

Definition. The plot of stress, usually on the ordinate or y-axis, versus strain, usually on the abscissa or x-axis. The relationship represents mechanical behavior of a *material.*

Examples. The stress-strain diagram of cancellous bone under compression, taken from the middle of the vertebral body along the direction of the longitudinal axis of the spine, serves as an example. First a suitable specimen is prepared, and its length and cross-sectional area are measured (Fig. A-59A). In a testing machine, an axial compressive load is applied. The load applied and the deformation produced are continuously measured and plotted on a graph paper. This is the *load-deformation* curve. Stress is obtained by

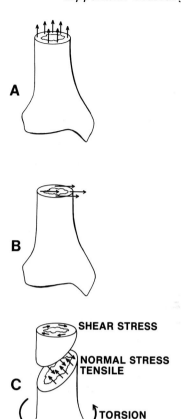

Fig. A-58. (A) Normal stress. (B) Shear stress. (C) Stresses during a ski fracture of the tibia.

dividing the load with the original cross-sectional area. Strain is obtained by dividing the deformation with the original length. Thus, the load-deformation curve is converted to the stress-strain diagram shown in Figure A-59B. Segment OA is the linear elastic range within which stress and strain are proportional. Also, in this range, on removal of the load, the specimen returns to its original length and shape. The segment AB is the nonlinear elastic range within which stress and strain are no longer proportional to each other. However, the specimen still returns to its original shape on removal of the load. Segment BC is the plastic range in which excessive deformation takes place for very small increase in load, and the specimen no longer goes back to its original

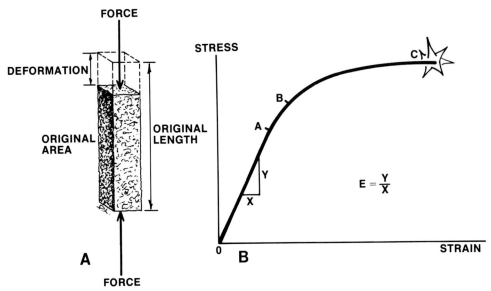

Fig. A-59. Stress-strain diagram. OA = Linear elastic range; AB = nonlinear elastic range; BC = plastic range; E = modulus of elasticity.

shape on removal of the load; a residual permanent deformation is produced. At point C there is sudden decrease in stress without additional strain, representing failure.

One of the important characteristics of a stress-strain diagram is the slope of its linear elastic range. It is called the modulus of elasticity (E) and is depicted in Figure A-59.

Stress and Strain Rates

Definition. The rate of change of load per unit area with time is called the stress rate. Similarly, the rate of change of deformation per unit length with time is called the strain rate. The respective units of measure are newtons per square meter per second (poundforce per square foot per second) for the stress rate and per second (per second) for the strain rate.

Examples. All materials are sensitive to the rate of loading to a certain degree. This phenomenon is more predominant in viscoelastic materials like plastics and biological tissue than in metals. "Silly Putty" is a plastic of chewing gum consistency, and its inherent sensitivity to loading rates is meant to intrigue both the child and the adult. A slow and mild pull on the putty can produce a deformation of as much as several

thousand per cent before fracture. However, a quick, strong pull will break the putty with less than 10 per cent deformation. So, if one were to describe the mechanical properties of "Silly Putty", or for that matter, any viscoelastic material, it would be silly not to mention the rate of loading.

It has been well established in the biomechanics literature that bone, ligaments, tendons, and passive muscles are viscoelastic, and therefore sensitive to the rate of loading. Nevertheless, one still finds data published on the mechanical properties of vertebrae, discs, and various ligaments, with no mention of the rate of loading. Such data is not of much use.

An example of the dependency of energy absorption capacity of a rabbit femur on the rate of deformation is shown in Figure A-60. Note that the bone strength increases with the rate of deformation, and seems to reach a maximum at about 1 rad/s.[12]

Stress Concentration

Definition. Any localized stress peak that cannot be predicted by simple strength of material theory.

Examples. Take two strips of metal, as shown

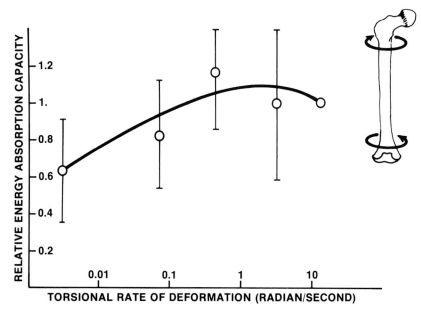

Fig. A-60. Rate of stress and strain.

in Figure A-61. Strip II has a small hole but is wider than Strip I, so that they both have the same net cross-sectional area. Now apply tensile forces. The resulting stress in Strip I is uniform and equal to the force divided by the area. Strip II has a local high stress at the edge of the hole, nearly three times in magnitude as compared to Strip I.[17] This high stress cannot be predicted by the simple strength of material theory. However, it is calculable by the so-called "Theory of Elasticity." If the strips are made of a ductile material, and the load is increased gradually, the strength of the two strips is found to be about the same. This is due to the fact that although the material at the hole edge does yield at one-third the load for Strip I, the effect is only local. However, if the load is cyclic or the material is brittle, there is a different situation. Under these circumstances the failure load for Strip II will actually be one-third of that for Strip I.

There are many instances of stress concentration in orthopaedic constructions. An example of a fixation plate is shown in Figure A-61B. Three possible causes of stress concentration, of the plate system, are depicted: (1) sudden change in the cross-section of the plate, (2) junction of two or more dissimilar components of the system with

mismatch of their mechanical properties, and (3) local stress at the points of application of loads.

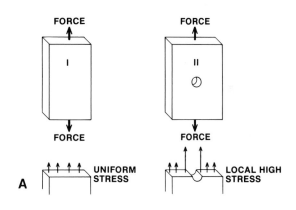

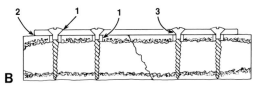

Fig. A-61. (A) Stress concentration in two strips of metal. (B) Stress concentration in a boneplate system due to (1) sudden change in cross-section, (2) mismatch of material properties, and (3) load application points.

Subluxations and Dislocations

Definition. A subluxation may be defined as a partial dislocation.

It is any pathological situation in which there is not a normal physiological juxtaposition of the articular surfaces of a joint. Such situations should be reliably demonstrable radiographically.

Dislocation is the term that is employed when there is no longer any degree of contact between the articulating surfaces.

Example. A femoral head that is totally out of the socket and lying posterior to the acetabulum is completely dislocated.

These clinical terms are employed frequently but are not always clearly defined.

Tangent

See *Trigonometric Functions.*

Tangential

See *Joint Reaction Force.*

Tensile Stress

See *Stress.*

Tension

Definition. A normal force that tends to elongate the fibers of a material. The unit of measure is newtons (poundforce).

Examples. When a rubber band is stretched, tension is applied. The rubber fibers are elongated. If there are any cuts or other weak spots on the surface, fracture cracks will initiate from these. If sufficient tension is applied, these cracks increase in size until the rubber band fails.

Tension is also manifested in the fibers on the convex side of a long structure when the structure is bent (see *Normal Stress*), as well as in fibers at 45 degrees to the long axis when torsion is applied (see *Shear Stress*).

When the spine is flexed, ligaments posterior to the instantaneous axis of rotation are subjected to tension. When axial rotation occurs in the spine, the disc is subjected to torsion and some fibers of the annulus are subjected to tension.

Three-Dimensional Motion

Definition. The most general kind of motion of a rigid body.

The body may move in any direction. It has all of the possible six degrees of freedom. The motion is a combination of translation along any direction and rotation about any axis in space. Most of the human body joints have three-dimensional motion.

Examples. A body performing plane motion may always be brought from one position to another by pure rotation about an axis, the so-called instantaneous axis of rotation. Similarly, a body performing three-dimensional motion may always be moved from one position to another by defined amounts of rotation about and translation along an axis, called the helical axis of motion (HAM). Thus, a step of three-dimensional motion is fully defined by the position and direction of the instantaneous helical axis of motion and the magnitude of translation along and rotation about this axis (see *Helical Axis of Motion*).

Lateral bending produces translation and rotation of the vertebrae in the coronal plane as well as axial rotation, due to inherent properties of the motion segment. This is not plane motion because various points on the vertebrae do not travel in parallel planes. It is a three-dimensional motion. Vertebrae in a scoliotic spine have undergone three-dimensional displacement from a normal spine to a scoliotic curve.

Three-Element Model

Definition. A mathematical model consisting of a spring-element connected in parallel with a dashpot-element. The two are then further connected in series with a second spring-element. The three-element model is shown in Figure A-62A. It is used to symbolize and mathematically simulate time-dependent mechanical behaviour of certain viscoelastic materials.

Examples. The creep phenomenon is often used to test viscoelastic behavior of biological materials. The behavior of the three-element model under creep is studied here in detail and to see if it can mimic the actual viscoelastic behavior. The creep phenomenon may be defined as a sudden application of a *constant* force as

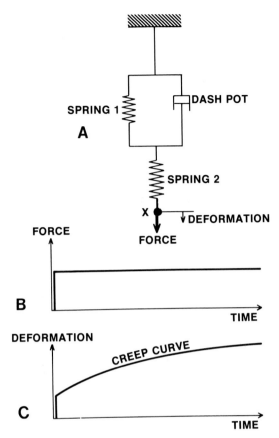

Fig. A-62. Three-element model. (*A*) Representation of a three-element model. (*B, C*) Creep behavior.

Most biological materials are viscoelastic in nature and their uniaxial behavior is adequately simulated by a single mathematical three-element model. By assigning different values to the stiffness coefficients of the two springs and the damping coefficient of the dashpot, time-dependent mechanical behavior of ligaments, tendons, skin, cancellous and cortical bone, and cartilage can be simulated.

During traction application to a scoliotic spine, immediate deformation of the spine may be represented by Spring 2 and the additional time-dependent deformation by a combination of Spring 1 and the dashpot. If suitable values are assigned to the three elements to represent the spine behavior, then it is theoretically possible to estimate the optimum time duration for traction.

Three-Point Bending

Definition. A structure is loaded in three-point bending with a single force applied on one side and two forces applied on the other side acting in the opposite direction.

Examples. A femur being subjected to three-point bending for determining its strength is shown in Figure A-63A. The bending moment produced varies along the length of the structure, being zero under the end forces and maximum under the middle force. This is represented by the triangular bending moment diagram (Fig. A-63B). The quantitative expression for maximum bending moment is given below.

When the archer draws the bow string, the bow is loaded in three-point bending (Fig. A-63C). The bow has maximum cross-section at its middle because the bending moment is highest under the middle force.

The Milwaukee brace is an example in which three-point bending forces are employed in addition to axial tension to obtain angular correction of the spine.

Explanatory Notes. The maximum bending moment is given by the following equation:

$$M = \frac{F \times A \times B}{A + B}$$

where F is the middle force and A and B are the distances of the two end forces from it (Fig. A-63B).

shown in Figure A-62B. After the force is applied the deformation as a function of time is measured. Two things happen when creep is performed on the three-element model by applying sudden force. Referring to Figure A-62A, with the sudden application of force the dashpot produces infinite resistance and locks in, but Spring 2 elongates, which produces immediate displacement of point X. Secondly, as time passes, with the force being held constant, the resistance of the dashpot decreases. This lets Spring 1 elongate at a rate defined by the dashpot and the stiffness properties of Spring 1. Thus, there is immediate elastic deformation with the application of a sudden force followed by an additional deformation as a function of time. The rate of deformation decreases with time, producing the characteristic creep curve (Fig. A-62C).

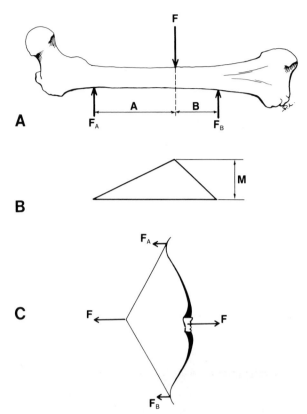

Fig. A-63. (*A*) A femur being subjected to three-point bending. (*B*) Triangular bending moment diagram. (*C*) A bow loaded in three-point bending.

Torque

See *Couple* and *Torsion.*

Torsion

Definition. A type of load that is applied by a couple of forces (parallel and directed opposite to each other) about the long axis of a structure.

The load is called torque. It produces relative rotation of different axial sections of the structure with respect to each other. For a straight structure, all the sections are subjected to the same torque. However, in a curved structure, loaded by a torque on its ends, each cross-section is subjected not only to torque, but also to bending. The magnitude of bending depends upon the orientation of the particular cross-section with respect to the torque axis.

Examples. In a straight bar (Fig. A-64A) shearing stress is produced in cross-sections that are perpendicular and parallel to the torque axis. These are called circumferential and longitudinal shear stresses, respectively. On the other hand, normal stresses, tension, and compression are produced at ±45 degrees with respect to the torque axis. These four stresses at a point are shown in Figure A-64A. The results are based upon stress analysis of a cylindrical structure. All four stresses are equal in magnitude. The relationships between the stresses and the dimensions of the structure are given below.

A piece of ordinary chalk, when subjected to torque, breaks along a plane about 45 degrees to the long axis where tensile stresses are maximum. From Figure A-64A, it is known that all four stresses produced at a point are equal in magnitude. Therefore, tensile stress failure indicates that the chalk material is weakest in tension, as compared to shear and compression.

According to some researchers, disc failure in low back pain is due to the combined torsion and bending loads.[6] Since the lumbar spine is a curved structure, it may be shown to be subjected

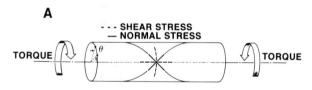

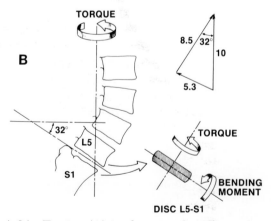

Fig. A-64. Torsion. (*A*) Application of torque produces shear and normal stresses. (*B*) Rotation of the trunk produces torsion and bending of the L5-S1 disc.

to these combined torsion and bending loads by simple axial rotation of the trunk with respect to the pelvis. The L5-S1 disc typically has an angle of 32 degrees with the vertical axis (Fig. A-64B). Therefore, when an axial torque of 10 N m (7.3 ft lbf) is applied about the vertical axis to the spine, the disc is subjected to a torque of 8.5 N m (6.2 ft lbf) and a lateral bending moment of 5.3 N m (3.9 ft lbf). These numbers were obtained by a free-body analysis (see *Free-Body Analysis*) of the disc and are shown in Figure A-64B.

Explanatory Notes.   When a straight structure is subjected to a torque, the shear and normal stresses (Fig. A-64A) are manifested and the two ends of the structure rotate with respect to each other. These stresses in newtons per square meter or pascals (poundforce per square foot) and the angular deformation are given by the following formulas:

$$\text{shear stress} = \text{normal stress} = \frac{T \times R}{J}$$

$$\text{deformation angle in radians} = \frac{T \times L}{G \times J}$$

where T = torque in N m (lbf ft)
     R = cylinder radius in m (ft)
     J = polar moment of inertia in m⁴ (ft⁴)
     L = cylinder length in m (ft)
     G = shear modulus of the material in N/m² (lbf/ft²)

where T = torque in N m (lbf ft)
R = cylinder radius in m (ft)
J = polar moment of inertia in m^4 (ft^4)
L = cylinder length in m (ft)
G = shear modulus of the material in N/m^2 (lbf/ft^2)

Torsional Rigidity

Definition.   The torque per unit of angular deformation. The unit of measure is newton meters per radian (foot poundforce per degree).

Examples.   Torsional rigidity means rotatory stiffness. An example of this is the resistance felt when turning the steering wheel of an automobile (Fig. A-65). The torsional rigidity of the steering wheel system can be measured by applying a defined torque and recording the angular displacement of the steering wheel before the tires turn on the pavement.

Torsional rigidity is an important quantity in characterizing body joints. For the analysis of the mechanism of ski fractures, it is essential to know the values of torsional rigidity of the joints involved. These values may be obtained by experi-

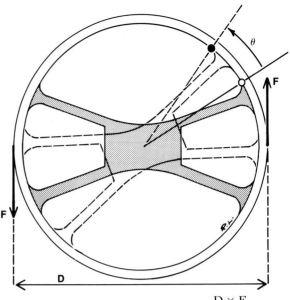

Fig. A-65.   Torsional rigidity $= \dfrac{D \times F}{\theta}$.

ments. To calculate torsional rigidity of simpler structures, such as a cylindrical specimen of bone, the formula given below may be used.

Average values of torsional rigidity of the joints of the lower extremity have been measured:[15]

Hip	1.3 N m/rad	(230 in lbf/rad)
Knee	2.0 N m/rad	(350 in lbf/rad)
Ankle	2.1 N m/rad	(360 in lbf/rad)

Explanatory Notes.   Mathematically, the following formulas apply:

$$\text{torsional rigidity} = \frac{T}{\theta}$$

where T = torque in N m (ft lbf)
θ = angular displacement in rad

For a cylindrical structure, the torsional rigidity in terms of its basic structural properties can be described:

$$\text{torsional rigidity} = \frac{G \times J}{L}$$

where G = shear modulus of the material in N/m^2 (lbf/ft^2)
J = polar moment of inertia in m^4 (ft^4)
L = cylinder length in m (ft)

Translation

Definition. Motion of a rigid body in which a straight line in the body always remains parallel to itself. The unit of measure is meters (feet).

Examples. If a boat is smoothly pushed straight from position 1 to position 2 without pitching or rolling, it moves in pure translation (Fig. A-66A). A straight line joining two points X and Y will always remain parallel to itself in any two instantaneous positions of its motion. The line joining the two positions of the same point is the translation vector of the body.

During gait, the head moves forward, sideways, and up and down with respect to the ground. Neglecting any minor angular motions, the head may be said to go through translatory motions in the three-dimensional space throughout its gait cycle.

Translation is a vector quantity. It has magnitude as well as direction. Motion of a point in space may be represented by a single translation vector. The motion of a rigid body may require one translation vector, if the body is undergoing pure translation. For a rigid body moving in a plane, the translation vectors of two points must be known. Finally, for a rigid body performing three-dimensional motion, translation vectors of three points are required.

Trigonometric Functions

Examples. There are three basic trigonometric functions: sine, cosine, and tangent. Their short forms are sin (A), cos (A) and tan (A), where A is a given angle in degrees or radians.

The functions are best described by referring to a right angle triangle, one with one 90-degree angle (Fig. A-66B).

Definition. Sin (A), the sine of angle A, is the ratio of length BC to length AB.

Cos (A), the cosine of angle A, is the ratio of length AC to length AB.

Tan (A), the tangent of angle A, is the ratio of length BC to length AC.

Explanatory Notes. From the above definitions, tan (A) can be obtained by dividing sin (A) by cos (A).

Because the trigonometric functions are ratios of one length to the other, they have no units of measure.

Ultimate Load

Definition. The final load reached by a structure subjected to failure. The unit of measure is newtons (poundforce) if the load is a force and newton meters (foot poundforce) if the load is a torque or moment.

Examples. For a simple structure subjected to a uniaxial load exemplified by a well machined tensile test specimen of bone, there is a well-defined unambiguous point of failure. This is the maximum load point on the load-deformation curve (Fig. A-67A). For complex structures subjected to a simple uniaxial load, the maximum load may not be called the ultimate load. This is well illustrated by the compressive load-deformation curve of an intact spine motion segment.

The tracing of an actual experiment carried out in a testing machine is shown in Figure A-67B.)* The compressive load increased and reached a maximum at point X and then decreased to Y and started increasing again. At point Z the load reached the limit of the transducer measuring load, but it was still increasing. What is the ultimate load? For the purpose of this experiment,

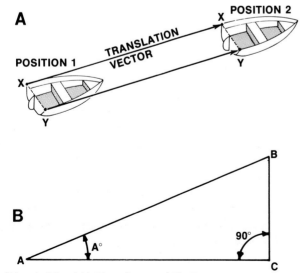

Fig. A-66. (*A*) Translation. (*B*) Trigonometric functions.

---

* Unpublished data. Engineering Laboratory for Musculoskeletal Diseases, Yale Medical Center, New Haven, Connecticut.

point X was selected because certain structures (probably the end-plates) within the motion segment failed and caused the decrease in the load-sustaining capacity. After the point X, the motion segment is not and can never be the same as it was in its initial pretest state. Therefore, any load that peaks after point X does not belong to the original motion segment. The actual ultimate load was 3700 N (811 lbf). It is important in reporting load bearing capacity to indicate exactly where on the load-deformation curve the actual failure point was read.

Ultimate load divided by the original cross-sectional area is called ultimate stress. In the case of force, the ultimate stress is a normal stress if the area under consideration is normal to the force, and a shear stress if the area is parallel to the force. The units of measurement are newtons per square meter (poundforce per square foot).

Units

See *Conversion Table.*

Unit Vector

Definition. A vector with unit magnitude. It is a mathematical quantity and is used to define a direction.

In three-dimensional space, a unit vector is made up of three numbers representing the inclination of its direction with respect to the three axes of a coordinate system.

Examples. Figure A-68A shows a sailboat in rough sea. How can one make use of this concept in defining the orientation of a sailboat? As shown in Figure A-68A, let vector N be parallel to the mast. It makes three angles with the axes: θ_x, θ_y, θ_z. The vector N is made up of these three angles, or rather the cosines of these angles, as shown in Figure A-68A (see *Trigonometric Functions*).

Facet orientation of the vertebrae varies with the level of the spine. In the cervical spine, the plane of the facets is approximately perpendicular to the sagittal plane and tilted about 45 degrees to the vertical direction. Knowing these two angles one can calculate, by the formula given below, the angles as shown in Figure A-68B. In the lumbar region (around L3) the orientation of the facets is more complex. The facet joints are not simple planes, but they describe moderately

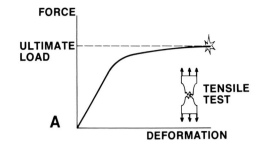

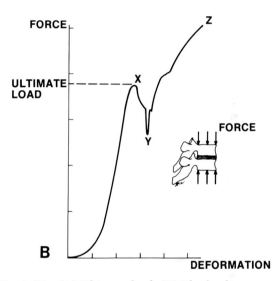

Fig. A-67. (*A*) Ultimate load. (*B*) The loading pattern observed in a real compression test situation.

curved surfaces. However, the unit vector concept can still be utilized to represent slopes of this complex surface at different points. For one such point in the middle of the facet, measured on a cadaver specimen, the angles of the unit vector components were found to have the following values: $\theta_x = 150°$, $\theta_y = 80°$, and $\theta_y = 118°$.

Explanatory Notes. Referring to Figure A-68A, if θ_x, θ_y, θ_z are the angles made by the direction of the unit vector N with the respective axes x, y, z, then the three components of the unit vector N are as follows:

$$N = \begin{bmatrix} \cos \theta_x \\ \cos \theta_y \\ \cos \theta_z \end{bmatrix}$$

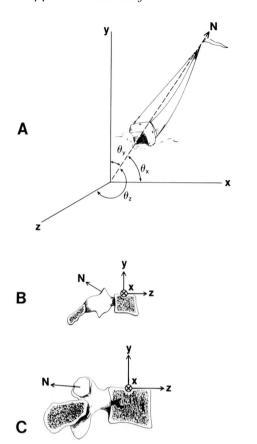

Fig. A-68.   Unit vector. The concept of the unit vector helps define orientation of (*A*) a boat mast, (*B*) the facet plane of a cervical vertebra, and (*C*) the surface of a lumbar facet.

Further, because the length of the unit vector is unity, the following applies:

$$(\cos \theta_x)^2 + (\cos \theta_y)^2 + (\cos \theta_z)^2 = 1$$

The two equations above define the unit vector completely once two of the three angles are known.

Vector

Definition.   A quantity that possesses both a magnitude and a direction.

All vectors obey the parallelogram rule of addition, which states the following: If a parallelogram is constructed so that the two vectors to be added are adjacent sides, then the resultant is represented by a certain diagonal of the parallelogram (Fig. A-69A).

Examples.   All traction techniques in orthopaedics are based upon the fundamental rule of the parallelogram. Traction forces may be represented by vectors. By single or multiple application of the rule, one can precisely determine the resulting force and its direction applied to the body part.

Weather vanes are mounted atop old farm houses to indicate wind direction (Fig. A-69B1). Vector V represents the wind and its force acting at the centroid of the vane (Fig. A-69B2). The centroid is eccentric with respect to the axis of rotation. Therefore, the wind velocity vector V produces a torque about the rotation axis. The weather vane will rotate, due to this torque, until it is in line with the wind velocity. This reduces the torque to zero, producing a stable direction

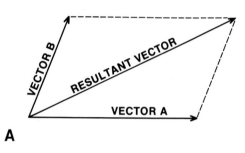

A

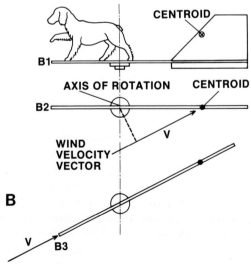

Fig. A-69.   Vector. (*A*) Parallelogram rule. (*B1*) Side view of a weather vane. (*B2*) Top view. (*B3*) Vector diagram.

for the weather vane. When the wind changes direction, the stable direction of the weather vane will also change. Thus, the weather vane always indicates the direction of the wind velocity vector. How does the dog distinguish if the wind is coming from the front or the back? Consider it as an exercise.

A mathematical definition of a vector in three-dimensional space is extremely useful in analysis of complex loads or motions and is described below.

Explanatory Notes. In a three-dimensional space, with respect to a Cartesian coordinate system, a vector has three components and they are depicted as follows:

$$V = \begin{bmatrix} V_x \\ V_y \\ V_z \end{bmatrix}$$

where V, the vector, is generally written in bold letters, and V_x, V_y, and V_z are its components or projections along the three coordinate axes. The magnitude of the vector (written with two vertical bars) is given by the following equation:

$$|V| = \sqrt{V_x^2 + V_y^2 + V_z^2}$$

Its direction is given by another set of equations:

$$\cos \theta_x = \frac{V_x}{|V|}$$
$$\cos \theta_y = \frac{V_y}{|V|}$$
$$\cos \theta_z = \frac{V_z}{|V|}$$

where θ_x, θ_y, and θ_z are the angles made by the vector with the respective coordinate system axes.

Velocity

Definition. The rate of change of position of a point with respect to a coordinate system. It is a vector quantity. Its magnitude is called speed. The velocity may be linear or angular, depending upon the type of motion. Correspondingly, the unit of measure is meters per second (feet per second) or radians per second.

Examples. A tennis ball traveling in mid-air, at any instant, has linear velocity. It may also have angular velocity if it spins.

The femur of a person running changes its

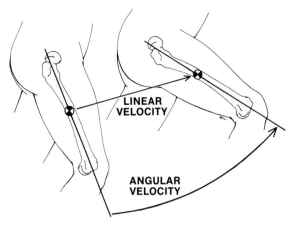

Fig. A-70. Velocity. During walking, the femur has linear as well as angular velocity.

linear and angular positions with time (Fig. A-70). Therefore, the femur has linear as well as angular velocities. (See also *Instantaneous Velocity.*)

Viscoelasticity

Definition. The property of a material to show sensitivity to rate of loading or deformation.

Examples. As the name suggests, two basic components of viscoelasticity are viscosity and elasticity. The behavior of a viscoelastic material is a combination of these two fundamental properties. Creep and relaxation are two phenomenological characteristics of viscoelastic materials and are utilized to document their behavior quantitatively. During creep tests, the load is suddenly applied and is kept constant thereafter; the resulting displacement is recorded against time. In relaxation tests, a deformation is produced and then fixed; the resulting decrease in load is recorded as a function of time.

There are two other practical phenomena that are typical of viscoelastic materials. A load-deformation curve of a viscoelastic material is dependent upon the rate of loading. The higher is the rate of loading, the steeper is the resulting curve. The other phenomenon involves the loading and unloading cycle. A viscoelastic material shows hysteresis (loss of energy in the form of heat during each cycle).

It has been experimentally determined that bone, ligaments, tendons, and passive muscles are viscoelastic, and their behavior can be reasonably simulated by the three-element model.

Explanatory Notes. Actual behavior of real life materials such as bone, soft tissue, and plastics is very complex. However, their main characteristics can be simulated mathematically and represented by models that combine the basic elements of mathematical modeling (spring and dashpot) in a well-defined manner. Three of these basic combinations are the Maxwell, Kelvin, and three-element models. The models and their corresponding creep and relaxation curves are shown in Figure A-71.

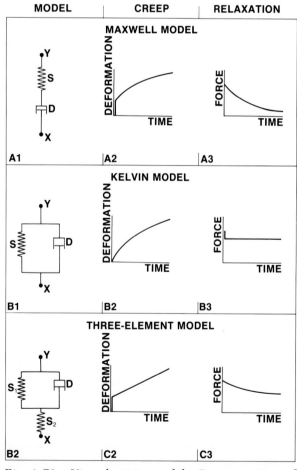

Fig. A-71. Viscoelasticity models. Representation of the model and its creep and relaxation behaviors are shown. (*A*) Maxwell model for fluids. (*B*) Kelvin model for solids. (*C*) Three-element model for most biological tissues.

The Maxwell model is a *series* combination of a spring S and a dashpot D (Fig. A-71A1). If a creep test is performed on it, then the motion of the point X, with point Y being fixed, as a function of time is given by the graph shown in Figure A-71A2. There is an immediate displacement followed by a proportionately increasing displacement with time. Results of the relaxation test are shown in Figure A-71A3. The force decreases exponentially (continuously at an ever decreasing rate, to zero).

The Kelvin model is a *parallel* combination of a spring S and a dashpot D (Fig. A-71B1). The creep curve shows that the displacement of the point X is continuously increasing, but with an ever decreasing rate (exponentially; Fig. A-71B2). The relaxation is immediate but incomplete (Fig. A-71B3). In other words, the force immediately decreases and then remains constant, never becoming zero.

The three-element model derives its name from the three mathematical components it is made of: two springs, S_1 and S_2, and a dashpot, D (Fig. A-71C1). Results of the creep test are an immediate displacement followed by an exponential displacement with time (Fig. A-71C2). The relaxation is exponential with time but is not complete (force never becomes zero; Fig. A-71C3; see also *Three-Element Model*).

Viscoelastic Stability

Definition. The type of stability in which the critical load is a function of time as well as the geometric and material properties of the structure.

Examples. Certain structures made of viscous and elastic elements when subjected to constant load may exhibit accelerating deformation behavior with time. Like a purely elastic structure, a viscoelastic structure does not have a critical load. It has a critical time period for a given load. Within this time period the system is stable, and beyond it, unstable. This phenomenon is called the viscoelastic stability, and it is in contrast to the elastic stability, in which the critical factor is the load, with no dependency on time whatsoever.

There are plastics and organic materials that exhibit viscoelastic instability. Glue is one of these. When a heavy piece of material like a picture frame is fixed to the wall with a piece of tape and falls off after a few hours or days, time-dependent stability has been exemplified.

Biological structures are viscoelastic and therefore have time-dependent stability. Living bodies are much more complex. They are able to respond to unstable situations by altering the structure so as to recreate structural stability.

Viscosity

Definition. The property of materials to resist loads that produce shear. Viscosity is the ratio of shearing stress to shearing strain rate, or shearing stress to velocity gradient. It is commonly represented by η (eta) or μ (mu). The units of measure are newton seconds per square meter (poundforce per square foot) and poise (1 poise = 0.1 newton seconds per square meter).

Examples. In lubrication of joints, the viscosity of the fluid plays a very important role. If it is too high, it will resist motion. If it is too low, it will have less friction, but it can support only small loads before the thin lubricating film breaks down.

Viscosity of water does not vary with the rate of shear strain or the velocity gradient. The synovial fluid, on the other hand, has viscosity that varies inversely with the velocity gradient: 100 poise at velocity gradient of 0.1 per second and 1 poise at 100 per second. Figure A-72A shows the variation of viscosity of water as well as the synovial fluid as functions of the velocity gradient. The two variables are plotted on logarithmic scales.

Explanatory Notes. Mathematically the viscosity (η) is as follows:

$$\eta = \frac{\text{shear stress}}{\text{shear strain rate}}$$

$$\eta = \frac{\text{shear stress}}{\text{velocity gradient}}$$

The former definition is used with viscous solids, while the latter is used with fluids. Stress and strain rates are defined elsewhere (see *Stress and Strain Rates*). Velocity gradient is the variation of fluid velocity with fluid depth. Take two glass plates with a fluid between them (Fig. A-72B). If one plate is moved with respect to the other a velocity gradient is created. The fluid layer at-

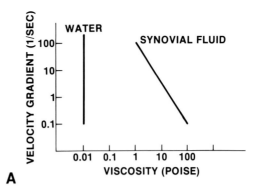

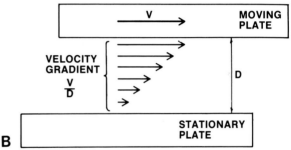

Fig. A-72. Viscosity. (*A*) The viscosity of water remains constant, while that of the synovial joint decreases with an increase in joint velocity. (*B*) Interpretation of the velocity gradient.

tached to the moving plate has velocity V, the same as the moving plate, while the fluid layer attached to the stationary plate is at rest. The layers between have intermediate velocities. If D is the distance of the plates, then V divided by D is the velocity gradient, assuming that the variation is linear.

Work

Definition. The amount of energy required to move a body from one position to another. Mechanical work is defined as the product of force applied to the distance moved in the direction of the force. The unit of measure for work is newton meters or joule (foot poundforce).

Examples. A girl weighing 60 kg (132 lb) climbs a flight of stairs that is 3 m (9.8 ft) high (Fig. A-73A). How much work did she do? She worked 1766 N m (1302 ft lbf) against earth's gravity. This is the amount of potential energy

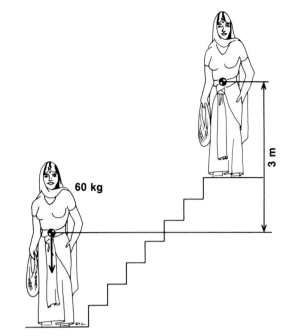

$$W = F \times D$$

where W = work N m (ft lbf) or joule
     F = force in N (lbf)
     D = distance moved in the direction of force in m (ft)

Here, the assumption of constant force is made. If the force varies, then $W = \int F \, dD$.

In the above example of a girl weighing 60 kg and climbing 3 m, the amount of work is as follows:

$$W = (60 \times 9.81) \times 3 = 1766 \text{ N m or Joule}$$
$$= 1302 \text{ ft lbf}$$

The amount of energy expanded during a gait cycle is as follows:

$$W = (60 \times 9.81) \times 0.6 = 35 \text{ N m}$$
$$= 26 \text{ ft lbf}$$

Note that 9.81 is the value of the gravitational acceleration in meters per second per second.

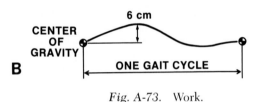

Fig. A-73. Work.

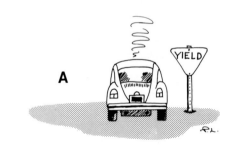

she possesses. To return back to the ground floor, the energy may be utilized positively to do some useful work, or it may be dissipated as heat.

During normal gait, the center of gravity of a person goes up and down approximately 6 cm (2.4 in; Fig. A-13B).[14] The energy expanded by a 60-kg (132-lb) person is about N m (26 ft lbf) per gait cycle. Fifty such gait cycles will be required to equal the energy expanded in climbing the stairs. Actual energy loss will be higher as additional energy is needed to accelerate and decelerate other parts of the body due to inertia effects. A person with abnormal gait may have to move his center of gravity up and down a larger amount. He would then consume energy at a higher rate.

Explanatory Notes. The mathematical definition of work is as follows:

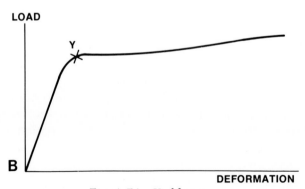

Fig. A-74. Yield stress.

Yield Stress

Definition.   That point of stress on the load-deformation curve at which appreciable deformation takes place without any appreciable increase in load. The unit of measure is newtons per square meter (poundforce per square foot).

In other words, yield stress is the stress of a material subjected to a load when plastic deformation has just started. It is not the stress one feels while approaching the YIELD traffic sign (Fig. A-74A).

Beyond the yield stress, the load-deformation curve is nearly a horizontal line. All deformation after the yield stress is permanent and is manifested at the time of removal of the load. Figure A-74B shows a tracing of an actual load-deformation curve of a bone specimen.[3] Yielding probably started at point Y. In this test, special care was taken to keep the specimen moist at all times.

REFERENCES

1. American Society for Testing and Materials: Standards for Surgical Implants. Tab. 2. Philadelphia, 1971.
2. Anderson, B. J. G., Örtengren, R., Nachemson, A., and Elfstrom, G.: Lumbar disc pressure and myoelectric back muscle activity during sitting. Part I and II. Scand. J. Rehabil. Med., 3 [Suppl.]:73, 1974.
3. Burstein, A. H., Currey, J. D., Frankel, V. H., and Reilly, D. T.: The ultimate properties of bone tissue: The effects of yielding. J. Biomec., 5:35, 1972.
4. Dohrmann, G. J., and Panjabi, M. M.: "Standardized" spinal cord trauma: Biomechanical parameters and lesion volume. Surg. Neurol., 6:263, 1976.
5. Evans, F. G.: Mechanical Properties of Bone. Springfield, Charles C Thomas, 1973.
6. Farfan, H. F.: Mechanical Disorders of the Low Back. Philadelphia, Lea & Febiger, 1973.
7. Frankel, V. H., Burstein, A. H., and Brooks, D. B.: Biomechanics of internal derangement of the knee. J. Bone Joint Surg., 53A:945, 1971.
8. Lucas, D. B., and Bresler, B.: Stability of the Ligamentous Spine. Biomechanics Laboratory, University of California, San Francisco, Tech. Rep. Series 11, No. 40, 1961.
9. Panjabi, M. M., Brand, R. A., and White, A. A.: Three Dimensional Flexibility and Stiffness Properties of the Human Thoracic Spine. J. Biomech., 9:185, 1976.
10. Panjabi, M. M., Conati, F., Aversa, J. A., and White, A. A.: Motion axes of M-P joint. To be published.
11. Panjabi, M. M., White, A. A., and Brand, R. A.: A note on defining body parts configurations. J. Biomech., 7:385, 1974.
12. Panjabi, M. M., White, A. A., and Southwick, W. O.: Mechanical properties of bone as a function of rate of deformation. J. Bone Joint Surg., 55A:322, 1973.
13. Paul, J. P.: Biomechanics and Related Bio-engineering Topics. p. 367. New York, Pergamon, 1965.
14. Perry, J.: The mechanics of walking. Phys. Ther., 47: 778, 1967.
15. Piziali, R. L.: The Dynamic Torsional Response of the Human Leg Relative to Skiing Injuries. Mechanics and Sports. New York, The American Society of Mechanical Engineers, 1973.
16. Pope, M. H., and Outwater, J. O.: Mechanical properties of bone as a function of position and orientation. J. Biomech., 7:61, 1974.
17. Timoshenko, S. P., and Goodier, J. N.: Theory of Elasticity. New York, McGraw-Hill, 1970.
18. Tkaczuk, H.: Tensile properties of human lumbar longitudinal ligaments. Acta Orthop. Scand., 115 [Suppl.], 1968.
19. Viidik, A.: A rheological model for collagenous tissue. J. Biomech., 1:3, 1968.
20. White, A. A.: Analysis of the mechanics of the thoracic spine in man. Acta Orthop. Scan., 127 [Suppl.], 1969.
21. ——: Kinematics of the normal spine as related to scoliosis. J. Biomech., 4:405, 1971.
22. White, A. A., Panjabi, M. M., and Brand, R. A.: A system for Defining Position and Motion of the Human Body Parts. Medical and Biological Engineering, 261:5, 1975.

Author Index

Subject Index